The Broad Range of Clinical Use of Phenytoin

Bioelectrical Modulator

BIBLIOGRAPHY AND REVIEW

Barry H. Smith, M.D., PH.D.
Samuel Bogoch, M.D., PH.D.
Jack Dreyfus

DREYFUS MEDICAL FOUNDATION

"The greatest crisis facing us is a crisis in the organization and accessibility of human knowledge. We own an enormous 'encyclopedia' which isn't even arranged alphabetically. Our 'file cards' are spilled on the floor. The answers we want may be buried somewhere in the heap."

—*Robert Heinlein*

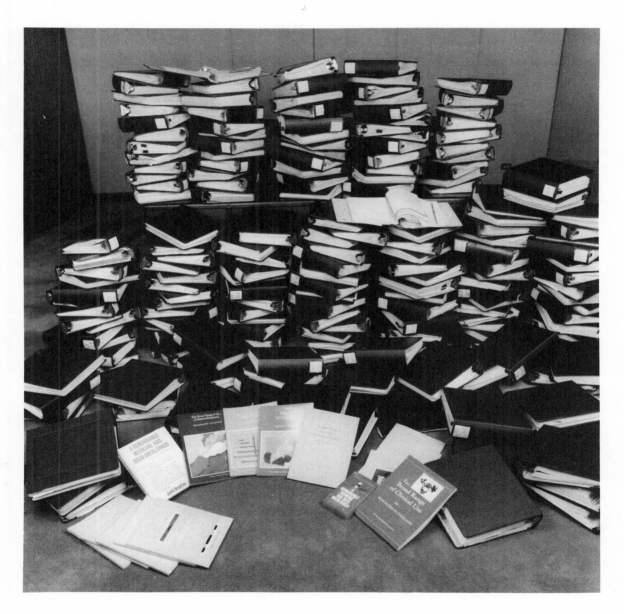

Photograph of over 10,000 studies from 38 countries,
published in over 250 medical journals,
that form the basis of this Bibliography and Review.

Prefatory

If one looks at the Physicians' Desk Reference, one will find that phenytoin's only listing with the FDA is as an anticonvulsant. This is a narrow description of a drug that has been reported by thousands of physicians throughout the world to be useful for over fifty symptoms and disorders.*

The misunderstanding of the broad clinical usefulness of phenytoin amounts to a great catastrophe. Millions of people—in this country alone—suffer because of it. This is not the fault of the FDA. It is not the fault of our physicians. There is a flaw in our system of bringing prescription medicines to the public.

The purpose of this Bibliography and Review is to put together, in one place, for the convenience of the physician and the government, a comprehensive summary of the world medical literature on phenytoin.†

* See Table of Contents.

† Other than in epilepsy.

A Personal Note

DEAR PHYSICIAN:

In 1963, a great piece of luck led me to ask my physician to allow me to try phenytoin for depressed moods. He had not heard of such a use, but allowed me to try it. It worked promptly. At first, we both attributed my recovery to coincidence. It seemed almost impossible that uses of a drug could have been overlooked for twenty-five years.

In the course of the next year I saw six other people, in succession, have similar benefits. The probabilities had changed. From being almost impossible, it became highly probable that PHT had been overlooked. PHT had taken me out of a miserable condition, and I had an obligation to investigate its potential for others.

I thought it would be easy to sponsor studies on phenytoin, and that the medical profession would then take over. I was mistaken. It became necessary to leave my businesses in Wall Street to spend full time in research on this matter.

The evidence about PHT is no longer at issue. Since its first clinical use, thousands of physicians, in hundreds of medical journals, have reported its usefulness for a broad range of disorders. Only a fraction of this work could be seen by a single physician, unless his or her life were spent reading over 3,000 medical journals.

Accompanying this Bibliography is *A Remarkable Medicine Has Been Overlooked,* a narrative of my experiences with PHT. I think you will enjoy reading it.

With the publication of this Bibliography, and the narrative, I have done what I can to discharge my obligation. The matter is now in the hands of our fine physicians.

I wish you the best of health, and good luck,

Jack Dreyfus

Brief History

In 1908, a German chemist, Heinrich Biltz, synthesized diphenylhydantoin (phenytoin). He sold PHT, along with other compounds, to Parke-Davis. The company did not patent it, nor did they find a use for it. It sat on their shelves for twenty-nine years.

In 1937, Putnam and Merritt, two doctors outside Parke-Davis, discovered phenytoin's first clinical use, in epilepsy. PHT was more effective than phenobarbital and, unlike that drug, it achieved its therapy without sedation.

That being the day of a single drug for a single disorder, phenytoin was tagged an anticonvulsant. On the basis of clinical experience, it was approved for safety by the FDA.

From its earliest use, there was evidence that phenytoin was more than an anticonvulsant. Reports started to appear in the medical literature of marked improvement in mood, emotional stability, and sense of well-being in the patients who took PHT. Since that time, an ever increasing number of reports and studies, by physicians from at least thirty-eight countries, have demonstrated that PHT is useful for a broad range of symptoms and disorders.

Basic mechanism studies have kept apace of the clinical studies, and make clear how one drug can have so many uses.

Today, fifty years after its first use, phenytoin's only listed indication with the FDA is still "anticonvulsant." There is a flaw in our system of bringing prescription medicines to the public.*

* The "flaw" is discussed in *A Remarkable Medicine Has Been Overlooked*, which accompanies this Bibliography.

Evidence

It is customary for a drug company to sponsor new uses for a drug. That hasn't happened in the case of phenytoin. This doesn't make the evidence less evidential.

Physicians around the world, with no interest but the scientific and a desire to help others, have reported PHT useful for a wide range of disorders. Published in more than 250 medical journals,* the reports and studies have many forms of control:

1. Double-blind studies with placebo or other drugs as controls.
2. Studies in which PHT has been found effective when other drugs have failed.
3. Trials in which PHT is found effective—withdrawn and symptoms return, reinstituted and symptoms disappear.
4. Promptness of action.
5. Clinical studies in which improvements are confirmed by laboratory means.

The most important control is the fact that the evidence comes from thousands of impartial observers. So many independent reports are like strands in a rope, each adding to its strength.

• • •

Basic mechanism studies confirm the clinical observations. They demonstrate that phenytoin corrects inappropriate electrical activity at the level of the single cell— with little or no effect on normal cell function. This fundamental property makes understandable how PHT can have so many uses.

* For list of medical journals, see p. 251.

Use of Approved Drugs for Unlabeled Indications

FDA Drug Bulletin, April 1982

"The appropriateness of prescribing approved drugs for uses not included in their official labeling is sometimes a cause of confusion among practitioners.

"The Federal Food, Drug and Cosmetic Act does not limit the manner in which a physician may use an approved drug. Once a product has been approved for marketing, a physician may prescribe it for uses or in treatment regimens or patient populations that are not included in approved labeling. Such 'unapproved' or, more precisely, 'unlabeled' uses may, in fact, reflect approaches to drug therapy that have been extensively reported in medical literature." (Excerpted—full text, p. 175.)

Terminology

The drug that is the subject of this book is known by two generic names, diphenylhydantoin and phenytoin. Phenytoin (PHT) is used in this book.

PHT's best known trade name in the United States is Dilantin. Other trade names, outside the United States, include Aleviaton, Dintoina, Epamin, Epanutin, Epelin, Eptoin, Hidantal, Idantoin, Phenhydan, Solantyl.

Prescription Medicine

PHT is a prescription medicine, which means it should be obtained through a physician.

Table of Contents

Clinical Uses of Phenytoin

Basic Mechanisms of Action

Clinical Uses of Phenytoin

Distinctive Characteristics of Phenytoin

Phenytoin has distinctive characteristics which, when viewed together, set it apart from other substances.

1. PHT regulates bioelectrical activity at the individual cell level. This action, at a level fundamental to all body functions, helps explain how PHT achieves its therapeutic effects in a wide range of disorders.

2. PHT corrects inappropriate electrical activity, but does not affect normal function. It has been found effective in both hyperexcitable and hypoexcitable conditions.

3. PHT has a corrective effect on post-tetanic potentiation and post-tetanic afterdischarge. This action seems to explain how repetitive and uncontrolled thinking is decreased and repetitive messages of pain are modified.

4. PHT has regulatory effects on endocrine and metabolic processes, and on stress. It has been demonstrated to have anti-anoxic effects, anti-toxic properties, and to promote healing.

5. PHT's action is prompt. Taken orally, it is effective within an hour, intravenously within a few minutes. Used topically, its effect against pain is rapid.

6. In therapeutic doses PHT has a calming effect without being sedative, and an energizing effect without being a stimulant.

7. PHT is effective for a wide range of symptoms and disorders. In addition to being useful for a target symptom, PHT can be therapeutic for many other symptoms—in effect have beneficial "side effects."

8. PHT is not habit-forming.

9. PHT's parameters of safety have been established over a fifty-year period by extensive and intensive use.

THOUGHT, MOOD
AND BEHAVIOR DISORDERS

Summary

Phenytoin has been found useful for so many symptoms and disorders (see Table of Contents) that an overall summary is impractical.

The section on Thought, Mood and Behavior Disorders deserves special attention—not only for the benefits in these disorders themselves, but because of the resultant lessening of tension and stress, associated with many other disorders.

Soon after phenytoin's introduction, in 1938, reports started to appear in the medical literature of patients' improvement in mood, concentration, cooperativeness and sense of well-being. By now, extensive published evidence from widely separated sources has established PHT's usefulness for thought, mood and behavior disorders.

. . .

Phenytoin has been shown to have a calming effect on the overactive brain. Symptoms of this condition are preoccupation, multiple thinking, and flashes and fragments of thoughts coming and going. PHT reduces this uncontrolled activity enabling more normal thinking processes to be restored. This effect is usually achieved within an hour, without sedation.

Anger and fear and related emotions are usually found in combination with the overactive brain. Emotional states related to anger for which PHT is therapeutic are impatience, impulsiveness, irritability, aggression, hostility, rage and violence. Emotional states related to fear for which PHT is therapeutic are worry, anxiety, guilt, pessimism and depression. Although excessive anger and fear states are decreased or eliminated by PHT, realistic reactions of anger and fear are not interfered with.

Sleep disturbances found in combination with the overactive brain fall into two general categories. The first and most frequent category is symptomatized by difficulty in falling asleep because of over-thinking, light sleep accompanied by unpleasant dreams and frequent nightmares, and insufficient sleep. A less frequent category is symptomatized by excessive sleep, so-called avoidance sleep. Relief from both types of sleep disturbances is usually prompt with PHT.

PHT is effective with extremes of mood ranging from depression to the hyperexcitable state. These apparently disparate effects are observed in the overactive, impatient individual who is calmed by PHT, and the tired, energyless individual who has a return to normal energy levels.

Somatic symptoms frequently associated with thought, mood and behavior disorders are usually relieved by PHT within an hour. Among them are headaches, pain, stomach discomfort, dizziness, trembling, excessively cold or warm hands or feet, and shortness of breath.

Stress. When the brain becomes overactive and the emotions of fear and anger appear, the body goes on alert, and a state of vigilance develops. For short periods this can be normal. But, if this is a chronic condition , there is constant stimulation of the hypothalamic-pituitary-adrenal (HPA) axis, resulting in the release of the chemicals of fight and flight. A cycle is created, the chemicals keeping the brain overactive and the overactive brain stimulating release of the chemicals. A condition of stress develops. By correcting the overactive brain, PHT seems to break this cycle, causing a more normal state to return—and stress, commonly associated with a wide range of disorders, is diminished or eliminated.

Basic mechanism studies are consistent with the clinical observations of the effectiveness of PHT. Of particular relevance are the studies in the section, Stabilization of Bioelectrical Activity.* They show that PHT, without affecting normal function, corrects hyperexcitability, as in post-tetanic potentiation or post-tetanic repetitive discharge. This would seem to be the mechanism by which PHT corrects the overactive brain.

* See p. 89.

Thought, Mood and Behavior

From the outset, in its use with epileptics, side benefits of PHT were noted. Improvements in thought, mood and behavior were observed.

"Salutary effects of PHT on personality, memory, mood, cooperativeness, emotional stability, amenability to discipline, etc., are also observed, sometimes independently of seizure control."—GOODMAN AND GILMAN (1955).[703]

BENEFITS IN EPILEPTICS

MERRITT AND PUTNAM, *Journal of the American Medical Association* (1938),[557] in the earliest clinical report on PHT observed: "In addition to a relief or a great reduction in the frequency of attacks, it was frequently noted by the parents of children that they were much better behaved, more amenable to discipline and did better work in school."

McCARTAN AND CARSON, *Journal of Mental Science* (1939),[556] while reporting on the efficacy of PHT in controlling seizures in a group of twenty patients, noted: "Irritability and violent episodes are markedly diminished in frequency and severity. The patients are bright and alert, and there is a subjective feeling of well-being.

"Patients comment on their increased efficiency, and the absence of drowsiness which they experienced on bromide and phenobarbital treatment."

KIMBALL AND HORAN, *Annals of Internal Medicine* (1939),[535] in a study of 220 children treated with PHT, reported that apart from the influence on convulsions, there are other benefits from the use of PHT.

The authors noted that there is a marked change in mental state and personality, evidenced by a definite improvement in memory, concentration, and sense of composure, with a return of social interest.

ROSS AND JACKSON, *Annals of Internal Medicine* (1940),[313] noted that in consonance with the alleviation of seizures almost all reports on PHT remark on the improvement in behavior, well-being, cooperation, alertness, general attitude, irritability, temperament, and personality of many patients. Their findings in a study of seventy-three patients were consistent with these reports.

FRANKEL, *Journal of the American Medical Association* (1940),[106] in a study involving forty-eight patients reported that, besides being an effective anticonvulsant, PHT has the advantage of not producing the sedative effect of the other anticonvulsants.

The author noted that the personality of the epileptic patient treated with PHT is remarkably improved.

FETTERMAN AND SHALLENBERGER, *Diseases of the Nervous System* (1941),[95] observed that an outstanding feature of the benefit of PHT is an amazing improvement in personality.

BAKWIN AND BAKWIN, *Journal of Pediatrics* (1951),[539] found PHT beneficial for irritability, hypermotility and variability of behavior in epileptic children, even when seizures were not the major problem.

IN NON-EPILEPTICS

LINDSLEY AND HENRY, *Psychosomatic Medicine* (1942),[225] in an early study, observed that problem children given PHT showed behavioral improvement.

BROWN AND SOLOMON, *American Journal of Psychiatry* (1942),[38] reported that delinquent boys committed to a state training school showed important behavioral improvement on PHT therapy.

Improvement was seen in a reduction in extreme hyperactivity, excitability and temper "flare-ups" and in attention span and more efficient work patterns.

SILVERMAN, *Criminal Psychopathology* (1944),[716] in what appears to be the first reported study on the use of PHT in prisoners, found PHT to be superior to all other agents tested. The study was done with sixty-four prisoners at the Medical Center for Federal Prisoners, Springfield, Missouri.

Improvements were noted in sleep, sense of well-being and cooperativeness. These observations were made in a double-blind crossover study with placebo.

BODKIN, *American Journal of Digestive Diseases* (1945),[25] reporting on his ten years of successful treatment of pruritus ani with PHT, noted that all the patients had one thing in common—they were highly nervous. (See p. 59.)

GOODWIN, *Journal of the National Proctologic Association* (1946),[127] reporting the successful treatment of patients with pruritus ani with PHT, agreed with BODKIN[25] that

nervousness was a factor common in the vast majority of these patients. (See p. 59.)

WALKER AND KIRKPATRICK, *American Journal of Psychiatry* (1947),[373] treated ten behavior problem children with abnormal EEG findings with PHT. None of the children had clinical evidence of seizures, and physical and neurological examinations were all negative.

All of these children showed definite clinical improvement under PHT treatment.

FABRYKANT AND PACELLA, *Annals of Internal Medicine* (1948),[92] in discussing the effects of PHT in labile diabetes, noted that PHT alleviated anxiety, nervous tension and irritability. In addition, the ability to concentrate and to work increased and the patients exhibited a general feeling of well-being.

ZIMMERMAN, *New York State Journal of Medicine* (1956),[395] gave PHT to a group of two hundred children having severe behavior disorders. Improvement was seen in 70% of the cases.

The use of PHT resulted in reduced excitability, less severe and less frequent temper tantrums, reduced hyperactivity and distractibility, fewer fears, and less tendency to go out of contact.

CHAO, SEXTON AND DAVIS, *Journal of Pediatrics* (1964),[51] conducted an extensive study of 535 children classified as having convulsive equivalent syndrome characterized by autonomic disturbances and dysfunction in behavior and communication. A majority of these patients had 14- and 6-EEG patterns. PHT was used alone with 296 of these children and in combination with other drugs in 117 children.

The symptoms benefited included headache, abdominal pain, vasomotor disturbances, nausea, dizziness or syncope, fever and/or chills, shortness of breath, eye pain, photophobia, sweating, weakness, pain in extremities and chest pain.

Behavioral and emotional problems, retardation, school problems in non-retarded, sleep disturbances, speech problems and neurological deficits also responded to treatment. The response was rapid and often striking.

JONAS (1965),[432] in his book *Ictal and Subictal Neurosis,* based on observations of 162 patients over a twelve-year period, found PHT of benefit in a wide range of nonconvulsive disorders.

Among the symptoms which the author noted were helped by PHT were anxiety, depression, agitation, irritability, violence, headache, sleep disturbances, abdominal symptoms, sexual disturbances, hypochondria, visual and auditory phenomena and body image distortion.

LYNK AND AMIDON, *Michigan Medicine* (1965),[576] studied the effect of medication with severely disturbed delinquents under court jurisdiction. The number of patients who received PHT (out of a total of 125) was not given.

They found that some of the children with borderline EEGs but no epilepsy had markedly aggressive behavior. These children responded to PHT when no other drug seemed to help.

DREYFUS (1966)[707] reported on "The Beneficial Effects of PHT on the Nervous System of Nonepileptics—As Experienced and Observed in Others by a Layman."

The author observed that multiple simultaneous thoughts as well as obsessive and preoccupied thinking were relieved by PHT. Coincident with this, marked improvements were noted in symptoms of anger and related conditions of impatience, irritability, agitation and impulsiveness. Also, there was marked improvement in symptoms of fear and the related emotions such as worry, pessimism, anxiety, apprehensiveness and depression.

He noted that the ability to fall asleep more promptly and to sleep more soundly, without nightmares, occurred in the majority of cases. However, with a minority who slept excessively (so-called avoidance sleep) duration of sleep tended to be beneficially reduced.

Based on his observations, the author formed the impression that excessive bioelectrical activity in the nervous system causes unfavorable emotional responses, anger and fear being chief among them. PHT corrects this excessive bioelectrical activity, causing excessive anger and fear to be eliminated.

ROSSI, *New York State Journal of Medicine* (1967),[314] stated that PHT is clinically effective in impulsivity and behavior in hyperactive children and particularly effective in controlling nightmares.

RESNICK, *International Journal of Neuropsychiatry* (1967),[297] reported a double-blind controlled study with crossover and placebo involving eleven inmates at a prison, selected from a group of forty-two volunteers. The entire study (RESNICK AND DREYFUS, 1966)[704] was recorded on tape. The beneficial effects of PHT were reported in connection with overthinking, anger and fear, tension, irritability and hostility. There was marked improvement in ability to concentrate and in sleep problems. Improvement was also observed in headaches, gastrointestinal disturbances and, in one case, phantom limb pain.

Subsequently similar observations were made at a reformatory in six juvenile delinquents ranging in age from twelve to fifteen. With the administration of 100 mg PHT daily, prompt relief in anger and fear was noted and clearly expressed in marked diminution in fighting by five of the boys. The sixth boy, who was withdrawn and passive, became more outgoing, talkative and had an occasional fight. General improvements in overthinking, tension, impatience, impulsiveness, irritability, anger, fear, sleep difficulties and headaches were also observed.

TURNER, *International Journal of Neuropsychiatry* (1967),[364] studied the effect of PHT on patients seen in psychiatric practice during an eighteen-month period. They suffered from a wide variety of emotional and behavioral disorders. Forty-six of fifty-six neurotic patients improved. Improvement was observed in relation to anger, irritability, tension, sleep disturbances, ruminations, anxiety, depression, feelings of guilt and withdrawal, regardless of diagnostic category or EEG findings.

Because of the lack of sedation or stimulation, the author suggested that PHT might be called a normalizer.

JONAS, *International Journal of Neuropsychiatry* (1967),[181] found that over half of 211 patients seen in general psychiatric practice had a therapeutic response to PHT, ranging from reduction to complete reversal of symptoms in the following conditions: anxiety and tension states, reactive depressions, certain cognitive disturbances, obsessive-compulsive manifestations, hypochondria, psychopathy, obesity, and addiction to alcohol and to cigarette smoking.

Many patients reported favorable reactions within one hour after intake of PHT.

The author suggested that the action of PHT placed it in a category separate from the tranquilizers or stimulants and agreed with TURNER[364] that the term normalizer seemed appropriate.

AYD, *International Drug Therapy Newsletter* (1967),[538] in a summary of the clinical psychopharmacological value of PHT entitled "New Uses for an Old Drug," pointed out the effectiveness of PHT for psychic overactivity, distractibility, short attention span, irritability, impulsiveness, insomnia and behavioral disorders in children.

ITIL, RIZZO AND SHAPIRO, *Diseases of the Nervous System* (1967),[178] studied the effect of PHT, combined with thioridazine, on twenty behaviorally disturbed children and adolescents. Eleven patients had personality disorders; five schizophrenic reactions; and four chronic brain syndrome, two with convulsions.

These patients showed low frustration tolerance, hyperactivity and restlessness, aggressive destructive behavior, impulsiveness, poor school or work performance, antisocial acts, sexual acting out, irritability and stubbornness.

After three months of treatment, fifteen of the twenty patients showed moderate to marked improvement and fourteen of them were discharged.

TEC, *American Journal of Psychiatry* (1968),[355] reviewed his fifteen years' experience with PHT in the treatment of behavior disorders in children.

The author reported that PHT improved disruptive behavior in the large majority of the children seen during that period and emphasized that PHT often helped when the phenothiazines and amphetamines failed.

BOELHOUWER, HENRY AND GLUECK, *American Journal of Psychiatry* (1968),[27] in a double-blind study with crossover features and placebo, reported that PHT alone or in combination with thioridazine (Mellaril) was effective at a statistically significant level in a group of seventy-eight patients, ranging in age from fourteen to thirty. Forty-seven of these patients showed 14- and 6-per second positive spiking, whereas no such abnormality was present in thirty-one.

The thirty-one patients without EEG abnormality responded best to PHT alone. The positive spike group responded better to PHT in combination with thioridazine than to either drug alone.

Significant changes were observed for the following factors with PHT alone: disturbance of affect, lack of social conformity, lack of insight, hostile aggressive behavior, dissociative tendency, thinking disorder, self-destructive tendency, and guilty self-concept. In addition to the above, significant changes were observed for the following factors with PHT and Mellaril combined: overt anxiety symptoms, dissociative concern, paranoid thinking, and depression.

BALDWIN, *Maryland Medical Journal* (1969),[706] reported on the treatment with PHT of behavior disorders in children (see also BALDWIN AND KENNY, 1966).[8] The most consistent complaint was hyperactivity. Other important problems were temper tantrums or rage reactions, impulsive behavior and social adaptation. Attention span was short and concentration poor. Of 300 cases treated during a six-month period, it was found that 109 had improved so markedly

that they were able to return to school. Of the 109 who showed marked improvement, 78 had received PHT—48 of them had behavior problems not associated with seizures.

CASE, RICKELS AND BAZILIAN, *American Journal of Psychiatry* (1969),[46] reported that anxious-neurotic psychiatric clinic outpatients were treated over a four-week period with PHT (100 mg twice daily). While some improvement was observed in this patient group, no statistically significant difference was noted between the PHT and a comparable placebo group.

However, the authors reported an interesting finding, namely, "a paucity of side effects in the PHT-treated group (only one patient reported mild dizziness), while our placebo control group had the usual variety of side effects . . . in twelve of the twenty patients." If the only variable in these two groups was that one took PHT and one took placebo, then the probability that PHT was effective in preventing the placebo "side effects" in these anxious-neurotic patients was at the level of significance of $p < 0.001$.

STEPHENS AND SHAFFER, *Psychopharmacologia* (1970),[700] in a double-blind study with thirty adult outpatients, found PHT to be markedly effective in reducing symptoms relating to anger, irritability, impatience and anxiety.

The therapeutic effectiveness of PHT was demonstrated at statistically high levels by both self-ratings and physician ratings of change. This double-blind study was done on a crossover basis with placebo. The dosage of PHT was 100 mg t.i.d.

When compared to placebo, such standard scale factors as "anger," "furious," and "impatience" improved with PHT at p levels between 0.01 and 0.001. Standard scale factors of "worried," and "angry" improved at levels of p<0.01. Factors of "tension," "grouchy," "ready for a fight," "nervous," "nervousness and shakiness," "trembling," and "quarrelsomeness" improved at levels of p<0.05.

In the crossover analysis, PHT improved "tension," "worried," "uncertain about things," "resentful," "bad tempered," "angry," "impatience," and global change rated by patient all at the level of p<0.01; PHT improved "bewildered," "nervous," "ready for a fight," "confused," "anxious," "irritability," "quarrelsomeness," "heart pounding," "temper outbursts," "trembling," "nervousness and shakiness," all at levels of p<0.05; and the factors of "furious," "grouchy," and global change rated by physician all were improved by PHT at levels of p<0.001.

The patients' feelings of tranquility, composure, relaxation, optimism and cheerfulness also showed statistically significant improvement with PHT.

No undesirable side effects were encountered.

LOOKER AND CONNERS, *Archives of General Psychiatry* (1970), [1304] conducted a double-blind study with PHT on seventeen subjects, ranging in age from five to fourteen years, who had periodic episodes of misbehavior. Although no statistically significant group changes were attributable to drug effect, it was the impression of the authors that among the patients "there were some who responded rather dramatically."

The authors also reported on three children in whom PHT had a marked effect in the treatment of severe temper tantrums. In each case the response to PHT was prompt.

The children were followed-up six months later and the marked improvement had persisted. In two of the cases, when the parents forgot to give PHT, deterioration

was noted within two days. This deterioration was promptly corrected with PHT.

GOLDBERG AND KURLAND, *Journal of Nervous and Mental Diseases* (1970), [713] in a double-blind study, reported the effectiveness of PHT on the emotional, cognitive and social behavior of forty-seven hospitalized retardates, ages nine to fourteen.

Patients treated with PHT showed strong improvement in ability to maintain attention, in self-control, and in improved interpersonal relationships with adults.

There was marked improvement in logical thinking, and decreased temper outbursts, impulsivity and aggression. There were also trends toward increased ability to concentrate and better visual-motor organization.

The effective dose of PHT was 100 mg twice daily. Neither toxicity nor side effects were observed.

DANIEL, *Geriatrics* (1970), [938] states that symptoms of confusion, which are so common in the aged, often are caused by underlying physical illness, frequently cardiac and respiratory disorders resulting in cerebral hypoxia. He states that PHT is therapeutically useful in this group, yet it is often overlooked.*

Among the symptoms of confusion so common in the aged are: disorientation; lack of attention and concentration; fluctuation in state of consciousness; memory loss, particularly of current events; and impairment of conventional judgment.

The author states that although problems of insufficient cerebral blood flow are well known in the aged, direct measurement of cerebral blood flow is difficult. However, the author states that symptoms of insufficient cerebral blood flow are identifiable clinically. Among these symptoms are irritability, restlessness, mental confusion and sometimes severe depression. The author notes that after cerebrovascular accident the patient often has paresthesias and tingling. He states that PHT not only frequently gives relief from the paresthesias, but that mental symptoms also improve.

BOZZA, in a detailed paper presented at the *Fourth Italian National Congress of Child Neuropsychiatry* (1971),[863] reports on an individual basis on twenty-one slightly brain damaged retarded children who were observed for periods of from twelve to thirty-six months. In most of the cases PHT was tried. The author concludes that PHT and vitamins materially improved the expected intellectual growth rate of these retarded children. (See also Refs. 8, 355, 373, 1626.)

ALVAREZ, in a book titled *"Nerves in Collision"* (1972),[761] reviews his twenty-five years' experience in the use of PHT for a wide variety of disorders.

In his book, Alvarez reports on the successful use of PHT in the treatment of anxiety, nervousness, tension, fear, nightmares, depression, rage, violent outbursts, confusion, fatigue (extreme), abdominal pain, alcoholism, anorexia nervosa, bed wetting, blackouts, dizzy spells, head pain, involuntary movements, migraine-like headaches. (See also Ref. 4.)

STEPHENS AND SHAFFER, *The Journal of Clinical Pharmacology* (1973).[1592] In an earlier paper[700] the authors had reported on the successful treatment with PHT of thirty private psychiatric outpatients. This study had been done on a double-blind crossover basis.

About two years later, ten of this group of patients participated in a double-blind study of PHT for four consecutive two-week periods.

Consistent with the previous study, 100 mg t.i.d. of PHT proved significantly more effective than placebo in relieving symptoms of anxiety, anger and irritability as assessed both by self-ratings and physicians' ratings of change.

BRODSKY, ZUNIGA, CASENAS, ERNSTOFF AND SACHDEV, *Psychiatric Journal of the University of Ottawa* (1983),[2357] describe a group of ten patients with recurrent attacks of anxiety. Eight responded to PHT alone. The ninth patient responded to a combination of PHT and clonazepam, and the tenth to carbamazepine. All patients had normal routine EEGs, but abnormal twenty-four-hour sleep EEGs. (See also Ref. 2356.)

DE LA TORRE, NAVARRO AND ALDRETE, *Current Therapeutic Research* (1985),[2437] reported a controlled study of eighty patients with irritable bowel syndrome. Forty patients received PHT (100 mg t.i.d.) and forty received conventional treatment which included either a tranquilizer or an antidepressant.

In addition to greater relief of abdominal pain, diarrhea, constipation, nausea, vomiting and pyrosis, patients receiving PHT had a statistically significant greater number of complete remissions of depression, insomnia and anxiety than patients receiving conventional therapy.

Violent Behavior

Many of the preceding studies have reported PHT useful for anger and related symptoms. Expressions used are aggressive behavior, anger, hostile, temper tantrums, impulsivity, rage, assaultive behavior and violent behavior. The following studies have their main focus on violence.

MALETSKY, *Medical Times* (1972),[1329] states that it is currently fashionable to ascribe the roots of violence to social ills. The role of brain dysfunction has been relatively neglected until recently.

The author reports on a study of twenty-two patients with the syndrome referred to as episodic dyscontrol. In describing this syndrome he states that the subjects usually have a history of hyperactivity and poor school performance as children, aggression toward other children and animals and fire-setting. Truancy and petty stealing frequently lead them to grand larceny, assault and battery and even murder. Other typical symptoms are traffic violations and recklessness. The author states that central to this dyscontrol syndrome is the "storm of violence." Upon minimal or even no provocation these patients lose control, wrecking property and directing violence against anyone in their way.

Twenty-two patients with episodic dyscontrol were treated with PHT. Tabulation of the results of this treatment was based on the author's observations and on reports of relatives and friends of the patient. The author pointed out that the patients had all been through futile trials with other drugs.

Nineteen of the patients achieved a result equal to or better than "good response." Fifteen of these achieved an excellent response with virtually complete absence of attacks. This response usually occurred within the first two weeks. Data collected at twelve months showed that all cases responding to PHT remained free of violent outbreaks.

All of the patients said they had not lost the ability to feel anger, but they were better able to control its escalation.

MALETSKY AND KLOTTER, *Diseases of the Nervous System* (1974),[1328] in a controlled study, found PHT significantly effective (p<.01) in twenty-two patients with episodic dyscontrol syndrome.

The authors state that this study, with placebo, confirms the earlier work of Maletsky in which he found PHT highly effective in the treatment of this syndrome. As a result of these studies, the authors conclude that PHT should be tried in patients with episodic dyscontrol.

DIAMOND AND YARYURA-TOBIAS, *Paper presented at the Fifth World Congress of Psychiatry* (1971),[961] found PHT effective in the treatment of violent and aggressive behavior in schizophrenics. Twenty-two patients were studied.

With PHT, in doses up to 300 mg a day, violent behavior was well controlled in all cases, eleven with excellent results and seven with moderate results.

The authors state that all therapeutic methods used by the patients prior to PHT administration were ineffective.

SOLOMON AND KLEEMAN, *California Medicine* (1971),[1569] in reporting seven cases of episodic dyscontrol syndrome, comment separately on the only two in which PHT was given. In both cases the patient's behavior was markedly improved.

In a case detailed, a thirty-nine-year-old woman entered the hospital because of repeated attacks of uncontrolled behavior. Without warning, she would be assailed by intense feelings of either rage or sexual excitement. Tranquilizing medication proved ineffective. PHT caused a remarkable improvement in this patient's behavior.

BACH-Y-RITA, LION, CLIMENT AND ERVIN, *American Journal of Psychiatry* (1971),[787] reported that in the course of two years they had seen 130 patients with assaultive and destructive behavior.

PHT was found useful whether or not EEG abnormalities were found.

Psychoses

PHT has been reported useful in decreasing irritability and improving sense of well-being in psychotics. In some cases where the psychosis has occurred in association with metabolic disorders or brain injury, the use of PHT has been reported to correct the psychotic state.

KALINOWSKY AND PUTNAM, *Archives of Neurology and Psychiatry* (1943),[186] reported on the treatment with PHT of sixty psychotic patients. Improvement occurred in over half of the patients during the period of treatment and usually consisted of diminution of excitement and irritability, almost irrespective of the type of psychosis.

Although PHT did not change the basic psychosis, the patients' mood, behavior and emotions were improved.

FREYHAN, *Archives of Neurology and Psychiatry* (1945),[110] reported on a group of forty psychiatric patients. PHT therapy, 300–600 mg/day, resulted in positive behavioral changes in certain excited patients.

KUBANEK AND ROWELL, *Diseases of the Nervous System* (1946),[201] used PHT in the treatment of prolonged chronic disturbed behavior in seventy-three psychotic patients unresponsive to other drugs. They found PHT unquestionably valuable for some of these patients.

HAWARD, *Proceedings of the Symposium on Aggressive Behavior* (1969),[697] reported that PHT was effective in reducing aggressive behavior in a double-blind study involving twenty chronic psychotic patients. Although the basic psychoses were not changed, important benefits in mood were noted.

PINTO, SIMOPOULOS, UHLENHUTH AND DEROSA, *Comprehensive Psychiatry* (1974),[1415] in a study of thirty-two severely regressed chronic schizophrenic patients, found that PHT in doses of 250–350 mg per day, when added to a phenothiazine, improved conditions such as irritability, aggression and negative behavior. (See also Ref. 1551.)

BELLAK, *American Journal of Psychotherapy* (1976),[2320] in summarizing thirty years of clinical experience, describes the usefulness of PHT in a subgroup of schizophrenics with minimal brain dysfunction. The author noted that these patients do not do well with phenothiazines, but that PHT, alone or in combination with methylphenidate and imipramine, is frequently effective.

SURMAN AND PARKER, *Psychosomatics* (1981),[2995] reported three patients with episodic psychotic disturbances associated with renal disease. All responded to PHT with resolution of the psychotic behavior and/or hallucinations.

Hypoglycemia

STAMBAUGH AND TUCKER, *Diabetes* (1974),[1583] describe the successful treatment, with PHT, of five patients with symptomatic hypoglycemia previously unresponsive to dietary management.

Among the symptoms, typical of the hypoglycemic patient, were chronic anxiety, extreme lethargy, chills, frequent nausea, sensory deficits and other neurological complaints. These symptoms disappeared during PHT therapy, and clinical reversal of hypoglycemia was observed in all of the five cases.

Six-hour glucose tolerance and radioimmunoassays of insulin levels, before and after PHT, demonstrated PHT's regulatory effects and confirmed the clinical observations (see below).

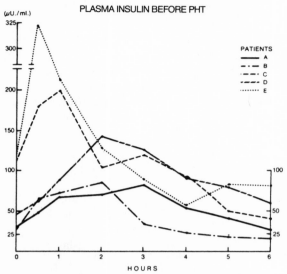

Abnormally large insulin response to a glucose load in hypoglycemic patients.

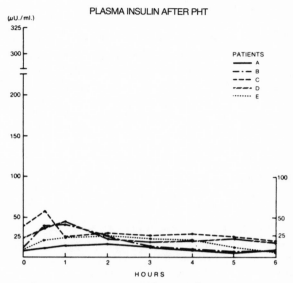

The same patients, with PHT, have an insulin response in the normal range.

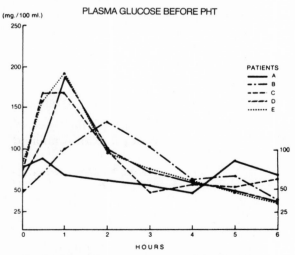

In the hypoglycemic patients, blood sugar falls to abnormally low levels in response to a glucose load.

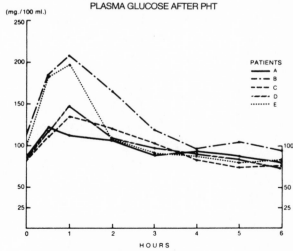

In the same hypoglycemic patients, with PHT, the blood sugar returned to normal levels.

Cognitive Function

HAWARD, *Portsmouth Journal of Psychology* (1968),[585] found PHT effective in the improvement of concentration. This was demonstrated in a performance test designed to simulate air traffic control tower conditions.

Twelve volunteers, nineteen to twenty-one years of age, were introduced to an air traffic control task requiring a high degree of concentration. The test was done with placebo, on a double-blind basis, and the essential variable was number of errors made. On this basis, improved efficiency was demonstrated by PHT at the significant level of $p<0.01$.

No individual felt a drug effect of any sort. The author stated that this subtlety of action was consistent with what frequently had been observed in the clinical use of PHT.

The author says that because of its high level of safety and its nonaddictive character, PHT has none of the negative qualities of the amphetamines, which have in the past been used for similar purposes.

HAWARD, *Drugs and Cerebral Function* (1970),[1139] studied the effect of PHT upon performance in a complex task, subject to fatigue, in twelve college students who had concentration difficulties. A double-blind crossover procedure was followed.

PHT was found to be significantly effective in delaying the onset of fatigue and accompanying errors.

The author notes that these findings are in accord with the observations of DREYFUS[707] that poor concentration can result from forced ruminative thinking, or the "turned-on mind," and that this can be corrected by PHT. (See also Ref. 527.)

GOLDBERG AND KURLAND, *Journal of Nervous and Mental Disease* (1970),[713] in a double-blind study, reported strong improvement in ability to maintain attention and concentration with PHT. (For more complete summary, see p. 8.)

DANIEL, *Geriatrics* (1970),[938] reported PHT useful for symptoms of confusion in the aged, including lack of attention and concentration. (For more complete summary, see p. 8.)

SMITH AND LOWREY, *Drugs, Development and Cerebral Function* (1972),[1564] suggest that improvement in cognitive performance can be due to improved concentration. Using standard IQ tests, the authors compared PHT to placebo on twenty hospital employee volunteers.

The test was done on a double-blind crossover basis. PHT, 100 mg three times daily, improved Verbal Scale and Full Scale scores at highly significant levels and the Performance Scale improvement was also significant.

The authors state that their findings are consistent with those obtained by HAWARD.[1139]

HAWARD, *Revue de Medicine Aeronautique et Spatiale* (1973),[1140] found that PHT significantly improved the performance of three separate groups of pilots in simulated flying and radar target-fixing tasks.

Three groups of pilots, twenty-two commercial pilots, eighteen military pilots and nineteen private pilots were studied. Two absorbing tasks were required of the pilots in an attempt to reach their full channel capacity. The first was a standard flight simulation procedure. The second task consisted of monitoring and responding to a new type of radar.

The pilots were scored on their ability to bring the simulated aircraft into position to correctly intercept a moving target. Sixty minutes before each task 150 mg of PHT was given.

With PHT the test results showed significant improvement in performance both in terms of lessened time spent and the increased number of correct responses. In all three groups the improvement was significant.

The author states that he chose PHT because other substances which have been tried for this purpose, such as amphetamine, pemoline and prolintane, can have undesirable side effects.

SMITH AND LOWREY, *Journal of the American Geriatrics Society* (1975),[1565] observed the beneficial effect of PHT upon cognitive function in a group of elderly normal subjects.

In the present study ten volunteers, four male and six female, average age sixty-nine years, were studied in a double-blind crossover test with placebo control. This crossover design was used to eliminate possible practice effects on performance.

With PHT significant improvement in scores occurred in information, comprehension, digit symbol and full scale IQ. The authors conclude that these significant improvements illustrate the effectiveness of PHT in improving generalized mental functions.

Speech Disorders

SCHÖNHÄRL, *Medicina Experimentalis* (1960),[331] reported that hydantoin therapy was helpful in a series of one hundred and forty patients treated for speech and voice disorders. The author did not specify which hydantoin was used.

SACK, *University of California, Doctoral Thesis* (1968),[320] conducted a double-blind study with PHT in twenty-four stutterers.

Statistically significant reduction of stuttering intensity was found with PHT (100 mg). The intensity of the stuttering was significantly reduced although the frequency of stuttering was not changed.

RILEY AND MASSEY, *Headache* (1980),[2047] report on three patients with aphasia and headache, and left temporal spikes, all of whom were successfully treated with PHT.

The authors note that in one case, when the patient "ran out" of PHT, headaches and slowing of speech returned.

For other reports on a variety of speech disorders, see Refs. 1763, 1821, 1911, 2029, 2154, 2172, 2198, 2206, 2208, 2243, 2568.

Alcoholism and Drug Addiction

PHT has been found useful in alcohol and drug withdrawal, not only for seizure control, but also for mood and behavioral problems.

Problems of the nervous system are frequent causes of drug and alcohol addiction. For this reason PHT's use as a preventive should be considered. In addition to its regulatory effect on the nervous system it has the advantage of being non-addictive.

WILHOIT, *Journal of the Florida Medical Association* (1965),[383] reported that one of the most important steps taken in the treatment of acute alcoholism and delirium tremens is the prophylactic use of PHT. With PHT patients tended to have a much easier and quicker recovery from acute alcoholism.

The author also noted that with PHT treatment, by the fourth to the seventh day, there was a marked improvement in sense of well-being, sleep pattern, appetite and motivation.

Fox, *Modern Treatment* (1966),[105] recommended PHT (100 mg four times a day) for five to ten days for prevention of convulsions due to alcohol withdrawal. The author stated that frequently convulsions due to withdrawal from alcohol are mistaken for epilepsy and the patient is sent home on PHT and phenobarbital. PHT offers no problem, but, in the case of phenobarbital, the danger exists that the patient may gradually increase it to the point of addiction.

Ramirez, *Personal Communication* (1967),[290] described the effective use of PHT during withdrawal of patients with various forms of addiction including heroin.

During a three-year period of clinical study it was found that after physical detoxification most patients went through a stormy period of behavioral difficulties which lasted from seven to ten days on the average. Patients were irritable, intolerant, and frequently showed temper tantrums. In addition, they were insomniac and depressed.

On PHT there was a rapid change in the over-all behavior patterns of the patients. Acting out behavior was much less frequent. Sleeplessness, which is a very difficult problem with addicts, was also modified favorably.

After a preliminary study with thirty patients, the author used PHT routinely, 100 mg three times a day.

Chafetz, *Journal of the American Medical Association* (1967),[571] stated that PHT is most effective in the treatment and prevention of convulsions associated with alcoholic withdrawal. He pointed out that PHT is a desirable medication because it lacks the hypotensive effect sometimes found with the phenothiazines.

Thurlow and Girvin, *Canadian Medical Association Journal* (1971),[1616] reported the successful treatment with PHT of two cases of flashbacks (recurrent visual hallucinations after LSD).

In one of the cases the patient had been suffering from flashbacks five months after the discontinuance of all hallucinogenic drugs. She was given chlorpromazine, 25 mg t.i.d., with moderate diminution in the intensity, frequency and affective component of her flashbacks. Hallucinations continued to occur, but were less terrifying. Chlorpromazine was discontinued and the previous level of flashbacks returned within twenty-four hours.

PHT was instituted, 100 mg t.i.d. Within forty-eight hours she noted a very marked reduction in all types of flashbacks.

In the other case, 100 mg of PHT intravenously terminated a flashback while in progress. Before injecting PHT, saline solution was injected, as a control, with no effect. (See also Ref. 1988.)

Adams, *Journal of the American Medical Association* (1971),[2141] states: "In more than 500 cases of acute alcohol withdrawal, I have yet to see a patient suffer delirium tremens or convulsions when PHT, 100 mg orally four times daily, is given . . ."

Finer, *Journal of the American Medical Association* (1971),[2182] reporting on the experience in a 1400-bed hospital, states that it is their belief that the tremors, apprehension and psychomotor excitation experienced in withdrawing alcohol should not be subdued by another depressant drug. The author states that it is their practice to give PHT orally, 100 mg four times a day.

Out of 735 admissions and 565 readmissions over a three-year period, no seizures occurred in alcoholic patients who received PHT.

FISHER AND DIMINO, *British Journal of Addiction* (1975),[1033] in discussing their clinical experience, report that they found PHT to be useful in their over-all therapeutic approach to withdrawal from addictive agents, including heroin, amphetamines, and alcohol.

IFABUMUYI AND JEFFRIES, *Canadian Psychiatric Association Journal* (1976),[1904] describe the successful use of PHT in treating several cases of drug-induced psychosis and detail three cases which had previously been unsuccessfully treated with major tranquilizers. All patients had taken hallucinogenic drugs for over five years.

PHT, 100 mg two or three times a day, resulted in prompt improvement in symptoms of psychotic behavior, bizarre visual, auditory and tactile hallucinations, feelings of derealization, fragmented thinking, and lack of concentration.

The authors state that PHT was dramatically effective in treating these refractory cases.

Sleep Disorders

Many of the preceding studies emphasize the benefits of PHT in sleep,* but few studies have been done on sleep disturbances alone. However, reports are consistent that people fall asleep more easily, sleep longer, and are less troubled with unpleasant dreams and nightmares. A less common sleep disturbance, too much sleep (avoidance sleep), is also reported helped by PHT.

* See Refs. 4, 51, 297, 314, 364, 538, 704, 707, 713, 716, 761, 1841, 2037.

BJERK AND HORNISHER, *Electroencephalography and Clinical Neurophysiology* (1958),[835] refer to generalities in the literature that anticonvulsants are not effective for narcolepsy.

The authors present a case, which they consider typical narcolepsy, that showed excellent response to treatment with PHT. The patient, a thirty-seven-year-old female, had overpowering attacks of sleep and other typical symptoms of narcolepsy.

On 100 mg of PHT t.i.d. the patient's symptoms left her on the seventh day. The improvement was marked by a complete loss of symptoms, appetite improved and the patient said that she had not felt so well in a long time.

When the patient stopped taking the medication the symptoms recurred.

ZUNG, *Psychophysiology* (1968),[397] studied the effect of PHT on sleep. Ten adults, between the ages of twenty and forty-six, were studied with all night EEG and electrooculogram recordings. With PHT the time spent in REM sleep was significantly decreased compared to control. Non-REM (deeper) sleep was increased.

BOLLER, WRIGHT, CAVALIERI AND MITSUMOTO, *Neurology* (1975),[1753] reported the complete relief with PHT in a sixty-five-year-old man from paroxysmal nightmares, a sequel to a stroke. These nightmare-like episodes gradually increased in frequency (twenty per day) to a point where the patient had to be hospitalized.

During an episode the patient would suddenly bolt upright, pace around with a terrified expression on his face, and shout in a dysarthric voice. At times he related fright visions.

PHT was given, with a loading dose of 300 mg intravenously, followed by 900 mg orally over the next twenty-four hours. Thereafter the patient received daily doses of 300 mg/day. The episodes ceased and the patient remained symptom-free when followed up six months later.

PEDLEY AND GUILLEMINAULT, *Annals of Neurology* (1977),[2014] described six patients, between the ages of seventeen and thirty-two years, who had been experiencing unusual sleepwalking episodes characterized by screaming or unintelligible vocalizations, complex and often violent automatisms, and ambulation.

All patients were treated with either phenytoin or carbamazepine, with cessation of the abnormal behavior during follow-up periods ranging from nine to forty-eight months.

FUKUYAMA, OCHIAI, HAYAKAWA AND MIYAGAWA, *Neuropadiatrie* (1979),[1841] describe the successful use of PHT in treating an eight-year-old male with choreoathetoid activity. In addition to eliminating the abnormal movements, behavior improvements were noted, and the patient's sleep patterns were improved.

Sleep patterns were evaluated before and after PHT. Increase in sleep time, decrease in number of stages, and disappearance of interrupting awakening were noted.

WOLF, RODER-WANNER AND BREDE, *Epilepsia* (1984),[3080] studied polygraphic (EEG, EOG or electrooculogram, ECG and respiration) sleep patterns in forty untreated epileptic patients. They compared phenobarbital and PHT in a randomized cross-over design. With both phenobarbital and PHT sleep onset came sooner, but with PHT light sleep was decreased and deep sleep increased. The authors state, "The decrease of light sleep to the benefit of deep sleep, together with the rapid sleep onset, make PHT look like an excellent sleeping medication." In addition, they comment that few patients report sleep "hangovers" with PHT.

See also Refs. 2626, 2858, 2967, 2986.

Enuresis

CAMPBELL AND YOUNG, *Journal of Urology* (1966),[43] reported that twenty-nine patients having enuresis and evidencing EEG abnormalities were treated with PHT, alone or in combination with other anticonvulsant medication.

Only twenty-two of these patients could be followed up. Eleven were reported to be cured or improved and eleven showed no change.

BALDWIN, *Maryland Medical Journal* (1969),[706] in a study of seventy-eight behavior problem children, noted that among the symptoms helped by PHT was enuresis.

Anorexia, Bulimia and Binge Eating

GREEN AND RAU, *American Journal of Psychiatry* (1974),[1097] found PHT highly effective in treating ten patients who had three distinct types of symptoms of compulsive eating.

One group was extremely underweight. Sometimes they ate nothing, yet they constantly thought about food. Frequently they would overeat and then would overcorrect this condition by forcing themselves to vomit. Thus they stayed underweight. These patients were considered by the authors to come under the category of primary anorexia nervosa.

The second group consisted of persons of normal weight. They were also preoccupied with food and they had a compulsive wish to eat. Their entire lives were structured to avoid exposure to food through various and complicated maneuvers. They occasionally went on eating binges that lasted for hours or days. They would then diet back to normal, unlike group one, who always dieted back to below normal.

Group three consisted of patients who gave in to their strong compulsion to eat. They became overweight over a period of years, some rapidly, some slowly. They were from 150 to 250 pounds above normal weight.

Of the ten patients, nine had abnormal EEGs but none was epileptic. PHT was highly effective in nine of these patients, including the one with normal EEG. In two cases PHT was withdrawn and symptoms returned. When PHT was reinstated, the symptoms disappeared.

The authors say that compulsive eating is usually accompanied by other undesirable symptoms, including depression. Improvement in these other symptoms was usually observed.

RAU AND GREEN, *Comprehensive Psychiatry* (1975),[2037] report on an additional eight patients with the syndrome of compulsive eating. These patients had abnormal EEGs. They were treated with PHT and five of them responded dramatically. Three had questionably positive responses.

The authors give as an example the case of an emaciated twenty-five-year-old female who weighed seventy-nine pounds. Her

compulsive eating episodes were followed by feelings of guilt, vomiting and sleeping difficulties. She was a compulsive stealer.

After two weeks' treatment with PHT, 100 mg t.i.d., she reported a "miracle." She had no further episodes of compulsive eating, was less obsessed with thoughts of food and there were no episodes of stealing. After six months she remained symptom-free and was approaching normal weight.

The authors state that their investigations suggest that compulsive eating has a neurologic etiology.

In a further study, RAU, STRUVE AND GREEN (1979),[2896] report that twenty-seven of forty-seven patients (some without abnormal EEGs) responded to PHT therapy. (See also Ref. 2038.)

WERMUTH, DAVIS, HOLLISTER AND STUNKARD, *American Journal of Psychiatry* (1977),[2117] based on the findings of GREEN AND RAU conducted a double-blind crossover study, using placebo, to test the efficacy of PHT in treating "binge eating."

After careful screening, medical, psychiatric and EEG evaluations, nineteen female patients, who had suffered for two to twenty-four years with episodes of binge eating, were selected for study.

Six patients markedly improved, two moderately improved, and six slightly improved during PHT treatment. Improvement in six of the patients who had EEG abnormalities was similar to that observed in other patients, and the authors concluded that treatment response did not correlate with EEG abnormalities.

Subjects whose binge eating was markedly reduced during PHT treatment reported better self-control, marked improvement in self-esteem, less preoccupation with eating, and more normal eating habits.

SZYPER AND MANN, *Neurology* (1978),[2100] reported a case of classical anorexia nervosa in a sixteen-year-old girl whose weight loss was greater than 16 kg (30% of body weight) over a two-year period. The patient also suffered partial complex seizures uncontrolled by barbiturates.

PHT treatment was begun, resulting in seizure control, EEG improvement and dramatic weight gain.

MOORE AND RAKES, *Journal of Clinical Psychiatry* (1982),[2804] describe a twenty-one-year-old student with disabling symptoms of binge eating, difficulty in concentrating and feelings of frustration and guilt.

PHT, 100 mg t.i.d., was started and, by the fourth day, the compulsion to eat had entirely disappeared. Problems with concentration and feelings of guilt and frustration also disappeared. The patient remained symptom-free for a year. PHT was discontinued and another episode of binge eating developed, which again responded to PHT. The patient remained symptom-free on 300 mg of PHT a day.

PARSONS AND SAPSE, *Journal of Ortho-molecular Psychiatry* (1985),[2849] treated forty-two patients with anorexia nervosa with PHT along with psychotherapy and other medications considered cortisol antagonists. After four to five days the patients exhibited marked improvement in attitudes towards food and they started eating more normally. Feelings of hostility and fear were diminished and feelings of confidence were improved.

For further references see 1869, 2116, 2304, 2556, 2625, 2656, 2800.

STUDIES IN WHICH SIGNIFICANT RESULTS WERE NOT OBSERVED

PASAMANICK, *Archives of Neurology and Psychiatry* (1951),[560] found that PHT, methylphenylethylhydantoin, trimethadione and phenobarbital caused no significant improvement in behavior in children with EEG abnormalities.

KLEIN AND GREENBERG, *American Journal of Psychiatry* (1967),[196] in a pilot study of the effectiveness of PHT on thirteen severely psychotic patients, found no general beneficial effect of PHT.

KANZLER, MALITZ AND HIGGINS, *Journal of the American Medical Association* (1968),[651] in a double-blind study, evaluated six "commonly prescribed antidepressants," including PHT. They did not find any of the drugs significantly different than placebo.

LEFKOWITZ, *Archives of General Psychiatry* (1969),[218] in a double-blind study with PHT and placebo, found "marked diminution in the disruptive behavior in both groups." Placebo results were better than with PHT.

CARDIOVASCULAR DISORDERS

Summary

Recognition of phenytoin's basic property, stabilization of bio-electrical activity, led to its therapeutic use in cardiology. The first evidence was provided by Harris and Kokernot in 1950 in a basic mechanism study showing that PHT reversed cardiac arrhythmias after coronary occlusion in dogs. The first evidence of its clinical usefulness in cardiac arrhythmias in man was presented, in a detailed paper, by Leonard in 1958.

Subsequent studies have shown that PHT is useful in a wide range of cardiovascular disorders. It is effective in the treatment of a variety of cardiac arrhythmias, including ventricular arrhythmias associated with hypokalemia, digitalis toxicity, ischemia and myocardial infarction, surgical procedures and myopathic processes; paroxysmal atrial tachycardia and atrial extrasystoles; and as prophylaxis against anesthesia- and cardioversion-induced arrhythmias.[1] PHT's ability to offset the toxic effects of digitalis without impairing its inotropic benefits allows larger amounts of digitalis to be given before toxic levels are reached.

PHT has been shown to have beneficial effects on the cardiac conduction system. These effects are an example of PHT's biphasic actions since, dependent on the initial state of the tissue, it can either increase or decrease conduction.[2] PHT does not alter normal sinus node function or rate, atrial refractoriness, intra-atrial conduction velocity, or prolong Q-T interval. PHT has been found beneficial in the treatment of the prolonged Q-T interval syndrome, torsade de pointes arrhythmias and tricyclic antidepressant induced arrhythmias.[2]

PHT has been shown to decrease sympathetic nervous system activity with resultant reduction in cardiac contractile force, blood pressure and heart rate. It has been reported to be useful in hypertension.[3]

Both clinical and laboratory studies have shown PHT to be useful in hypoxic-ischemic states. Clinically, PHT has been reported to reduce the frequency and severity of anginal attacks,[4] improving ST depression on the electrocardiogram. It controls ischemia-induced arrhythmias; and improves brain function in ischemic states, including reduction of neurological deficits after cardiac arrest.[5] In the laboratory, PHT has been demonstrated to increase cerebral and cardiac blood flow and to have anti-anoxic and anti-ischemic effects in brain, nerve, heart and lung.

PHT has been reported to increase high-density lipoprotein-cholesterol (HDL-C) levels. Since there is evidence that there is an inverse relationship between HDL-C levels and atherosclerotic problems such as myocardial infarction and stroke, the use of PHT as a preventive against these disorders is suggested.[6]

In addition to its specific cardiovascular actions, PHT has general properties relevant to the treatment of cardiovascular disorders. These include its usefulness against pain, anxiety, fear, anger and stress, without sedative effect.[7]

---

[1] *Cardiac arrhythmias (various):* Refs. 18, 61, 141, 166, 187, 221, 248, 310, 418, 517, 720, 721, 753, 987, 1052, 1121, 1214, 1264, 1339, 1390, 1488, 1847, 2058, 2083, 2251, 2331, 2390, 2528, 2569.

Cardioversion-induced arrhythmias: Refs. 248, 720, 923, 936, 1264, 1289.

Arrhythmias associated with myocardial infarction: Refs. 221, 248, 516, 987, 1120, 1705, 2150, 2151, 2478, 2649, 2650, 2729.

[2] *Conduction defects:* Refs. 22, 154, 158, 327, 753, 764, 816, 826, 830, 831, 832, 833, 884, 935, 1114, 1120, 1264, 1390, 1434, 1450, 1488, 1562, 1590, 1645, 1776, 1804, 1822, 2069, 2163, 2223, 2296, 2348, 2361, 2376, 2377, 2478, 2558, 2565, 2664, 2695, 2799, 2883, 2992, 3037, 3052, 3066.

Prolonged Q-T interval: Refs. 764, 1776, 1972, 2069, 2071, 2094, 2223, 2328, 2361, 2370, 2376, 2462, 2558, 2695, 2807, 2837, 2895, 2951, 2957, 3066.

Torsade de pointes: Refs. 158, 764, 816, 935, 2069, 2296, 2478, 2664, 2799, 2883, 2992, 3052.

Tricyclic antidepressant overdose: Refs. 2348, 2377, 2565.

[3] *Hypertension:* Refs. 414, 1480, 1717, 1797, 2090, 2316, 2668.

[4] *Angina pectoris:* Refs. 18, 1611, 2667.

[5] *Cerebrovascular insufficiencies:* Refs. 938, 1216, 1560, 1718, 1719, 2142, 2768. See also Anti-anoxic Effects of PHT.

[6] *High-density lipoproteins (HDL):* Refs. 1893, 1961, 2002, 2162, 2235, 2318, 2319, 2323, 2428, 2542, 2649, 2650, 2652, 2734, 2741, 2813, 2814, 2827, 2897, 2946.

[7] See also Thought, Mood and Behavior section—beneficial effects of PHT on fear, anxiety, anger and stress; and Pain section.

Cardiac Arrhythmias

The first use of PHT in cardiac disorders was reported by LEONARD in 1958. Since it was the pioneer paper in this field, it will be summarized in some detail. It brings into focus three important points which develop throughout the literature: 1) PHT is an effective antiarrhythmic, prompt in its action; 2) PHT has a high margin of safety; 3) In the acute stage, substantial amounts of PHT may be required, adjusted to the severity of the condition.

LEONARD, *Archives of Internal Medicine* (1958),[221] demonstrated the beneficial effect of PHT in controlling ventricular hyperirritability complicating myocardial infarction in a patient.

The patient was gravely ill with cardiographic findings of typical ventricular tachycardia. In spite of the previous history of complete heart block, it was felt that intravenous procainamide, if carefully controlled, was the treatment of choice. The patient was receiving Arterenol to maintain his blood pressure at 110/70. Procainamide was given intravenously. During a period of approximately two hours, 2300 mg of procainamide was given, in spite of several episodes of marked hypotension, but finally discontinued because of disturbing widening of the QRS complex without reversion to a normal sinus mechanism.

The patient's condition remained critical, and it was considered advisable to investigate the therapeutic potential of intravenous PHT. PHT was administered slowly intravenously in a dose of 250 mg. A cardiogram recorded approximately two minutes later revealed a normal sinus mechanism coupled with premature auricular contractions. In twenty minutes ventricular tachycardia had recurred. An immediate additional dose of 250 mg of PHT was given and within moments a normal sinus mechanism appeared.

Four hours later ventricular tachycardia returned and was again successfully reverted to a normal sinus rhythm with 250 mg of intravenous PHT. Because the duration of effectiveness of PHT was unknown, a constant, slow intravenous infusion of 250 mg of PHT was started. The normal sinus mechanism was maintained in this fashion for successive periods of six and four hours. At these intervals ventricular tachycardia returned, but was promptly reverted with additional intravenous doses of 250 mg of PHT.

At this time it was considered advisable to supplement the intravenous therapy with 3 grains of PHT and 500 mg of procainamide every four hours orally. Eighteen hours after its initiation the intravenous PHT was discontinued. An electrocardiogram at this time showed posterior myocardial infarction with a normal sinus mechanism.

On the following day procainamide was discontinued, and the patient was maintained with 3 grains of PHT orally every six hours. There was no recurrence of signs of ventricular irritability.

The patient made an uneventful recovery.

The author suggests that PHT may represent a drug with a wide margin of safety that is effective in controlling serious ventricular hyperirritability.

BERNSTEIN, GOLD, LANG, PAPPELBAUM, BAZIKA AND CORDAY, *Journal of the American Medical Association* (1965),[18] used oral PHT in the treatment and prevention of recurring cardiac arrhythmias in a group of sixty patients, who had been refractory to or intolerant of conventional medication.

In thirty-seven patients with premature ventricular contractions, twenty-six returned to normal sinus rhythm, and seven had a decrease in the number of ectopic beats. In thirteen patients, who had atrial tachycardia, ten had excellent response and two had moderate improvement. Six patients with paroxysmal atrial fibrillation responded. Two patients with premature atrial contractions and one with premature nodal beats had excellent response. One patient with recurrent atrial flutter did not respond. The patients had been evaluated for periods up to nineteen months, the time the study was reported.

CONN, *New England Journal of Medicine* (1965),[61] found that PHT, administered intravenously to twenty-four patients with a variety of cardiac arrhythmias, was particularly effective in supraventricular and ventricular arrhythmias resulting from digitalis excess. It was also of benefit in controlling paroxysmal atrial and ventricular arrhythmias. In three cases of atrial fibrillation and two with atrial flutter no therapeutic effect was noted. Toxicity consisted of transient bradycardia and hypotension in one patient and short-term atrioventricular block with bradycardia in another.

The author stated that PHT appears to be a significant addition to the drug therapy of cardiac arrhythmias.

LUGO AND SANABRIA, *Acta Medica Venezolana* (1966),[517] reported the effectiveness of oral PHT, 100 mg q.i.d., in eleven patients with chronic Chagasic cardiac disease, with multifocal ventricular extrasystoles.

In eight cases response was excellent with conversion to normal sinus rhythm which continued up to the eight months the patients were followed. In two cases there was excellent response, but the drug had to be discontinued because of skin rash. In one case with ventricular extrasystoles and atrial fibrillation, the extrasystoles were controlled.

HOLECKOVA, *Vnitrni Lekarstvi* (1967),[166] reported that in a group of thirty patients showing various forms of cardiac arrhythmias an improvement in nineteen was achieved using PHT.

KARLINER, *Diseases of the Chest* (1967),[187] described fifty-four patients who received intravenous PHT on fifty-seven occasions for abnormal cardiac rhythm. Nineteen of twenty-three who had digitalis-induced arrhythmias responded with abolition or marked suppression of a ventricular ectopic focus, or with conversion of supraventricular arrhythmias to a regular sinus mechanism. Of twenty-eight patients whose arrhythmias were unrelated to digitalis, seven responded favorably.

As a result of this study the author confirmed the usefulness of PHT in a variety of cardiac arrhythmias, especially those which appear to be related to digitalis excess. Rapidity of action and relative paucity of side effects make PHT an effective antiarrhythmic agent.

MERCER AND OSBORNE, *Annals of Internal Medicine* (1967),[248] reported on their six years' experience in the treatment, with PHT, of 774 cases of cardiac arrhythmias.

The authors state that intravenous PHT is highly efficacious in the treatment of ventricular arrhythmias associated with anesthesia, cardioversion, cardiac catheterization, and cardiac surgery. On the basis of their experience they consider PHT to be superior to quinidine and procainamide in these arrhythmias.

PHT also had a good effect against digitalis-induced ventricular arrhythmias and an even better effect against digitalis-induced atrial tachycardia.

The authors reviewed the literature, including their own series, on the oral use of PHT. There were reported successes in twenty out of twenty-four cases of supraventricular arrhythmias, twenty-six out of thirty-eight cases of ventricular arrhythmias and five out of eight cases of unclassified paroxysmal tachycardia.

BASHOUR, EDMONSON, GUPTA AND PRATI, *Diseases of the Chest* (1968),[418] reported on twelve patients who were treated with PHT, all of whom had clinical evidence of digitalis toxicity. Most patients had more than one type of arrhythmia.

During intravenous administration of PHT, continuous electrocardiographic monitoring was usually performed, and after conversion to sinus rhythm or subsidence of the arrhythmia, monitoring of the cardiac rhythm was continued for a period of ten minutes.

In five of the cases, atrial fibrillation was present with other arrhythmias. Two of these arrhythmias were of recent origin and were restored to normal sinus rhythm by PHT. Three cases of chronic atrial fibrillation did not respond to treatment.

Four of the patients were uremic. The successful termination of their cardiac arrhythmias, especially ventricular tachycardia, with PHT, was of special interest. In uremic patients with arrhythmias the usual therapeutic measures are both less effective and more hazardous.

EDDY AND SINGH, *British Medical Journal* (1969),[987] treated thirty-seven patients with cardiac arrhythmias with intravenous PHT. Twenty-one had acute myocardial infarctions and sixteen had other conditions. There was a favorable response in eighteen of the twenty-one cases of myocardial infarction and in six of the other sixteen cases.

GATTENLOHNER AND SCHNEIDER, *Munchener Medizinische Wochenschrift* (1969),[1052] reported fifteen patients in whom they studied cardiac hemodynamics. PHT, in doses of 125 and 250 mg, did not alter or interfere with cardiac output or stroke volume. In the eight patients with digitalis-induced arrhythmias, they noted return to normal sinus rhythm. They conclude that PHT is not only effective but may be life-saving in digitalis-induced arrhythmias. (See also Ref. 2230.)

HELFANT, SEUFFERT, PATTON, STEIN AND DAMATO, *American Heart Journal* (1969),[720] report on the use of intravenous PHT in a variety of cardiac arrhythmias.

In a controlled study, eight of eleven patients treated with PHT prior to cyclopropane anesthesia did not develop arrhythmias; whereas, in the control group, eight of nine patients did develop arrhythmias. In another phase of the study, PHT restored sinus rhythm in all eight patients who developed arrhythmias during the administration of various anesthetics.

In a second group with ventricular arrhythmias, unresponsive to procainamide, PHT abolished or decreased the ectopia in ten of twelve patients.

In a third group of twelve patients given prophylactic PHT prior to DC countershock, none developed arrhythmias.

In patients on digitalis, twenty-one of twenty-four with ventricular arrhythmias, and six of eleven with supraventricular arrhythmias responded to PHT.

The authors confirmed PHT's effectiveness and safety in prevention and treatment of cardiac arrhythmias.

LESBRE, CATHALA, SALVADOR, FLORIO, LESCURE AND MERIEL, *Archives des Maladies du Coeur et des Vaisseaux* (1969),[1264] investigated the antiarrhythmic value of PHT in a variety of arrhythmic disturbances with the following results:

	Patients	Successes
Atrial tachysystole	3	2
Atrial extrasystole	3	3
Ventricular extrasystoles	17	16
Bouts of tachycardia	3	3
First-degree block	8	5
Second-degree block	6	5

In another study, they compared forty patients with atrial fibrillation given PHT before cardioversion with a similar group of forty patients given a beta-blocking agent. The results with PHT were better.

GAUTAM, *British Heart Journal* (1969),[721] reports on the use of intravenous PHT in treating serious cardiac arrhythmias following open heart surgery in fourteen patients. PHT was rapidly and highly effective in abolishing supraventricular and ventricular arrhythmias in thirteen of these patients. Higher doses were required for the more serious arrhythmias.

The author states that the rapidity of its action and the relative paucity of side effects make PHT an effective antiarrhythmic agent.

BIELAK AND POKORA, *Polski Tygodnik Lekarsky* (1970),[2331] report their experience in 106 patients with either oral or intravenous PHT for various arrhythmias caused by infarction, digitalis toxicity, valvular heart lesions, chronic cardiopulmonary disease and myocarditis as follows:

	Patients	Successes
Ventricular extrasystole	73	63
Ventricular tachycardia	4	2
Supraventricular extrasystole	12	9
Paroxysmal atrial flutter	6	4
Paroxysmal atrial fibrillation	1	1
Paroxysmal supraventricular tachycardia	10	5
TOTAL	106	84

The authors also evaluated the prophylactic use of PHT, 300 mg/day. No arrhythmias were recorded in sixty-three of 125 patients with acute myocardial infarction. Twenty-two patients with ectopic ventricular beats were successfully treated with PHT. In twelve of these patients, ectopic beats returned when PHT was discontinued. In a group of ten patients with recurring atrial arrhythmias, five had no recurrences.

HANSEN, *Medizinische Klinik* (1970),[2569] reported the use of PHT in 150 patients who developed arrhythmias during digitalis treatment. One hundred and three of 115 with ventricular arrhythmias responded favorably. Seventy-nine of these converted to normal sinus rhythm. In twenty-four patients who had atrial fibrillation and extrasystoles, the ventricular extrasystoles disappeared, but the fibrillation was not affected.

Seven patients with supraventricular extrasystoles were successfully treated with PHT. Eight of nine patients with paroxysmal atrial fibrillation and five of seven patients with supraventricular tachycardia were also controlled.

In seven of twelve patients with partial second-degree heart block of Wenckebach type, conduction irregularity was reversed by PHT.

CHICHE, BENAIM AND CHESNAIS, *Annales de Cardiologie et D'Angeiologie* (1971),[2390] reported that thirteen of twenty-six patients with atrial arrhythmias, other than atrial fibrillation and flutter, responded to intravenous PHT. In eight patients with atrial flutter or fibrillation, PHT slowed the ventricular response without change in the atrial arrhythmia. Fourteen out of seventeen patients with ventricular arrhythmias responded to PHT. Seven patients undergoing DC cardioversion were pretreated with PHT and there were no arrhythmias.

In the group treated with oral PHT, seven of thirteen patients with atrial arrhythmias and nine of fifteen with ventricular arrhythmias were successfully treated.

HANSEN AND WAGENER, *Deutsche Medizinische Wochenschrift* (1971),[1121] in a controlled study of 200 patients with PHT and 300 patients without PHT, evaluated the effect of PHT when added to cardiac glycoside administration.

By combining PHT and glycosides, the incidence of arrhythmias was reduced from 21% in the non-PHT group to 2.5% in the PHT-treated group.

The authors state that this clinical experience indicates that PHT administration reduces the toxic effect of glycosides in man without affecting their inotropic benefits. Thus, the use of PHT improves the chance of effective treatment in heart failure.

KEMP, *Journal of the American Geriatrics Society* (1972),[1214] studied the effect of PHT on ventricular ectopic rhythms. These arrhythmias were not caused by digitalis. PHT was given to five patients and five patients were given placebo.

For the first three weeks the dosage of PHT was 100 mg q.i.d. During the rest of the three-month study the dosage was reduced to 100 mg t.i.d. The numbers of premature ventricular contractions during a five-minute continuous ECG monitoring period were recorded before therapy, after three weeks of therapy, and after three months of therapy.

At the end of the three-month period, premature ventricular contractions were abolished in two of the PHT patients and almost eliminated (165 to 1, 100 to 2, and 80 to 3) in three patients. On the other hand, in the control group, contractions increased in two patients, and were moderately decreased in three.

O'REILLY AND MACDONALD, *British Heart Journal* (1973),[1390] reported on the successful use of PHT in treating two cases of ventricular arrhythmia induced by hypokalemia.*

The authors emphasize the usefulness of PHT in the management of the notoriously resistant and malignant arrhythmias associated with hypokalemia, where the usual antiarrhythmic agents are at best ineffective and may even be dangerous.

* Hypokalemia results in below normal potassium in nerve and muscle cells. Relevant to the above paper is the fact that PHT has been demonstrated to have a regulatory effect on low potassium in cells. (See "downhill movement" of ions, Refs. 157, 387, 728, 731, 1012, 1025, 1225, 1379, 1418, 1642, 1662, 2224, 2374, 2458.)

RUMACK, WOLFE AND GILFRICH, *British Heart Journal* (1974),[1488] detailed the successful treatment with PHT of a patient who attempted suicide with a massive digoxin overdose.* Serum digoxin levels reached 35 ng/ml. Pronounced hyperkalemia was noted fourteen hours after ingestion.

The patient responded to seven doses of 25 mg intravenous PHT over a period of thirty-six hours. The patient had complete heart block and PHT improved this to a first-degree block.

The authors note that low doses of PHT were effective in this case and they suggest that it should be used early in the treatment of acute digoxin overdose.

* In addition to the digoxin, seventeen 400 mg tablets of meprobamate had also been ingested.

ROTMENSCH, GRAFF, AYZENBERG, AMIR AND LANIADO, *Israel Journal of Medical Sciences* (1977),[2058] reported on three cases of suicide attempt with massive digoxin overdoses.

Intravenous PHT was dramatically effective in controlling digitalis arrhythmias in these three patients. The authors suggest PHT's early use in the treatment of this type emergency.

CARDIAC ARRHYTHMIAS IN CHILDREN

GARSON, KUGLER, GILLETTE, SIMONELLI AND MCNAMARA, *The American Journal of Cardiology* (1980), [1847] reported the use of PHT in treating six young patients with chronic post-operative ventricular arrhythmias and abnormal hemodynamics following surgery for congenital cardiac defects. Arrhythmias varied from ten or more premature ventricular complexes per hour to bigeminy and ventricular tachycardia.

PHT alone controlled the arrhythmias in five patients. In the sixth, a combination of PHT and disopyramide was effective.

GARSON AND GILLETTE, *Pacing and Clinical Electrophysiology* (1981),[2528] studied the effects of PHT in fifty-one young patients with chronic arrhythmias consisting of multiform premature ventricular contractions (PVCs), couplets and ventricular tachycardia. The patients were divided into three groups according to hemodynamics. PHT was the initial drug used, followed by the addition or substitution of other drugs if effective response was not obtained. Five patients were not responsive to any treatment.

PHT alone corrected the arrhythmias in thirty-nine patients: twenty-two with severe, and sixteen with moderate hemodynamic abnormalities, and one with normal hemodynamics.

The authors observed that PHT was most effective in patients with the most abnormal hemodynamics, and say that PHT is the drug of choice for children with ventricular dysrhythmias.

ROCCHINI, CHUN AND DICK, *American Journal of Cardiology* (1981),[2251] reviewing their records on treatment and follow-up of children with ventricular tachycardias of various etiologies, report that PHT abolished arrhythmias in four patients with ventricular tachycardia following tetralogy of Fallot repair. A combination of PHT and propanolol effectively controlled symptoms and abolished ventricular tachycardias in two patients with prolonged Q-T interval.

KAVEY, BLACKMAN AND SONDHEIMER, *American Heart Journal* (1982),[2654] reported the effects of oral PHT in nineteen patients, seen consecutively, who developed ventricular premature complexes (VPCs) late after surgery for congenital heart disease. Arrhythmias included ventricular tachycardia, couplets and frequent multiform or uniform VPCs, documented by twenty-four-hour ambulatory ECG. Sixteen had undergone previous repair of the tetralogy of Fallot and three had had aortic valve surgery. Nine of these children had been unresponsive to previous treatment.

PHT decreased ventricular dysrhythmias in all nineteen patients. The arrhythmias were completely suppressed in fifteen, and in four they were reduced to uniform VPCs.

The authors state that the high rate of success in treating these patients, who are at particular risk for sudden death, and the relative lack of side effects suggest that PHT is the drug of choice for this patient group.

Conduction

HELFANT, LAU, COHEN AND DAMATO, *Circulation* (1967),[158] studied the effects of intravenous PHT on atrioventricular conduction in fourteen patients at constant heart rates in digitalized and nondigitalized states. In both groups, PHT was found to decrease P-R interval with the changes highly significant (p<0.001). It was suggested that when digitalis excess is manifested by both ectopia and incomplete heart block, PHT would have special utility. In contrast to the commonly used antiarrhythmic agents, PHT enhances A-V conduction in addition to suppressing ectopia.

DAMATO, BERKOWITZ, PATTON AND LAU, *American Heart Journal* (1970),[935] in thirteen patients, showed that PHT enhanced atrioventricular conduction (i.e., shortened the P-H interval) over various paced heart rates. Also PHT did not prolong intraventricular conduction as measured by H-Q interval.

These observations were made while studying His-bundle activity with an electrode catheter technique.

REIMANN, LEMMEL AND THEISEN, *Munchener Medizinische Wochenschrift* (1971),[1450] found that, in forty-seven of fifty patients, PHT eliminated extrasystoles and tachycardias of both atrial and ventricular origin. They noted that A-V conduction was not delayed.

Intravenous PHT, 125–375 mg, was usually promptly effective.

BENAIM, CHAPELLE AND CHICHE, *Annales de Cardiologie et d'Angeiologie* (1972),[816] reported fifteen patients with arrhythmias, who were injected with doses of 5 to 10 mg/kg of PHT. Recordings of the His-potential achieved during the therapeutic test showed that PHT does not usually alter the frequency of the sinus node; and it definitely improves atrioventricular conduction. In fact, a shortening of the P-H interval was obtained eight times out of eleven in conducted sinus rhythms. In most cases it did not alter intraventricular conduction:

H-V remained constant eleven times out of fifteen. In four cases, a depression in intraventricular conduction was noted with a lengthening of the H-V interval.

In conclusion, the authors emphasize how valuable PHT is in arrhythmias accompanied by atrioventricular conduction defects.

ANDERSON, DAVIS, DOVE AND GRIGGS, *Neurology* (1973),[764] studied the effect of PHT on cardiac conduction in patients who suffered from myotonic dystrophy. They found that PHT was beneficial, not only for the myotonia, but also for cardiac conduction defects common in this disease.

In five of eight patients treated with oral PHT the P-R interval was shortened by 5 to 35 msec. This was in marked contrast to quinine and procainamide. Quinine produced P-R interval prolongation in four of ten patients, and procainamide produced P-R interval prolongation in nine of ten patients.

The authors' studies indicate diffuse involvement of the His-Purkinje system in myotonic dystrophy. They note that studies by others in normal subjects have shown a depression of His-Purkinje conduction with procainamide and quinine, but not with PHT.

BISSETT, DESOYZA, KANE AND MURPHY, *The American Journal of Cardiology* (1974),[831] directly measured conduction in the His-Purkinje system in fourteen patients and found that PHT improved intraventricular conduction.

Utilizing the introduction of premature atrial beats, the relative refractory period of the His-Purkinje system and the functional refractory period of the atrioventricular (A-V) node were measured in the fourteen patients before and after administration of PHT. Before infusion of PHT, His-Purkinje conduction delay occurred with right bundle branch block in nine patients, and with left bundle branch block in five patients. After intravenous PHT (5 mg/kg at a rate of 50 mg/min) the onset or degree of His-Purkinje delay was improved in all patients. In the nine patients, PHT reduced the relative refractory period of the His-Purkinje system to a value of less than that of the functional refractory period of the A-V node, so that His-Purkinje conduction delay no longer occurred after PHT.

In the five patients with left bundle branch block, PHT also reduced the relative refractory period of the His-Purkinje system or altered the degree of aberrant conduction, or both.

The authors note that the present study demonstrates that PHT improves intraventricular conduction in man.

QUIRET, BENS, DuBOISSET, LESBRE AND BERNASCONI, *Archives des Maladies du Coeur et des Vaisseaux* (1974),[1434] studied the cardiovascular effects of PHT in 105 patients.

The authors say that PHT appears to have the following properties. It favors, or in any case does not adversely affect, atrioventricular conduction as well as intraventricular conduction. It checks manifestations of atrial and/or ventricular hyperexcitability secondary to organic cardiopathy or an excess of digitalis and has little or no effect on sinoatrial automatism.

DHATT, AKHTAR, REDDY, GOMES, LAU, CARACTA AND DAMATO, *Circulation* (1977),[1804] studied effects of PHT on macro-re-entry within the His-Purkinje system in ten patients. In seven patients, PHT modified determinants of re-entry and abolished re-entry in three patients. In all patients PHT significantly shortened functional and effective refractory periods of the His-Purkinje system, without affecting the ef-

fective refractory period of the ventricular muscle. PHT either abolished or significantly shortened the retrograde gap zones in the His-Purkinje system.

Q-T Interval Syndrome

LIPP, PITT, ANDERSON AND ZIMMET, *The Medical Journal of Australia* (1970),[2223] describe a twenty-year-old male with recurrent syncopal episodes as well as two documented episodes of ventricular fibrillation associated with prolongation of Q-T interval. After the patient was stabilized following a severe episode of fibrillation, he was placed on oral PHT and had no further arrhythmias. He remained free of syncope during the eighteen-month follow-up period.

The authors conclude that PHT is probably the most effective drug for the management of this syndrome since it suppresses myocardial irritability as well as reducing paroxysmal autonomic discharge.

COCHRAN, LINNEBUR, WRIGHT AND MATSUMOTO, *Clinical Research* (1977),[1776] did electrophysiologic studies of three patients with hereditary long Q-T interval syndrome. When admitted to the hospital these patients had ventricular tachyarrhythmias unresponsive to maximum doses of intravenous lidocaine. At this point DC countershock was used to terminate ventricular tachycardia in two patients. In the third patient, intravenous PHT promptly terminated the tachyarrhythmia.

Intravenous PHT shortened the Q-T interval in all three patients.

SCHNEIDER, BAHLER, PINCUS, STIMMEL, *Chest* (1977),[2069] describe a forty-five-year-old patient with congenital prolongation of the Q-T interval and recurrent ventricular arrhythmias. After numerous efforts to stabilize the patient, a transvenous pacemaker was inserted to suppress ectopic activity. Attempts to decrease the pacemaker rate below 150 per minute resulted in recurrence of ventricular arrhythmias and the Q-T interval remained prolonged.

The patient was placed on oral PHT (200 mg t.i.d.), the Q-T interval decreased and her ECG returned to normal. She had no further episodes of premature ventricular systoles or syncope, and was subsequently discharged on 200 mg PHT twice daily.

BROWN, LIBERTHSON, ALI AND LOWENSTEIN, *Anesthesiology* (1981),[2361] report a post-operative patient with prolonged Q-T interval and episodes of ventricular ectopic beats progressing to ventricular tachycardia. Oral PHT was started after numerous medications had been unsuccessful over a thirty-hour period. With PHT, no further ectopic beats were observed, even after discontinuation of lidocaine. Maintained on PHT and examined four weeks later, she had normal sinus rhythm and no ectopic activity.

See also Refs. 1972, 2071, 2094, 2223, 2328, 2370, 2376, 2462, 2558, 2695, 2807, 2837, 2895, 2951, 2957, 3066.

Torsade de Pointes

PUCCINELLI, CECCARELLI, MUCCI AND LANDUCCI, *Minerva Cardioangiologica* (1981),[2883] described two coronary care unit patients hospitalized for torsade de pointes ventricular tachycardia whose arrhythmias were promptly corrected by intravenous PHT.

The authors point out the electrophysiologic properties and molecular actions of PHT and suggest its utilization as a rapid and safe therapy in this kind of rhythm disturbance.

SUNG, LIANG, WANG, SHIEH AND LU, *Chinese Medical Journal* (1982),[2992] report a seventy-nine-year-old patient with complete A-V block, syncope and torsade de pointes ventricular tachycardia. Electric shock and intravenous lidocaine and isoproterenol were given without success. With PHT, the arrhythmia disappeared.

MISSRI AND SHUBROOKS, *Connecticut Medicine* (1982),[2799] describe a patient with rheumatic heart disease, cardiomyopathy and torsade de pointes ventricular arrhythmias, including fibrillation. Quinidine and procainamide exacerbated the arrhythmias. PHT (100 mg every six hours) was given with no further episodes of tachycardia. The authors recommend the use of PHT in patients with this type of arrhythmia.

ELDAR, MOTRO, YAHINI AND NEUFELD, *American Heart Journal* (1983),[2478] report a patient with acute myocardial infarction complicated by left heart failure, multiple premature ventricular contractions and A-V block requiring a pacemaker. After the pacemaker was discontinued, he developed a run of ventricular tachycardia of torsade de pointes type. Quinidine was stopped. He was placed on PHT (200 mg/day) and the ventricular ectopy immediately subsided. (See also Ref. 2664.)

Tricyclic Antidepressant Overdose

HAGERMAN AND HANASHIRO, *Annals of Emergency Medicine* (1981),[2565] demonstrated the effectiveness of intravenous PHT in reversing cardiac conduction abnormalities due to severe tricyclic antidepressant overdose in ten patients. Eight of the patients had combined first degree A-V block and intraventricular conduction delay; one had A-V block alone; and one had intraventricular conduction delay alone.

With PHT (5–7 mg/kg), five patients had complete normalization within forty-six minutes, and the remaining five showed immediate improvement in conduction with complete normalization within fourteen hours.

BOEHNERT AND LOVEJOY, *Veterinary and Human Toxicology* (1985),[2348] reported the intravenous use of PHT in the treatment of conduction delay and ventricular arrhythmias in seven patients with tricyclic antidepressant overdose, and compared the results with seven matched controls. All fourteen patients had QRS of at least 0.10 sec.

In the seven patients treated with PHT (average dose 900 mg infused at rates up to 25 mg/min), the QRS duration narrowed by an average of 55% within twenty to ninety-six minutes. Three of these patients had ventricular arrhythmias which resolved during PHT infusion. In the control group there was no change in QRS duration in the first three hours and only slight narrowing by 5.7 hours.

The authors conclude that PHT is rapidly effective and appears safe in the treatment of tricyclic antidepressant overdose.

Cardioversion

MERCER AND OSBORNE, *Annals of Internal Medicine* (1967),[248] in an extensive study of 774 patients with a variety of cardiac arrhythmias, reported the effectiveness of intravenous PHT in the treatment of twenty-one of twenty-three patients with postcardioversion arrhythmias. (For a more full review, see p. 23.)

LESBRE, CATHALA, SALVADOR, FLORIO, LESCURE AND MERIEL, *Archives des Mala-* *dies du Coeur et des Vaisseaux* (1969),[1264] as part of an extensive study to investigate the antiarrhythmic value of PHT in a variety of cardiac disturbances, gave PHT to forty patients with atrial fibrillation, prior to cardioversion. A beta-blocking agent was given to a similar group of forty patients. Comparison of the two groups showed to the advantage of PHT. (For a more full review, see p. 24.)

DAMATO, *Progress in Cardiovascular Disease* (1969),[936] pretreated ten digitalized patients, undergoing elective cardioversion, with intravenous PHT (5 mg/kg) fifteen minutes prior to procedure. None of the patients developed ventricular arrhythmias following cardioversion.

HELFANT, SEUFFERT, PATTON, STEIN AND DAMATO, *American Heart Journal* (1969),[720] reported that in twelve patients, pretreated with PHT, DC countershock produced regular sinus rhythm with no immediate postshock arrhythmias.

CUAN-PEREZ AND ORTIZ, *Archivos del Instituto de Cardiologia de Mexico* (1971),[923] found PHT effective in preventing recurrence of fibrillation after cardioversion.

The study included 230 cases. PHT was compared with quinidine and propranolol.

PHT and the other two drugs acted in similar fashion with regard to percentage of recurrence. However, the authors found PHT the drug of choice because no toxic complications were observed with it, and this was not the case with quinidine and propranolol.

LINDE, TURNER AND AWA, *Pediatrics* (1972),[1289] in a review, suggest that because of the increased risk in cardioversion following digitalis administration, cardioversion should be preceded by PHT (5 mg/kg) administered intravenously over ten minutes, monitoring the electrocardiogram and blood pressure.

Myocardial Infarction

LEONARD, *Archives of Internal Medicine* (1958),[221] was the first to report the use of PHT for the control of ventricular hyperirritability complicating myocardial infarction. (See p. 22.)

MERCER AND OSBORNE, *Annals of Internal Medicine* (1967),[248] reported the effectiveness of PHT in treating ventricular arrhythmias in 67 of 101 patients with acute myocardial infarction complicated by arteriosclerotic heart disease. (See p. 23.)

BASHOUR, JONES AND EDMONSON, *Diseases of the Chest* (1967),[2150] in a controlled study, report the preventive use of PHT in acute myocardial infarction. In the treated group of thirty patients, PHT reduced both the incidence and severity of ventricular arrhythmias. Twenty did not develop ventricular arrhythmias. In the ten who did have ventricular tachycardia, the episodes were less severe when compared with the control group and only one persisted as long as eight hours.

In the control group of nineteen patients, twelve developed ventricular tachycardia and two ventricular fibrillation. (See also Ref. 2151.)

HANSEN AND WAGENER, *Munchener Medizinische Wochenschrift* (1969),[1120] reported the effective use of PHT in the treatment of cardiac arrhythmias following myocardial infarction.

In fifty patients who had a fresh myocardial infarction, PHT was slowly injected intravenously with excellent tolerance.

EDDY AND SINGH, *British Medical Journal* (1969),[987] reported the successful use of intravenous PHT in the treatment of cardiac arrhythmias in eighteen of twenty-one patients who suffered acute myocardial infarction.

LUCKMANN, HOSSMANN, DORNER, ROTHENBERGER AND WICHERT, *Presented at the Third Konigsteiner Symposium in Hamburg* (1973),[2729] used intravenous PHT in twenty-six patients with either ventricular or supraventricular extrasystoles resulting from acute myocardial infarction. Of the twenty patients with ventricular extrasystoles, fourteen had elimination of the arrhythmia and three had reduction in extrasystoles.

In six patients, supraventricular extrasystoles were eliminated in two and reduced in three.

YANG, *Journal of the Kansas Medical Society* (1973),[1705] states, "When faced with an intractable ventricular tachycardia and bewildered by the failure of treatment, try PHT; it could be life saving."

The author reports on a case of intractable ventricular tachycardia following acute myocardial infarction. Procainamide, large doses of lidocaine, repeated DC countershock, and propranolol failed to convert this life-threatening cardiac arrhythmia.

PHT abolished the persistent ventricular tachycardia, and also permitted continuous digitalization when digitalis was so critically needed.

Angina Pectoris

BERNSTEIN, GOLD, LANG, PAPPELBAUM, BAZIKA AND CORDAY, *JAMA* (1965),[18] as part of a larger study (see p. 22), reported the effectiveness of PHT in the treatment of angina pectoris of six years' duration in a sixty-seven-year-old female.

With PHT (100 mg three times a day), there was a marked improvement in the frequency and severity of the attacks, a decrease in the frequency of palpitations, and a dramatic decrease in need for nitroglycerin. Before PHT, she required twelve to sixty nitroglycerin tablets per week; and with PHT, she required none to four tablets per month.

TAYLOR, *Chest* (1974),[1611] reports the effectiveness of PHT in angina pectoris, based on a double-blind crossover study with sixteen patients.

The patients had typical symptoms of angina pectoris including chest pain, discomfort and tightness, radiating to arm, neck or jaw, precipitated by exertion, emotion and cold, and accompanied by dyspnea.

No drug therapy, apart from glyceryl trinitrate, was taken in the two-week period prior to the trial. The double-blind study showed that oral PHT used as a prophylactic significantly reduced the frequency of the attacks and the severity of symptoms in patients with angina pectoris.

KOTIA, HALDIA AND GUPTA, *Clinician* (1980),[2667] report a controlled study, with PHT and placebo, in thirty patients with ischemic heart disease and angina pectoris. All patients had stable effort-induced angina and all had ST changes at rest and on exertion. Fifteen patients were treated with PHT, 100 mg three times a day, and fifteen patients received placebo.

PHT markedly reduced the incidence of anginal attacks (p<0.01). ST depression was also significantly improved (p<0.05) in the treated group.

Hypertension

STARKOVA, MAROVA, LEMESHEVA, GONCHAROVA, ATAMANOVA AND SEDYKH, *Problemy Endokrinologii* (1972),[2090] reported PHT decreased or normalized blood pressure in fifteen hypertensive patients with Cushing's syndrome. (See p. 67.)

DE LA TORRE, MURGIA-SUAREZ AND ALDRETE, *Clinical Therapeutics* (1980),[1797] compared PHT with conventional therapy in two groups of forty mildly hypertensive patients and found PHT useful in the reduction of both systolic and diastolic blood pressure. The authors also found PHT more effective in relieving symptoms such as anxiety, headaches, tinnitus, palpitations, chest pain, and dyspnea than the conventional therapy.

The authors suggest that PHT provides an alternative antihypertensive therapy, simple compared with most conventional therapies, and with fewer side effects.

ALDRETE AND FRANATOVIC, *Archives of Surgery* (1980),[1717] studied changes of arterial blood pressure and heart rate occurring during anesthesia and in the immediate post-operative period in three groups (30 patients each) of hypertensive patients. One group was untreated. A second group received 100 mg of PHT, and the third 200 mg of PHT, the evening before and the morning of surgery.

The administration of 200 mg the evening before and on the morning of surgery provided significantly improved hemodynamic stability during surgery.

KOTOVSKAYA AND ERINA, *Biulleten Vsesoiuznogo Kardiologicheskogo Nauchnogo Tsentra AMN SSSR* (1982),[2668] studied the effects of PHT, pyrroxan and placebo in preventing hypertensive crises in thirty-five patients. In the PHT group (ten patients) there were no crises in five and in three a reduction of frequency and severity of crises was noted.

BECHTEREVA, NIKITINA, ILIUCHINA, DAMBINOVA AND DENISOVA, *European Journal of Clinical Investigation* (1984),[2316] discussed the use of PHT in treating 120 patients with hypothalamic syndrome. With PHT, blood pressure and body temperature were normalized. In addition there was marked improvement in symptoms such as headache, irritability and feelings of fear. Sleep was also improved.

Cerebrovascular Insufficiencies

KENNEDY, ANDERSON AND SOKOLOFF, *Neurology* (1958),[1216] studied cerebral blood flow in four epileptic children, before and after PHT for one week, using a modified nitrous oxide test. Although the group was small, the authors found the increase in mean blood flow to be statistically significant (from 85 to 102 cc per 100 gram per minute).

SLOSBERG, *Mount Sinai Medical Journal* (1970),[1560] reports on his eight years of experience with medical therapy for cerebrovascular insufficiencies in a series of sixty-one elderly patients. Among these were patients with occlusive disease of the neck arteries; occlusive disease of the intracranial arteries; hypoplastic arteries; vascular anomalies of the circle of Willis; patients with reaction to compression of the common carotid arteries or of the carotid sinus areas; and patients with postural hypotension.

The author found a simple and effective method for treating cerebrovascular insufficiencies of diverse origins. This method consists of the use of PHT in conjunction with carotid sinus therapy and support stockings.

The author found that this method was both applicable and safe in this heterogeneous group of patients with cerebrovascular insufficiency, and has been well tolerated in the acute stages and on long-term follow-up.

DANIEL, *Geriatrics* (1970),[938] says that symptoms of confusion which are so common in the aged often are caused by underlying physical illness, frequently cardiac and respiratory disorders resulting in cerebral hypoxia or ischemia. He states that PHT is therapeutically useful in this group, yet it is often overlooked. (See p. 8.)

ALDRETE, ROMO-SALAS, MAZZIA AND TAN, *Critical Care Medicine* (1981),[2142] studied the cerebral protective effects of PHT in ten patients who suffered cardiac arrest during or after anesthesia.

PHT was given after spontaneous heartbeat and systolic blood pressure greater than 100 mm Hg had been restored and the diagnosis of neurological deficit had been established on the basis of unconsciousness, dilated and areflexic pupils and rigid and/or decerebrate posture.

With PHT (7 mg/kg) nine of the ten patients recovered nearly complete neurological function; the other patient had partial recovery but succumbed to other complications.

The authors note that laboratory studies of anti-anoxic protective effects of PHT support their clinical findings that PHT may have a reversing effect on post-ischemic brain injury. (See also Refs. 1718, 1719.)

MASSEI, DE SILVA, GROSSO, ROBBIATI, INFUSO, RAVAGNATI AND ALTAMURA, *Journal of Neurological Science* (1983),[2768] report twelve patients treated with intravenous

PHT prior to clamping during carotid thromboendarterectomy. During and after surgery no neurological complications or alterations in cardiac function were observed.

Prompt awakening, absence of neurologic deficits, and absence of side effects supported their hypothesis that PHT provides cerebral protection during carotid surgery.

High-Density Lipoproteins—Atherosclerosis

NIKKILA, KASTE, EHNHOLM AND VIIKARI, *Acta Medica Scandinavica* (1978),[2002] measured serum high-density lipoprotein-cholesterol (HDL-C) levels in twenty-eight epileptic patients who received PHT. These were compared with ninety healthy controls, forty-four men and forty-nine women. The patients treated with PHT had significantly higher HDL-C levels than the controls.

The authors say that serum HDL-C shows an inverse correlation with the risk of coronary heart disease, and note that some clinicians taking care of epileptic patients have been impressed by the low incidence of myocardial infarction.

HENRY, BELL AND GLITHERO, *New England Journal of Medicine* (1979),[1893] report that nineteen patients on long-term PHT therapy had significantly higher HDL-C levels (p<0.01) as compared to twenty-seven controls.

LUOMA, MYLLYLA, SOTANIEMI, LEHTINEN AND HOKKANEN, *European Neurology* (1980),[2734] in a study of HDL-C levels in patients on anticonvulsive therapy, reported that forty patients on PHT alone, and thirty-nine on PHT in combination with carbamazepine, all had increased levels of HDL-C as compared to controls. It was noted that patients on PHT alone had significantly higher levels.

MURPHY, REDDY AND MARQUARDT, *Annals of Neurology* (1981),[2813] in a study of HDL-C levels in children on various anticonvulsants, report that in eleven children on PHT the HDL-C levels were significantly elevated (p<0.001) compared to controls. The authors suggest that PHT may protect against atherosclerosis.

KASTE, MUURONEN, NIKKILA, AND NEUVONEN, *Stroke* (1982),[2649] and (1983),[2650] measured serum HDL-C and other lipoproteins before and during PHT therapy (200–300 mg/day) in twenty-seven patients with a history of transient ischemic attacks. Nine of these patients had arterial hypertension; seven, heart disease; and four, diabetes. Three had suffered myocardial infarction and two, brain infarction. Before PHT, HDL-C levels were lower in these patients than in normal healthy controls.

After one month's treatment with PHT, HDL-C concentrations reached normal levels. After nine months of therapy, there was a mean increase in HDL-C of 42% in the males and 68% in females. Low-density lipoproteins (LDL) did not increase, so that HDL/LDL cholesterol ratios improved.

Only seven patients had recurrent transient ischemic attacks. None had brain or myocardial infarction over the two-year period of PHT treatment.

The authors conclude that low serum HDL-C can be increased with PHT and this could retard the development of atherosclerotic disorders such as myocardial infarction or stroke.

O'NEILL, CALLAGHAN, STAPLETON AND MOLLOY, *Acta Neurologica Scandinavica* (1982),[2235] measured serum total cholesterol and HDL-C in fifty-two epileptic patients taking either PHT or carbamazepine. Total cholesterol concentrations did not differ significantly from controls, but the percentage of HDL-C and its ratio to total cholesterol increased in both groups. The increase was significant for PHT.

The authors point out that the change in this ratio is of particular significance because HDL facilitates the uptake of cholesterol from peripheral tissues and transports it to the liver for breakdown and excretion.

DANILENKO AND IVANIV, *Vrachebnoe Delo* (1983),[2428] reported the effects of PHT (300–450 mg/day for twenty days) on lipid metabolism and microsomal enzyme activity in twelve patients with atherosclerosis, mostly of the pelvis and lower extremities. PHT caused an increase in HDL-C concentrations (average 18% in arterial blood and 15% in venous blood). The ratio of HDL-C to total cholesterol also increased. The arteriovenous differences in concentration for total cholesterol, LDL and very low density lipoproteins decreased significantly.

Based on their data, the authors suggest that the PHT-induced rise in HDL-C results in a decrease in cholesterol and atherogenic lipoproteins in the peripheral vessels and that this may slow the development of the atherosclerotic process.

BELL AND DITTMEIER, *Arteriosclerosis* (1985),[2319] in a controlled study, investigated the effects of PHT (200 mg/day for three months) on HDL-C subfractions (HDL$_2$ and HDL$_3$) in forty-five patients, forty-one with angiographic confirmation of coronary artery disease. All had HDL-C to total cholesterol ratios of less than 20%.

During PHT treatment, the HDL$_2$ subfraction increased significantly in twenty-five patients. Total HDL-C also increased in twenty-nine of the forty-five patients, while mean subfraction HDL$_3$ increased only slightly.

The authors note, that since HDL$_2$ is associated with reduced coronary heart disease, PHT may be beneficial in preventing the progression of coronary artery disease.

MUURONEN, KASTE, NIKKILA, AND TOLPPANEN, *British Medical Journal* (1985),[2814] evaluated all deaths (1399) among epileptic patients in Finland from 1978 to 1980, and compared them with those in a control group, also 1399, matched for age, sex and date of death. Autopsies had been performed on 695 in the epileptic group and 734 in the control group.

There was a 29% (p <0.001) lower mortality rate due to deaths from ischemic heart disease (258) among epileptics who had been treated with PHT, phenobarbital and/ or carbamazepine compared with controls (382). Total cardiovascular mortality was also lower in the treated epileptics.

In a discussion of the reasons for the lower cardiovascular mortality seen in the epileptic patients, the authors point out that PHT, carbamazepine, and barbiturates all raise plasma concentrations of high density lipoproteins and induce microsomal liver enzymes. They note that PHT's ability to reduce hyperinsulinemia, an independent positive risk factor in ischemic heart disease, and its antiarrhythmic actions may contribute to its protective effects.

See also Refs. 1961, 2162, 2318, 2323, 2542, 2652, 2741, 2827, 2897, 2946.

NEUROMUSCULAR DISORDERS

Summary

The effectiveness of PHT in a variety of neuromuscular disorders has been observed clinically and, in many cases, demonstrated by quantitative electrophysiology. Some of these disorders cause much suffering and are frequently disabling or incapacitating.

Neuromuscular disorders for which PHT has been reported useful include continuous muscle fiber activity syndromes, such as Isaacs' syndrome and myotonic dystrophy; Sydenham's chorea; paroxysmal choreoathetosis; "restless legs"; muscle spasms; abnormal movements associated with Parkinsonism; intractable hiccups; palatal and respiratory myoclonus; and tetanus.

In muscle, as in nerve, PHT corrects inappropriate electrical activity without interfering with normal function. PHT does not sedate, and does not compromise respiratory function.

Choreas

SYDENHAM'S CHOREA
(CHOREA MINOR)

SHAPERA, *Pittsburgh Medical Bulletin* (1940),[338] discussed the narrowness with which new drugs are frequently viewed and suggested that PHT might have broader uses than that of an anticonvulsant. The efficacy of PHT in conditions of involuntary movements, such as tremors, rigidity and spasticity, was studied. The author found PHT effective in treating involuntary movements in ten of fifteen patients with Sydenham's chorea.

GINABREDA, *Revista Espanola De Pediatria* (1945),[421] reported on the effectiveness of PHT in six cases of chorea minor in children between the ages of five and twelve years. Improvement occurred in all of the cases in an average of fifteen to sixteen days. (See also Ref. 114.)

DE LA VEGA, *Revista Clinica Espanola* (1947),[75] reported on an epidemic of chorea minor or Sydenham's chorea. PHT was used in thirty-four cases with excellent results. In twenty-six cases there was complete elimination of symptoms in three weeks of treatment. There were four relapses when PHT was discontinued, which were corrected with the renewal of treatment.

Not only did PHT shorten the duration of the disease, but there was a marked reduction of complications—even those of cardiac lesions, a frequent and serious sequel to chorea minor.

SCHWARTZMAN, McDONALD, PERILLO, *Archives of Pediatrics* (1948),[591] in a study of Sydenham's chorea in which many medications were tried, reported that of eight patients given PHT, six were improved and two were cured.

ATHETOSIS

KABAT AND McLEOD, *Connecticut Medicine* (1959),[185] reported the successful use of PHT in five of six athetosis patients. Treatment with PHT resulted in prompt and striking improvement in neuromuscular performance.

STEVENS, *Archives of Neurology* (1966),[351] reported that PHT treatment was usually promptly effective in the relief of symptoms of paroxysmal choreoathetosis.

HUDGINS AND CORBIN, *Brain* (1966),[549] treated a mother, son and daughter suffering from familial paroxysmal choreoathetosis with PHT and mephobarbital. The relief was prompt and lasting with continued treatment.

KERTESZ, *Neurology* (1967),[191] reported on ten patients with paroxysmal kinesigenic choreoathetosis as an entity within the paroxysmal choreoathetosis syndrome. The attacks consisted of athetoid movements or tonic posturing of limbs, trunk and face. Duration was usually fifteen to thirty seconds. Paroxysms were precipitated by sudden movements, associated with surprise or haste.

The author reported that the majority of patients responded well to PHT.

JUNG, CHEN AND BRODY, *Neurology* (1973),[1200] reported ten cases of paroxysmal choreoathetosis in two families. The authors state that, to their knowledge, this is the first report of its occurrence among the Chinese. Episodes may occur several times daily with varying degrees of bizarre posturing, which can reach such intensity that the patient is hurled to the floor.

The authors state that the therapeutic effect of PHT is so prompt and so dramatic that there is little doubt as to the effectiveness of the treatment. They state that, except for one early report, PHT has been the drug of choice for this disorder.

ZENTENO VACHERON, CARRASCO ZANINI AND RAMOS RAMIREZ, *Epilepsy Abstracts* (1977),[2137] described the successful use of PHT in treating two patients with paroxysmal dystonic choreoathetosis.

WALLER, *American Journal of Psychiatry* (1977),[2111] described a case of paroxysmal kinesigenic choreoathetosis in a twenty-two-year old female whose condition was markedly improved by PHT.

GOODENOUGH, FARIELLO, ANNIS AND CHUN, *Archives of Neurology* (1978),[1866] reported the complete cessation of symptoms of from two to eight years duration in three cases of familial kinesigenic dyskinesia treated with PHT. The authors state that the response to PHT was prompt.

FUKUYAMA, OCHIAI, HAYAKAWA AND MI-YAGAWA, *Neuropadiatrie* (1979),[1841] reported the complete elimination of choreoathetoid attacks in an eight-year-old boy with PHT. Marked improvement in sleep was also observed.

HOMAN, VASKO AND BLAW, *Neurology* (1980),[1899] report on the use of PHT in the treatment of five patients with paroxysmal kinesigenic choreoathetosis. The patients, two children and three adults, experienced episodes of choreoathetoid posturing without alteration of consciousness.

PHT controlled these symptoms in all cases. Discontinuation of PHT resulted in a return of symptoms.

FRANSSEN, FORTGENS, WATTENDORFF AND VAN WOERKOM, *Archives of Neurology* (1983),[2508] report a study of an eighteen-year-old male patient with paroxysmal kinesigenic choreoathetosis of a year's duration. Attacks were precipitated by anticipated movements, confirmed by enhancement of the slow negative wave component of the contingent negative variation.

With PHT, the attacks of paroxysmal choreoathetosis disappeared and the slow negative wave amplitude became normal.

PLANT, *Journal of Neurology, Neurosurgery and Psychiatry* (1983),[2875] presented three cases of unilateral and one case of bilateral paroxysmal kinesigenic choreoathetosis.

In all four patients the attacks were completely abolished by PHT. There were no recurrences during an eighteen-month follow-up.

ZACCHETTI, SOZZI AND ZAMPOLLO, *Italian Journal of Neurological Sciences* (1983),[3098] report the treatment of a patient with paroxysmal kinesigenic choreoathetosis. Treatment with PHT, 200 mg/day, led

to complete disappearance of the attacks, confirmed in follow-up. It was of interest that symptoms were controlled with PHT blood levels of 3 μg/ml.

WANG AND CHANG, *Therapeutic Drug Monitoring* (1985),[3058] reported the effectiveness of PHT at varying therapeutic blood levels in the control of paroxysmal choreoathetosis in eight patients. Successful treatment in all eight patients was defined as complete control of attacks within six months, at which time blood levels were measured. The doses used ranged from 50 to 200 mg per day. Effective blood levels ranged from 1.1 to 10.9 μg/ml. The authors emphasize that, in the treatment of disorders other than epilepsy, lower doses of PHT are often effective.

See also Refs. 718, 1305, 1431, 1610, 2339, 2366, 2721, 2809.

Continuous Muscle Fiber Activity

ISAACS, *Journal of Neurology, Neurosurgery and Psychiatry* (1961),[176] describes the syndrome of continuous muscle fiber activity in two patients, marked by progressive muscle stiffness increased by voluntary muscle contractions and accompanied by fasciculation and weakness. Electromyography recorded a state of constant rapid dysrhythmic discharge of independent muscle fibers. The author defined the state as myotonic afterdischarge and likened it to post-tetanic afterdischarge. Neither patient showed response to numerous medications including quinidine, procainamide, cortisone, and atropine.

Treatment with PHT (100 mg q.i.d.) resulted in dramatic improvement in symptoms and electromyographic changes both at rest and on voluntary effort.

In a five-year follow-up,[1183] the author reported that both patients were still well and had lost their abnormal stiffness. He noted that on the occasions when PHT had been stopped, the symptoms returned.

ISAACS, *Journal of Neurology, Neurosurgery and Psychiatry* (1967),[1183] reports on another patient with continuous muscle fiber activity, a twenty-year-old Indian male. The rapid effectiveness of PHT was apparent. See also Ref. 2612.

MERTENS AND ZSCHOCKE, *Klinische Wochenschrift* (1965),[251] report on three cases of neuromyotonia. Each patient had in common a continuous spastic contraction of the entire skeletal musculature, which did not even diminish while asleep or under anesthesia. Extensive electromyographic, histologic and other laboratory studies confirmed the electrophysiological abnormality. Quinine, quinidine, novocamid, steroids and diuretics had little or no effect.

PHT and mephenytoin were tried. PHT was far more effective. With two injections of PHT, 250 mg, at sixty-minute intervals it was possible to obtain significant elimination of spastic contractions and inhibition of movement in all muscle groups within two to four hours.

The authors state that with oral PHT they were able to maintain this astonishing effect. A trial of discontinuing the PHT resulted in recurrence or rapid increase of the abnormal contraction.

LEVY, WITTIG AND FERRAZ, *Arquivo de Neuro Psiquiat* (1965),[1280] describe a case of continuous muscle fiber activity at rest, diagnosed by electromyography. The condition showed some clinical improvement with corticosteroids, although this improvement was not reflected on the electromyogram.

The authors report that PHT, 300 mg/day, markedly improved both the clinical picture and the abnormal electrical tracing in a few days.

HUGHES AND MATTHEWS, *Journal of Neurology, Neurosurgery and Psychiatry* (1969),[1171] described a patient who for thirty-two years had suffered from a form of muscular rigidity clinically resembling myotonia but, in fact, identical with continuous muscle fiber activity.

The patient was treated with 100 mg of PHT q.i.d., which produced immediate and continuing benefits. If he stopped taking PHT, for as short a period as twenty-four hours, the symptoms returned.

BUSCAINO, CARUSO, DE GIACOMO, LABIANCA AND FERRANNINI, *Acta Neurologica* (1970),[881] describe a case of continuous muscle fiber activity syndrome (neuromyotonia).

The man, age forty-five, had suffered for twenty years from stiffness of all muscles, wide-spread fasciculations, myokymia and excessive sweating. The muscular stiffness was present even during sleep. The nature of the electrical abnormality was documented on the electromyogram.

This condition, present for twenty years, had been treated with a variety of substances without success. The authors state that the condition was dramatically resolved by the use of PHT or carbamazepine.

WALLIS, VAN POZNAK AND PLUM, *Archives of Neurology* (1970),[1658] report on two cases involving generalized muscular stiffness, fasciculations and myokymia of peripheral nerve origin. Electromyographic and other laboratory findings were consistent with the clinical diagnosis.

In one case the authors state PHT, 100 mg t.i.d., provided dramatic relief. In the other case it was not found effective. In the successful case, when PHT was discontinued, within three days, all pretreatment symptoms returned. Prompt relief recurred with the reinstitution of PHT.

WELCH, APPENZELLER AND BICKNELL, *Neurology* (1972),[1676] report a case of peripheral neuropathy with myokymia, sustained muscular contraction and continuous motor unit activity in a twenty-two-year-old female.

The patient was tried with quinine for one month without success. The patient was then given PHT, 300 mg/day, with almost immediate remission of symptoms. This remission continued with daily PHT.

KOSTOV, TACHEV AND NASTEV, *Zhurnal Nevropatologii i Psikhiatrii imeni S.S. Korsakova* (1973),[1231] report on a patient with pseudomyotonia (Isaacs' syndrome) characterized by hypertonia of the distal extremities. Spontaneous electromyographic activity was present at rest, and did not disappear even after novocaine blockade of the peripheral nerve.

PHT and carbamazepine each had favorable therapeutic effect. Withdrawal of the medications resulted in a return of the disorder.

LEVINSON, CANALIS AND KAPLAN, *Archives of Otolaryngology* (1976),[1954] reported an unusual case of continuous muscle activity complicated by airway obstruction secondary to laryngeal spasm.

Treatment with PHT, 300 mg/day, resulted in rapid improvement of the peripheral symptoms and the laryngeal spasms.

IRANI, PUROHIT AND WADIA, *Acta Neurologica Scandinavica* (1977),[1907] reported prompt and remarkable improvement upon administration of PHT in three of four patients with continuous muscle fiber activity.

LUTSCHG, JERUSALEM, LUDIN, VASSELLA AND MUMENTHALER, *Archives of Neurology* (1978),[1970] reported the successful treatment with PHT of a seven-year-old boy who had suffered for two years with the syndrome of continuous muscle fiber activity.

JACKSON, SATYA-MURTI, DAVIS AND DRACHMAN, *Neurology* (1979),[1910] report on a case of Isaacs' syndrome with laryngeal involvement, confirmed by clinical, pharmacologic and electrophysiologic findings.

The patient responded well to treatment with a combination of PHT and carbamazepine.

LUBLIN, TSAIRIS, STRELETZ, CHAMBERS, RIKER, VANPOZNAK AND DUCKETT, *Journal of Neurology, Neurosurgery and Psychiatry* (1979),[1967] report two cases of continuous motor activity with impaired muscular relaxation. EMG showed continuous motor activity at rest. Treatment with PHT, 500 - 700 mg/day, resulted in marked diminution in myokymia and continuous motor activity. Clinical improvement persisted in two-year follow-up.

REEBACK, BENTON, SWASH, SCHWARTZ, *British Medical Journal* (1979),[2040] report a patient treated for rheumatoid arthritis with penicillamine who developed muscle contractions and weakness suggesting neuromyotonia. EMG showed continuous motor firing at rest. The patient was treated with PHT with marked improvement in three days, which was confirmed by EMG studies six weeks later.

GRASSA, FIGA-TALAMANCA, LORUSSO, GIACANELLI AND PONTESILLI, *Italian Journal of Neurological Science* (1981),[2553] report a thirty-four-year-old woman with diffuse muscle contractions and other symptoms of continuous muscle fiber activity syndrome, confirmed by EMG. With oral PHT, 400 mg/day, improvement, which included cessation of the painful muscle spasms and excessive sweating, occurred. EMG, nine months later, showed almost complete disappearance of the abnormal activity.

VASILESCU AND FLORESCU, *Journal of Neurology* (1982),[3047] report a case of a male alcoholic who developed continuous muscle fiber activity. Electrophysiologic studies and muscle biopsy confirmed mixed sensorimotor polyneuropathy.

PHT, 400 mg/day, was started and the clinical symptoms and EMG activity at rest disappeared within two days. This result persisted at follow-up six months later.

MARIA AND PISANELLI, *Rivista di Neurologia* (1983), [2763] report a fifty-three-year-old male patient with neuromyotonia (Isaacs' syndrome), who had been treated unsuccessfully with dopamine and benzodiazepines. Carbamazepine was tried with partial success. Treatment with PHT, 600 mg/day, resulted in remarkable improvement. When PHT was discontinued, the symptoms reappeared.

ZISFEIN, SIVAK, ARON AND BENDER, *Archives of Neurology* (1983),[3100] report a sixteen-year-old boy with severe episodic muscle cramps and generalized myokymia (Isaacs' syndrome), associated gastrocnemius hypertrophy and ankle areflexia. The patient was treated with PHT, 300 mg/day, with total relief of cramps, marked decrease in myokymia and return of ankle reflexes. There was marked reduction in the muscle hypertrophy after three months.

BROWN, *Archives of Physical Medicine and Rehabilitation* (1984),[2363] reports a twenty-year-old male patient with myokymia in all four extremities, hyporeflexia and hypertrophy of thenar musculature,

who presented with cramping pain in both thighs and difficulty releasing grip. EMG revealed continuous motor unit activity at rest.

The patient was treated with PHT and showed almost complete resolution of symptoms within twenty-four hours. The author states that rapid response to PHT, in conjunction with clinical and EMG findings, are diagnostic of Isaacs' syndrome.

See also Refs. 836, 1549, 1758, 2016, 2124, 2146, 2147, 2298, 2302, 2312, 2397, 2407, 2409, 2448, 2456, 2572, 2612, 2683, 2692, 2780, 2850, 2920, 3003, 3043, 3057.

Myotonias

DYSTROPHIC AND CONGENITA

MUNSAT, *Neurology* (1967),[262] reported a double-blind crossover study of seven patients with dystrophic myotonia and two with myotonia congenita. The authors found both PHT and procainamide effective in treatment of the myotonic symptoms. PHT was better tolerated and did not increase the preexisting cardiac conductive defects, which were made worse by procainamide.

BHATT, VIJAYAN AND DREYFUS, *California Medicine* (1971),[825] in a review of clinical and laboratory aspects of myotonia, state that of treatments which have been used successfully for myotonia, including PHT, procainamide, quinine, and adrenocorticotropic hormone, PHT appears to be the most effective, the safest and the best tolerated.

THOMPSON, *New England Journal of Medicine* (1972),[1614] in a letter to the editor wrote:

"In three members of a family in my practice with myotonia congenita, PHT, 100 mg three times a day, was started. The patients were sixteen, twenty and twenty-three years of age. Their disabilities included inability to dance, difficulty getting up from a sitting position, difficulty relaxing grips, and some falling because of inability to relax the muscles.

"On PHT therapy they are all much improved. The sixteen-year-old girl is particularly delighted because she can now dance. No side effects have occurred and the improvement is dramatic."

GRIGGS, DAVIS, ANDERSON AND DOVE, *American Journal of Medicine* (1975),[2558] studied the effect of PHT on cardiac conduction in patients who suffered from myotonic dystrophy. They found that PHT was beneficial, not only for the myotonia, but also for cardiac conduction defects common in this disease.

In seven of ten patients treated with oral PHT the P-R interval was shortened by 5 to 50 msec. This was in contrast to quinine and procainamide. Quinine produced P-R interval prolongation in six of thirteen patients, and procainamide produced P-R interval prolongation in eleven of twelve patients.

The authors state that since they and others have found that PHT is an effective antimyotonic agent and since their own findings have shown that it does not have negative effects on cardiac conduction abnormalities as do quinine and procainamide, PHT is the treatment of choice in myotonic dystrophy. (See also Ref. 764.)

BIRYUKOV, *Zh Nevropatol Psikhiatr* (1976), [1752] compared the effects of PHT and novocainamid in two groups of myotonic patients.

With PHT, 400–500 mg/day for a period of three to four weeks, there was a significant improvement in nine of the fourteen patients treated. The myotonic contractures

disappeared almost completely in six with myotonia congenita, and the myotonic component was significantly reduced within two weeks in three with myotonic dystrophy.

Sixteen patients were treated with novocainamid, 0.75–1.5 g/day. In two, treatment had to be stopped because significant bradycardia developed. There was some improvement in six of fourteen patients, four with myotonia congenita and two with myotonic dystrophy.

The author notes that PHT was not only more effective, but also better tolerated than novocainamid. Its lack of adverse effects on cardiac function distinguished it from novocainamid.

DURELLI, MUTANI, SECHI, TRACCIS, MONACO AND GLORIOSO, *Electroencephalography and Clinical Neurophysiology* (1982),[2469] compared PHT, carbamazepine and placebo in a double-blind study of eight patients with dystrophic myotonia (Steinert's disease). Criteria included subjective and objective clinical findings as well as EMG evaluation. Both drugs were found to be effective.

STRIANO, MEO, BILO AND VITOLO, *Encephalography and Clinical Neurophysiology* (1983),[2986] report a patient with typical Thomsen's disease (myotonia congenita), who also had evidence of sleep-induced apnea and excessive daytime somnolence. All-night polysomnography demonstrated obstructive and central apneas with accompanying cardiac arrhythmias.

PHT improved not only the myotonia, but also the breathing patterns, sleep soundness and excessive daytime somnolence.

See also Refs. 1073, 1939, 2446, 2867.

SCHWARTZ-JAMPEL SYNDROME

TAYLOR, LAYZER, DAVIS AND FOWLER, JR., *Electroencephalography and Clinical Neurophysiology* (1972), [3007] reported on three patients with Schwartz-Jampel syndrome, a rare autosomal recessive disease consisting of generalized myotonia and bone abnormalities, including dwarfism. PHT improved muscle contractions in two of the patients.

BROWN, GARCIA-MULLEN AND MURAI, *Neurology* (1975),[2362] reported two patients with myotonic chondrodystrophy (Schwartz-Jampel syndrome) which had progressed to marked limitation of joint mobility in adulthood.

PHT resulted in such improvement in ambulation that both patients were able to return to gainful employment.

CRUZ MARTINEZ, ARPA, PEREZ CONDE AND FERRER, *Muscle and Nerve* (1984),[2418] reported a seven-year-old girl with Schwartz-Jampel syndrome. EMG showed persistent continuous electrical activity and high frequency discharges. Treatment with PHT, 200 mg/day, resulted in improvement in muscle relaxation and motor ability, including gait.

Stiff-Man Syndrome

NEVSIMAL, SUTA AND TUHACEK, *Cheskoslovenska Neurologie* (1967)[1998] describe a case of Stiff-man syndrome of fifteen years duration in a fifty-year-old female patient. Treatment with PHT decreased muscular spasms and rigidity.

GOBERNADO, ORTIN, RODRIGUEZ DE CASTRO AND GIMENO, *Prensa Medica Argentina* (1981),[2543] describe a patient with severe leg muscle contractions consistent with Stiff-man syndrome. The patient had had progressive symptoms for twenty years. Sodium valproate was unsuccessful. Initial treatment with diazepam had to be discontinued due to side effects. A combination of PHT and diazepam produced both clinical and electrophysiological improvement.

Parkinson's Syndrome

SHAPERA, *Pittsburgh Medical Bulletin* (1940),[338] reported on the treatment with PHT of twenty-two patients with Parkinson's syndrome. These patients had received other medication with little or no beneficial effect. With PHT improvement in involuntary movements was observed.

The author noted that there was a psychic improvement in some of these patients and that this alone made PHT therapy worthwhile.

KABAT, *Annals of Internal Medicine* (1959),[184] reported the therapeutic effectiveness of PHT in seven cases of Parkinson's syndrome.

Three of these patients, who had been taking the maximal tolerable dose of anti-Parkinson drugs, still showed rigidity, tremor and poor isotonic function. With the addition of PHT isotonic and isometric function improved. Rigidity disappeared in one case and was reduced in the other two cases. Improvement in ambulation and in use of the upper extremities was also noted on addition of PHT.

The other four patients, who had not previously taken any anti-Parkinson drugs, were treated with PHT alone. In each case, prompt improvement in isotonic contraction of the muscles resulted. Rigidity disappeared in one case and was significantly reduced in the others. Tremor was moderately improved. Voluntary motion of the affected extremities was improved significantly in all cases.

DOMZAL, *Neurologia i Neurochirurgia Polska* (1972),[971] reported on the use of PHT in treating fourteen patients with Parkinson's syndrome. Eight of these patients had received synthetic anticholinergic drugs, and six had not received any previous anti-Parkinsonism medication.

With PHT, 300–400 mg/day, over a two-week period, eleven patients reported marked improvement in sense of well-being; ten reported improvement in muscle tone; and six exhibited improvement in general tremor, which disappeared entirely in three. Steadier mobility, better expression and improved gait were observed in three patients.

Other Muscular Disorders

RESTLESS LEGS

HOGG, *Practitioner* (1972),[1155] describes the successful treatment of seven cases of "restless legs," or Ekbom's syndrome, with PHT. For this syndrome, of unknown etiology, vasodilators, intravenous iron and Dextran have been tried with only partial success.

The syndrome, he states, derives its name "restless legs" from the fact that the majority of these patients are unable to rest in bed at night and take to moving their legs sometimes vigorously because of the gnawing aches and "crawling pains."

In each of the seven patients, 100 mg of PHT daily resulted in cessation of symptoms. Since the symptoms occurred at night, and interrupted sleep, PHT was given before going to bed.

STEROID MYOPATHY

STERN, GRUENER AND AMUNDSEN, *JAMA* (1973),[1594] report on a forty-seven-year-old man suffering with steroid myopathy, who was successfully treated with PHT.

The patient required steroids (prednisolone) for his rheumatoid arthritis. Without changing the regimen of prednisolone, two six-week trial periods of PHT and placebo capsules were instituted with crossover every three weeks. The results of the two trials revealed that while on PHT there was a significant improvement in hip flexor strength, as contrasted to placebo. Muscle strength was measured with a dynamometer.

The authors state that although this was only one case, the results suggest that PHT might be used along with steroids to decrease the risk of steroid myopathy. (See also Ref. 1103.)

INTRACTABLE HICCUPS

PETROSKI AND PATEL, *Lancet* (1974),[1411] in a letter to the editor, report on a patient with refractory hiccups and an old right hemiparesis. He was mentally alert, but repetitive attacks of hiccups seriously interfered with his feeding and sleep and left him exhausted. The hiccups did not respond to pharyngeal stimulation by catheter or parenteral prochlorperazine.

On the sixth day, the frequency of hiccups increased to more than thirty per minute. PHT (200 mg), given intravenously over five minutes, completely eliminated hiccuping within an hour. Then 100 mg q.i.d. orally was continued until the eleventh day without any recurrence of hiccups.

RESPIRATORY MYOCLONUS

PHILLIPS AND ELDRIDGE, *New England Journal of Medicine* (1973),[1414] describe a case of abnormal repetitive diaphragmatic contractions, which they refer to as respiratory myoclonus.

In the case reported, treatment with quinidine had been ineffective. Because of PHT's membrane stabilizing and synaptic effects, it was tried. A dose of 400 mg of PHT daily was sufficient to inhibit the abnormal muscle activity as demonstrated by diaphragmatic, scalene and intercostal muscle electromyography.

PHT was discontinued on three occasions with a return of symptoms. At the time of the writing the patient had taken PHT daily for a year with no recurrence.

The authors state that in the past the only effective form of therapy for this disorder has been phrenicectomy. They suggest a trial of PHT first.

PALATAL MYOCLONUS

FERRO AND CASTRO-CALDAS, *Annals of Neurology* (1981),[2181] report on a case of palatal myoclonus observed in a hypertensive sixty-five-year-old male. Neurological examination, electroencephalogram and CT scan were performed. The lower half of the right side of the face, both eyelids, the tongue, lower jaw, soft palate, and posterior pharyngeal wall showed a rhythmic myoclonus that disturbed speech and swallowing, and persisted during sleep.

Clonazepam improved the myoclonus but caused intolerable drowsiness and confusion. Sodium valproate had no effect, and carbamazepine worsened the condition.

PHT (600 mg/day) improved the myoclonus, reducing its amplitude and the area of the body it affected.

FITZGERALD, *Laryngoscope* (1984),[2500] presented a case of palatal myoclonus related to acoustical stimulation and tinnitus. Diazepam was tried with little effect. The patient was switched to carbamazepine without change. He was then placed on a combination of PHT and phenobarbital with remarkable improvement in tinnitus and myoclonus.

SPASMS IN MULTIPLE SCLEROSIS

MATTHEWS, *Brain* (1958),[1342] reported the effectiveness of PHT in the treatment of frequent painful spasms in a patient with multiple sclerosis. When PHT, 100 mg t.i.d. was prescribed, the attacks stopped within two days. The author did not claim that PHT had a primary beneficial action on multiple sclerosis itself, but that it was useful in the treatment of the painful spasms.

JOYNT AND GREEN, *Archives of Neurology* (1962),[1192] found that PHT had definite suppressing effects on muscle spasms in three patients with multiple sclerosis.

KUROIWA AND SHIBASAKI, *Folia Psychiatrica et Neurologica Japonica* (1968),[1243] found that PHT and/or carbamazepine were useful in suppressing the painful tonic spasms in four patients with multiple sclerosis.

The authors noted that, before PHT, a wide variety of drugs had been tried in all four cases, without success. (See also Ref. 1541.)

WEINTRAUB, MEGAHED AND SMITH, *New York State Journal of Medicine* (1970)[710] describe three patients with multiple sclerosis presenting with spasticity affecting the flexor muscles of the forearm.

In two patients, the use of PHT resulted in increased strength and ability to move the extremities. In the third case quinine resulted in slight improvement in strength.

BERGER, SHEREMATA AND MELAMED, *Archives of Neurology* (1984),[2322] report the use of PHT in the treatment of four patients in whom paroxysmal dystonia was the initial manifestation of multiple sclerosis. Three of the patients had a good response to PHT.

HYPOCALCEMIA

SCHAAF AND PAYNE, *New England Journal of Medicine* (1966),[326] studied the effect of PHT and phenobarbital in ten patients with overt and latent tetany. Phenobarbital was relatively ineffective alone. PHT eliminated tetany, tetanic equivalents and a strongly positive Trousseau test in six of these patients with hypocalcemia due to hypoparathyroidism or pseudo-hypoparathyroidism. PHT was also effective in one patient with hypocalcemia and hypomagnesemia due to malabsorption. Chvostek's sign became negative in five of these patients. Serum calcium, phosphorus and magnesium were unchanged by treatment. PHT was not effective in three patients with idiopathic latent tetany.

The authors cited extensive studies that have confirmed that calcium is a critical stabilizer of neuromuscular membranes. In their study they found that PHT in doses therapeutic in man can counteract the increased nervous excitability in hypocalcemic patients.

TETANUS

RODRIGUEZ, PEREZ, QUINTERO, HERNANDEZ, MACIAS, CHAPA AND ANDRADE, *European Journal of Clinical Investigation* (1984),[2913] reported that intravenous PHT was rapidly effective as antispasm therapy in eighteen patients with severe tetanus. Substantial amounts of PHT were used in combination with the usual antibacterial and antitoxin measures. After the spasms were under control, the patients were watched, carefully, twenty-four hours a day, and additional intravenous PHT was given promptly to keep the spasms under control.

The authors noted that PHT did not sedate the patients or depress respiratory function, as did other drugs they used to control spasms, and the need for respiratory support was decreased. No cardiovascular, sympathetic or autonomic disturbances, frequently seen in these patients, occurred. Compared with the authors' experience, tetanus related mortality decreased markedly, as did hospitalization time.

Additional unpublished data from Mexico, Brazil and India give further indication of the usefulness of PHT against this disease. It is reported that large amounts of intravenous PHT may be needed in the acute stage (1500 mg a day or more in an adult is not unusual). Dosage depends on patient condition. When contractions recur, more PHT is indicated promptly. Later, when the bacteria and toxin are under control, less PHT should be needed.

It is reported that PHT can be used in combination with other medications commonly used in the treatment of tetanus.

See also Basic Mechanisms of Action-Muscle section, p. 138.

TREATMENT OF PAIN

Summary

Phenytoin has been found effective in the treatment of so many types of pain that it is useful as a general pain medication. PHT's usefulness in pain is enhanced by the fact that it is not sedative and it is not habit-forming. It can be used alone or in combination with narcotics and other pain medications.

PHT's first use in pain, for trigeminal neuralgia, was reported in 1942 by Bergouignan. Since then, PHT has been reported useful for facial and head pain, including trigeminal and glossopharyngeal neuralgia; peripheral nerve neuralgias and neuropathic pain, including that of polyneuritis, late-stage syphillis, diabetic neuropathy, Fabry's disease, and post-herpetic and post-sympathectomy pain states; migraine and other headache; post-operative pain; phantom limb pain; pain of skeletal muscle spasms; post-stroke pain; and pain caused by malignant disease.

In recent years, used topically, in addition to speeding healing, PHT has been shown to rapidly decrease pain of ulcers, burns and wounds.

Initial messages of pain are necessary protective mechanisms. PHT does not interfere with these initial bioelectrical impulses, but it does reduce repetitive neuronal activity, as in post-tetanic afterdischarge.

Trigeminal Neuralgia

Bergouignan, *Revue de Laryngologie* (1942),[15] reported the complete cure of essential facial neuralgia in three patients treated with PHT, 200–300 mg/day.

Bergouignan and D'Aulnay, *Revue d'Oto-Neuro-Ophtalmologie* (1951),[16] reported on the treatment with PHT of seventeen patients with trigeminal neuralgia. On PHT therapy, 300–600 mg/day, sixteen were benefited.

The rapidity of the drug's action was noted. The effects usually were felt within twenty-four hours.

Jensen, *Arztliche Wochenschrift* (1954),[180] reported on the use of PHT, 300–600 mg/day, in treating forty-five cases of trigeminal neuralgia. Sixteen patients showed complete cessation of pain, which lasted after discontinuance of PHT. Nineteen patients experienced distinct improvement during PHT treatment. Pain recurred when PHT was withdrawn. Four patients showed slight improvement and five patients did not improve.

The author pointed out the desirability of PHT to relieve pain, as opposed to the potent pain relievers and opiates which all too easily lead to addiction.

Jensen, *Therapiewoche* (1955),[518] in a subsequent study of fifty-nine typical cases of trigeminal neuralgia treated with PHT, reported that fifty-seven were completely freed of pain. Twenty remained so after medication was discontinued; but with thirty-seven pain returned when PHT was withdrawn. Only two cases showed no improvement.

Winiker-Blanck, *Deutsche Stomatologie* (1955),[384] reported that of twenty-seven cases of genuine trigeminal neuralgia treated with PHT, 300–600 mg/day, fifteen remained completely free of pain and seven showed lasting improvement making the condition entirely bearable for the patient. After the pain was under control, the patients were maintained on 100 mg/day.

Because of its safety, PHT therapy was recommended as the treatment of choice.

Ende, *Virginia Medical Monthly* (1957),[605] reported that over a period of two years he had successfully treated nine consecutive cases of trigeminal neuralgia with PHT.

The author found that not only was PHT effective, but frequently relief began with the first capsule. These patients had been subjected previously to nearly every form of therapy recommended.

Bergouignan, *Revue Neurologique* (1958),[14] reported that twenty-six of thirty patients who had been treated for trigeminal neuralgia were relieved of their attacks during the first three days of treatment with PHT. Ten of these patients had previously had peripheral or deep alcohol injections with transient or incomplete results and two had neurotomy.

Iannone, Baker and Morrell, *Neurology* (1958),[175] reported that with PHT definite relief of pain was obtained and paroxysms of pain were controlled in all of four patients with trigeminal neuralgia and one with glossopharyngeal neuralgia.

Lamberts, *Journal of the Michigan State Medical Society* (1959),[214] reported on thirty patients with trigeminal neuralgia treated with PHT, 200–400 mg/day. In almost every instance relief from pain was complete within forty-eight hours, but usually not before twenty-four hours after treatment commenced. The dosage had to be increased in two of the patients before the pain disappeared.

KUGELBERG AND LINDBLOM, *Journal of Neurology, Neurosurgery and Psychiatry* (1959),[202] in a study of fifty patients with trigeminal neuralgia, investigated the relationship between stimuli applied to the trigger zone and the pain paroxysm. Intravenous PHT, 3–5 mg/kg, was found to raise the attack threshold as well as to shorten the duration of the attack.

BRAHAM AND SAIA, *Lancet* (1960),[31] used PHT, 300 mg/day, in twenty cases of trigeminal neuralgia. Relief of pain was complete in eight and partial in six.

REEVE, *Lancet* (1961),[611] reported that PHT was effective in nine cases of trigeminal neuralgia and recommended that a trial of PHT precede more radical treatment.

LINDBLOM, *Svensk Lakartidningen* (1961),[224] reported that of thirty cases of trigeminal neuralgia treated with PHT, 300–600 mg/day, complete relief or considerable reduction of the symptoms occurred in seventeen cases. Improvement lasted as long as the drug was administered.

BAXI, *Antiseptic* (1961),[9] reported that eleven of fifteen patients with trigeminal neuralgia, treated with PHT, obtained relief within a week.

The author stated that PHT not only gave lasting relief of pain but also relieved the apprehension of an impending attack.

VON ALBERT, *Munschener Medizinische Wochenschrift* (1978),[2109] reported on twelve cases of typical trigeminal neuralgia and two cases of glossopharyngeal neural-

gia. Neither oral carbamazepine nor PHT had produced sufficient results. However, intravenous PHT, in some cases up to 750 mg over three to six hours, followed by oral PHT (200–400 mg/day), achieved freedom from pain in the fourteen patients. It was not found effective in four patients with herpetic neuralgia.

VON ALBERT, *Advances in Epileptology* (1983),[3051] reviewing eight years experience with PHT, states that intravenous PHT is very effective, not sedative, has only mild side effects, and is the therapy of choice for trigeminal neuralgia in elderly patients.

Glossopharyngeal Neuralgia

KONG, HEYMAN, ENTMAN AND MCINTOSH, *Circulation* (1964),[583] reported the successful use of PHT in treating a patient who had been suffering for ten years with glossopharyngeal neuralgia associated with disturbances of cardiac and cerebral function.

At the time of admission to hospital the patient was experiencing between ten and twenty attacks a day. Treatment with 500 mg PHT a day completely relieved the pain. On 300 mg/day the patient remained symptom-free.

LEE, LEE AND TSAI, *Journal of Formosan Medical Association* (1975),[1949] reported the successful use of PHT in treating a case of glossopharyngeal neuralgia. The paroxysms of pain, about thirty a day, were so unbearable that the patient was afraid to swallow or talk. On 400 mg PHT a day the patient became symptom-free.

RUSHTON, STEVENS AND MILLER, *Archives of Neurology* (1981),[2253] reported eighteen patients with glossopharyngeal neuralgia, who were treated with PHT. Four patients had good relief for periods up to several months. Five additional patients had good relief, sufficient to avoid surgery.

See also Refs. 2978, 3056.

Migraine and Other Headaches

SHAPERA, *Pittsburgh Medical Bulletin* (1940),[338] reported that two of four cases of migraine were improved with PHT.

McCULLAGH AND INGRAM, *Diseases of the Nervous System* (1956),[235] in their paper "Headaches and Hot Tempers," reported that their experience showed that PHT was by far the most useful medication in the treatment of a syndrome in which migraine headaches were related to familial cerebral dysrhythmias.

KELLAWAY, CRAWLEY AND KAGAWA, *Epilepsia* (1959–1960),[551] in a report on 459 children, found PHT one of the drugs of choice in the treatment of headache accompanied by 14- and 6-per-second positive spike patterns.

HIRSCHMANN, *Therapeutische Umschau* (1964),[161] reported on a study of forty-four patients with migraine not relieved by ergot preparations alone. Of these, thirty-two remained in treatment. When they were treated with a combination of PHT, caffeine and ergot, nineteen were either completely relieved or had less frequent or milder attacks.

WIEDEMANN, *Medizinische Monatsschrift* (1966),[380] in a series of studies on migraine, found preparations containing PHT and caffeine useful in the treatment of a variety of neuralgias and cephalalgias. This treatment was particularly suitable for patients with true migraine and trigeminal neuralgia.

JONAS, *Headache* (1967),[693] administered PHT to eighteen migraine sufferers. Nine patients afflicted with paroxysmal migraine experienced complete relief. Of six non-paroxysmal patients, four benefited by the use of PHT.

CAPLAN, WEINER, WEINTRAUB, AUSTEN, *Headache* (1976),[1763] reported the successful use of PHT in the treatment of a fifty-five-year-old male patient with neurological dysfunction accompanied by classic migraine headaches following cardiac surgery.

The patient was experiencing episodes of neurological dysfunction manifested by tingling, numbness, weakness and pain in the hands, arms, thighs and face, inability at times to find words, slow speech, and dysarthria with repetitive speech.

With PHT, 100 mg t.i.d., no further episodes occurred. On follow-up three years later, the patient continued to do well on PHT.

MILLICHAP, *Child's Brain* (1978),[1987] found PHT effective in relieving severe recurrent headaches associated with other symptoms, including nausea, vomiting, dizziness and vertigo, in forty-seven of seventy children.

SWANSON AND VICK, *Neurology* (1978),[2096] treated three cases of basilar artery migraine with PHT, 300 mg daily. In two cases the attacks were completely relieved. In the third case the frequency and severity of the attacks were reduced.

Post-Stroke or Brain Injury

FINE, *British Medical Journal* (1967),[2496] reported five patients with post-stroke hemiplegia and pain in part or all of the affected side of the body. Three of the patients received PHT alone, one received a combination of PHT and phenobarbital, and one phenobarbital alone. All responded dramatically with complete resolution of pain.

CANTOR, *British Medical Journal* (1972),[883] reports two patients with thalamic pain who experienced good relief with PHT.

The author states that the treatment of the painful, burning dysesthesias which can occur after thalamic infarction has been a particularly vexing problem, in that a variety of drugs have been tried with variable but generally ineffective results.

The author reports that in each of the cases, when PHT treatment was stopped, the painful dysesthesia recurred. Reinstitution of PHT again resulted in alleviation of the pain.

MLADINICH, *JAMA* (1974),[1369] reported successful use of PHT for relief of facial pain associated with Wallenberg syndrome.

A forty-year-old man was afflicted with ipsilateral burning facial pain around the eye. Ordinary analgesics did not relieve this pain. PHT, 1000 mg in divided doses the first day and then 300 mg daily, was tried. Symptoms of facial pain were considerably relieved within several days.

AGNEW AND GOLDBERG, *Bulletin of the Los Angeles Neurological Societies* (1976),[1715] tried PHT in a group of ten patients with chronic, severe, intractable thalamic pain, unresponsive to previous treatment. Three patients were markedly improved and two were slightly improved.

Other Pain and Neuralgias

DIABETIC NEUROPATHY

ELLENBERG, *New York State Journal of Medicine* (1968),[431] in a study of sixty diabetic patients, reported that PHT was effective in the treatment of pain and paresthesias associated with neuropathy. Good to excellent results were observed in forty-one, fair results in ten, and none were worse.

KANNAN, DASH AND RASTOGI, *Journal of Diabetic Association of India* (1978),[1920] in a double-blind crossover study of sixteen patients with diabetic neuropathy, found that thirteen had significant relief of pain and/or paresthesia on 100 mg PHT t.i.d.

CHADDA AND MATHUR, *Journal of the Association of Physicians in India* (1978),[1767] in a double-blind study with PHT found significant improvement in pain and paresthesia in twenty-eight of thirty-eight patients with diabetic neuropathy.

The authors conclude that PHT is an effective and well-tolerated drug for the relief of pain in diabetic neuropathy, and is preferable to narcotics.

FABRY'S DISEASE

LOCKMAN, HUNNINGHAKE, KRIVIT AND DESNICK, *Neurology* (1973),[1299] based on a double-blind study, report the effectiveness of PHT in the relief of the pain of Fabry's disease, a rare lipid storage disorder.

The authors state that the single most debilitating and morbid aspect of Fabry's disease is the pain. Excruciating crises of abdominal, chest and muscle pain, as well as arthralgias and fever, may occur episodically and last several days.

A double-blind crossover study with eight patients was conducted comparing PHT with aspirin and placebo. In the comparison, relief with PHT was statistically significant ($p < 0.001$).

The authors note that the pain in Fabry's disease is only partially relieved by narcotics at soporific doses.

DUPERRAT, PUISSANT, SAURAT, DELANOE, DOYARD AND GRUNFELS, *Annales de Dermatologie et de Syphiligraphie* (1975),[1813] described a twenty-three-year-old male patient who from birth had suffered from angiokeratomas and Fabry's disease. Pain progressed in intensity over the years. PHT (200 mg/day) resulted in complete disappearance of pain in less than a week. (See also Ref. 2352.)

DYSESTHESIA (PAINFUL TOUCHING)

GERZ, *Physicians' Drug Manual* (1972),[1066] reports an unusual case of "painful touching" (dysesthesia) in which a forty-year-old male patient showed dramatic response to PHT.

The patient reported that a painful, intolerable, cold stream would run all over his body when touched by human hands. Because of the extreme pain on being touched, he frequently became dangerous and violent, and wanted a certificate from the clinic stating that he suffered from a "mental problem."

He was tried on a variety of medications without success. Finally he was given PHT, 100 mg t.i.d. Within two weeks he was completely free of disturbing symptoms.

TABES

DATTNER, in the course of a discussion of a paper by CAVENESS, ADAMS, POPE AND WEGNER, *Transactions of the American Neurological Association* (1949),[48] said that some patients with lightning pains in tabes showed a favorable response to PHT or Tridione.

BRAHAM AND SAIA, *Lancet* (1960),[31] reported PHT effective in treating lightning pains in two cases of tabes.

GREEN, *Neurology* (1961),[129] reported that PHT was administered to two patients with severe lightning pains due to tabes dorsalis. Remarkable relief was obtained in both cases.

POST-HERPETIC NEURALGIA

REEVE, *Lancet* (1961),[611] reported that PHT was effective in four cases of post-herpetic neuralgia, and recommended that a trial of PHT precede more radical treatment.

HALLAQ AND HARRIS, *Journal of American Osteopathic Association* (1969),[1116] give a detailed report on the successful use of PHT in a case of post-herpetic neuralgia, with motor paralysis of an extremity, a rare complication. The patient, a seventy-six-year-old woman, had persistent pain in the right upper extremity, causing the entire limb to assume a semiflexed and adducted position. Diagnosis after examination was post-herpetic right brachial neuralgia and monoparesis.

After seven days in the hospital the patient was placed on PHT, 100 mg t.i.d. Within three days she was free of pain and remained so when narcotic analgesics were withdrawn and an extra 100 mg of PHT was added. The patient continued free of pain as long as she took PHT.

REFRACTORY CHRONIC PAIN

GABKA, *Medizinische Monatsschrift* (1963),[113] reported PHT (100–300 mg/day), combined with 0.025 g of caffeine, as the most effective treatment for the relief of pain in 115 out of 142 patients. The painful conditions included recurring headaches, migraine, genuine and symptomatic trigeminal neuralgia, post-operative jaw and facial pain, and pain following extensive facial tumor surgery.

The authors state that PHT was by far the best conservative therapy in the treatment of these types of recurring head and facial pain.

RASKIN, LEVINSON, PICKETT, HOFFMAN AND FIELDS, *American Journal of Surgery* (1974), [1444] as part of a larger study, reported that two of the patients with post-sympathectomy neuralgia, unresponsive to meperidine, had immediate relief with intravenous PHT.

TAGUCHI, WATANABE AND IOKU, *Neurologia Medico Chirurgica (Tokyo)* (1981), [2998] reported a patient with bulbar syringomyelia who developed severe, intractable pain and paresthesias in her legs, abdomen and chest after cervical laminectomy. She also developed muscle spasms of her upper body. PHT, 250 mg/day, stopped both the pain and muscle spasms.

SWERDLOW, *Clinical Neuropharmacology* (1984), [2997] reviewed a series of 200 patients with various types of refractory chronic lancinating or paroxysmal pain. The etiologies of the pain included post-laminectomy, post-traumatic, post-herpetic, post-operative, and post-amputation neuralgias, as well as pain secondary to nerve or plexus injury or operation, atypical facial pain, and central pain syndromes. Of fifty-two patients who received PHT as their first drug, twenty-four found it effective. This success rate was higher than that achieved with carbamazepine, clonazepam, and valproate.

PAIN IN MULTIPLE SCLEROSIS

MATTHEWS, *Brain* (1958), [1342] reported the effectiveness of PHT in the treatment of painful spasms in a patient with multiple sclerosis. When PHT, 100 mg t.i.d., was prescribed, the attacks stopped within two days.

KUROIWA AND SHIBASAKI, *Folia Psychiatrica et Neurologica Japonica* (1968), [1243] found that PHT and/or carbamazepine were useful in suppressing the painful tonic spasms in four patients with multiple sclerosis. In a further study, SHIBASAKI AND KUROIWA, *Archives of Neurology* (1974), [1541] reported the successful treatment of five of seven patients with PHT alone or in combination with carbamazepine.

SKILLRUD AND GOLDSTEIN, *Journal of the American Medical Association* (1983), [2963] reported in detail the case of a twenty-seven-year-old male physician with multiple sclerosis and paroxysmal limb hemiataxia and crossed facial paresthesias who became symptom free on 500 mg of PHT per day.

CLIFFORD AND TROTTER, *Archives of Neurology* (1984), [2396] reviewing the records of 317 multiple sclerosis patients with a wide variety of painful syndromes and therapies, reported PHT's usefulness in the treatment of limb, facial, head, and thoracic pain.

ABDOMINAL PAIN

KELLAWAY, CRAWLEY AND KAGAWA, *Epilepsia* (1959–1960), [551] in a review of experience with a group of 459 children who had consistent 14- and 6-per-second spike patterns on the EEG and whose primary complaints were headache and abdominal pain, found the most effective treatments were PHT and Diamox, alone or in combination.

PEPPERCORN, HERZOG, DICHTER AND MAYMAN, *JAMA* (1978), [2018] found PHT useful in the treatment of three patients with paroxysmal abdominal pain. When two of the patients stopped their medication the symptoms returned. With the resumption of the medication symptoms disappeared.

SCHAFFLER AND KARBOWSKI, *Schweizerische Medizinische Wochenschrift* (1981),[2928] reported six cases of paroxysmal abdominal pain occurring in association with cerebral dysrhythmias. PHT controlled or reduced the severity of the attacks in the four cases in which it was used alone. In one case, PHT, in combination with carbamazepine, was used successfully and, in another case, carbamazepine was used alone.

WOUNDS, ULCERS, BURNS

The topical use of PHT to promote healing of skin ulcers, burns and other wounds is reviewed in the Clinical Healing section. The important benefit of topical PHT, prompt relief of pain, is discussed here.

CHIKHANI, *Actualites Odonto-Stomatologiques* (1972),[894] in a study of fifty-eight patients, with periodontal disease, reported the beneficial effects of topical PHT on gingival pain as well as bleeding.

LUDWIG AND OTTO, *Russian Pharmacology and Toxicology* (1982),[2730] in a controlled study of sixty patients with atrophic gingivitis, found topical application of PHT (1% gel) controlled gum pain and heat sensitivity. Edema and gum bleeding disappeared. No effects were seen in the control group.

RODRIGUEZ-NORIEGA, ESPARZA-AHU-MADA, ANDRADE-PEREZ, ESPEJO-PLASCENCIA AND CHAPA-ALVAREZ, *Investigacion Médica Internacional* (1983),[2911] reported a group of twenty patients with venous stasis or diabetic ulcers treated with topical PHT powder. All patients experienced rapid improvement in local pain. In the control group, pain persisted until the lesion was completely healed.

MENDIOLA-GONZALES, ESPEJO-PLASCEN-CIA, CHAPA-ALVAREZ AND RODRIGUEZ-NORIEGA, *Investigacion Médica Internacional* (1983),[2788] reported a group of eighty patients with second-degree burns. Twenty patients were treated topically with PHT powder, ten with oral PHT, and ten with both topical and oral PHT. Bilateral burns provided control and treatment sites for the topical applications. Pain improved in five to twenty-five minutes at the treated sites, compared to twelve to fifteen hours at control sites.

Other clinical reviews and studies on the use of PHT in pain: facial pain including trigeminal neuralgia, glossopharyngeal neuralgia, and temporomandibular joint syndrome, Refs. 2470, 2472, 2492, 2523, 2593, 2619, 2801, 2847, 2943; headache including migraine, Refs. 2317, 2492; postherpetic neuralgia, Refs. 2474, 2657; reflex sympathetic dystrophy and post-sympathectomy pain, Refs. 2492, 3040; pain in multiple sclerosis, Refs. 2601, 2929; central and other chronic pain syndromes, Refs. 2452, 2460, 2492, 2756, 2784, 2997.

HEALING

Summary

Phenytoin, used orally and/or topically, promotes healing. The healing properties of oral PHT were first reported by Bodkin in 1945 in an extensive study of pruritus ani. Subsequently, oral PHT has been reported useful in the treatment of periodontal disease, scleroderma, epidermolysis bullosa, peptic ulcers, and a variety of skin and soft tissue wounds and ulcers.

Topical PHT has been demonstrated to relieve the pain and promote the healing of chronic soft tissue ulcers, including venous stasis, diabetic and decubitus ulcers, and also burns. Recently, PHT has been found effective in healing the chronic trophic ulcers of leprosy.

Relief of pain with topical PHT is prompt, usually occurring in a matter of minutes.

Biopsies of PHT-treated ulcers show increased formation of new blood vessels and increased collagen content. In addition, the scar tissue that forms is more flexible in PHT-treated wounds. Extensive laboratory studies have shown that PHT accelerates the healing and tensile strength of various wounds and fractures, stimulates fibroblast proliferation, increases collagen synthesis, content, and maturation in granulation tissue, and inhibits collagenase and collagen peptidase activity.

Periodontal

SHAPIRO, *Experimental Medicine and Surgery* (1958),[339] conducted a double-blind study of the effects of PHT on healing in patients with various degrees of periodontal disease. Thirty-three patients received oral PHT and nineteen received placebo.

Sections of gingiva were surgically removed and the wounds were covered with protective packs. When the packs were changed at the end of one week, the PHT-treated group exhibited less erythema, less pain and advanced wound healing. On histological section, there was marked acceleration of fibroblastic activity, clot organization, and epithelial proliferation as compared to the control group.

The author stated that PHT may be useful to increase the rate of wound healing in other areas of the body, as in burns.

SAVINI, POITEVIN AND POITEVIN, *Revue Francaise d'Odontostomatologie* (1972),[1504] presented a study of the use of PHT locally in the treatment of periodontal disease in 118 cases.

The authors examined the effect of PHT in a gingival paste-type ointment which was applied by the patient with massage to the gingival mucosa inside and outside after normal tooth brushing, morning and evening, and left for about five minutes before rinsing.

The findings were based both on the patient's observations and on physical examination, x-rays and, in forty-six cases, by biopsy.

With PHT, total resolution of pain occurred in most cases. Rapid regression of gingival bleeding and inflammation, increased healing, and decreased dental mobility were also seen. Although lesions were stabilized, there was no periodontal restoration.

The authors conclude that PHT is an effective aid in the treatment of periodontal disease.

PAYEN, *Revue d'Odontostomatologie du Midi de la France* (1972),[1403] studied the effect of a topical preparation of PHT for gingival massage in seventy-five patients with periodontal disease. Twenty-nine of the patients were hospitalized and forty-six were outpatients.

With PHT, decreased inflammation and increased production of collagen in the healing process were observed in twenty of the hospitalized patients and in forty-five of the outpatients.

CHIKHANI, *Actualites Odontostomatologiques* (1972),[894] in a study of fifty-eight patients, reported clinical and histological effects of daily PHT gingival massage in periodontopathies. The author states that the study demonstrates the beneficial effect of PHT, particularly on bleeding gums and on pain; and histological findings confirmed the fibroblastic action of PHT and the healing with sclerosis which accompanied the decrease in inflammatory infiltration.

The author states that beneficial effects were clear after forty to sixty days of treatment.

GOEBEL, *Journal of Oral Surgery* (1972),[1080] reported a controlled study of the effects of PHT, before and after surgery, on wound healing of extraction sockets. As controls, eighteen patients were given chlorpromazine, and fifteen were untreated.

Compared with controls, significant improvement was observed in wound healing in the nine patients who received PHT.

OTTO, LUDEWIG AND KOTZSCHKE, *Stomatologie der DDR* (1977),[2009] in a double-blind study, treated eighty patients with complex periodontal disease with a local application of PHT gel. Compared with the control group, there was marked subjective and objective improvement in the group treated with PHT.

LUDEWIG AND OTTO, *Russian Pharmacology and Toxicology* (1982),[2730] studied the effects of topical PHT in the treatment of atrophic gingivitis. Sixty patients were divided into three groups. Two groups were treated with topical PHT in a 1% gel applied twice a day for six and twelve weeks, respectively. A third group was treated with the gel alone and served as control.

The PHT-treated patients ceased to complain of gum pain and heat sensitivity. Edema and gum bleeding disappeared. On biopsy, improvement was evidenced by decrease in inflammatory infiltration and regeneration of connective tissue. No benefits were seen in the control group.

CARIES

APTON, *Dental Hygiene* (1977),[1724] conducted a study to determine if there was a difference in the incidence of decayed, missing and filled surfaces of teeth (DMFS) in patients with PHT therapy, versus those without it.

The author compared the incidence of DMFS in forty-five patients taking PHT for at least one year with national statistics from HEW as controls.

Acknowledging that the study was imperfectly controlled, and complicated by the introduction of fluoride, the author says that there was enough evidence that PHT was effective against DMFS to recommend that further work be done in this field.

The author's recommendation is supported by the controlled laboratory study of ROVIN, et al.[1485] in which it was found that PHT was useful against caries in mice (see p. 161).

Ulcers

SIMPSON, KUNZ AND SLAFTA, *New York State Journal of Medicine* (1965),[344] reported that PHT promoted the healing of leg ulcers. The study contained double-blind and crossover controls.

Thirty hospitalized psychiatric patients (age range forty to seventy-seven years) were chosen for the project. The sole criterion for the patient selection was that all had chronic leg ulceration. The ulcers had been present for from two to fifteen years. Occasional healing had taken place but this was minimal and most of the patients had an area of ulceration present at all times despite the fact that they received standard topical treatment and occasional bed rest.

Repeated measurements were carried out under double-blind conditions. Measurements were made by means of a planimeter reading of the ulcer area as well as the actual scaling area around the ulcer. A clinical rating was also given.

All three indices measured showed improvement in the PHT group compared with the placebo group. Statistical analysis of the actual ulcer areas demonstrated a difference at better than the 0.05 level of significance between the two groups.

Small doses such as 200 mg a day were found to be associated with better healing than were larger doses.

STREAN, *Chemical Abstracts* (1966),[669] reported PHT effective in promoting the complete healing of an antecubital ulcer, a diabetic ulcer and two peptic ulcers, all of long duration. It was found that PHT provided for the regeneration of healthy tissue in the denuded zone.

TAYLOR, *Personal Communication* (1969),[730] reported a twenty-four-year-old patient with typical oral and genital ulcerations of Behcet's syndrome. The patient also had involvement of the temporomandibular joints (Costen's syndrome). Clenching the jaw produced pain typical of the syndrome. In addition, she suffered with conjunctivitis, urethritis, vaginitis and arthritis.

By the sixth day, with treatment with PHT, 100 mg/day, the ulcerated areas had healed and all other symptoms disappeared. The patient remained symptom-free when seen five months later.

RODRIGUEZ-NORIEGA, ESPARZA-AHUMADA, ANDRADE-PEREZ, ESPEJO-PLASCENCIA AND CHAPA-ALVAREZ, *Investigacion Médica Internacional* (1983),[2911] studied forty patients with venous stasis, diabetic and other soft tissue ulcers. They compared the use of PHT, topically, in twenty patients with conventional treatment in a control group of twenty patients. The average time to healing or grafting in the PHT-treated group was twenty-one days, compared to forty-five days in the control group.

Biopsy of the PHT-treated ulcers showed more rapid infiltration of fibroblasts and greater collagen deposition, as well as increased new blood vessel formation. Bacterial cultures of the ulcer surface improved more rapidly, and more stable scar formation was also seen in the PHT group. (See also Ref. 2690).

BARBA RUBIO, *Presented at the XII Mexican Congress of Dermatology* (1985),[2308] presented a report on the use of topical PHT in the treatment of trophic lower extremity ulcers in seven leprosy patients. The ulcers were chronic and had been refractory to previous forms of treatment for up to fifteen years.

With PHT, three of the patients had complete healing of their ulcers within six weeks. The remaining four patients had good results consisting of diminished exudate, appearance of healthy granulation tissue, reduction in ulcer size, and suitability for skin grafting.

Burns

MENDIOLA-GONZALEZ, ESPEJO-PLASCENCIA, CHAPA-ALVAREZ AND RODRIGUEZ-NORIEGA, *Investigacion Médica Internacional* (1983),[2788] reported the topical use of PHT powder in the treatment of second-degree burns. The study included eighty patients. Forty, given conventional treatment, were used as controls. Twenty were treated with topical PHT, ten with oral PHT, and ten with a combination of topical and oral PHT.

In the control group, the average time to healing or grafting was thirty days. In the oral PHT group, it was twenty-three days. In the topical group and the combined treatment group, the time to healing or grafting was sixteen days.

Topical PHT resulted in rapid elimination of pain at the burn site. Biopsy of the PHT-treated burns showed increased collagen, decreased inflammation, and more capillaries compared to controls. Bacterial burn-surface cultures in the PHT groups became negative after five to ten days of treatment. The bacterial cultures remained positive in the conventional treatment group, until healing or grafting.

Pruritus Ani

BODKIN, *American Journal of Digestive Diseases* (1945),[25] described the successful treatment of forty-one of forty-two cases of pruritus ani upon the addition of PHT to oral therapy.

In this series of forty-two cases, only one showed no improvement and another recovered rather slowly. Almost all of the others responded in a surprisingly short time.

The author stated that, "Pruritus ani has always been a difficult and baffling problem to the proctologist . . . It is notable for its chronicity and resistance to treatment. No one form of therapy has been effective, as is evidenced by the lengthy list of measures employed. It is therefore most interesting to come upon a method of treatment, mainly oral, that gives prompt symptomatic relief and which produces clearly visible results in the skin. It is aimed at the most likely site of origin of the condition—the nervous system . . . The one definite and positive finding that stood out in all the cases that I have carefully studied for the past ten years or more was this: every one of them was highly nervous."

The duration of the symptoms in the group studied was from one to thirty years and included three cases that also had pruritus vulvae. The author had previously used takadiastase, novatropin and phenobarbital. When PHT was added, the results were rather striking. Even long standing cases obtained marked symptomatic relief within a few days.

GOODWIN, *Journal of the National Proctologic Association* (1946),[127] described the successful treatment of twenty cases of pruritus ani treated with PHT and a starch digestant. The results obtained were superior to any therapy previously employed. The author stated that this study confirmed the work of BODKIN.[25]

Length of treatment varied. Usually the physical signs of bleeding, maceration, leathery appearance, moist skin, fissures, cracked skin and itching began to disappear from one to three weeks after institution of therapy. The patients usually volunteered before they were examined that they were much better after two or three weeks' treatment.

One severe case of pruritus was observed in which there was extensive maceration and bleeding of the anus, scrotum and groin. So intense was the pruritus that nothing seemed of value in bringing even tem-

porary relief. With PHT and a starch digestant, the patient showed marked improvement to the point that treatment was discontinued at the end of six weeks.

Recurrence was observed in one patient. Reestablishing treatment effected prompt relief.

In the author's experience the rapid relief of symptoms acheived with PHT had not been obtained with the use of any local treatment.

BODKIN, *American Journal of Digestive Diseases* (1947),[26] in an expanded series of 111 cases of pruritus ani, again reported excellent results with PHT. Of the 111 cases treated, only six failed to respond. Five patients discontinued medication and their outcome was unknown.

The author stated that it was a pleasant surprise to find that recurrences were not too numerous and that they were rather easily controlled by reinstitution of PHT.

Scleroderma

MORGAN, *Cutis* (1971),[1371] reports that patients with scleroderma, treated with PHT, showed marked improvement when compared with patients treated by conventional therapy.

The study consisted of sixty-five patients with two general types of scleroderma, morphea and systemic. Twenty-nine were treated with PHT and thirty-six were treated by conventional means.

The attention of the author was brought to the use of PHT in scleroderma in an unusual way. A sixty-seven-year-old woman had progressive generalized morphea. For over a year, a wide variety of medications had been tried and failed to halt progression of the disease. Then the patient had a mild stroke and was placed on PHT by her neurologists. Progressive improvement in scleroderma was evident three weeks after she began PHT. Two years later her skin showed no evidence of scleroderma and has remained clear to date.

Because of the unexpected improvement in this case, the author decided to explore the possibility that PHT might be effective in the treatment of scleroderma. In his study the author used PHT in twenty-nine patients and conventional therapy in thirty-six patients. The results follow:

	With PHT	Other Therapy
Number of Patients	**29**	**36**
Worse	0	11
No change	2	10
Improved (patient and doctor agree)	12	9
Complete clearing of sclerosis	12	4
Complete clearing of sclerosis, atrophy and pigment	3	2

The author concludes that in this series of patients with scleroderma, the administration of PHT appeared not only to prevent progression of sclerosis but also to aid in its resolution.*

* In a smaller group of patients, the author also investigated the use of PHT in a less serious disorder, lichen sclerosis et atrophicus, and found PHT as effective as conventional therapy.

Localized Linear Scleroderma

NELDNER, *Cutis* (1978),[1994] reported significant reversal of localized linear scleroderma in five patients treated with 100–300 mg PHT daily.

The duration of the disease prior to PHT treatment was one to sixteen years. Morbidity included arthralgia and joint stiffness, decreased range of motion, gait disturbances, inability to grasp or throw, alopecia, headache, neuralgias, and neuroses. The most distressing complication was that of deep atrophy beyond the area of linear sclerosis, which produced facial hemiatrophy or

atrophy of an entire limb with varying degrees of permanent joint fixation and deep sclerotic bands underlying cutaneous hyperpigmentation.

The author states that the response to PHT treatment, and the recurrence of the condition when PHT was prematurely discontinued, point towards the true pharmacologic effect of PHT in the treatment of this disorder.

See also Refs. 1729, 2097, 2297, 2360, 2784, 2953, 3030.

Epidermolysis Bullosa

EISENBERG, STEVENS AND SCHOFIELD, *Australian Journal of Dermatology* (1978),[1817] studied the effects of PHT on the collagenolytic system in tissue samples from patients with dystrophic epidermolysis bullosa. The collagenolytic system is known to be excessive in this disorder. PHT was found to inhibit the excessive activity.

As a result of these findings, two children with dystrophic epidermolysis bullosa were given PHT. Marked improvement in skin fragility resulted. The authors concluded that the clinical effects of PHT on both blister formation and collagenase activity are consistent with the protective effect observed *in vitro* and suggested that PHT is useful in the management of this disease.

BAUER, COOPER, TUCKER AND ESTERLY, *The New England Journal of Medicine* (1980),[1738] citing the work of EISENBERG, STEVENS AND SCHOFIELD,[1817] studied the effect of PHT on the collagenolytic system *in vitro*, and clinically in seventeen patients with recessive dystrophic epidermolysis bullosa.

With PHT there was a significant decrease in blistering in all patients. In twelve patients the reduction was from 46% to

90%. The clinical study was controlled in that all patients underwent a period without PHT during which they experienced a notable exacerbation in blistering.

The authors state that the correlation of the clinical responsiveness and *in vitro* inhibition of collagenase indicates that PHT represents a therapeutic option of relatively low risk in a disease for which there has been no rational method of therapy.

BAUER AND COOPER, *Archives of Dermatology* (1981),[2153] reported an extended study (76 to 99 weeks) of nine patients with moderate or severe recessive dystrophic epidermolysis bullosa. In seven of the nine patients, the decrease in blisters and erosion with PHT was 70%. In the other two patients, blistering decreased 24% to 40%. (See also Refs. 2176, 2188, 2247.)

BANDMANN AND PERWEIN, *Zeitschrift fur Hautkrankheiten* (1982),[2306] in a detailed case report, describe a patient with the rare Gedde-Dahl type of epidermolysis bullosa, with severe blistering, erosions, and dysphagia due to esophageal stenosis.

With PHT, fewer blisters developed, and blisters and erosions already present healed more quickly. (See also Ref. 2863.)

WIRTH, NESCH, OSTAPOWICZ AND ANTON-LAMPRECHT, *Zeitschrift fur Hautkrankheiten* (1983),[3075] state that they have used oral PHT in the treatment of eleven patients with recessive dystrophic epidermolysis bullosa (Hallopeau-Siemens and Inversa type) since 1978. The authors detail six of their cases, ages six weeks to sixty-one years. Treatment with PHT, at blood levels of 8–15 μg/ml, resulted in definite reduction in blistering and lessened skin fragility.

The authors report that four of their patients had esophageal stenosis, one with complete obstruction. With PHT, improve-ment was such that esophageal dilation could be performed in all four.

COOPER AND BAUER, *Archives of Dermatology* (1984),[2406] studied the effects of PHT in twenty-two patients with recessive dystrophic epidermolysis bullosa. Therapeutic response was defined as mean decrease in blistering of more than 40%. The authors stated that, with this strict criterion, fourteen of the twenty-two patients had 46% or more reduction of blistering. PHT, 100–300 mg/day, was adjusted to maintain blood levels of at least 8 μg/ml.

To determine if prolonged treatment altered response, nine of the patients were studied for periods longer than seventy-five weeks. Seven of these patients continued to have a mean decrease in blistering of at least 40%.

The authors noted that with PHT patients had an enhanced sense of well-being.

See Refs. 2247, 2491, 2532, 2546, 2560, 2602, 2617, 2643, 2658, 2793, 2818, 2876, 3009, 3087. Also, regulatory effect of PHT on collagen synthesis and breakdown, Refs. 172, 501, 502, 811, 1867, 1882, 2107, 2571, 2581.

Pachyonychia

BLANK, *British Journal of Dermatology* (1982),[2156] reported his experience with PHT in treating a patient with pachyonychia.

The patient had been incapacitated by blisters and erosions of her feet and hands, and painful lesions in her mouth.

She was treated with oral PHT with dramatic results. She became able to walk for many blocks. Although many of the hyperkeratotic lesions persisted, her mouth and hands were greatly improved. After three years of this treatment she felt so well that she planned to marry.

TREATMENT OF OTHER DISORDERS

Asthma

The three papers which follow furnish strong evidence that phenytoin is useful in asthma.

Consistent with these findings are basic mechanism studies which show PHT's ability to relax bronchial smooth muscle, to regulate the autonomic nervous system, and to prevent the effects of hypoxia.

SHULMAN, *New England Journal of Medicine* (1942),[341] selected seven cases of severe bronchial asthma, which were considered intractable because they had not responded to conventional treatment. These cases were treated with PHT. In a detailed study the author reported marked relief of asthma in six of seven cases and partial relief in the seventh.

In this study PHT was used exclusively and was not begun until all other medications were eliminated. With the application of PHT six of the patients were consistently free of attacks of bronchial asthma and the seventh showed some improvement. Two of the patients had stubborn eczema which cleared to a remarkable degree with PHT.

The author notes that the efficacy of PHT was further evidenced by the fact that the patients were able to successfully engage in situations and environments which formerly precipitated attacks of bronchial asthma.

SAYER AND POLVAN, *Lancet* (1968),[401] described sixteen patients with bronchial asthma, with frequent asthmatic crises. Fourteen had abnormal EEGs and two had EEGs within normal limits.

All patients were taken off other medications and given PHT for an average of forty-five days. Ten patients were closely followed up during this period. Seven had neither asthmatic crises nor wheezing. One patient had occasional wheezing and in the other two cases the frequency of crises was greatly diminished.

SHAH, VORA, KARKHANIS AND TALWALKAR, *Indian Journal of Chest Diseases* (1970),[1535] conducted a study of the usefulness of PHT in bronchial asthma in twenty-seven patients. Both clinical and laboratory observations were made.

The authors state that the prevention of the spread of electrical discharge is one of the most important, interesting and unexploited pharmacological properties of PHT. Noting that other paroxysmal disorders have responded to PHT, they felt that its use in the paroxysmal spasms of asthma should be explored.

In the study of the twenty-seven patients, careful histories were recorded, including the severity of asthma, graded by age at onset, frequency of attacks during past twelve months, absenteeism from work, number of days absent in the last month, and number of sleepless nights in the last month.

Effort tolerance tests were performed during and between attacks. Appraisal of previous therapy during the last month was noted by the number of adrenaline and/or aminophylline injections and oral drugs (bronchodilators and steroids). Each patient had laboratory investigations, chest x-ray and electrocardiogram to exclude any cardiopulmonary disease simulating bronchial asthma. Ventilation studies, including maximum breathing capacity, were carried out initially and repeated at weekly follow-up examinations. At the end of the treatment period all examinations were repeated.

Before starting patients on PHT all other medicines were discontinued. Dosage was 100 mg PHT t.i.d. The trial was for one month. Assessment of subjective and objective results was verified by all participating physicians.

While on PHT, twenty-five of the twenty-seven patients experienced impressive relief. Fifteen of these patients showed improved ventilation tests. Although some wheezing persisted in twelve patients, the distress was less evident. As a whole, the patients were more relaxed.

The results of this study led the authors to suggest that PHT would seem to be a useful anti-asthmatic agent.*

* A number of people with emphysema have reported to the Dreyfus Medical Foundation that since taking PHT for other reasons they had experienced improvement in their breathing. We are not aware of published work on the use of PHT for emphysema. It would seem an area for research. (See Anti-anoxic Effects of PHT.)

Gastrointestinal Disorders

IRRITABLE BOWEL SYNDROME

CHADDA, JOSHI AND CHADDA, *Journal of the Association of Physicians in India* (1983),[2380] reported a randomized double-blind crossover trial of PHT (100 mg t.i.d.) versus placebo in twenty-five patients with irritable bowel syndrome. Seven had spastic colitis; eight, alternating diarrhea and constipation; and ten, mucous colitis. Twenty-two of the patients also suffered abdominal pain. Trials were for three weeks each, with a ten-day drug-free interval between crossover.

Improvement was observed in twelve of the patients while on PHT. Five improved in the placebo group.

DE LA TORRE, NAVARRO AND ALDRETE, *Current Therapeutic Research* (1985),[2437] compared PHT with conventional treatment in a study of eighty patients with irritable bowel syndrome. Forty patients received PHT, 100 mg t.i.d., and forty patients received an anticholinergic, an antacid, and either a tranquilizer or an antidepressant.

With PHT, thirty of the forty patients had an excellent to satisfactory response, compared to eighteen in the group that received conventional treatment.

Abdominal pain, diarrhea, constipation, nausea, vomiting and pyrosis were among the symptoms that responded. In addition, PHT treatment resulted in a statistically significant greater number of complete remissions of depression, insomnia and anxiety.

ULCERATIVE COLITIS

SCHAERRER, *Personal Communication* (1963),[2927] reported observations of forty-six patients with chronic idiopathic ulcerative colitis. Nineteen patients responded to treatment with PHT, 150–300 mg/day. Patients were classified as responding only if they remained symptom-free for a period of at least one year. All patients responding to PHT returned to normal or near-normal bowel habits, had a normal mucosal pattern, and gained weight.

DIABETIC DIARRHEA

THOMAS AND VERGES, *La Presse Medicale* (1985),[3012] report the use of PHT (300 mg daily) to treat severe motor diarrhea in five diabetic patients. The patients had been insulin-dependent for two to seventeen years and had advanced neuropathy. With PHT the diarrhea ceased in all five patients within twenty-four to forty-eight hours.

The effectiveness of PHT was further established by the fact that the diarrhea recurred in four patients when PHT was stopped and disappeared when PHT was given again.

With maintenance PHT treatment there were no relapses in the three-month to five-year follow-up.

See also Basic Mechanisms — Smooth Muscle section, p. 142.

Endocrine Disorders*

LABILE DIABETES

FABRYKANT AND PACELLA, *Annals of Internal Medicine* (1948),[92] detailed the use of PHT in the treatment of three cases of labile diabetes. In each case, PHT stabilized insulin requirements and reduced negative reactions. In addition, the patients showed remarkable improvement in mood.

As a control, when PHT was discontinued for periods of from five to thirty-three days, the patients reverted to frequent reactions and nervousness.

WILSON, *Canadian Medical Association Journal* (1951),[382] described three cases of labile diabetes whose control was unsatisfactory and not compatible with life outside

the hospital. In all instances abnormal electroencephalograms were found. Prior to PHT treatment, these patients presented extremely labile diabetes, characterized by frequent reactions, uncontrollable glycosuria, and personality changes.

The institution of PHT therapy resulted in a marked improvement in diabetic control and enabled these individuals to lead a relatively normal life, not necessitating a return to the hospital.

FABRYKANT, *Annals of Internal Medicine* (1953),[91] again reported the effectiveness of PHT therapy in the management of labile diabetes associated with electrocerebral dysfunction. In this study of seven patients, five showed an appreciable diminution in the frequency and severity of insulin reactions along with a decrease in insulin requirement. This resulted in better control of diabetes and psychologic improvement. The other two patients did not adhere to therapy, but the author noted that in one case there was a marked improvement while on PHT. (See also Ref. 430.)

ROBERTS, *Journal of the American Geriatrics Society* (1964),[429] reported an extensive study entitled, "The Syndrome of Narcolepsy and Diabetogenic ('Functional') Hyperinsulinism."

Although the use of PHT was not the major focus of his work, the author stated that with regard to the symptoms of labile diabetes his experiences with PHT confirm those of others who have observed clinical and electroencephalographic improvement following its administration.

AV RUSKIN, TIO AND JUAN, *Clinical Research* (1979),[2149] demonstrated that PHT

---

* PHT has been shown to influence endocrine function in a number of ways (see Metabolic and Endocrine Regulatory Effects, p. 121). It modulates the hypothalamic and other neuronal systems that regulate pituitary function. It alters hormone release directly by its effects on calcium-dependent secretion processes, and can alter hormone metabolism and protein binding.

has a modulating effect on basal glucagon in eight type-1 juvenile diabetes mellitus patients. PHT lowered arginine-induced blood glucose and glucagon responses.

The authors suggest that PHT be considered as adjunctive therapy in diabetes mellitus when hyperglucagonemia is present.

See also Basic Mechanisms — Metabolic and Endocrine Regulatory Effects, p. 121.

DIABETIC NEUROPATHY

ELLENBERG, *New York State Journal of Medicine* (1968),[431] recognized the urgent need for a beneficial therapeutic agent in diabetic neuropathy and stated that this need was underscored by the frequent use of narcotics to control the severe pain, with the ever-present threat of addiction. The author noted that PHT was not addictive, did not sedate and, on the assumption that the symptoms of diabetic neuropathy might have a similar background to tic douloureux in which PHT was used with success, a therapeutic trial was undertaken.

PHT was used to treat painful diabetic peripheral neuropathy in sixty patients. Based on symptomatic relief of pain and paresthesias, excellent results were obtained in forty-one patients and fair response in ten patients. Improvement was noted in from twenty-four to ninety-six hours. As a feature of control, when the drug was discontinued, symptoms frequently recurred. A salutary response was uniformly repeated on reinstitution of PHT.

In two of the sixty cases skin rash occurred, one associated with fever. These reactions disappeared upon withdrawal of the medicine.

Nine years later, in *JAMA*,[1819] ELLENBERG repeated his recommendation of the use of PHT in the treatment of painful diabetic neuropathy, eliminating the use of narcotics.

KANNAN, DASH AND RASTOGI, *Journal of Diabetic Association of India* (1978),[1920] in a double-blind crossover study of sixteen patients with diabetic neuropathy, found that thirteen had significant relief of pain and/or paresthesias with 100 mg PHT t.i.d.

CHADDA AND MATHUR, *Journal of the Association of Physicians in India* (1978),[1767] in a double-blind study with PHT found significant improvement in pain and paresthesias in twenty-eight of thirty-eight patients with diabetic neuropathy.

The authors conclude that PHT is an effective and well-tolerated drug for the relief of pain in diabetic neuropathy, and is preferred to narcotics.

See also Treatment of Pain, p. 48.

HYPOGLYCEMIA

KNOPP, SHEININ AND FREINKEL, *Archives of Internal Medicine* (1972),[1222] reported that PHT inhibited the stimulated insulin release in a patient with an islet cell tumor. They noted that their observations indicate that PHT may warrant consideration as a safe therapeutic adjunct in inoperable or poorly controlled islet cell tumors.

COHEN, BOWER, FIDLER, JOHNSONBAUGH AND SODE, *Lancet* (1973),[909] reported the effect of PHT on a patient with a benign insulinoma. PHT was found effective in raising the mean fasting plasma glucose concentration and improved the immunoreactive insulin to glucose ratio.

The authors conclude that PHT appears to be a promising agent in the treatment of certain patients with insulinoma.

STAMBAUGH AND TUCKER, *Diabetes* (1974),[1583] describe the successful use of PHT in the treatment of five patients with functional hypoglycemia previously unresponsive to dietary management.

Clinical reversal of hypoglycemia, including marked improvement in mood and emotional stability, was observed in all five cases. Laboratory tests were confirmatory in both six-hour glucose tolerance and insulin level tests, performed before and after PHT therapy.

BRODOWS AND CAMPBELL, *Journal of Clinical Endocrinology and Metabolism* (1974),[872] describe the successful control of refractory hypoglycemia with therapeutic doses of PHT in a patient with a suspected functional islet cell tumor. The authors state that the adequacy of the control of the hypoglycemia by PHT was evidenced by normal overnight fasting glucose levels and the absence of hypoglycemia during total fasting up to twenty-four hours. They note that it is of interest that there was a high degree of correlation between post-absorptive glucose and serum PHT levels and also a significant lowering of basal insulin levels during PHT therapy.

HOFELDT, DIPPE, LEVIN, KARAM, BLUM AND FORSHAM, *Diabetes* (1974),[1154] reported on the use of PHT in three patients with surgically proven insulinomas, tested with oral and intravenous glucose.

The authors found that PHT had no significant effect on basal glucose or insulin values, but was useful in reducing insulin secretion after stimuli.

BRICAIRE, LUTON, WECHSLER, MESSING AND HALABY, *Annales de Medecine Interne* (1976),[1756] reported the successful use of PHT in a case of organic hypoglycemia due to insulinoma for a period of five months prior to surgical removal of tumor.

AGAPOVA AND MIKHALEV, *Therapeutic Archives* (1977),[1714] reported the control with PHT of hypoglycemia attacks in a patient with an adenoma of the pancreas during the preoperative period until the adenoma was surgically removed.

See also Refs. 2533, 2610, 2925, 2932.

CUSHING'S SYNDROME

STARKOVA, MAROVA, LEMESCHEVA, GONCHAROVA, ATAMANOVA AND SEDYKH, *Problemy Endokrinologii* (1972),[2090] studied fifteen patients with Cushing's syndrome given PHT, 300 mg per day, for a period of three weeks.

This treatment led to normalization of the urinary excretion of ketosteroids and of aldosterone and pregnanediol, and to a normalization of the content of 17-hydroxyketosteroids in blood. There was also an increase in the potassium content in blood. The rate of secretion of cortisol decreased for all patients.

The authors noted that all the patients displayed a reduction or normalization of blood pressure and body weight, and a decrease in headaches and in weakness. (See also Ref. 427.)

FRENKEL, SAFRONOVA, MAROVA AND LEMESHEVA, *Problemy Endokrinologii* (1976),[2510] treated nine Cushing's syndrome patients with PHT, 300 mg/day, for three weeks.

With PHT, reduction or normalization of blood pressure, decrease in headaches, decrease in fatigue, and reduction in excretion of 17-hydroxyketosteroids and ketosteroids were observed. In seven of the patients, there was also normalization of the EEG parameters, especially those indicating diencephalic disturbances.

INAPPROPRIATE ANTIDIURETIC HORMONE SYNDROME

LEE, GRUMER, BRONSKY AND WALDSTEIN, *Journal of Laboratory Clinical Medicine* (1961),[219] using acute water loading as a diagnostic test for the inappropriate antidiuretic hormone (ADH) syndrome in hyponatremia, treated two patients with confirmed inappropriate ADH syndrome with intravenous PHT (250 mg).

Both patients showed an increase in free-water clearance. In one patient with tuberculous meningitis, a normal response to acute water loading was noted after one month of therapy.

FICHMAN, KLEEMAN AND BETHUNE, *Archives of Neurology* (1970),[97] studied the effect of intravenous PHT on antidiuretic hormone (ADH) activity in six patients with inappropriate ADH syndrome. PHT markedly increased the excretion of a 20 ml/kg water load and markedly decreased minimum urine osmolality in four of the patients in three hours. Two of the patients with bronchogenic carcinoma did not respond.

The authors state that their data suggests that, in man, PHT affects water balance by inhibiting ADH release.

LANDOLT, *Acta Endocrinologica* (1974),[1256] reported an eight-year-old patient who, following surgery for craniopharyngioma, developed diabetes insipidus followed by inappropriate ADH secretion. Intravenous PHT resulted in an increase in urine output. Serum sodium values returned to normal and the patient became more alert. During a subsequent recurrence of inappropriate ADH secretion, PHT again increased the urine output.

The author concludes that PHT regulates water metabolism during periods of inappropriate ADH secretion, but has no effect in patients with normal water balance.

TANAY, YUST, PERESECENSCHI, ABRAMOV AND AVIRAM, *Annals of Internal Medicine* (1979),[2101] reported on the use of PHT in the treatment of a sixty-eight-year-old female who had been admitted to hospital because of precordial pain, headache, nausea, and blurring of vision. In addition, confused behavior and diminished orientation in time and place were observed. A diagnosis of inappropriate antidiuretic hormone secretion was made and confirmed by laboratory findings.

The authors state that treatment with PHT, 100 mg t.i.d., resulted in reversal of the clinical and laboratory findings and demonstrated the effectiveness of PHT in treating this syndrome.

SORDILLO, MATARESE, NOVICH, ZABETAKIS AND MICHELIS, *Clinical Nephrology* (1981),[2971] report two patients with inappropriate ADH syndrome who were successfully treated with PHT.

The authors state that PHT can suppress drug-induced, as well as excess endogenous, ADH secretion.

HYPERTHYROIDISM

ROMERO, MARANON AND BOBILLO, *Revista Iberica de Endocrinologia* (1970),[1479] describe a variety of treatments for hyperthyroidism including thyroidostatic therapy, surgical resection, and radioisotope therapy, noting these methods have complications and side effects.

The authors state that about twenty years ago they started using PHT, 50 mg t.i.d., in combination with hydrazides. The treatment consisted of alternating PHT one week with hydrazides the next week.

As a result of their long experience with PHT, the authors initiated a detailed study of nineteen patients. Eight patients showed very favorable improvement; four, moderate improvement; one, slight improvement; and two, no improvement. Marked relief of nervousness, characteristic of this disorder, was observed.

The authors state that in some patients treated with PHT there was decrease in size of goiter and exophthalmus. (See also Refs. 1125, 2499, 2846, 2964.)

MENSTRUAL DISTURBANCES

MICK, *JAMA* (1973),[1359] reported the case of a girl who had edema of the legs, fingers and puffiness of the face, accompanied by dizzy spells. These symptoms occurred about ten days before each menstrual cycle.

Diuretics had been tried without success. On 100 mg of PHT, twice daily, the patient became completely free of her episodic edema. Improvement in dizziness was also noted.

KRAMER, *American Journal of Diseases of Children* (1977),[1936] described a thirteen-year-old girl with a pattern of recurrent psychotic episodes, which seemed to coincide with her menstrual periods. After four to seven days of bizarre, catatonic behavior, the patient would return to a normal state.

The episodes were virtually eliminated by treatment with PHT, 400 mg a day. During a three-and-a-half year follow-up, the patient continued to be symptom-free, as long as she was maintained on adequate PHT.

Fever and Temperature Regulation
RECURRENT FEVER

SNYDER, *Pediatrics* (1958),[2967] reported on the use of PHT (100–200 mg/day) in eight children with a variety of paroxysmal symptoms including headache, migraine, vertigo, abdominal pain and nightmares. All experienced prompt relief from these symptoms with PHT.

In two cases, intermittent fevers of unexplained origin were eliminated by PHT.

BERGER, *Postgraduate Medicine* (1966),[819] reported on an unusual case of recurrent fever, successfully treated with PHT.

A sixteen-year-old boy had irregular attacks of fever for eight years. These attacks would last from four to twenty-four hours, and disappear abruptly, regardless of treatment. His temperature would rise to 102°F and stay within a degree of this reading until the attack was terminated. Headache, vertigo, weakness, irritability, and sometimes violent rages accompanied the fever.

Over a four-year period the patient missed 260 days of school because of these attacks of fever. Extensive tests for causes of fever proved negative. Penicillin, tetracycline and sulfadimethoxine were tried without effect.

The patient was treated with 400 mg of PHT per day and the attacks stopped. Subsequently, on a dose of 25 mg q.i.d., he had been free of fever, and the symptoms that accompanied it, for four years.

On four occasions PHT was withdrawn. Each time the fever and other symptoms returned within a few days.

FAMILIAL MEDITERRANEAN FEVER

HAMED, ABDEL-AAL, ABDEL-AZIZ, NASSAR, SWEIFY, ATTA, EL-AWADY, EL-AREF AND EL-GARF, *Journal of the Egyptian Medical Association* (1975),[1879] stated that since 1966 they have used PHT to treat forty-seven children for a periodic disease of unknown etiology, which has many names and which they refer to as familial Mediterranean fever. Thirty-one of the children were available for follow-up. Twenty-two had improvement in the severity and frequency of attacks, six were unimproved and three became worse.

The authors conclude that PHT significantly reduces the frequency and severity of attacks of familial Mediterranean fever.

TRANSFUSION REACTION

RICEVUTI, MAZZONE, DANESINO, TOSCANO AND RIZZO, *Lancet* (1984),[2907] in a study of granulocyte transfusion reactions, noted that six patients pretreated with PHT did not develop fever; whereas, ten of fifteen non-treated patients did have fever. (see Granulocyte Transfusion Reaction, below.)

HYPOTHALAMIC SYNDROME

BECHTEREVA, NIKITINA, ILIUCHINA, DAMBINOVA AND DENISOVA, *European Journal of Clinical Investigation* (1984),[2316] reported on the use of PHT in 120 patients with hypothalamic syndrome of varying etiologies. PHT (50–100 mg b.i.d. or t.i.d.) resulted in stabilization of body temperature as well as cardiovascular function (including blood pressure) and improvements in mood, sleep and headaches.

In the laboratory, PHT was found to inhibit glutaminergic receptor function. The authors suggest that these findings are related to PHT's clinical actions.

. . .

A number of individuals taking PHT have reported to the Dreyfus Medical Foundation that their usual attacks of "flu," "virus," etc., have been accompanied by less fever than they would have expected. Research in this area seems indicated.

Granulocyte Transfusion Reaction

RICEVUTI, MAZZONE, DANESINO, TOSCANO AND RIZZO, *Lancet* (1984),[2907] reported

twenty-five patients who received granulocyte transfusions. To control common transfusion reactions, including fever, malaise, nausea and vomiting, six were pretreated with PHT (10 mg/kg). Four received hydrocortisone, and fifteen received no pretreatment.

None of the patients who received PHT had any of these reactions. The four who received hydrocortisone had slight fever. Ten of the fifteen nontreated patients had fever. Four of these were subsequently treated with PHT with gradual, but definite, reduction of fever. In addition, the patients treated with PHT had similar neutrophil function before and after the transfusion; whereas, both the untreated and hydrocortisone groups showed decreased function after transfusion.

Head Injuries and Surgery

HOFF AND HOFF, *Monatsschrift Psychiatrie and Neurologie* (1947),[2599] reported a controlled study of the effectiveness of PHT in the prevention of post-traumatic seizures. One hundred World War II veterans with head injuries were randomized into two groups of fifty. One group received 200 mg PHT daily, while the other group, serving as controls, received no treatment unless seizures developed. During the first four years, only two patients (4%) from the PHT-treated group developed seizures, (one after he had become a heavy drinker), while seventeen (38%) developed seizures in the control group.

Four years later, BIRKMAYER, *Wiener Klinische Wochenschrift* (1951),[2340] reported additional results of this study. Six percent of the patients in the PHT-treated group had seizures compared to 51% in the control group.

The author concludes that small doses of PHT are sufficient to protect against post-traumatic epilepsy.

THE CZECHOSLOVAKIA HEALTH MINISTRY, *Medical World News* (1968),[70] issued a directive requiring doctors to give PHT and phenobarbital to every trauma victim who remains unconscious for more than three hours. After six months, if no signs of epilepsy have appeared, the drugs are phased out over the next nine to eighteen months.

This directive was based upon work by DR. KAREL POPEK, chief neurologist at the Neurological Clinic of the University Medical Faculty in Brno, Czechoslovakia. Dr. Popek conducted a controlled clinical study of PHT and phenobarbital in patients with cerebral concussion or other serious head injuries.

He considered the results of the study persuasive enough to warrant routine use of the drugs as preventive therapy. (See also SERVIT AND MUSIL, Ref. 2256.)

WOHNS AND WYLER, *Journal of Neurosurgery* (1979),[2122] reported on sixty-two patients whose head injuries were sufficiently severe to cause high probability of post-traumatic seizures. Of fifty patients treated with PHT, 10% developed late onset seizures. Twelve patients not treated with PHT, but who had head injuries of equal magnitude, had a 50% incidence of seizures.

YOUNG, RAPP, BROOKS, MADAUSS AND NORTON, *Epilepsia* (1979),[2134] in a study involving eighty-four patients with head injuries, reported the beneficial use of PHT for post-traumatic seizure prophylaxis.

With PHT only five of eighty-four individuals had seizures within a year after severe head injury, and only one of these patients had more than one seizure.

The authors concluded that the greatly reduced incidence of post-traumatic seizures in these patients demonstrates the prophylactic effect of PHT.

SERVIT AND MUSIL, *Epilepsia* (1981),[2256] reports the results of a long-term study of prophylactic treatment of post-traumatic epilepsy performed in Czechoslovakia during the years 1963 through 1980. The prophylactically treated group of 144 patients with severe brain injuries was compared with a control group of twenty-four equally damaged cases without prophylactic treatment.

Prophylactic treatment consisted of PHT (160–240 mg/day) and phenobarbital (30–60 mg/day) administered for periods of two years in the majority of cases. The incidence of late post-traumatic epilepsy was 25% in the control, compared with 2.1% in the prophylactically treated group.

WHITE, PENRY, BRACKET, LISCO, ART, NEMORE, MANN, MUMAW AND WHITLEY, *NINCDS* (1982),[3068] in a double-blind study of forty-nine severely head-injured patients, compared the combination of PHT and phenobarbital to placebo in preventing post-traumatic seizures. Groups were matched for severity of injury. PHT levels were maintained at 10–20 μg/ml and phenobarbital levels at 20–30 μg/ml.

Patients treated with PHT and phenobarbital had a significantly lower incidence of post-traumatic epilepsy than the placebo group.

NORTH, PENHALL, HANIEH, FREWIN AND TAYLOR, *Journal of Neurosurgery* (1983),[2833] reported a double-blind study of PHT versus placebo as prophylaxis against post-craniotomy seizures in 281 patients. One hundred forty patients received PHT and 141, placebo. Patients were followed for one year. PHT significantly reduced the incidence of post-craniotomy seizures in comparison to placebo. For the entire group of PHT-treated patients, this reduction was greatest within the first three months, when the risk of seizures was greatest. In certain high-risk patients (following operations for aneurysm, head injury and meningioma) there was a significantly lower incidence of seizures at both one month and approximately one year.

Glycogen Storage Disease

JUBIZ AND RALLISON, *Archives of Internal Medicine* (1974),[1193] report on four patients with glycogen storage disease, two with debranching enzyme system deficiency, one with phosphorylase deficiency and one with glucose-6-phosphatase deficiency.

These patients were treated with PHT for more than two years and there was a good response. This was evidenced by a reduction in liver size and hepatic glycogen content. Hyperlacticacidemia improved.

Ophthalmology

ACCOMMODATIVE ESOTROPIA

GALIN, KWITKO AND RESTREPO, *Proceedings of the International Strabismological Association* (1969),[746] found PHT useful in the treatment of accommodative esotropia.

A study with thirty-five children was completed. Their ages ranged from two-and-a-half to fourteen years. Children less than six years of age were given 30 mg PHT twice daily, then increased to three times daily if after two days it was well tolerated. Standard orthoptic studies were performed before and after PHT.

Of twenty-five patients with abnormal near-point accommodation, twenty improved with a decrease of three diopters and ten of these had a concomitant decrease in esotropia. Because they were too young, the near point of accommodation was not obtained in ten patients.

Nine out of twenty-one patients responded to PHT in the combined accommodative groups (including thirteen accommodative and eight partial accommodative).

Accommodative convergence/accommodation (AC/A) ratios were most favorably influenced by PHT in those patients having high ratios. PHT had little effect on normals. Phospholine iodide, which had a greater effect on AC/A ratios than PHT, was not selective and had an effect on normals as well as abnormals.

GLAUCOMATOUS FIELD LOSS

BECKER AND PODOS, *Symposium on Ocular Therapy* (1973),[812] in earlier studies had found that PHT partly protected the optic nerve *in vitro* when subjected to anoxia, cyanide or ouabain. They decided to explore the possibility that PHT might reverse some of the effects of ischemia on the optic nerve in humans.

The authors instituted a study to examine the effects of PHT in glaucomatous field loss. This study involved fifty patients who were given 100 mg PHT t.i.d. for two to five months. The effects on visual fields were quantitatively recorded.

When treated with PHT, only one of the fifty patients had a worsening of visual fields, twenty-nine showed no worsening, and twenty patients showed improvement in visual fields. This salutary effect in visual fields occurred despite the fact that intraocular pressures, which previously had been deleterious, persisted.

In seven of the patients that showed improvement, PHT was discontinued and worsening of visual fields occurred. The authors found of considerable interest the fact that when PHT was reinstituted in five of these seven patients, improvement in visual fields again occurred.

The authors conclude that this pilot study suggests that where the blood supply is decreased, PHT may be able to protect optic nerve function.

Arthritis

BOBROVE, *Arthritis and Rheumatism* (1983),[2345] reported three patients with inflammatory arthritis, two with rheumatoid arthritis and one with psoriatic arthropathy, who developed seizure disorders necessitating treatment with PHT. Within six months of instituting PHT, all three patients had definite sustained improvement in their joint disease. There was a reduction in morning stiffness, intensity and frequency of clinical flare-ups, as well as reduction in the number of painful and swollen joints. Prior to PHT, all had been taking a nonsteroidal anti-inflammatory drug with only modest benefit.

GRINDULIS, NICHOL AND OLDHAM, *The Journal of Rheumatology* (1986),[2559] reported a thirty-two week study on the use of PHT in eighteen patients with active rheumatoid arthritis. The patients, thirteen females and five males, ages thirty-five to seventy-two, had arthritis of three-month to ten-year duration. Two of the patients withdrew from the study because of mild side effects, and one because of lack of effect.

The starting dose of PHT was 100 mg/day which was increased to 300 mg/day during the course of the study. Clinical and laboratory measurements were made at frequent intervals throughout the study, and during an eight-week period when PHT was withdrawn. Clinical assessments included articular index, clinical score and visual analog pain score. Laboratory measures included serum C-reactive protein, plasma viscosity and hemoglobin.

With PHT there was significant clinical improvement. Laboratory improvements attained significance occasionally. There was

no relapse of the clinical or laboratory measurements during the eight-week period when PHT was withdrawn.

MACFARLANE, CLARK AND PANAYI, *Annals of Rheumatic Diseases* (1986),[2749] reported on the use of PHT (100-300 mg daily) in eleven patients with active rheumatoid arthritis (mean duration 12.4 years). Two patients were withdrawn from the study because of other illness and surgery, and two, because of a mild rash.

Seven patients completed a twenty-week course of PHT treatment. All showed continuous clinical improvement. Laboratory improvement (erythrocyte sedimentation rate, C-reactive protein and IgM rheumatoid factor) was also observed at twelve and twenty weeks. When PHT was withdrawn for eight weeks, all patients showed clinical and laboratory deterioration.

The authors note that the usefulness of drugs such as gold, penicillamine, azathioprine and cyclophosphamide in rheumatoid arthritis is seriously limited by side effects. Based on their study, the authors suggest that PHT may be an alternative safe therapy for rheumatoid arthritis.

See also Refs. 2816 and 2979 for laboratory studies.

Rabies

HATTWICK, WEIS, STECHSCHULTE, BAER and GREGG, *Annals of Internal Medicine* (1972),[1138] give an extensive and detailed report on their successful treatment of a six-year-old boy with clinical rabies, with complete recovery. The authors comment that this is extremely rare, and possibly the first documented case of recovery from rabies in humans.

Many conventional and other measures

were used to offset this desperate condition. Special attention was given to the prevention of hypoxia, cardiac arrhythmias and seizure.* Approximately forty days after the infection occurred and while the boy had been in a comatose condition for several days, PHT was administered, 150 mg daily. Four days later recovery started and progressed steadily to complete recovery.‡

* The role, if any, that PHT played in this recovery is not known. However, since no remedy for clinical rabies is known, this case is of interest. It is well established that PHT is effective against seizures and cardiac arrhythmias, and it is also reported to have antianoxic effects. Of possible relevance is the evidence that PHT has antitoxic effects against a wide variety of substances. See p. 165–166.

‡ See also Pollen,[1424] reporting the use of PHT in the successful treatment in a case of cat-scratch encephalitis.

Tinnitus

HALMOS, MOLNAR AND KORMOS, *HNO-Praxis* (1982),[2567] compared the effects of PHT and carbamazepine (CBZ) in the treatment of 138 patients with tinnitus and sensorineural hearing loss. Seventy-two of the patients received PHT, 100 mg t.i.d., and seventy-five received CBZ, starting with 200 mg b.i.d. and gradually increasing to 400 mg t.i.d.

The severity of tinnitus diminished in thirty-eight of the seventy-two patients treated with PHT. Their hearing loss improved by 5 to 25 decibels. Classified according to etiology, thirty-two of fifty tinnitus patients with eighth-nerve lesions improved, as did two of three cases with otologic defects. Four of fifteen patients with presbycusis improved. There was no improvement in the four patients who developed tinnitus after head injury. No adverse effects were observed in the PHT group.

Improvement was observed in only twelve of the sixty-six carbamazepine-treated patients. It had to be stopped in nine patients because of side effects.

The authors state that they found PHT superior to CBZ for tinnitus. PHT had the additional advantage of being better tolerated. (See also Ref. 2500.)

SURGERY

Summary

Phenytoin has been reported useful prior to, during and after surgery. Among its uses are relief of apprehension and anxiety, prevention and treatment of cardiac arrhythmias, prevention of ischemic brain damage and relief of pain.

PHT, in therapeutic doses, does not depress respiration or cerebral function, thus optimizing pre-operative state and post-operative recovery. PHT's ability to relieve pain, without sedation, reduces the need for narcotics.

JAFFE, *Personal Communication* (1966),[747] found PHT useful in the pre-operative and post-operative periods and during the course of cataract surgery.

PHT replaced large doses of barbiturates previously used pre-operatively to combat apprehension. PHT replaced Demerol and opiates pre-operatively and was especially useful in cases where unpredictable or aggressive behavior was anticipated.

During the course of surgery where intravenous Demerol had previously been required to control violent outbursts in the operating room, intravenous PHT was successfully substituted.

MERCER AND OSBORNE, *Annals of Internal Medicine* (1967),[248] reported on the use of intravenous PHT in the treatment of 259 patients who developed arrhythmias during and after cardiac surgery. With PHT, complete control of the arrhythmias was achieved in 164 patients and partial response (at least 50% reduction of arrhythmias) was observed in sixty-five patients.

SEUFFERT, HELFANT, DANA AND URBACH, *Anesthesia and Analgesia* (1968),[409] report on the use of PHT, prophylactically and therapeutically, in the treatment of arrhythmias which develop and persist during surgery.

Twenty patients undergoing elective surgery, scheduled to receive cyclopropane anesthesia, were divided into two groups: eleven were pretreated with PHT (5 mg/kg) intravenously, and nine received an equivalent amount of lactated Ringer's solution with or without propylene glycol solvent for PHT, serving as controls.

Eight of the nine patients in the control group developed arrhythmias, whereas only three of the eleven patients pretreated with PHT developed arrhythmias during the entire anesthesia procedure. During "maintenance," eight of the nine in the control group developed arrhythmias, in contrast to only one of eleven pretreated with PHT. The authors pointed out that this difference was statistically significant.

PHT was also given to ten other patients under general anesthesia, who developed arrhythmias which did not respond to standard treatment. PHT promptly restored regular sinus rhythm in eight patients who developed ventricular arrhythmias. It was not effective in two of the patients who developed supraventricular arrhythmias. (See also Ref. 720).

GAUTAM, *British Heart Journal* (1969),[721] reported on the use of intravenous and oral PHT in treating a variety of cardiac arrhythmias following open heart surgery (thirteen Starr-Edwards prosthetic valve replacements and one atrial septal defect closure). The arrhythmias, which included multiple ventricular extrasystoles, recurrent ventricular tachycardia and nodal tachycardia, appeared within two to thirty hours after surgery. PHT was rapidly and highly effective in abolishing the arrhythmias in thirteen patients.

The author states that the rapidity of its action and the relative paucity of side effects make PHT an effective antiarrhythmic agent.

BARASCH, BARAS AND GALIN, *Personal Communication* (1970),[732] found that PHT replaced all pre-operative and post-operative medication in cataract surgery other than the local anesthetic. The authors previously had used barbiturates, Demerol, Compazine, codeine and aspirin.

Because PHT does not impair normal function, its use instead of narcotics and sedatives permitted the prompt ambulation of patients. For this reason the use of PHT enabled the discharge of patients within twenty-four hours, in a series of 100 consecutive uncomplicated cases of cataract surgery.

The authors state that since this study, they now use PHT routinely in cataract surgery.

CHAMBERLAIN, *Personal Communication* (1970),[744] reported on the therapeutic value of PHT in a series of 200 surgical cases.

The ages of the patients varied from six months to ninety years.

Dosage of PHT: 25 mg to 600 mg depending on age of patient and severity of symptoms and surgical procedure used.

PHT was successfully employed as follows:

1. As pre-operative medication for anxiety.
2. As post-operative medication for anxiety and pain.
3. In the agitated, depressed and alcoholic surgical patient.
4. In long-term treatment of both the operable and inoperable patient with malignant disease.

Certain trends presented themselves with the use of PHT:

(a) In children, PHT (25 mg q.i.d. to 100 mg t.i.d.) reduced or eliminated the use of pre- and post-operative narcotics.
(b) In adults, 200 mg of PHT prior to surgery reduced the need for pre-operative narcotics.

(c) In adults, post-operative use of PHT (500–600 mg daily) relieved pain, making it possible to do away with practically all post-operative narcotics. PHT also decreased anxiety and promoted a general feeling of well-being in most cases.

(d) Elderly agitated and difficult patients became much calmer with PHT.

(e) In the inoperable malignant cases, PHT in doses up to 600 mg daily relieved pain, making it possible to greatly cut down on the amount of narcotics used. PHT definitely improved the mental outlook of these forlorn patients.

(f) In post-operative malignant cases undergoing radiation and other forms of treatment, the use of PHT, 400–600 mg daily, relieved pain and allowed for a marked decrease or elimination of the need for narcotics.

The author notes that, in general, there was marked improvement of mental outlook in patients receiving PHT.

WINTER, *International Surgery* (1972),[1692] presents a detailed study on surgery in patients with asthma and emphysema.

In this study the author says that severe respiratory problems require careful pre-operative and post-operative medical treatment. He states that in patients with severe respiratory problems he does not use narcotics and that, in his opinion, they should never be used in such cases. He further says that barbiturates and tranquilizers should only be used in small doses.

The author states that he has found PHT of considerable value in severe respiratory problems, both pre-operatively and post-operatively. He notes that PHT appears to have special value in patients with bronchospastic problems. (See also Refs. 341, 401, 1535, and Anti-anoxic Effects of PHT, p. 131.)

LANDOLT, *Acta Endocrinologica* (1974),[1256] reported a patient who developed the syndrome of inappropriate ADH secretion following surgery for craniopharyngioma.

Intravenous PHT, during two such episodes, promptly increased urine output. Serum sodium values returned to normal and the patient became more alert. (See Inappropriate ADH Syndrome, p. 68).

ALDRETE AND FRANATOVIC, *Archives of Surgery* (1980),[1717] studied the effects of PHT on changes of arterial blood pressure and heart rate occurring during anesthesia and in the immediate post-operative period.

In a controlled study, ninety hypertensive patients were separated into three groups. One group was untreated. One group received 100 mg of PHT, and another group received 200 mg, the evening before and the morning of surgery. Both groups receiving PHT had better hemodynamic stability than the non-treated group. The group receiving 200 mg had statistically significant improvement.

ALDRETE, ROMO-SALAS, MAZZIA AND TAN, *Critical Care Medicine* (1981),[2142] studied the effect of intravenous PHT in ten patients who suffered cardiac arrest during or after anesthesia.

PHT was given after spontaneous heartbeat and systolic blood pressure greater than 100 mm Hg had been restored and the diagnosis of neurological deficit had been established on the basis of unconsciousness, dilated and areflexic pupils and rigid and/or decerebrate posture.

With PHT (7 mg/kg) nine of the ten patients recovered nearly complete neurological function. The other patient had partial recovery but succumbed to other complications.

GARSON AND GILLETTE, *PACE* (1981),[2528] reported the use of oral and intravenous PHT for the treatment of chronic ventricular dysrhythmias in fifty-one young patients, thirty-five of whom had previously undergone corrective surgery for cardiac malformations including ventricular septal defect, tetralogy of Fallot, and valvular insufficiency.

Overall, PHT was the most effective drug, controlling the arrhythmias in thirty-nine of the fifty-one patients.

The authors conclude that PHT is the drug of choice for children with ventricular dysrhythmias, especially those with abnormal hemodynamics. (See also Ref. 1847.)

ROCCHINI, CHUN AND DICK, *American Journal of Cardiology* (1981),[2251] reported the elimination of ventricular tachycardia by PHT in four children who had undergone repair of the tetralogy of Fallot.

The authors state that PHT appears to be the antiarrhythmic agent of choice after repair of the tetralogy of Fallot.

KAVEY, BLACKMAN AND SONDHEIMER, *American Heart Journal* (1982),[2654] reported the effects of oral PHT in nineteen patients, seen consecutively, who developed ventricular premature complexes (VPCs) late after surgery for congenital heart disease. Arrhythmias included ventricular tachycardia, couplets and frequent multiform or uniform VPCs, documented by twenty-four hour ambulatory ECG. Sixteen had undergone previous repair of the tetralogy of Fallot and three had had aortic valve surgery. Nine of these children had been unresponsive to previous treatment.

PHT decreased ventricular dysrhythmias in all nineteen patients. The arrhythmias were completely suppressed in fifteen, and in four they were reduced to uniform VPCs.

The authors state that the high rate of success in treating these patients, who are at particular risk for sudden death, and the relative lack of side effects suggests that PHT is the drug of choice for this patient group.

MASSEI, DESILVA, GROSSO, ROBBIATI, INFUSO, RAVAGNATI AND ALTAMURA, *Neurosurgical Science* (1983), [2768] reported on the use of PHT for cerebral metabolic protection during carotid thromboendoarterectomy (TEA).

PHT was chosen because of its known therapeutic properties in reducing cerebral metabolic oxygen consumption, preserving energy compounds, increasing cerebral blood flow, and in regulating intra- and extracellular cerebral ion content.

Twelve patients undergoing TEA were given intravenous PHT (15–17 mg/kg), fifteen minutes before clamping. EEG and PHT blood levels were monitored during and after surgery at fixed intervals over a twenty-four-hour period.

The authors stated that patients awakened promptly and did not require intensive care. This was in contrast to their experience with other methods of cerebral protection, including barbiturates. Also, with PHT, no postoperative neurological complications were observed.

PEREZ-RUVALCABA, QUINTERO-PEREZ, CAMPA-URIBE, CHAPA-ALVAREZ, RODRIGUEZ-NORIEGA, *European Journal of Clinical Investigation* (1984),[2858] reviewed the multiple uses of PHT in their general hospital. Their review included the use of 100 mg of PHT, as sole preoperative medication the evening before surgery, in fifty patients. Treatment with PHT resulted in excellent control of apprehension and sleep disturbances usually encountered preoperatively.

The authors state that these beneficial effects of PHT were achieved without the undesirable sedative effects experienced with many commonly used sedatives and/or tranquilizers.

PHENYTOIN AS A PREVENTIVE

PHT has been found useful for over fifty symptoms and disorders, and this suggests a broad potential for preventive medicine. There are numerous examples in the clinical and basic mechanisms literature of PHT's effectiveness as a preventive.[1]

PHT's established ability to calm the overbusy brain and modify or eliminate excessive emotions of fear and anger, and to improve duration and quality of sleep are consistent with the general principle of good health.

PHT's therapeutic effect on blood pressure, its anti-ischemic effects, its ability to stabilize bioelectrical activity, and its ability to increase HDL levels, are indications of protection against cardiac disorders and stroke.

By its regulatory effect on the HPA axis, PHT decreases excessive levels of epinephrine, norepinephrine and cortisol. Since these chemicals are closely associated with stress, this action of PHT could be protective against a wide variety of stress-related disorders.

PHT is not habit-forming. Its long-term safety has withstood the test of millions of people taking it daily for decades. PHT's use in preventive medicine, particularly when people are susceptible to serious disorders, deserves consideration.

[1] *Clinical:* Refs. 91, 92, 105, 161, 290, 338, 341, 382, 383, 401, 409, 429, 571, 697, 701, 720, 819, 923, 943, 944, 998, 999, 1033, 1121, 1140, 1253, 1264, 1289, 1328, 1329, 1349, 1359, 1388, 1415, 1510, 1535, 1565, 1583, 1594, 1666, 1717, 1724, 1738, 1817, 1847, 1879, 1893, 1926, 1961, 2002, 2114, 2122, 2134, 2141, 2142, 2149, 2150, 2182, 2223, 2235, 2256, 2306, 2318, 2319, 2340, 2342, 2406, 2428, 2431, 2465, 2528, 2532, 2542, 2599, 2617, 2649, 2652, 2709, 2734, 2741, 2768, 2813, 2814, 2827, 2833, 2868, 2882, 2897, 2907, 3009, 3054, 3060, 3068.

[2] *Basic mechanisms:* Refs. 37, 56, 99, 118, 155, 163, 164, 171, 213, 233, 263, 392, 419, 482, 483, 520, 529, 685, 717, 739, 790, 804, 914, 921, 1015, 1027, 1058, 1071, 1092, 1122, 1160, 1208, 1267, 1279, 1354, 1374, 1419, 1485, 1507, 1509, 1525, 1529, 1591, 1668, 1718, 1781, 1791, 1806, 1822, 1828, 1864, 1875, 1878, 1932, 1958, 1969, 2004, 2013, 2024, 2062, 2088, 2144, 2157, 2177, 2185, 2192, 2193, 2195, 2200, 2213, 2229, 2263, 2269, 2272, 2279, 2280, 2281, 2291, 2311, 2349, 2420, 2445, 2502, 2516, 2525, 2571, 2583, 2609, 2623, 2627, 2628, 2682, 2698, 2701, 2707, 2708, 2732, 2739, 2740, 2741, 2742, 2743, 2757, 2820, 2844, 2854, 2855, 2900, 2977, 3001, 3005, 3017, 3039, 3063.

SAFETY AND TOXICOLOGY

Background and Perspective

Since its introduction, in 1938, millions of people have taken phenytoin on a daily basis for long periods of time. The world use of PHT is estimated to have been the equivalent of one hundred fifty to two hundred million patient-years. This translates into an estimated one-and-a-half to two trillion 100 mg doses. Thus PHT has been subjected to the important tests of time, volume of use, number of individuals who have used it, and continuous use over long periods.

With this in perspective, reports of serious side effects associated with PHT have been extremely rare. As a point of reference, only six deaths associated with PHT alone have been reported to the FDA's Adverse Drug Experience Monitoring Program in the last eighteen years.

Because it has been in use for such a long time, the literature of PHT's safety and toxicology is extensive. No single reviewer can presume to have all of this information. For this reason, we refer the reader to other reviews.*

* Examples: Refs. 1075, 1586, 1700, 1836, 1884, 1891, 1923, 1940, 2043, 2189, 2244, 2249, 2288, 2423, 2427, 2463, 2467, 2607, 2655, 2845, 2874, 2890, 2903, 2934, 3041, 3048, as well as the Physicians' Desk Reference.

Clinical

PHT's first use was in epilepsy and at that time it was classified as an anticonvulsant. This classification is narrow and misleading. The world medical literature describes PHT more broadly as a bioelectrical stabilizer or normalizer.

Since 1938, PHT has been reported in the world literature to be therapeutic for a wide range of symptoms and disorders. Among them are uncontrolled thinking, occupied with negative feelings of anger and fear and related emotions; bad mood; depression; sleep disturbances; poor concentration; muscle disorders; migraine, trigeminal neuralgia, and other pain; asthma; and cardiac disorders.[1]

The topical use of PHT is a rapidly expanding field. Used topically, in a variety of conditions including skin ulcers and burns, PHT is effective against pain and promotes healing.

PHT has unusual properties. It calms without sedation. It effects an improvement in energy without being an artificial stimulant. And it is not habit-forming.[2]

The basic mechanisms findings explain how PHT can have such broad clinical usefulness.

[1] See this Bibliography.
[2] This is not to be confused with the well-known fact that epileptics should *not* be suddenly withdrawn from PHT.

Basic Mechanisms of Action

In the basic mechanism literature PHT has been referred to as a stabilizer of bioelectrical activity or as a membrane stabilizer.

PHT has been shown to have a stabilizing effect on bioelectrical activity in tissues, groups of cells, and in single cells. This ability to regulate bioelectrical activity has been demonstrated in brain, spinal cord, ganglia, peripheral nerve, cardiac, skeletal and smooth muscle.

PHT reduces or eliminates excessive potentiation and repetitive afterdischarge. In therapeutic amounts, it has little or no effect on normal cell function. These properties could account for many of PHT's therapeutic applications.

Dosage

The adult dosage of PHT used in non-epileptic disorders tends to be lower (100–300 mg/day) than that used in epilepsy (300–600 mg/day). Dosage depends on the type and severity of the condition. Acute conditions may temporarily require higher doses.

The usual therapeutic blood level range in epilepsy is 10–20 μg/ml. In other disorders, therapeutic effects are frequently achieved at lower blood levels. Clinical observation is usually the best guide to dosage.

The liver is the chief site of PHT metabolism. Patients with disease-impaired liver function, or patients who metabolize the drug slowly, may require lower doses of PHT. Patients who have lower serum protein binding, such as those with kidney disease, may also require lower doses because the free fraction of PHT in the blood can be higher.

It has been recommended that intravenous PHT be administered slowly—at a rate of 50 mg/min. or less.

Abrupt discontinuance of other medication, on which the patient may have become dependent, is usually not advisable when PHT therapy is instituted.

Possible Interactions

PHT is compatible with most drugs and drug combinations. Interactions with other drugs have been reported. They vary from individual to individual and are difficult to generalize. In some cases, adjustment of the dosage of PHT, the other drug, or both may be necessary. Such adjustments may be guided by clinical observations or, where necessary, by monitoring blood levels.

For information on drugs for which interactions have been reported, we refer the reader to the Physicians' Desk Reference, as well as Refs. 2338, 2422, 2680, 2681, 2824, 2859, 2861, 2862, 2877.

Safety

LIVINGSTON AND WHITEHOUSE, *Modern Treatment*,[227] stated that in their experience with PHT in many thousands of epileptic patients, some of whom have taken it continuously for more than twenty years, "We have not encountered a single instance of a serious untoward reaction to phenytoin which was not reversible on withdrawal of the drug."

GAUTAM, *British Heart Journal*,[721] reporting on the use of intravenous PHT in the treatment of cardiac arrhythmias following open heart surgery, states, "Rapidity of action and the paucity of side effects make the drug an effective antiarrhythmic agent."

CHUNG, *Modern Treatment*,[905] stated "Toxic manifestations of PHT are usually rare and not serious . . . PHT is probably the safest and most effective drug in the treatment of all types of digitalis-induced tachyarrhythmias." (See also Ref. 923.)

BHATT, VIJAYAN, AND DREYFUS, *California Medicine*,[825] in a review of clinical and laboratory aspects of myotonia, state, "Of the various drugs used, PHT appears to be the most effective, the safest and best tolerated."

FISHER AND DIMINO, *British Journal of Addiction*,[1033] discussing their clinical experience with PHT in the treatment of drug and alcohol withdrawal, state, "Because PHT is nonaddictive, is not a sedative, and has a wide range of safety, it is particularly well-suited for use in addicted persons."

SCHMIDT, *Adverse Effects of Antiepileptic Drugs*,[2933] in an extensive review of forty-four years of world experience with PHT, reports that side effects of PHT are usually mild and transient, and serious adverse effects are very rare.

DELGADO-ESCUETA, WASTERLAIN, TREIMAN AND PORTER, *Advances in Neurology*,[2447] report the special usefulness of PHT in the treatment of head trauma and other neurological disorders in which "alteration of the patient's state of consciousness is contraindicated."

TOMAN, *The Pharmacological Basis of Therapeutics*,[359] states, "Doses totaling many grams have occasionally been ingested by accident or taken with suicidal intent . . . deaths have been rare. Fortunately, PHT is a very poor drug with which to commit suicide." (See also Refs. 134, 216, 283, 357, 537, 565, 1870, 2118, 2989.)

Toxicology

Skin Rash/Hypersensitivity: Skin rash, either local or generalized, can occur with PHT. The incidence is estimated to be in the range of 2 to 4%. These reactions, some of which may be dose related, most frequently appear within the first few weeks of therapy, occasionally later. The most common form is the morbilliform (measlelike) rash. If such a rash appears, the medicine should be stopped. The rash usually disappears in a few days. After disappearance of the rash, reintroduction of the medicine may be tried, but only with careful observation and starting with tiny doses.

Serious allergic reactions, extremely rare, are usually symptomatized by severe rash and/or fever. PHT should be stopped promptly and not reintroduced. Failure to do so could lead to serious hypersensitivity reactions such as Stevens-Johnson syndrome, erythema multiforme, hepatitis and blood dyscrasias.

Nervous System: Side effects of PHT

therapy referable to the central nervous system are generally dose related and usually disappear on reduction of dosage. These include nystagmus, ataxia, slurred speech and confusion, and, very rarely, dyskinesias. (See Refs. 359, 666, 1075, 1178, 1586, 1700, 2288, 2423, 2463, 2467, 2845, 2890, 2935, 3041, 3048.)

There are reports that at substantial or excessive doses of PHT there may be impairment of some cognitive functions. (See Refs. 2902, 3013, 3025, 3026.) However, extensive evidence has demonstrated that, in therapeutic doses, PHT has a beneficial effect on cognitive function including concentration, memory, and ability to perform in school. (See Refs. 38, 527, 538, 556, 557, 585, 707, 713, 863, 938, 1139, 1140, 1564, 1565, 1808, 2311.)

There have been occasional reports of peripheral neuropathy related to long-term, high-dose use of PHT. (See Refs. 232, 470, 829, 897, 933, 950, 2423, 2534, 2890, 2934, 2935, 3006.)

Connective Tissue: Gingival hyperplasia has been reported during PHT treatment of epileptics. The hyperplasia usually occurs in the presence of gingivitis and can be decreased or eliminated with good oral hygiene. (See Refs. 307, 547, 607, 612, 627, 629, 634, 1074, 1115, 1294, 2463, 2581, 2845, 2890, 2934, 2935.)

The effect of PHT on gum tissue seems to be a stimulation of healing processes. In 1958, SHAPIRO[339] reported accelerated gingival wound healing in non-epileptics treated with PHT. Since then, systemic and topical PHT have been found effective in the treatment of periodontal disease, and in the healing of chronic ulcers and burns. (See Clinical—Healing section, p. 56.)

Skeletal: Lowered levels of vitamin D and calcium and, in rare cases, osteomalacia have been reported in some epileptic patients on PHT. (See Refs. 851, 989, 1296, 1318, 1321, 2423, 2463, 2845, 2890, 2934.) There is laboratory evidence that PHT promotes bone healing and reduces bone resorption. (See Refs. 343, 1104, 1131, 1840, 1878, 2088, 2281, 2571, 2574, 2613, 2623, 2708, 2854, 2855, 2980.)

Hematologic: Low serum folate and macrocytosis, usually not clinically significant, have been reported in patients taking PHT. In rare cases megaloblastic anemia has occurred. It is responsive to folate replacement and usually does not require discontinuance of PHT. (See Refs. 349, 1460, 2043, 2874, 2890, 2903.)

Since 1938, there have been a few reports of pancytopenia, hemolytic anemia, thrombocytopenia and granulocytopenia. These seem to have been related to hypersensitivity reactions. (See Refs. 203, 253, 295, 1460, 2427, 2874, 2903, 2935, 3049.)

Lymphadenopathy, including benign lymphnode hyperplasia and pseudolymphoma have been reported in patients taking PHT. These appear to be related to a hypersensitivity reaction and regress when PHT is discontinued. (See Refs. 217, 294, 322, 615, 620, 632, 736, 874, 1884, 2423, 2467, 2874, 2903, 2935.)

Although lymphoma and Hodgkin's disease, on rare occasions, have been reported in patients taking PHT, a causal link is not established. In an extensive survey, CLEMMESEN[1773] states that he did not find a higher incidence of Hodgkin's disease in PHT-treated patients as compared with the general population.

Lowered serum IgA levels have been reported in some patients taking PHT. (See Refs. 1102, 1572, 1940, 2305, 2642, 2812, 2845, 3002.)

Gastrointestinal: Feelings of nausea and stomach discomfort may occasionally occur when PHT is first taken. They usually disappear by themselves, but taking PHT with food may be useful.

There have been rare reports of constipation, but the general experience has been that patients taking PHT have improvement in bowel habits.

Hepatic: Although abnormal liver function tests, such as gamma glutamyltransferase levels, have been reported, these are generally not clinically significant. Hepatotoxicity is rare and usually due to a hypersensitivity reaction. (See Refs. 1884, 2551, 2588, 2607, 2974.)

Endocrinology: In some diabetic patients receiving PHT, moderate increases in blood glucose levels have been reported, but adjustment of the diabetic therapy has not been necessary in most cases.

With toxic levels of PHT, there have been reports of temporary hyperglycemic effects in non-diabetic patients. In normals and non-diabetic patients taking therapeutic doses of PHT, glucose tolerance is normal. (See Refs. 924, 1327, 1330, 1762, 1809, 2646.)

PHT has been reported to increase steroid metabolism in patients on steroid therapy. Adjustment of the steroid dose may be required. (See Refs. 377, 896, 1128, 1627, 1679, 2382, 2485, 2633.) Because PHT may increase the metabolism of androgens and estrogens, oral contraceptive dose may need adjustment. Hypertrichosis has been reported in epileptic patients taking PHT.

Pregnancy: Although there have been reports that children of epileptic women taking PHT have a higher incidence of birth defects than children of normal mothers, the evidence that PHT is the cause of these defects is not clear. The reported defects are frequently associated with developmental abnormalities from other causes. Many variables including use of other drugs, and the reported increase of birth defects in children born to epileptic mothers who took no medication, make the data difficult to interpret. (See Refs. 606, 737, 1298, 1401, 1484, 1575, 1586, 1587, 1836, 1891, 2189, 2432, 2621, 2655, 2803, 2934, 2935, 2987, 2988.) Coagulation defects, which have been reported in neonates born to epileptic mothers taking PHT, can usually be prevented by adequate diet and supplemental vitamin K. (See Refs. 2903, 2935.)

Basic Mechanisms of Action of Phenytoin

Basic Mechanisms of Action
of Phenytoin

Summary

The evidence which has accumulated on phenytoin's basic mechanisms of action, from the earliest studies to the present, is extensive and consistent.

PHT has been shown to have a modulatory effect on bioelectrical activity in single cells, groups of cells and physiological systems. This ability to regulate and/or to correct abnormal membrane function has been demonstrated in brain, spinal cord, autonomic ganglia, peripheral nerve, skeletal muscle, cardiac muscle and conduction systems, and intestinal and vascular smooth muscle.

In the nerve and muscle cell, PHT reduces or eliminates excessive potentiation and hyperexcitability, as in post-tetanic potentiation and afterdischarge. If the cell is depolarized and firing rapidly, PHT normalizes it, reducing the firing. The more rapid the firing, the greater the effect. PHT has little or no effect on normal bioelectrical function at therapeutic levels. In the nerve cell, neither the resting potential nor single impulse transmission is altered.[1]

The basis for PHT's selective effects in neurons and muscle cells is found in its action on the cell membrane—its ability to regulate transmembrane ionic fluxes and also intracellular distribution of sodium, potassium, and calcium.[2] Recent work in neurons suggests that PHT binds to active sodium channels and delays their return from the inactivated, unusable state. This results in a decrease of sodium influx and correlates with PHT's frequency-dependent effects on the sodium-dependent action potential. Similar effects on calcium flux have also been reported. At the synapse PHT influences both calcium-dependent neurotransmitter release and postsynaptic response. Acetylcholine, norepinephrine, dopamine, GABA, and serotonin release, uptake and/or binding may all be regulated, dependent on the state of the neuron or circuit.[3]

The functions of other cell types such as glia, endocrine cells and fibroblasts are also modulated by PHT. Examples of PHT's actions include stimulation of glial cell potassium uptake;[2] modulation of hypothalamic-pituitary adrenal function, including ACTH release and cortisol metabolism;[4] and modulation of thyroid stimulating hormone, thyroxine, insulin, vasopressin, oxytocin, calcitonin and other hormone release and metabolism.[5] PHT stimulates hepatic enzyme metabolizing systems (cytochrome P-450);[6] increases high-density lipoprotein levels;[7] and stimulates healing processes (formation of granulation tissue and neovascularity).[8]

PHT has protective effects on cells. It preserves energy compounds and decreases "downhill movement" of ions, characteristic of energy depletion in neurons, whether such depletion is induced by physiological hyperactivity or chemical, electrical, or anoxic/ischemic injury.[9]

PHT has been reported to diminish or counteract, in animals or in man, the toxic effects of over thirty therapeutic and poisonous substances, as diverse as steroids, cyanide, DDT, digitalis, methaqualone, morphine, ouabain, reserpine and strychnine, and of radiation.[10]

The broad range of clinical use of PHT is best understood in the light of its ability to maintain normal bioelectrical activity. A rational basis for the clinical use of PHT takes into account its basic mechanisms of action, which indicate that it may be useful wherever stabilization or modulation of bioelectrical activity can have a therapeutic effect.

---

[1] See Stabilization of Bioelectrical Activity, p. 89–97 and Sodium, Potassium and Calcium Regulation, p. 99–109.

[2] See Sodium, Potassium and Calcium Regulation, p. 99–109.

[3] See Neurotransmitter Regulatory Effects of PHT, p. 110–120.

[4] See Pituitary-Adrenal Hormones, p. 125–126.

[5] See Pituitary-Thyroid Function and Other Hormones, p. 126–130.

[6] Enzyme regulation: see Refs. 296, 442, 450, 451, 771, 772, 896, 915, 998, 1003, 1004, 1128, 1130, 1208, 1251, 1573, 1740, 2128, 2129, 2334, 2335, 2336, 2564, 2587, 2732, 2735, 2739, 2740, 2742, 2873, 2891.

[7] See Lipid Metabolism—HDL, p. 123–125.

[8] See Healing, p. 158–162.

[9] See Anti-Anoxic Effects of PHT, p. 131–137.

[10] See Anti-Toxic Effects of PHT, p. 165–166.

STABILIZATION
OF BIOELECTRICAL ACTIVITY

From the earliest studies to the latest, the evidence is consistent that phenytoin (PHT) selectively corrects hyperexcitability as in post-tetanic potentiation and post-tetanic afterdischarge. This normalization of hyperexcitability is achieved without interfering with initial single impulses, and without impairment of normal transmission of nerve impulses. PHT's effects are in direct proportion to the frequency of axonal firing or synaptic transmission: the more the system fires, the greater PHT's effects. Mechanisms by which this selective action may be achieved, including effects on the sodium and calcium channel and glial cell ion homeostasis, are discussed in Sodium, Potassium and Calcium Regulation. See also Neurotransmitter Regulatory Effects of PHT, Muscle, and Cardiovascular Basic Mechanisms sections.

The following studies are in chronological order.

PUTNAM AND MERRITT, *Science* (1937),[11] *Archives of Neurology and Psychiatry* (1938),[250] and *JAMA* (1938),[557] were the first to discover that PHT was a therapeutically effective substance when they demonstrated that it counteracted electrically-induced hyperexcitability and convulsions in the cat. Others had previously tested PHT and, finding that it was not a sedative, had not investigated its properties further.

The authors demonstrated that PHT was much more effective in controlling convulsions than the bromides and phenobarbital. They also observed that PHT, unlike these other substances, did not sedate.

The authors applied their laboratory findings to clinical use and with PHT treated a group of 118 patients with chronic grand mal attacks who had not responded to treatment with bromides and phenobarbital. The results were dramatic. Fifty-eight percent of these intractable cases became free of attacks and twenty-seven percent showed marked improvement, without sedation. Although Putnam and Merritt were focusing on epilepsy at the time, they suggested that PHT might be useful for a broad range of dysrhythmias.

TOMAN, *Electroencephalography and Clinical Neurophysiology* (1949),[458] studied the effect of PHT on isolated frog sciatic nerve. The frog sciatic nerve was electrically stimulated and the action potential, with and without PHT, was recorded.

PHT was found to have little effect upon the membrane threshold for single shocks. However, PHT increased membrane stability when repetitive shocks were used. The author noted that these findings might explain PHT's effectiveness in preventing abnormal spread of electrical discharge, without affecting normal function.

The author stressed the fact that these stabilizing effects were achieved with low concentrations of PHT, without interfering with normal function. He suggested that the protective properties of PHT could have broad applicability when neurons are more sensitive than normal, such as the conditions brought on by injury or ischemia.

KOREY, *Proceedings of the Society of Experimental Biology and Medicine* (1951),[472] studied the effect of PHT on the giant axon of squid. The nerve and its ganglion were dissected and kept in a solution of artificial sea water to maintain ionic equilibrium. The nerve was then exposed to other solutions and electrical recordings were made.

When PHT was added to the "normal" artificial sea water, no appreciable effect on the electrical activity of the giant axon was observed. When the sea water was changed by reducing calcium and magnesium, but without PHT, a hyperexcitable state of spontaneous firing occurred. When the sea water was brought back to normal by adding calcium and magnesium, it took ten to fifteen minutes to reverse the spontaneous firing. However, when PHT was added to the solution from which calcium and magnesium had been withdrawn, it took only two or three minutes to correct the excessive firing.

The author concludes that PHT does not affect normal nerve function. However, in an abnormal condition of hyperexcitability, induced by withdrawal of calcium and magnesium, PHT corrects hyperexcitability.

ESPLIN, *Journal of Pharmacology and Experimental Therapeutics* (1957),[90] studied the effect of PHT on post-tetanic potentiation in cat spinal cord, stellate ganglion and vagus nerve C fibers.

The author found that PHT reduced or abolished post-tetanic potentiation but only slightly affected single impulses in spinal cord and stellate ganglion.

The author states that post-tetanic potentiation may be a significant factor in all functions of the nervous system characterized by repetitive activity.

MORRELL, BRADLEY AND PTASHNE, *Neurology* (1958),[257] examined the effects of PHT on the peripheral nerve in rabbit. Hyperexcitability was induced by both chemical and electrical methods.

The authors found that PHT (10–25 mg/kg) raised the resistance of the peripheral nerve to being made hyperexcitable by repetitive electrical stimulation. In a separate experiment they showed that when the nerve was made hyperexcitable by the removal of calcium, PHT corrected this hyperexcitability.

MORRELL, BRADLEY AND PTASHNE, *Neurology* (1959),[258] found that PHT limited the spread of seizure activity from an epileptogenic focus induced in rabbit visual cortex.

STILLE, *Nervenarzt* (1960),[352] in a study of the basis for the beneficial effect of PHT on pain, found that PHT (20 mg/kg) reduced the cortical response to single or low-frequency electrical stimulation of the reticular formation in rabbits. The author notes that PHT differs from the barbiturates and chlorpromazine in that it does not interfere with the arousal reaction produced by electrical stimulation of the mesencephalic reticular formation, or by sensory stimulation.

ASTON AND DOMINO, *Psychopharmacologia* (1961),[6] found, in the rhesus monkey, that the effective elevation of motor cortical thresholds could be accomplished by PHT without markedly altering the reactivity of the reticular core to electrical stimulation and without significant anesthetic effect.

NAKAMURA AND KUREBE, *Japanese Journal of Pharmacology* (1962),[264] using concentric bipolar stimulating and recording electrodes, demonstrated, in cat, that PHT (5–20 mg/kg) elevated hippocampal seizure threshold and suppressed propagation, with no effect on afterdischarge pattern. At doses sufficient to prevent hippocampal seizure PHT did not interfere with reticular arousal thresholds.

TUTTLE AND PRESTON, *Journal of Pharmacology and Experimental Therapeutics* (1963),[365] studied the influence of PHT (10–60 mg/kg) on neural pathways in the cat. They state that, confirming previous studies, PHT was found to have no apparent effect on single-impulse transmission or monosynaptic reflex amplitude, whether initiated by dorsal root stimulation or by peripheral nerve stimulation. However, when post-tetanic potentiation was produced by repetitive electrical stimulation, PHT counteracted the abnormal state.

PARISI AND RAINES, *Federation Proceedings* (1963),[1400] studied the effect of PHT on the soleus nerve of the cat, and on neuromuscular transmission via this nerve.

In this study the effect that PHT had on neuromuscular transmission was gauged by its effect on twitch response to repeated nerve volleys and also on the twitch response to single impulses. Repeated nerve volleys caused post-tetanic repetitive discharge of the motor nerve terminals which in turn caused a contractile post-tetanic potentiation in the muscle. Intravenous PHT (20 mg/kg) abolished this abnormal muscle post-tetanic potentiation. When a normal muscle was given a single volley, PHT did not affect the normal twitch.

The authors placed emphasis on this selective action of PHT which enables it to counteract post-tetanic repetitive activity without interfering with normal transmission or contraction.

TOMAN, *The Pharmacological Basis of Therapeutics* (1965),[359] noted that PHT modifies the pattern of maximal tonic-clonic electroshock seizures elicited by supramaximal current. The characteristic tonic phase, representing maximal interneuronal facilitation in the brain, can be abolished completely by PHT.

RAINES AND STANDAERT, *Journal of Pharmacology and Experimental Therapeutics* (1966),[289] found that intravenous PHT (10–20 mg/kg) abolished repetitive afterdischarges originating in the nerve terminals of soleus motor axons of the cat. The suppression of these afterdischarges markedly reduced post-tetanic potentiation of the soleus muscle.

BRUMLIK AND MORETTI, *Neurology* (1966),[469] found that PHT did not affect normal conduction velocities in human median and ulnar nerve.

RAINES AND STANDAERT, *Journal of Pharmacology and Experimental Therapeutics* (1967),[467] showed that PHT abolishes post-tetanic potentiation originating in the central terminals of dorsal root fibers of spinal cats.

ROSENBERG AND BARTELS, *Journal of Pharmacology and Experimental Therapeutics* (1967),[311] studying the effects of PHT on the spontaneous electrical activity of squid giant axon, found that at concentrations of PHT which do not affect the action potential response to stimulation, spontaneous activity is decreased. Resting potential was unaltered.

JULIEN AND HALPERN, *Journal of Pharmacology and Experimental Therapeutics* (1970),[1197] studied the effect of PHT on the electrical responsiveness of isolated rabbit vagus nerve after repetitive electrical stimulation. PHT did not affect the compound action potential produced by a single electrical stimulation. Conduction velocity of both the myelinated and nonmyelinated fibers was not affected by PHT. The authors noted that the effects of PHT were in contrast to those of barbiturates which depress axonal conduction. In addition, PHT markedly shortened the duration of post-tetanic hypoexcitability of C fibers. PHT enhanced this recovery without depressing conduction velocity or excitability thresholds.

RIEHL AND MCINTYRE, *Electroencephalography and Clinical Neurophysiology* (1970),[1467] studied the effect of intravenous PHT on the electroencephalogram analyzed quantitatively by frequency/voltage ratio.

In seven previously untreated epileptic patients with unilateral EEG abnormalities, PHT (250 mg) produced a decrease in abnormal EEG activity. The effect was observed within ten to fifteen minutes in the pathologically affected hemisphere. In the normal unaffected hemisphere of these same patients, and in three control normal subjects, no effect of PHT was observed. (See also Ref. 461.)

BAKER, OKAMOTO AND RIKER, *Pharmacologist* (1971),[789] found that, in a cat soleus nerve-muscle preparation, pretreatment with PHT counteracted abnormal excitability produced by exogenous acetylcholine. The authors note that PHT selectively suppresses the post-tetanic potentiation of motor nerve terminals without impairing single-impulse transmission.

RUTLEDGE, SOHN AND SARDINAS, *Pharmacologist* (1971),[1494] studied the effect of PHT on the hyperexcitability of a cat soleus nerve-muscle preparation. They found that PHT (20–40 mg/kg) counteracted succinylcholine-induced muscle fasciculation and twitch potentiation, but did not impair normal neuromuscular transmission.

JULIEN AND HALPERN, *Epilepsia* (1972),[1199] studied the effect of PHT on cerebellar Purkinje cell discharge rates and cerebral cortical epileptiform activity in cats with penicillin-induced foci in sensorimotor cortex.

In control experiments, using extracellular microelectrode recordings, Purkinje cell activity revealed characteristic low-frequency discharge rates during periods of cortical quiescence and discharge rates of 150 Hz occurring concomitant with focal cortical spike activity. Purkinje cell discharges abruptly ceased during development of cortical epileptiform bursts which became generalized and maximal in both cerebral hemispheres. Following intravenous PHT (10 mg/kg), cortical epileptiform burst frequency and duration were markedly reduced, and sustained Purkinje cell discharge rates of 140 Hz were recorded.

To establish that PHT's effect on the Purkinje cell was important in inhibition of the cortical epileptiform burst activity, the authors removed the cerebellum. Consistent with their hypothesis, PHT was less effective in reducing cortical bursts after cerebellectomy. (See also Refs. 1117, 1198.)

LIPICKY, GILBERT AND STILLMAN, *Proceedings of the National Academy of Sciences* (1972),[1291] studied the effect of PHT (5–50 μM) on the voltage-dependent currents of the squid giant axon. PHT did not change the resting membrane potential, but decreased the early transient sodium currents by 50% with little or no effect on potassium currents.

The authors suggest that this observation may be relevant to PHT's antiarrhythmic action in heart and its stabilizing effects in peripheral nerve.

Su and Feldman, *Archives of Neurology* (1973),[1602] in a microelectrode study of *in vivo* rat neuromuscular transmission, found that intravenous PHT (10–40 mg/kg) had no effect on normal muscle resting potential or miniature endplate potential (mepp) frequency or amplitude. However, when the neuromuscular junction was abnormally stimulated by depolarization with high potassium (35 mM), PHT increased the resting potential of the muscle membrane by 15% and decreased mepp frequency by 60%. The onset of PHT's effect was rapid, occurring within ten minutes.

The authors conclude that PHT stabilizes both the motor-nerve ending and the muscle membrane.

Delgado, Mora and Sanguinetti, *Personal Communication* (1973),[954] studied the effect of PHT on afterdischarge in the amygdala of the brain of awake active rhesus monkeys.

Earlier work[953] had shown that certain forms of abnormal spread of electrical afterdischarge could be induced in the monkey by intracerebral electrical stimulation in several areas of the brain, including the thalamus and amygdala. Electrical afterdischarge was decreased dramatically in the thalamus by PHT. It also markedly limited the spread of electrical afterdischarge in the cerebral cortex.

In the present study, with repeated electrical stimulation sufficiently close together, in this case ten minutes apart, repetitive afterdischarge could be obtained with 100% reliability. Certain abnormal behavioral sequences accompanied the measurable afterdischarges from the amygdala. Intramuscular or intracerebral injection of PHT was found to completely prevent these electrical afterdischarges.

PHT showed some effect in reducing afterdischarge fifteen to thirty minutes after injection, and produced complete abolition of afterdischarges by one hour.

The authors note that PHT did not change normal spontaneous electrical activity in any of the animals.

Carnay and Grundfest, *Neuropharmacology* (1974),[885] studied the effects of PHT and calcium on electrical properties of the pre- and postsynaptic membranes of frog neuromuscular junction. When muscle fibers were bathed in solutions either deficient in calcium or containing germine monoacetate, membrane instability and repetitive firing of the fibers were produced. PHT was effective in preventing this abnormal repetitive firing.

At concentrations of 10–20 μg/ml in normal media, PHT did not alter normal muscle fiber resting potential, effective membrane resistance, threshold membrane potential, and miniature endplate potential frequency and amplitude.

The authors conclude that PHT has a stabilizing effect similar to that of calcium on abnormal membrane states.

Matthews and Connor, *Pharmacologist* (1974),[1343] studied the effect of PHT on single impulse transmission and post-tetanic potentiation in rat brain. Post-tetanic potentiation was induced in the hippocampus by stimulating the commissural fibers with rapid repetitive impulses (10 Hz, five seconds duration). PHT (40 mg/kg) reduced the potentiated responses by 50%, without diminishing single impulse transmission.

ROSES, BUTTERFIELD, APPEL AND CHESTNUT, *Archives of Neurology* (1975),[2057] using electron spin resonance spectroscopy, substantiated the presence of membrane defects, increased membrane fluidity and decreased polarity, in red blood cells from patients with myotonic dystrophy. PHT caused the local increased fluidity near the surface of myotonic red blood cells to decrease to essentially that of normal controls. PHT did not significantly change parameters of the normal red blood cell membranes.

HANSOTIA, MAZZA AND GATLIN, *American Journal of Clinical Pathology* (1975),[1881] studied the effects of PHT on membrane function and fragility of red blood cells in normal subjects and in patients with hereditary spherocytic anemia.

Red blood cells from five normal individuals and from three patients with congenital spherocytic hemolytic anemia were incubated with PHT and osmotic fragility was measured. It was shown that PHT reduces the osmotic fragility of normal and spherocytic erythrocytes. In the presence of ouabain, which may induce hemolysis, PHT still had a protective effect on red blood cells.

RICHELSON AND TUTTLE, *Brain Research* (1975),[2045] found that PHT (20 μM) specifically inhibits the repetitive action potential discharge induced in single mouse neuroblastoma cells by low calcium and potassium medium. PHT's action was rapid (10 sec.) and reversible. Other compounds tested had no effect, even at high concentrations.

ROSEN, DANILO, ALONSO AND PIPPENGER, *The Journal of Pharmacology and Experimental Therapies* (1976),[2055] using intracellular microelectrode techniques, studied the effects of therapeutic concentrations of PHT on transmembrane potentials of normal and depressed canine Purkinje fibers. The authors state that their findings show that the electrophysiologic effects of PHT are determined by the condition of the cardiac fiber. Depending on the condition of the cardiac fiber, PHT either enhances or depresses conduction, in the direction of the normal.

AYALA, JOHNSTON, LIN AND DICHTER, *Brain Research* (1977),[1732] studied the effects of PHT (25–200 μM) on certain synapses of neurons in the abdominal ganglia of Aplysia and on the GABA-mediated inhibitory synapse of the crayfish stretch receptor neuron.

PHT decreased the amplitude of the excitatory postsynaptic potential and enhanced the "long" acetylcholine-mediated, potassium-dependent inhibitory postsynaptic potential (IPSP) at Aplysia synapses. PHT prolonged the stretch receptor IPSP up to ten times control values.

The authors suggest that these selective synaptic actions of PHT contribute to its regulation of neuronal hyperexcitability.

AYALA, LIN AND JOHNSTON, *Brain Research* (1977),[1733] studied PHT's effects on the membrane properties of crayfish stretch receptor neurons and Aplysia abdominal and buccal ganglia neurons. PHT (100–300 μM) decreased abnormal repetitive firing and membrane resistance, with little or no change in the resting potential. Effects on the action potential, which varied with the type of neuron being studied, included decreased overshoot and prolonged falling phase. Potassium conductance and post-tetanic hyperpolarization were also decreased.

The authors comment that the observed changes in membrane parameters are consistent with PHT's ability to reduce repetitive firing and the spread of abnormal electrical activity.

DEISZ AND LUX, *Neuroscience Letters* (1977),[1794] and AICKIN, DEISZ AND LUX, *Journal of Physiology* (1978),[1716] found that PHT (as low as 10^{-9} M) increased inhibitory synaptic conductance and prolonged inhibitory postsynaptic potentials of crayfish stretch receptor neurons. The authors conclude that PHT decreases the rate of closing of the GABA-activated chloride channel, thereby enhancing inhibition.

SCHWARZ AND VOGEL, *European Journal of Pharmacology* (1977),[2072] studied the excitability-reducing action of PHT in single myelinated frog nerve fibers.

PHT hyperpolarized the resting membrane potential, raised the threshold potential. It also reduced the peak sodium current by 45%. The onset of PHT's effect on the sodium current occurred within 3.8 seconds.

The authors suggest that the excitability-reducing action of PHT is mainly due to a potential-dependent blockage of the sodium channel.

POLLEN, *Brain Behavior and Evolution* (1977),[2024] working on a prosthesis for the blind, found PHT useful in minimizing the production of afterdischarges following electrical stimulation of the visual cortex in cats.

SELZER, *Annals of Neurology* (1978),[2073] in studies on a composite electrical-chemi-cal synapse in the lamprey spinal cord, found that PHT (20 μg/ml) reversibly reduced the chemical component of the excitatory postsynaptic potential by up to 70%. PHT also greatly reduced or eliminated post-tetanic potentiation of the chemical component, but produced little or no decrease in the size of the electrical component, which reflects the presynaptic spike.

TUTTLE AND RICHELSON, *Journal of Pharmacology and Experimental Therapeutics* (1979),[2105] studied the effect of PHT (40 μM) on passive and active membrane properties of mouse neuroblastoma cells. They found PHT's effect was greatest on the calcium-dependent components of the action potential. PHT reduced the hyperpolarization following an action potential and its potentiation under a repetitive stimulus.

GRAFOVA AND DANILOVA, *Bulletin of Experimental Biology and Medicine* (1980),[2202] demonstrated, in a rat model of generalized myoclonus, that PHT abolished the spontaneous clonic discharges from tetanus toxin-induced hyperexcitable generators in the ventral horns of the spinal cord. Evoked tonic activity was more resistant.

FROMM, CHATTHA, TERRENCE AND GLASS, *European Journal of Pharmacology* (1982),[2515] studied the effects of PHT and carbamazepine on segmental and periventricular inhibition elicited in cat spinal trigeminal nucleus by stimulation of the maxillary nerve. Therapeutic levels of PHT and carbamazepine facilitated the segmental inhibition, but depressed the periventricular inhibition, while also depressing the response of trigeminal nucleus neurons to maxillary nerve stimulation.

The authors suggest that PHT's ability to produce a relative facilitation of inhibitory feedback mechanisms is important to its regulation of abnormal electrical activity in the CNS.

MCLEAN AND MACDONALD, *The Journal of Pharmacology and Experimental Therapeutics* (1983),[2783] studied the concentration dependence of several actions of PHT in mouse spinal cord neurons in culture using intracellular microelectrode techniques. At 1–2 µg/ml (equivalent to therapeutic cerebrospinal fluid concentrations), PHT reduced high-frequency repetitive firing during long depolarizing current pulses. There was a progressive reduction of the maximal rate of rise of the action potential (V_{max}) during the train until firing failed. While PHT did not affect V_{max} of single action potentials, recovery of V_{max} after repetitive firing was prolonged.

PHT concentrations above 3 µg/ml reduced V_{max}, spontaneous neuronal firing, and calcium-dependent action potential amplitude. PHT abolished convulsant-induced paroxysmal bursting, and augmented postsynaptic responses to iontophoretically-applied GABA.

The authors conclude that, at therapeutic levels, PHT prolongs sodium channel recovery from inactivation, an effect which is critical to its ability to limit sustained high-frequency repetitive firing. (See also Refs. 2745, 2746, 2747, 2748, 2782.)

SELZER, DAVID AND YAARI, *The Journal of Neuroscience* (1985),[2945] reported that PHT (200–300 µM) dramatically reduced the early component of the post-tetanic potentiation (PTP) produced by a 30-second, 30-Hz tetanus at the frog neuromuscular junction. The late component of PTP was also reduced, although to a lesser extent. PHT reduced PTP even when there was no failure of the endplate potential during tet-

anus. The PHT effect did not require a complete block of the presynaptic action potential. PHT had no effect on PTP in the presence of tetrodotoxin.

The authors suggest that their results indicate that PHT reduces PTP by producing a graded reduction of sodium influx into nerve terminals during high rates of axonal stimulation.

YAARI, DAVID AND SELZER, *Personal Communication* (1985),[3089] utilizing a frog sciatic nerve preparation, reported that PHT has no effect at low-frequency stimulation but, at higher rates of stimulation, it produces a progressive decline in compound action potential amplitude and integral. They state that PHT's use- and frequency-dependent depression of axonal excitability is likely to account for its ability to suppress abnormal brain discharge, without significantly altering normal activity. (See also Refs. 3090, 3092, 3093.)

ADLER, YAARI, DAVID AND SELZER, *Brain Research* (1986),[2276] reported on the use- and frequency-dependent effects of PHT on the sodium-dependent action potential of lamprey spinal axons. Control lamprey action potential amplitude and conduction velocity showed little reduction during a 500-stimulus train at frequencies of 2 to 100 Hz. With 20 µg/ml PHT, there was a progressive attenuation of the action potential amplitude and velocity with the same stimulus conditions. The higher the frequency of stimulation, the greater PHT's effect.

PHT's effects at a given concentration were much greater when the extracellular potassium concentration was raised from 2.1 to 5 mM. The authors conclude that increased potassium may, in part, account for PHT's ability to distinguish between normal and abnormal neuronal excitability.

HARTMAN, FIAMENGO AND RIKER, *Anesthesiology* (1986),[2576] found that pretreatment with intravenous PHT (30 mg/kg) suppressed succinylcholine-induced motor nerve terminal repetitive firing and post-tetanic potentiation, as well as muscle fasciculations, in an *in situ* cat soleus neuromuscular preparation.

PHT was more effective than d-tubocurarine in suppressing the fasciculations. In addition, PHT enhanced succinylcholine's desired blocking effect, while d-tubocurarine reduced it.

The authors comment that succinylcholine, a depolarizing neuromuscular blocker used in anesthesia, has a number of undesirable side effects which can be reduced by suppressing fasciculations. They suggest that PHT may be clinically useful in preventing these side effects.

SODIUM, POTASSIUM AND
CALCIUM REGULATION

Sodium and Potassium

WOODBURY, *Journal of Pharmacology and Experimental Therapeutics* (1955),[387] demonstrated that in normal rats, PHT decreased both the total and the intracellular concentration of brain sodium and increased the rate of movement of radio-sodium into and out of brain cells. The net result was that the ratio of extracellular to intracellular brain sodium was increased. PHT also decreased intracellular sodium concentrations in skeletal and cardiac muscle, but to a lesser extent than in brain.

Acutely induced low sodium in blood was associated with an increase in intracellular brain sodium and a decrease in intracellular brain potassium. These changes from normal were largely prevented by treatment with PHT.

KOCH, HIGGINS, SANDE, TIERNEY AND TULIN, *Physiologist* (1962),[1225] studied the effect of PHT on the reabsorption of ions by kidney in dogs. PHT enhanced active sodium transport in the kidney.

FESTOFF AND APPEL, *Journal of Clinical Investigation* (1968),[94] studied the effects of PHT on sodium-potassium-ATPase in rat brain synaptosomes. With a ratio of 5–10 to 1 of sodium-to-potassium, PHT had no effect. When the ratio of sodium-to-potassium was raised to 50 to 1 or higher, PHT exerted an increasingly greater effect on enzyme activity, causing stimulation of synaptosome ATPase. Thus the authors observed a selectivity of action of PHT on ATPase, depending on whether the ratio of sodium-to-potassium is in the normal or abnormal range.

HELFANT, RICCIUTTI, SCHERLAG AND DA-MATO, *American Journal of Physiology* (1968),[157] demonstrated that PHT prevented the efflux of potassium from cardiac tissue pretreated with toxic doses of digitalis and reversed digitalis-induced ventricular arrhythmias.

VAN REES, WOODBURY AND NOACH, *Archives Internationales de Pharmacodynamie et de Therapie* (1969),[1642] found that in loops of intestine of intact rats, PHT increased the rate of absorption of both sodium and water from the lumen of the intestine.

PINCUS, GROVE, MARINO AND GLASER, *Archives of Neurology* (1970),[699] indicate that PHT (100 μM) does not affect intracellular sodium in normally functioning, oxygenated nerves, but that it tends to reduce the abnormal accumulation of intracellular sodium in hypoxic nerves. PHT was also found to limit the rise in intracellular sodium in nerves in which the sodium extrusion mechanism has been destroyed by ouabain, cyanide or both.

The authors state: "Phenytoin has been shown to have a stabilizing influence on virtually all excitable membranes. These effects have been seen in a wide variety of vertebrate and invertebrate species." (See also Refs. 285, 293.)

CRANE AND SWANSON, *Neurology* (1970),[728] showed that PHT (100–500 μM) prevents the loss of potassium and the gain in sodium by brain slices during repeated high-frequency electrical stimulation. Repeated depolarization of neuronal membranes makes it increasingly likely that the resting intra- and extracellular balance of ions will not be restored.

These "downhill movements" of sodium and potassium ions represent the failure of active transport to restore the resting balance of ions between intracellular and extracellular compartments. PHT, by preventing and reversing these shifts, tends to restore the balance toward the normal resting state.

FERTZIGER, LIUZZI AND DUNHAM, *Brain Research* (1971),[1025] studied the effect of PHT on potassium transport in lobster axons using radioisotopic potassium. The authors observed that PHT (100 μM) stimulated potassium influx. They postulated that this regulatory effect on potassium transport, in addition to the well-established regulation of intracellular sodium content of nerve, might relate to the stabilizing effect of PHT on hyperactive neurons.

DEN HERTOG, *European Journal of Pharmacology* (1972),[955] studied the basis for PHT's ability to inhibit post-tetanic potentiation and repetitive afterdischarge. The author found that PHT (20 μg/ml) did not alter the electrogenic component of the sodium pump or change normal membrane threshold or post-tetanic hyperpolarization in repetitively stimulated, non-myelinated axons of desheathed rat vagus nerve.

ESCUETA AND APPEL, *Archives of Internal Medicine* (1972),[1012] studied the effect of PHT (100 μM) on sodium and potassium levels in isolated brain synaptosomes. Rat brain rendered hyperexcitable by electrical stimulation resulting in seizure states was found to contain a decreased level of potassium and an increased level of sodium within the synaptic terminals.

The authors note that these changes reflected the "downhill movement" of ions in synaptic terminals. PHT corrected these changes through its effect on membrane function.

LIPICKY, GILBERT AND STILLMAN, *Proceedings of the National Academy of Sciences* (1972), [1291] studied the effect of PHT (5–50 μM) on the voltage-dependent currents of the squid giant axon. PHT did not change the resting membrane potential, but decreased the early transient sodium currents by 50%, with little or no effect on potassium currents.

The authors suggest that this observation may be relevant to PHT's antiarrhythmic action in heart and its stabilizing effects in peripheral nerve.

NASELLO, MONTINI AND ASTRADA, *Pharmacology* (1972),[1379] studied the effect of PHT on electrically stimulated rat dorsal hippocampus. When the hippocampus was constantly stimulated, potassium release was observed. PHT counteracted this release.

PINCUS, *Archives of Neurology* (1972),[1418] found that PHT (100 μM) reduced sodium influx by 40% in stimulated lobster nerves. Sodium influx was not found to be affected in the resting nerve. PHT did not affect the rate of stimulated or resting sodium efflux.

The author concludes that PHT acts primarily by limiting the increase in sodium permeability which occurs during stimulation. PHT appears to counteract "downhill" sodium movements in stimulated nerves without affecting normal sodium movements.

WATSON AND WOODBURY, *Chemical Modulation of Brain Function* (1973),[1664] studied the effect of PHT on sodium transport and membrane permeability of the epithelium of frog skin and toad urinary bladder preparations. PHT increased net sodium transport in both cases by increasing the permeability of the outer membrane to sodium. The authors suggest that these findings are consistent with PHT's action in stimulating sodium-potassium-ATPase, when the sodium-potassium ratio is high (25 to 1).

NOACH, VAN REES AND DE WOLFF, *Archives Internationales de Pharmacodynamie et de Therapie* (1973),[1385] found that when sodium is lacking from the intestinal lumen, PHT causes the sodium to increase in the lumen by active extrusion of sodium from the gut wall.

LOH, *Federation Proceedings* (1974),[2224] in studies of isolated frog atrial trabeculae, found that PHT reversed digitalis-induced potassium loss. The net gain of tissue potassium and the reduction of potassium efflux led the author to conclude that these changes might account for PHT's effects on transmembrane potentials and its stabilization of membranes.

JOHNSTON AND AYALA, *Science* (1975),[1917] demonstrated that PHT (20–200 μM) decreases the bursting pacemaker activity in certain Aplysia neurons. The sodium-dependent negative resistance characteristic, which is essential for bursting behavior, is reduced in the presence of PHT. The authors believe these findings may be applicable to PHT's inhibition of the downhill flux of sodium ions and paroxysmal depolarizing shifts in mammalian neurons.

O'DONNELL, KOVACS AND SZABO, *Pflugers Archives* (1975),[2006] noting that PHT is considered to exert a stabilizing effect on all excitable cell membranes, studied the influence of PHT on potassium and sodium movements in isolated frog skeletal muscle. They conclude that in this system PHT acts in a normal ionic environment to reduce the resting passive component of potassium exchange across the muscle fiber membrane, and that this might account for the membrane stabilizing action of PHT.

EHRING AND HONDEGHEM, *Proceedings of the Western Pharmacological Society* (1978),[1815] studied the effects of PHT on isolated guinea pig heart papillary muscle. PHT (60–100 μM) decreased action potential V_{max} only when stimulus frequency was high or when the cells were depolarized. PHT's effects were less when the cells were hyperpolarized.

Based on this evidence, the authors suggest that PHT achieves its antiarrhythmic effects by binding to open sodium channels, thus regulating sodium influx.

PERRY, McKINNEY AND DeWEER, *Nature* (1978),[2021] demonstrated that PHT (100 μM) does not affect active sodium transport, but regulates resting and excitable sodium channels in isolated squid giant axons.

By limiting sodium influx, in addition to

limiting calcium influx through the sodium channel, PHT raises the firing threshold, stabilizes excitable membranes and counteracts post-tetanic potentiation.

Nosek, *Epilepsia* (1981),[2233] studying the crayfish giant axon, found that PHT (110 μM) decreased both sodium and potassium conductances, but had no effect on chloride conductance or active transport of sodium and potassium.

The author suggests that PHT's ability to reduce potassium efflux from the neuron may be important in its selective effects on hyperexcitability.

Yeh, Quandt, and Kirsch, *Federation Proceedings* (1981),[2133] noting that PHT is used clinically in cardiac, nervous system and muscle disorders, sought to demonstrate common mechanisms of action of PHT in a variety of excitable membranes: perfused squid axons, single fibers of frog skeletal muscle and cultured neuroblastoma cells. In all three preparations, PHT (20–100 μM) decreased slow sodium currents. PHT also reduced calcium currents in neuroblastoma cells.

The more the depolarization of the membrane, the greater PHT's effect.

Grenader, Ponomareva, Zurabishvili and Vasiev, *Biofizika* (1982),[2557] report that PHT (2–8 μg/ml) causes a decrease in the fast inward sodium current in rabbit heart atrium and ventricular tissue. This leads to increased refractoriness and is one of the mechanisms by which PHT achieves its antiarrhythmic effects.

Courtney and Etter, *European Journal of Pharmacology* (1983),[2412] studying single myelinated sciatic nerve fibers with voltage clamp techniques, showed that PHT, carbamazepine and phenobarbital se-

lectively bind to the inactive state of the sodium channel. These agents also showed increased effects when the membrane was depolarized, indicating selectivity for the hyperactive state.

McLean and Macdonald, *The Journal of Pharmacology and Experimental Therapeutics* (1983),[2783] studied the concentration dependence of several actions of PHT in mouse spinal cord neurons in culture using intracellular microelectrode techniques. At 1–2 μg/ml (equivalent to therapeutic cerebrospinal fluid concentrations), PHT reduced high-frequency repetitive firing during long depolarizing current pulses. There was a progressive reduction of the maximal rate of rise of the action potential (V_{max}) during the train until firing failed. While PHT did not affect V_{max} of single action potentials, recovery of V_{max} after repetitive firing was prolonged.

PHT concentrations above 3 μg/ml reduced V_{max} and spontaneous neuronal firing, reduced calcium-dependent action potential amplitude, eradicated convulsant-induced paroxysmal bursting, and augmented postsynaptic responses to iontophoretically applied gamma-aminobutyric acid.

The authors conclude that, at therapeutic levels, PHT prolongs sodium channel recovery from inactivation, an effect which is critical to its ability to limit sustained high-frequency repetitive firing. (See also Refs. 2745, 2746, 2747, 2748, 2782.)

Matsuki, Quandt, Ten Eick and Yeh, *Journal of Pharmacology and Experimental Therapeutics* (1984),[2770] studied the interaction of PHT with membrane ionic channels of cultured mouse neuroblastoma cells, using voltage clamp and intracellular perfusion techniques. PHT (20–100 μM) inhibited inward sodium current in a dose-dependent manner, and slowed recovery from voltage-dependent inactivation of sodium current during conditioned block. Recovery was faster when the membrane was hyperpolarized. When the membrane was depolarized or stimulated at higher frequencies, PHT's inhibitory effects increased.

The authors conclude that PHT regulates membrane function both by increasing the fraction of sodium channels in an inactivated state and by delaying the transition from inactivated to closed but available channels.

NORRIS AND SAEZ, *IRCS Medical Science* (1984),[2832] compared the effects of PHT and carbamazepine on the electrical properties of isolated toad skin. Both agents increased sodium transport across the skin, but the stimulatory effect of carbamazepine was less than that of PHT. In some cases, carbamazepine had inhibitory effects in the same dosage range within which PHT was stimulatory.

WILLOW, KUENZEL AND CATTERALL, *Molecular Pharmacology* (1984),[2268] and WILLOW, GONOI AND CATTERALL, *Molecular Pharmacology* (1985),[3073] studied the effects of PHT on voltage-sensitive sodium channels in cultured neuroblastoma cells and rat brain synaptosomes using voltage clamp techniques and $^{22}Na^+$. In the neuroblastoma cells, PHT reduced sodium currents without effect on the voltage dependence of sodium-channel activation. Half-maximal inhibition was seen at 30 μM. Depolarization and repetitive stimulation increased PHT's inhibition of sodium current. Hyperpolarization decreased the effect.

In other experiments, PHT competitively inhibited batrachotoxin-activated $^{22}Na^+$ influx in both the neuroblastoma cells and the synaptosomes.

The authors suggest that PHT regulates electrical activity by binding to receptor sites associated with activation of voltage-sensitive sodium channels. (See also Refs. 2379, 3072.)

CALDWELL AND HARRIS, *European Journal of Pharmacology* (1985),[2374] evaluated the effects of anesthetics and anticonvulsants on the calcium-dependent efflux of potassium in human erythrocytes. PHT (30–100 μM) and phenobarbital were the only agents that inhibited the efflux process in a concentration-dependent manner.

DAVID, SELZER AND YAARI, *Brain Research* (1985),[2429] reported that PHT (100–300 μM) is able to block aminopyridine-induced afterdischarges at presynaptic nerve terminals. The authors suggest that this is due to PHT's ability to reduce sodium conductance at the synaptic terminal.

WADA, IZUMI, YANAGIHARA AND KOBAYASHI, *Archives of Pharmacology* (1985),[3053] showed that PHT (10–100 μM) reduced veratridine-induced influx of sodium and calcium, and secretion of catecholamines in cultured bovine adrenal medullary cells. PHT also abolished ouabain's potentiation of the veratridine-induced effects.

The authors conclude that PHT modulates the intracellular accumulation of sodium which, in turn, regulates calcium influx and secretion of medullary catecholamines.

WHITE, CHEN, KEMP AND WOODBURY, *Epilepsia* (1985),[3069] studied the effects of acute and chronic PHT on various parameters of anion and cation transport in the cerebral cortex of neonatal and adult rats.

Acute administration of PHT (20 mg/kg) inhibited sodium-potassium-ATPase activity in both neonates and adult rats. Chronic treatment (20 mg/kg b.i.d. or q.i.d. for seven days) in adult rats slightly decreased neuronal sodium-potassium-ATPase activity, while markedly increasing its activity in glia. Chronic PHT treatment also increased both DNA content and the activity of the glial enzyme carbonic anhydrase and the mitochondrial enzyme HCO_3^--ATPase. Both of these enzymes are involved in ionic regulation and are related to brain excitability.

The authors suggest that PHT's stimulation of glial uptake of extracellular potassium may be important in its regulatory effects on hyperexcitability. (See also Refs. 3084, 3085.)

WHITE, YEN-CHOW, CHOW, KEMP AND WOODBURY, *Epilepsia* (1985),[3070] studied the effects of PHT in primary rat glial cell cultures. PHT (1–100 μM) increased glial cell control of elevated extracellular potassium. The efficiency of glial sodium-potassium-ATPase was substantially enhanced by PHT over a wide range of extracellular potassium concentrations. Significant membrane hyperpolarization accompanied the marked increase in intracellular potassium which resulted from the PHT-induced increase in enzyme activity.

QUANDT AND YEH, *Society for Neuroscience Abstracts* (1986),[2885] found that PHT enhanced the slow inactivation of single sodium channels in excised patches of membrane from cultured N1E-115 neuroblastoma cells. PHT (100 μM) reduced the time to onset of slow inactivation. Under conditions of sustained depolarization, PHT reduced the duration of bursts of sodium channel opening; lengthened interval between bursts; and reduced the probability of a channel being open and the mean open-channel time.

The authors suggest that these actions could account for PHT's selective effects on repetitive neuronal firing.

Calcium

KOREY, *Proceedings of the Society of Experimental Biology and Medicine* (1951),[472] in a study of the isolated squid giant axon, found that PHT corrected the hyperexcitability induced by the withdrawal of calcium and magnesium from the bathing medium. PHT corrected this excessive firing within two to three minutes. When calcium and magnesium were added back into the medium, it took fifteen minutes for the axon to return to normal.

PINCUS AND LEE, *Archives of Neurology* (1973),[1417] found that, when PHT (50–500 μM) was added to rat brain slices, the uptake of calcium was decreased and there was a decrease in the release of norepinephrine from the cells. The authors state that it has been demonstrated that, in the absence of calcium, the electrical stimulation of brain slices does not result in norepinephrine being released from the cell. They note that when calcium concentration is reduced, norepinephrine release from the cells is also reduced.

Calcium and PHT were antagonistic with respect to their effect on norepinephrine release induced by potassium depolarization. Tetrodotoxin at high concentration had no effect on norepinephrine release. Thus the authors suggest that the effect of PHT on norepinephrine release was mediated entirely by its reduction of calcium uptake by depolarized brain slices.

The authors note that the effects of PHT upon calcium uptake may be relevant to the regulatory action of PHT in other situations, including the secretion of insulin and the contractile mechanisms in skeletal and cardiac muscle.

SOHN AND FERRENDELLI, *Neurology* (1973),[1567] studied the effect of PHT on calcium uptake by synaptosomes isolated from rat brain. PHT (200 μM or greater) consistently inhibited calcium uptake by potassium depolarized synaptosomes. Nondepolarized synaptosomes required higher concentrations of PHT (400 μM) for an inhibitory effect on calcium uptake.

These results support the concept that one pharmacological action of PHT is inhibition of calcium transport into stimulated neuronal tissue. The authors suggest that this may be a mechanism by which PHT inhibits neurotransmitter release and, in turn, suppresses post-tetanic potentiation.

PENTO, GLICK AND KAGAN, *Endocrinology* (1973),[1406] demonstrated the effect of PHT on calcitonin secretion in the pig. Normal basal levels of calcitonin secretion were not significantly changed by PHT. When extra calcitonin secretion was stimulated by means of glucagon or calcium administration, PHT reduced the rise in plasma calcitonin produced by these two stimuli.

The authors state that these findings are in accord with other demonstrations that PHT does not alter normal basal secretion of pituitary-adrenal hormones, or insulin; but when unusual stimuli are present, PHT exerts a regulatory influence.

CARNAY AND GRUNDFEST, *Neuropharmacology* (1974),[885] studied the effects of PHT and calcium on the electrical properties of the pre- and postsynaptic membranes of frog neuromuscular junction. When muscle fibers were bathed in solutions deficient in calcium, membrane instability and repetitive firing of the muscle fibers occured. Within five minutes after the addition of PHT (10–20 μg/ml), the abnormal repetitive activity and irritability were abolished, without affecting the threshold or amplitude of the stimulated single action potential or endplate potential. PHT reversed the abnormal membrane receptor desensitization that occurs in calcium-deficient media and, like calcium, corrected the membrane instability induced by germine monoacetate.

The authors conclude that PHT has a stabilizing effect similar to that of calcium on abnormal membrane properties.

HASBANI, PINCUS AND LEE, *Archives of Neurology* (1974),[1136] demonstrated that PHT (200 μM) reduced radioisotopic calcium uptake in rapidly stimulated lobster axons. The PHT metabolite, hydroxyphenyl-phenylhydantoin (HPPH), had no effect on calcium uptake.

RIDDLE, MANDEL AND GOLDNER, *European Journal of Pharmacology* (1975),[2046] studied the effects of PHT and calcium simultaneously on solute transport in frog skin. In the presence of external calcium, PHT (15–100 μg/ml) elicited a significant increase in active sodium transport, but in the absence of calcium, PHT had no effect. PHT also increased passive solute permeability, independent of calcium.

WATSON AND SIEGEL, *European Journal of Pharmacology* (1976),[2267] demonstrated that PHT inhibited calcium uptake, but not release, by submandibular microsomes. They also found, in *in vivo* experiments, that PHT decreased secretory response of the submandibular and parotid glands to intra-arterial methacholine.

The authors suggest that the reduction in secretory volume related to PHT's regulation of calcium uptake.

GOLDBERG, *Neurology* (1977),[1860] states that PHT, which acts on many levels of the nervous system as well as many non-neural sites, must affect some general membrane property, and only when the membrane is unstable.

The author found that binding of PHT to phospholipids is related to fatty acid composition in rabbit and human brain fractions. Dipalmitoyl and dioleoyl lecithins, the most abundant lecithins in brain, showed the greatest binding. PHT increased the binding of radioisotopic calcium to phospholipids up to five-fold.

The author suggests that this PHT-induced increase in calcium binding may explain PHT's membrane stabilizing action and its effectiveness in treatment of hypocalcemic symptoms. (See also Refs. 1859, 2547.)

PACE AND LIVINGSTON, *Diabetes* (1979),[2011] studied the effects of PHT on insulin release and metabolism of isolated rat islets of Langerhans. Glucose and veratridine were used to stimulate insulin release by activating the calcium and sodium channels. PHT (100 μM) inhibited the glucose-stimulated insulin release (77%) and glycolysis (74%). PHT also inhibited the veratridine-stimulated insulin release (60%) and glycolysis (100%). When extracellular calcium was raised from 2.5 to 5.0 mM, PHT's effects were less.

Noting that PHT has been reported to hyperpolarize the beta-cell membrane and to inhibit glucose-induced spike activity, the authors conclude that the inhibitory action of PHT on the pancreatic beta-cell is due to its regulatory effect on sodium and calcium channels.

YAARI, PINCUS, AND ARGOV, *Brain Research* (1979),[2130] showed a biphasic effect of PHT at the frog neuromuscular junction. PHT (200 μM) increased quantal content of acetylcholine in media containing low calcium concentrations, but decreased quantal

content in normal calcium. The authors suggest that PHT not only reduced calcium entry into axon terminals, but also reduced the activity of the intracellular calcium sequestration-extrusion system.

QUANDT AND NARAHASHI, *Neuroscience Abstracts* (1980),[2884] studied the effects of PHT (20–50 μM) on sodium and calcium voltage-dependent currents in neuroblastoma cells in culture. Peak inward calcium current was reduced 25%, whereas peak sodium-dependent current was reduced only 10%. The suggestion is that, at least in these cells, PHT's inhibition of calcium flux is more important than its effect on sodium.

STUDY, *Journal of Pharmacology and Experimental Therapeutics* (1980),[2093] reported that PHT inhibited the calcium-dependent increases in cyclic GMP induced by high-potassium depolarization and muscarinic receptor activation in N1E-115 neuroblastoma cells. PHT's inhibition of the cyclic GMP response to depolarization was half-maximal at 40 μM. Inhibition of the muscarinic receptor response by PHT could be overcome by increasing extracellular calcium.

The author suggests that reduction of calcium influx is the means by which PHT blocks cyclic GMP responses in these cells.

HERCHUELZ, LEBRUN, SENER AND MALAISSE, *European Journal of Pharmacology* (1981),[2589] investigated the mechanism by which PHT inhibits glucose-stimulated insulin release by studying its effects on calcium and rubidium fluxes in isolated pancreatic islets.

PHT inhibited both basal and glucose-stimulated calcium uptake by islet cells and markedly reduced the secondary rise in calcium efflux normally provoked by glucose. PHT also decreased the calcium exchange evoked by an increase in extracellular calcium concentration. Rubidium uptake was not affected, indicating that PHT's effects on insulin release were not attributable to activation of sodium-potassium-ATPase.

The authors conclude that PHT inhibits glucose-induced insulin release by limiting calcium entry into islet cells.

PINCUS AND HSIAO, *Experimental Neurology* (1981),[2241] demonstrated that PHT (200 μM) inhibits both depolarization-coupled synaptosomal calcium uptake and calcium efflux in rat brain. The authors specifically related PHT's effect on calcium efflux to modulation of calcium-sodium exchange. (See also Ref. 2240.)

FERENDELLI AND DANIELS-MCQUEEN, *Journal of Pharmacology and Experimental Therapeutics* (1982),[2490] studied the actions of PHT on veratridine-stimulated (sodium-dependent) and on potassium-stimulated (sodium-independent) calcium uptake in synaptosomes from rat cerebral cortex. PHT (15–300 μg/ml) inhibited both veratridine- and potassium-induced calcium uptake, but was more effective against veratridine. Inhibition of veratridine-stimulated calcium uptake by PHT appeared to be competitive, whereas the interaction between potassium and PHT was noncompetitive.

The authors conclude that PHT inhibits sodium and calcium conductances in nervous tissue by different mechanisms.

SIEGEL, JANJIC AND WOLLHEIM, *Diabetes* (1982),[2952] studied the inhibition of insulin release by PHT in rat pancreatic islet culture. PHT (80μM), added during the second phase of glucose-induced biphasic insulin release, resulted in marked and rapid inhibition. PHT also significantly reduced glucose-induced calcium uptake of islet cells. The authors suggest that PHT inhib-

its glucose-stimulated insulin release by regulating calcium uptake via voltage-dependent calcium channels.

DELORENZO, *Annals of Neurology* (1984),[2441] reviewed his own work and that of others on calmodulin systems in neuronal excitability. PHT has been found to inhibit calcium-calmodulin-regulated protein phosphorylation and neurotransmitter release by synaptic vesicles. The author suggests that this action of PHT is important in its ability to regulate abnormal neuronal excitability. (See also Refs. 2438, 2439, 2440.)

GREENBERG, COOPER AND CARPENTER, *Annals of Neurology* (1984),[2555] report that PHT (30–300 μM) inhibited binding of the calcium antagonist [^{3}H]-nitrendipine to voltage-dependent calcium channels in brain membranes. Phenobarbital, carbamazepine, valproic acid, and clonazepam failed to do so, or did so only at concentrations much higher than used clinically.

GUREVICH AND RAZUMOVSKAYA, *Farmakologii i Toksikologii* (1984),[2563] in a review of the world laboratory literature, conclude that most of PHT's membrane stabilizing effects are related to its modulation of transmembrane calcium flux. The authors suggest that PHT's inhibition of sodium entry into the cell may actually be secondary to its effects on calcium. In addition, they point out that PHT's effects on cyclic nucleotides, synaptic protein phosphorylation, transmitter release, and microtubule polymerization are calcium-dependent.

HARRIS, *Biophysical Journal* (1984),[2575] studied the effects of membrane perturbants on voltage-activated sodium and calcium channels and calcium-dependent potassium channels in mouse synaptosomes. PHT (200 μM) decreased synaptosomal uptake of sodium and calcium, while decreasing calcium-stimulated potassium efflux.

The author concludes that PHT's inhibition of sodium influx may be due to perturbation of membrane lipids, but that this effect is not sufficient to explain all of its effects on calcium and potassium channels.

PINCUS AND WEINFELD, *Brain Research* (1984),[2870] evaluated the effects of PHT on the release of acetylcholine (ACh) from rat brain synaptosomes. PHT (200 μM) reduced depolarization-linked ACh release in calcium-containing (1.0 mM) media. In nondepolarized synaptosomes, PHT increased basal ACh release irrespective of the external calcium concentration. The first effect, the authors suggest, is due to PHT's reduction of calcium influx, whereas the latter is due to an inhibition of intracellular calcium sequestration-extrusion mechanisms.

SUGAYA, MATSUO, TAKAGI, KAJIWARA AND KIDOKORO, *IRCS Medical Science* (1984),[2990] reported that PHT (10 μM) inhibits the hyperexcitability of frog sciatic nerve induced by low extracellular calcium. The authors suggest that PHT inhibits abnormal intracellular calcium release induced by the low-calcium medium.

SUGAYA, ONOZUKA, FURUICHI, KISHII, IMAO AND SUGAYA, *Brain Research* (1985),[2991] studied the effects of PHT on intracellular calcium and protein changes during pentylenetetrazol (PTZ)-induced bursting activity in snail neurons. They utilized computer-controlled electron probe x-ray microanalysis.

PHT inhibited the intracellular calcium shift induced by PTZ, as well as the calcium binding state change near the cell membrane. PHT also inhibited the intracellu-lar protein changes. These intracellular changes were produced without any effect on sodium, calcium, or potassium transmembrane ionic currents.

The authors suggest that PHT's actions on intracellular calcium movement and intracellular proteins are important to its ability to regulate abnormal excitability.

MESSING, CARPENTER AND GREENBERG, *Journal of Pharmacology and Experimental Therapeutics* (1985),[2790] evaluated the effects of PHT on potassium-stimulated calcium uptake and [³H]-nitrendipine binding in PC12 pheochromocytoma cells and compared these effects to those of a group of classical calcium channel antagonists including nimodipine, diltiazem, verapamil and flunarizine.

PHT inhibited calcium uptake at clinically relevant concentrations and this effect was not significantly modified by sodium or potassium channel blockage. PHT also inhibited binding of [³H]-nitrendipine to PC12 membranes. The authors suggest that PHT and the above calcium channel antagonists inhibit voltage-gated calcium flux by distinct, but functionally linked, mechanisms.

TWOMBLY AND NARAHASHI, *Society for Neuroscience Abstracts* (1986),[3036] in voltage-clamp studies of N1E-115 neuroblastoma cells, found that PHT (above 10 μM) interfered with type I calcium currents by favoring the inactivated state of the calcium channel. PHT shifted the voltage dependence of this steady-state inactivation in the hyperpolarizing direction, allowing fewer calcium channels to open during test pulses. PHT's effects were both use- and frequency-dependent.

YATANI, HAMILTON AND BROWN, *Circulation Research* (1986),[3094] using whole-cell patch-clamp techniques, studied the effects of PHT on calcium currents in single isolated guinea pig ventricular cells after suppression of sodium and potassium currents.

PHT produced a voltage- and concentration-dependent decrease in calcium currents without significant change in current-voltage relations. At low frequencies (0.1 Hz) and negative holding potentials (-50 mV), PHT's half-blocking effect occurred at 200 μM.

PHT prolonged the recovery of calcium currents from inactivation, bound selectively to the inactivated calcium channel state, and competitively blocked [^{3}H]-nitrendipine binding to ventricular membrane preparations.

Noting that PHT's effects on sodium and calcium channels are similar, the authors suggest that binding sites for PHT exist on both channels. (See Ref. 2922.)

YI, SEITZ AND COOPER, *Federation Proceedings* (1987),[3095] using a radioimmunoassay, found that PHT (100 μM) inhibited the release of calcitonin induced by high extracellular calcium (2.5 mM) in rat thyroparathyroid complexes *in vitro*. Release of calcitonin in normal (1 mM) calcium was unaffected.

The calcium channel blocker, nitrendipine, also inhibited calcium-stimulated calcitonin release. A calcium channel activator (BAY-K-8644) reversed the inhibitory effects of both nitrendipine and PHT.

The authors suggest that PHT inhibits stimulated calcitonin secretion by interacting with calcium channels in thyroid parafollicular cells.

Acetylcholine (ACh)

BOSE, SAIFI AND SHARMA, *Archives Internationales de Pharmacodynamie et de Therapie* (1963),[30] found that PHT lowered acetylcholine levels in rat heart by 9.6% at 4 mg/kg PHT and by 18.9% at 8 mg/kg.

AGARWAL AND BHARGAVA, *Indian Journal of Medical Research* (1964),[1] determined brain acetylcholine (ACh) levels in rat using a frog rectus abdominis muscle bioassay. PHT (100 mg/kg) intraperitoneally, lowered brain ACh levels 38%; methedrine lowered brain ACh by 42%; and pentamethylene tetrazol lowered brain ACh by 47%. In contrast, phenobarbital, pentobarbital, morphine, meprobamate and reserpine increased brain ACh, and chlorpromazine produced no change.

BAKER, OKAMOTO AND RIKER, *The Pharmacologist* (1971),[789] found that in a cat soleus nerve-muscle preparation, pretreatment with PHT counteracts the additional excitation produced by injecting acetylcholine. The authors note that PHT selectively suppresses the post-tetanic potentiation of motor nerve terminals without impairing single impulse transmission.

WOODBURY AND KEMP, *Psychiatria, Neurologia, Neurochirurgia* (1971),[1696] discuss the work of Van Rees, Woodbury and Noach at their laboratory in which small amounts of PHT (0.3–3 μg/ml) were found to increase the release of acetylcholine from parasympathetic nerve endings in the wall of the ileum and also from the intramural ganglia and thus have a stimulating effect on the contraction of the ileum. However, when the contraction of the ileum was made excessive by the addition of acetylcholine, PHT inhibited the contractions. Thus, a biphasic effect of PHT in this circumstance was referred to by the authors.

GILBERT AND WYLIE, *Advances in Epileptology* (1978),[2536] studied the effects of PHT and other drugs on magnesium-ATPase located in synaptic vesicles and on acetylcholine and norepinephrine release. They found that PHT (200 μM) can inhibit magnesium- and sodium-potassium-ATPase in the nerve terminal. PHT did not alter basal acetylcholine release, but increased basal norepinephrine release. PHT abolished the electrically-evoked release of acetylcholine and reduced the evoked release of norepinephrine.

VIZI AND PASZTOR, *Experimental Neurology* (1981),[3050] reported that PHT (1 μM) significantly reduced the ouabain-induced release of acetylcholine, without affecting resting release, in isolated human cortical brain slices. The authors suggest that PHT's ability to reduce repetitive firing and ACh release contributes to its therapeutic effects.

ALY AND ABDEL-LATIF, *Neurochemical Research* (1982),[2285] reported on the effects of PHT, carbamazepine, phenobarbital and valproate on acetylcholine-stimulated ^{32}P incorporation into phospholipids in rat brain synaptosomes. Of the four drugs studied, only PHT (10–100 μM) blocked the ACh-stimulated labeling of phosphatidylinositol and phosphatidic acid and breakdown of polyphosphoinositides. In the absence of acetylcholine, PHT had no effect on the ^{32}P labeling of phospholipids or ATP.

The authors suggest that PHT's regulation of sodium and calcium membrane permeability is important to its actions on ACh-stimulated phospholipid metabolism and, thus, synaptic function.

PRASAD AND KUMARI, *Indian Journal of Pharmacology* (1982),[2879] reported the effects of PHT on acetylcholine content of different areas of the dog brain and on the release of ACh from dog cerebral cortex. They found that intravenous PHT (30 mg/kg) increased ACh in the frontal cortex, hippocampus, corpus callosum and midbrain, but decreased it in the hypothalamus. PHT significantly reduced release of ACh from the cerebral cortex.

QUEST, BREED AND GILLIS, *Journal of Cardiovascular Pharmacology* (1982),[2887] found that PHT significantly reduced cardiac slowing produced by both vagus stimulation and injected acetylcholine in cats with cervical vagotomy and spinal cord transection. PHT's blockade of the ACh response suggested that it acts on the postsynaptic membrane.

DIAMOND, GORDON, DAVIS AND MILFAY, *Advances in Neurology* (1983),[2451] studied the effects of PHT on the phosphorylation of acetylcholine receptors (AChR) in the electric organ of the eel. They found that the membrane-bound AChR is reversibly phosphorylated by endogenous protein kinase and that PHT markedly inhibits this phosphorylation. Half-maximal inhibition occurred at 50 μM.

The authors suggest that PHT achieves this inhibition by its direct effects on the availability of postsynaptic protein substrates for the phosphorylation reaction and that PHT may modulate receptor sensitivity by this mechanism.

PINCUS AND WEINFELD, *Brain Research* (1984),[2870] studied the effect of PHT on acetylcholine release from rat brain synaptosomes. PHT (200 μM) reduced the depolarization-dependent release of ACh in media containing 1.0 mM calcium and 56 mM potassium-chloride. PHT increased ACh release in non-depolarized synaptosomes, irrespective of calcium concentration. PHT did not affect release of ACh from depolarized synaptosomes in calcium-free media.

The authors note that PHT has two effects. By limiting sodium-calcium exchange, it increases calcium concentration intracellularly, leading to an increase in spontaneous ACh release. By interfering with calcium uptake at the synaptosomal membrane during depolarization, PHT decreases depolarization-linked ACh release.

MILLER AND RICHTER, *British Journal of Pharmacology* (1985),[2795] reported that PHT, administered intraperitoneally prior to preparation of synaptosomes, increased high-affinity choline uptake (20–48%) in mouse hippocampal synaptosomes. This was in contrast to barbiturates, which inhibited choline uptake, and to carbamazepine, which had no effect.

Serotonin, Norepinephrine and Dopamine

Serotonin (5-HT) and norepinephrine (NE) levels in mouse brain were reported not to be affected by PHT (P'AN,

FUNDERBURK AND FINGER, 1961).[510] BONNYCASTLE, PAASONEN AND GIARMAN (1956)[575] and BONNYCASTLE, BONNYCASTLE AND ANDERSON (1962)[573] found that PHT significantly increased the concentration of serotonin in brain. By fluoroassay, PHT at 50 mg/kg produced a 32.7% elevation of brain serotonin in 30 minutes. This was similar to the effect produced by pentobarbital (31.5%), but less than that produced by harmaline (58.1%). FRANCIS AND MELVILLE (1959)[629] confirmed the increase of brain serotonin by PHT in the ferret.

The inhibition by reserpine of the effect of PHT on serotonin as reported by CHEN AND ENSOR (1954)[463] and confirmed by GRAY, RAUH AND SHANAHAN (1963),[545] is apparently not due to brain amine depletion (RUDZIK AND MENNEAR, 1965).[448]

CHASE, KATZ AND KOPIN, *Transactions of the American Neurological Association* (1969),[2161] observed that PHT produces concentrations of serotonin significantly above control levels in rat brain.

HADFIELD, *Archives of Neurology* (1972),[1109] studied the effect of PHT (1–100 μM) on the uptake and binding of norepinephrine and dopamine in rat brain synaptosomes and in brain slices. Different effects of PHT were observed depending on whether the preparations were anoxic or well-oxygenated. In anoxic synaptosome preparations PHT stimulated the uptake of norepinephrine, whereas in oxygenated preparations PHT reduced the uptake of norepinephrine.

PINCUS AND LEE, *Archives of Neurology* (1973),[1417] reported that PHT (100 μM) decreased potassium-stimulated, calcium-dependent release of norepinephrine from rat brain slices. PHT also reduced calcium uptake.

HADFIELD AND BOYKIN, *Research Communication on Chemistry, Pathology and Pharmacology* (1974),[1108] studied the effect of PHT, administered orally and intraperitoneally for fourteen days, on [³H]-norepinephrine uptake by isolated rat brain synaptosomes.

The authors observed that PHT stimulated the uptake of norepinephrine when the medium was anoxic. They note that these *in vivo* results are confirmatory of their earlier *in vitro* results in which PHT was added directly to the isolated synaptosomes.[1109]

The authors conclude that this provides further evidence for the regulatory effect of PHT on uptake, storage and release of neurotransmitters in brain.

LEW, *Proceedings of the Society of Experimental Biology and Medicine* (1975),[1282] found that PHT increased the concentration of norepinephrine in the hypothalamus, cerebellum and brainstem in a strain of naturally hypertensive rats.

The author notes that a deficiency of norepinephrine in the hypothalamus has been reported with hypertension.

HADFIELD AND WEBER, *Biochemical Pharmacology* (1975),[1875] in a study of fighting mice and non-fighting mice, found that the uptake of [³H]-norepinephrine was increased by fighting. PHT (100 μM) significantly decreased this uptake. The authors state that inhibition of norepinephrine uptake may explain PHT's effect on aggressive behavior in animals and humans.

HADFIELD AND RIGBY, *Biochemical Pharmacology* (1976),[1874] measured [³H]-dopamine uptake in striatal synaptosomes from fighting mice. They found that intense fighting produced virtually instantaneous increases in dopamine uptake and that PHT (100 μM) inhibited this uptake.

FRY AND CIARLONE, *Neuropharmacology* (1981),[2191] studied cerebellar levels of serotonin and norepinephrine, two to twenty-eight hours after a single intraperitoneal PHT injection in mice. PHT (20 mg/kg) increased levels of both norepinephrine and serotonin by up to 22%, with increases observed as early as four hours. Elevated levels were also seen at twenty-eight hours.

The authors suggest that the PHT may in part regulate hyperexcitability in the nervous system by increasing the levels of these inhibitory neurotransmitters in the cerebellum, thereby enhancing the effects of cerebellar inhibition on other brain regions. (See also Ref. 1839.)

QUATTRONE, CRUNELLI, AND SAMANIN, *Neuropharmacology* (1978),[2886] evaluated the possible involvement of neurotransmitters in the control of hyperexcitability in the rat central nervous system by PHT, phenobarbital and carbamazepine. Brain levels of norepinephrine and serotonin were selectively lowered, using 6-hydroxydopamine and raphe lesions, respectively, prior to measuring seizure threshold and PHT's antiseizure effects.

The authors found that lowered norepinephrine levels reduced seizure threshold and lessened PHT's effects. PHT's antiseizure actions, however, were less affected than those of phenobarbital and carbamazepine.

Raphe lesions, which were used to lower brain serotonin levels, did not change seizure threshold or alter the effectiveness of any of the drugs.

DE BOER, STOFF AND VAN DUIJN, *Brain Research* (1982),[2436] reported the effects of PHT and other drugs on potassium-induced presynaptic release of norepinephrine, serotonin, acetylcholine, GABA and glutamate in rat cortical slices. PHT reduced the release of norepinephrine and serotonin at concentrations as low as 8–20 μM. GABA and glutamate release was affected only at higher concentrations of PHT (100–200 μM). Acetylcholine release was not affected by doses up to 200 μM in these experiments.

While diazepam and sodium valproate had little effect on neurotransmitter release, phenobarbital and pentobarbital, especially at high concentrations, reduced release of all neurotransmitters. At concentrations which cause neuronal hyperexcitability, penicillin and pentylenetetrazol increased release of the excitatory neurotransmitter glutamate.

The authors suggest that PHT's ability to regulate neurotransmitter release is important in its effects on hyperexcitability and stress that these effects may be more prominent in abnormal membrane states.

MATSUMOTO, HIRAMATSU AND MORI, *IRCS Medical Science* (1983),[2771] evaluated the effects of PHT (40 mg/kg intraperitoneally for three days) on serotonin levels in the forebrain and cerebellum of mice with a hereditary susceptibility to seizures. PHT increased the levels of serotonin at both sites and completely prevented stimulation-provoked seizures.

MATSUMOTO, HIRAMATSU AND MORI, *Neurosciences* (1984),[2772] evaluated the effects of fourteen-day treatment of mice with intraperitoneal PHT (40 mg/kg) on brain norepinephrine, dopamine, and serotonin. Levels of norepinephrine and dopamine in the cerebrum increased from the first day, attaining a maximum on the fifth and sixth day (20–40% higher) and then decreased to above-baseline levels, which were constant from the seventh to the fourteenth day. The serotonin levels attained a maximum on the fourth day (30% above normal) and then decreased to constant above-baseline levels from the fifth to the fourteenth day.

Levels of norepinephrine and dopamine in the cerebellum attained a maximum on the third day.

PRATT, JENNER AND MARSDEN, *Neuropharmacology* (1985),[2881] found that PHT (40 mg/kg and above, 1.5 hours prior to measurements) caused a dose-related elevation of serotonin, 5-hydroxyindoleacetic acid (5-HIAA), and tryptophan in mouse brain. Their studies indicated that PHT did not affect synthesis, but rather decreased utilization of serotonin.

See also Refs. 1789, 2086, 2329, 2554, 2624, 2685, 2703.

Gamma-aminobutyric Acid (GABA)

VERNADAKIS AND WOODBURY, *Inhibitions of the Nervous System and Gamma-aminobutyric Acid* (1960),[532] demonstrated that PHT enhanced the conversion of free glutamic acid to glutamine and GABA in rat brain. This was in contrast to the effect of cortisol, which shunted free glutamic acid to the Krebs cycle and away from glutamine and GABA.

BHATTACHARYA, KISHOR, SAXENA AND BHARGAVA, *Archives Internationales de Pharmacodynamie et de Therapie* (1964),[522] demonstrated that PHT increased brain GABA in mice.

VERSTER, GAROUTTE, ICHINOSA AND GUERRERO-FIGUEROA, *Federation Proceedings* (1965),[454] observed that the uptake of [14C]-GABA by mouse brain was increased by 35% with PHT.

SAAD, EL MASRY AND SCOTT, *Communications in Behavioral Biology* (1972), [1495] studied the effect of PHT on the GABA content of normal mouse cerebral hemispheres and of cerebral hemispheres depleted of GABA. PHT (25–50 mg/kg) increased normal cerebral hemisphere GABA, and also increased cerebral hemisphere concentrations of GABA which had been previously reduced by isoniazid.

WEINBERGER, NICKLAS AND BERL, *Neurology* (1976),[2115] demonstrated in rat brain synaptosomes that PHT and pentobarbital facilitated glutamate uptake. However, PHT (10–100 µM) facilitated GABA uptake to a lesser extent than pentobarbital. The authors suggest that these differences of action may relate to PHT's lack of hypnotic effect.

AYALA, JOHNSTON, LIN AND DICHTER, *Brain Research* (1977),[1732] observed that PHT (25–200 µM) increases and prolongs GABA-mediated postsynaptic conductance in the crayfish stretch receptor.

DEISZ AND LUX, *Neuroscience Letters* (1977),[1794] and AICKIN, DEISZ AND LUX, *Journal of Physiology* (1978),[1716] found that PHT (as low as .001 µM) increased inhibitory synaptic conductance and prolonged inhibitory postsynaptic potentials of crayfish stretch receptor neurons. The authors conclude that PHT decreases the rate of closing of the GABA-activated chloride channel, thereby enhancing inhibition.

TUNNICLIFF, SMITH, AND NGO, *Biochemical and Biophysical Research Communications* (1979),[3031] found that PHT (10 µM) competitively inhibited the binding of [3H]-diazepam to rat cerebral cortex synaptic membranes. GABA increased the binding affinity of both drugs three- to four-fold.

From their data, the authors suggest that PHT and diazepam bind at the same GABA-related site and that PHT's ability to reduce neuronal hyperexcitability may be related to this effect.

ESSMAN AND ESSMAN, *Brain Research Bulletin* (1980),[2482] studied the effects of PHT, pentobarbital and diazepam (all at 100 μM) on GABA uptake by synaptosomes isolated from different rat brain regions in resting and post-convulsion states.

In the resting state, all three agents significantly increased GABA uptake by cerebral cortical nerve endings (74%), but decreased uptake in hippocampal synaptosomes. Only pentobarbital increased cerebellar synaptosome GABA uptake (28%).

In the post-convulsion state, GABA uptake was decreased in the cerebral synaptosomes and increased in the hippocampal synaptosomes by all three agents.

GALLAGHER, MALLORGA AND TALLMAN, *Brain Research* (1980),[2518] using extracellular unit recording and microionotophoretic techniques in rat brain, found that PHT enhanced benzodiazepine inhibition of neuronal firing. This increased effect correlated with enhanced specific binding of benzodiazepines due to an increase in the total number of binding sites in animals pretreated with intraperitoneal PHT (100 mg/kg) sixty minutes before testing. The effects of PHT on benzodiazepine binding were different from, and independent of, those of GABA. (See also Refs. 2519, 2520.)

ADAMS, CONSTANTI AND BANKS, *Federation Proceedings* (1981),[2274] studying the effects of GABA and inhibitory nerve cells on crayfish abdominal stretch receptor neurons, found that inhibitory postsynaptic current decay was prolonged by PHT (50 μM). They suggest that PHT slows the closing of channels opened by GABA, thus augmenting GABA's effect.

PATSALOS AND LASCELLES, *Journal of Neurochemistry* (1981),[2851] studied the effects of ten-day PHT treatment (50 mg/kg) on rat regional brain concentrations of GABA, glutamate, aspartate, and taurine in rats. PHT reduced cerebellar GABA, taurine and aspartate, and hypothalamic GABA and aspartate. Of the other agents tested, sodium valproate raised GABA and taurine, and phenobarbital raised GABA, in most brain regions.

BOWLING AND DELORENZO, *Science* (1982),[2351] reported PHT binding to micromolar affinity benzodiazepine receptors present in rat brain membrane. PHT, in therapeutic concentrations, exhibited specific, saturable membrane binding, which could be displaced by diazepam. This binding affinity was not significantly influenced by GABA or muscimol, a GABA agonist. The authors suggest that this receptor is important to the actions of both PHT and diazepam in reducing abnormal neuronal hyperexcitability. (See also Ref. 2350.)

CZUCZWAR, TURSKI AND KLEINROK, *Neuropharmacology* (1982),[2421] reported that PHT (8 mg/kg), intraperitoneally, potentiated the antipentylenetetrazol activity of clonazepam and nitrazepam in mice. The authors suggest that a PHT-induced increase in the number of benzodiazepine receptors accounts for this effect.

DE BELLEROCHE, DICK AND WYRLEY-BIRCH, *Life Sciences* (1982),[2435] found that PHT, diazepam, clonazepam and phenobarbital inhibited potassium-stimulated, but not resting, [^{14}C]-GABA release from tissue slices of rat cerebral cortex. Carbamazepine, at concentrations up to 100 μM, had no effect.

FILE AND LISTER, *Neuroscience Letters* (1983),[2493] found that, in rats, PHT (10 mg/kg) reversed the anxiogenic and convulsant effects of Ro 5-4864, a selective ligand for benzodiazepine micromolar receptors. The authors suggest that PHT has actions at central nervous system micromolar receptors.

POZDEEV, *Mediator Processes in Epilepsy* (1983),[2878] studied the effects of PHT (37.5–125 mg/kg), twice a day for three to seven days, on brain neurotransmitter systems. Whole brain analysis of rats treated with 37.5 mg/kg intraperitoneally for seven days showed increased levels of taurine (48%), glutamate (18%), glycine (63%), and aspartate (21%). GABA levels decreased by 15% and glutamic acid decarboxylase and GABA-transferase activities increased by 27% and 32% respectively. The author notes that animals treated with PHT at this dosage appeared well and their motor activity and appetite increased.

At higher dosage levels (for example, 75 mg/kg twice a day for three days), where there was evidence of toxicity, taurine levels decreased 50%; GABA levels increased by 11% with evidence of inhibition of GABAergic systems; glutamate levels increased 20%; and the metabolic inactivation of glutamate was decreased. Serotonergic and glycinergic systems showed increased activity. In some animals the neurotransmitter systems returned to normal with continued treatment.

The author concludes that PHT's effects cannot be explained by an influence on a single neurotransmitter, but rather by alterations in the balance of excitatory and inhibitory neurotransmitter systems.

SKERRITT AND JOHNSTON, *Clinical and Experimental Pharmacology and Physiology* (1983),[2961] evaluated the *in vitro* effects of phenobarbital, carbamazepine and PHT on potassium-stimulated release of [^{14}C]-GABA and D-aspartate from slices of rat cerebral cortex. PHT (25–200 μM) and phenobarbital, but not carbamazepine, selectively inhibited the release of the excitatory amino acid D-aspartate. There was also some inhibition of GABA release, but it was less than that for D-aspartate.

The authors note that interactions with both sodium and calcium appear necessary for PHT's effects.

MACDONALD, MCLEAN AND SKERRITT, *Federation Proceedings* (1985),[2747] reported that, at concentrations achieved in human cerebrospinal fluid, PHT, carbamazepine and valproic acid limited sustained repetitive firing, but did not alter postsynaptic GABA responses in primary dissociated cultures of mouse neurons. The barbiturates and benzodiazepines, on the other hand, increased postsynaptic GABA responses.

The authors conclude that PHT's primary effect in mouse spinal cord neurons is on repetitive firing, rather than postsynaptic GABA response.

See also Refs. 1780, 2273, 2307, 2389, 2399, 2494, 2645, 2670, 2686, 2745, 2748, 2797, 2798, 2864, 2921, 2954, 3004, 3046.

Excitatory Amino Acids

VERNADAKIS AND WOODBURY, *Inhibitions of the Nervous System and Gamma-aminobutyric Acid* (1960),[532] demonstrated that PHT enhanced the conversion of free glutamic acid to glutamine and GABA in rat brain.

PATSALOS AND LASCELLES, *Journal of Neurochemistry* (1981),[2851] reported that PHT (50 mg/kg), daily for ten days, reduced rat cerebellar and hypothalamic aspartate levels.

STONE, *Advances in Biochemical Psychopharmacology* (1981),[2983] reported that PHT reduced the response of rat somatosensory cortical neurons to iontophoretically applied glutamate and aspartate, but not acetylcholine.

GANKINA, AVDULOV AND MAISOV, *Farmakologiia i Toksikologiia* (1982),[2524] found that PHT stimulated glutamate uptake by rat brain synaptosomes, but only at very high concentrations (500 μM).

SKERRITT AND JOHNSTON, *Clinical and Experimental Pharmacology and Physiology* (1983),[2961] reported that PHT (25–200 μM) significantly inhibited potassium-evoked release of D-aspartate, in rat brain slices, which is consistent with its actions in reducing abnormal hyperexcitability. (See also Ref. 2962.)

STONE AND JAVID, *Brain Research* (1983),[2984] reported that PHT (40 mg/kg) was effective in preventing glutamate-induced seizures in mice. The authors suggest that PHT may act by reducing glutaminergic transmission.

BECHTEREVA, NIKITINA, ILIUCHINA, DAMBINOVA AND DENISOVA, *European Journal of Clinical Investigation* (1984),[2316] demonstrated the inhibitory effect of PHT on glutamate receptors in a cortical synaptic membrane preparation and suggest that this is an important mechanism by which PHT regulates neuronal excitability.

Taurine

BASKIN, LEIBMAN, DE WITT, ORR, TARZY, LEVY, KRUSZ, DHOPESH AND SCHRAEDER, *Neurology* (1978)[1735] examined platelet taurine levels, as a model for nerve-ending biochemistry, in epileptic patients. Patients whose seizures were controlled by PHT had significantly higher platelet taurine levels than patients not receiving PHT.

BASKIN AND FINNEY, *The Effects of Taurine on Excitable Tissues* (1981),[2152] studied the effect of PHT on taurine concentrations in the rat brain. They found that PHT (25 mg/kg), one hour prior to measurement, increased cerebellar, brainstem and cerebral taurine. At 50 mg/kg PHT and above, there was reduction in taurine levels.

The authors suggest that PHT exerts its therapeutic effect by increasing endogenous taurine levels.

POZDEEV, *Mediator Processes in Epilepsy* (1983),[2878] studied the effects of PHT on rat brain neurotransmitter systems. Whole brain analysis of rats treated with PHT, 37.5 mg/kg twice a day, intraperitoneally, for seven days, showed increased levels of taurine (48%).

Treatment with PHT, 75 mg/kg twice a day for three days, which led to toxicity in some animals, decreased taurine levels (50%). Taurine levels normalized in these animals with continued PHT treatment.

GUREVICH, MATVEEVA, OGURECHNIKOV AND KOROVKINA, *Farmakologiia i Toksikologiia* (1984),[2562] found that PHT increased incorporation of [14C]-taurine by rat cerebral cortex microsomes, suggesting the importance of PHT's effects on intracellular membranes. The greatest effect (doubling of incorporation) was seen at 400 μM PHT. Higher doses were inhibitory.

PHT (200 μM) increased [14C]-taurine uptake in cultured C1300 neuroblastoma cells. PHT had no effects on [14C]-glycine incorporation. Phenobarbital had no effects on either taurine or glycine incorporation.

The authors suggest that PHT's effects on taurine may be important in its modulation of nervous system hyperexcitability.

IZUMI, KISHITA, NAKAGAWA, HUXTABLE, SHIMIZU, KOJA AND FUKUDA, *Progress in Clinical and Biological Research* (1985),[2614] reported that treatment of mice with 1% guanidinoethane sulfonate for nine days lowered taurine levels by 24%. Under these circumstances, the effectiveness of PHT and phenobarbital against maximal electroshock seizures was less.

See also Refs. 2513, 2615, 2786, 2851.

Endorphin

LASON, PRZEWLOCKA AND PRZEWLOCKI, *Life Sciences* (1985), [2691] studied the effects of a group of substances, including PHT, on beta-endorphin and dynorphin levels in rat hypothalamus, pituitary, hippocampus and thalamus. PHT (10 mg/kg) decreased the concentrations of beta-endorphin, but not dynorphin, in the hypothalamus.

The authors suggest that the release of beta-endorphin induced by low doses of PHT may account for its therapeutic effects in affective disorders.

Adenosine

LEWIN AND BLECK, *Epilepsia* (1981), [2716] reported that, in mice, PHT (100 mg) intraperitoneally, ten minutes prior to convulsive electroshock, markedly reduced the seizure-induced rise in brain inosine and hypoxanthine, two metabolites of adenosine. The rise in adenosine resulting from a series of subconvulsive shocks was also reduced by PHT.

PHILLIS AND WU, *Comparative Biochemistry and Physiology* (1982), [2869] showed that PHT inhibited adenosine uptake by rat brain synaptosomes. PHT reduced this uptake by 20% at 1.5 μM and 50% at 200 μM. Phenobarbital and carbamazepine also inhibited adenosine uptake, but weakly.

The authors propose that PHT corrects abnormal neuronal hyperexcitability by inhibiting uptake, and increasing extracellular levels, of adenosine.

BERNARD, WILSON, PASTOR, BROWN AND GLENN, *Pharmacologist* (1983), [2324] noting

that PHT, as well as carbamazepine and phenobarbital, inhibit the binding of [³H]-phenylisopropyladenosine to rat brain membranes, reported that the adenosine antagonists, theophylline and caffeine, reduced the protective effects of PHT against maximal electroshock seizures in mice. The authors suggest that PHT may achieve some of its effects on neuronal hyperexcitability through adenosine receptors.

Cyclic AMP and GMP

THAMPI, MADER AND EARLEY, *Pharmacologist* (1974), [2103] demonstrated that PHT (5–15 μg/ml) produces an increase in cyclic AMP and a corresponding decrease in cyclic GMP in rat brain synaptosomes.

PULL AND McILWAIN, *Biochemical Pharmacology* (1975), [2027] observed that PHT (300 μM) decreased by 20% release of adenine derivatives, including adenosine, from electrically-stimulated guinea pig neocortical tissues. In unstimulated tissue, PHT increased the adenine derivative output. The authors suggest that PHT's inhibition of adenosine release reduces the rise in cyclic AMP caused by electric stimulation.

LEWIN AND BLECK, *Epilepsia* (1977), [1958] noting that increased cyclic AMP may have a role in abnormal neuronal excitability, demonstrated that PHT (300 μM) reduced the increase in cyclic AMP produced by the depolarizing agent ouabain, in rat brain cortex slices. The authors suggest that PHT reduces the increase in cyclic AMP by inhibiting stimulated adenosine release.

LEWIN, *Epilepsia* (1977), [1957] demonstrated that PHT significantly reduced the increase in release of adenine derivatives induced by depolarizing agents ouabain and veratridine in rat brain cortex slices, human astrocytoma cell cultures and mouse neuroblastoma cell cultures.

Ferrendelli and Kinscherf, *Epilepsia* (1977),[1830] demonstrated, in mouse cerebral cortex and cerebellum slices, that PHT (10–25 μg/ml) inhibited both ouabain- and veratridine-induced increases in cyclic AMP and cyclic GMP. Resting levels of cyclic AMP and cyclic GMP were not affected.

Dretchen, Standaert and Raines, *Epilepsia* (1977),[1811] evaluated the effects of PHT on the motor nerve terminal of an *in vivo* cat soleus nerve-muscle preparation. PHT, 10 mg/kg, reduced the repetitive afterdischarges in motor nerve endings due to tetanic conditioning. It also reduced the repetitive activity due to adenylate cyclase activation with sodium fluoride, or to exogenous dibutyryl cyclic AMP.

Lust, Kupferberg, Yonekawa, Penry, Passonneau and Wheaton, *Molecular Pharmacology* (1978), [1969] demonstrated, in mice, that PHT (25 mg/kg) decreases the cerebellar cyclic AMP increase induced by electroshock.

McCandless, Feusner, Lust and Passonneau, *Journal of Neurochemistry* (1979),[2229] found that PHT (25 mg/kg), administered twenty-five minutes prior to electroshock, protected mouse cerebellum from seizure-induced decreases in energy compounds and increases in cyclic AMP and cyclic GMP.

Palmer, Jones, Medina, Palmer and Stavinoha, *Epilepsia* (1979),[2013] observed that pretreatment with PHT (75 mg/kg) prevents the rise in cyclic AMP in mouse cerebrum and cerebellum following injection with pentylenetetrazol.

In mouse cerebral cortex slices, PHT reduced the increase in cyclic AMP induced by norepinephrine, adenosine and ouabain.

Ferrendelli, *Antiepileptic Drugs: Mechanisms of Action* (1980),[1828] reported that, in mouse cerebral cortex slices, PHT prevented cyclic AMP and cyclic GMP increases induced by ouabain or veratridine depolarization, but not potassium- or glutamate-induced depolarization. This inhibitory effect of PHT was dose-dependent, significant at 10 μg/ml.

In *in vivo* studies, PHT (25 mg/kg) produced a 50% reduction of basal cyclic GMP levels, but not cyclic AMP levels, in mouse cerebellum. In the cerebral cortex, striatum, thalamus and hippocampus, cyclic GMP and cyclic AMP were unchanged.

The authors suggest that these cyclic nucleotide changes produced by PHT relate to its regulatory effect on sodium channels.

Folbergrova, *Neuroscience Letters* (1980),[2502] reported that the administration of PHT (30 mg/kg) intraperitoneally, thirty minutes prior to seizure induction, markedly reduced the rise in cyclic AMP, but not cyclic GMP, in the cerebral cortex of mice during seizures induced by 3-mercaptopropionic acid.

Study, *The Journal of Pharmacology and Experimental Therapeutics* (1980),[2093] demonstrated that PHT (3–300 μM, half-maximal effect at 40 μM) inhibited calcium-dependent increases in cyclic GMP produced by potassium depolarization or muscarinic receptor activation in N1E-115 neuroblastoma cells. These results suggest that PHT inhibited the cyclic GMP increase by blocking calcium influx.

See also Refs. 1829, 1831, 2236, 2341, 2627, 2628, 2743, 2834.

Calmodulin

DeLorenzo, Emple and Glaser, *Journal of Neurochemistry* (1977),[2169] reported that therapeutic concentrations of PHT decreased the level of phosphorylation of two specific proteins present in rat brain synaptosomal preparations. The authors suggest that some of the stabilizing actions of PHT on neuronal tissue, including its inhibition of post-tetanic potentiation, may be due to its effect on synaptosomal protein phosphorylation.

DeLorenzo, *Antiepileptic Drugs: Mechanisms of Action* (1980),[1799] demonstrated that PHT, in therapeutic concentrations, inhibited the effects of calcium on calmodulin-dependent norepinephrine release, as well as phosphorylation of synaptic vesicle-associated proteins. Carbamazepine also inhibited neurotransmitter release and protein phosphorylation, but phenobarbital had no effect.

Lazarev, Chernokhvostov, Kokoz, Freydin, Kosarsky and Saxon, *Advances in Myocardiology* (1982),[2694] reported that PHT (5 μM) inhibited calcium activation of the inward rectifying potassium channels in frog atrium. The authors suggest that PHT's effect is due to inhibition of calcium-calmodulin-mediated protein phosphorylation.

DeLorenzo, *Annals of Neurology* (1984),[2441] reviewing and extending the study of calmodulin systems, reported that PHT, carbamazepine and the benzodiazepines all inhibit calcium-calmodulin regulated protein phosphorylation and neurotransmitter release through a common binding site.

The author suggests that calmodulin-mediated processes play a role in the development of abnormal excitability and that PHT and the other agents tested control hyperexcitability, including post-tetanic potentiation, by regulating these processes.

See also Refs. 2367, 2368, 2439, 2440.

METABOLIC AND ENDOCRINE
REGULATORY EFFECTS OF PHT

Carbohydrate Metabolism

LEVIN, BOOKER, SMITH AND GRODSKY, *Journal of Clinical Endocrinology and Metabolism* (1970),[1269] studied the effect of PHT on insulin secretion by the isolated perfused rat pancreas. PHT (300 μM) completely inhibited immunoreactive insulin release in response to a glucose stimulus.

KIZER, VARGAS-CORDON, BRENDEL AND BRESSLER, *Journal of Clinical Investigation* (1970),[1220] studied the effect of PHT on the secretion of insulin *in vitro* by isolated islets of Langerhans and 5-mg pieces of pancreatic tissue. PHT (30–160 μM) reduced the release of insulin in a dose-dependent manner. The effect was reversed by potassium and ouabain.

BIHLER AND SAWH, *Biochimica et Biophysica Acta* (1971),[1750] in a study of rat hemidiaphragm *in vitro,* demonstrated that PHT (100–500 μM) has a regulatory effect on sugar transport. The transport of the nonmetabolized glucose analog 3-0-methyl-D-(^{14}C)-glucose was inhibited by PHT when internal potassium was increased and sodium decreased. Conversely, sugar transport was stimulated by PHT following the opposite ionic changes.

GOSSEL AND MENNEAR, *Pharmacologist* (1971),[1092] studied the effect of pretreatment with PHT on the development of alloxan-induced diabetes in mice. PHT (20–45 mg/kg), administered one hour prior to alloxan, was found to prevent the development of alloxan-induced diabetes.

The authors note that the work of others [1220,1269] indicates that PHT has a regulatory effect on insulin secretion by the isolated pancreas and suggest that PHT binds to, and exerts a selective action on, these pancreatic cells. The authors conclude that PHT protects the pancreatic beta-cell binding sites from alloxan.

LEVIN, GRODSKY, HAGURA, SMITH, LICKO AND FORSHAM, *Clinical Research* (1972),[1272] and *Diabetes* (1972),[1273] studied the kinetics of PHT's regulation of insulin secretion in isolated perfused pancreas.

The authors conclude that PHT exerts its regulatory effect both on the labile compartment of insulin and on the supply of insulin to this compartment prior to secretion.

GERICH, CHARLES, LEVIN, FORSHAM AND GRODSKY, *Journal of Clinical Endocrinology* (1972),[1062] studied the effect of PHT on glucagon secretion in the isolated perfused rat pancreas. At 25 μg/ml, PHT markedly diminished glucagon release and had no effect on insulin release.

The authors note that this selective action of PHT in controlling glucagon release presumably reflects the special sensitivity to PHT of the alpha cells of the pancreas as compared with the beta cells. Since glucagon and insulin act in an opposite manner in the control of blood sugar, PHT's influence on the release of both hormones means that it has at least two potential regulatory actions on blood sugar.

KARP, LERMAN, DORON AND LARON, *Helvetica Paediatrie Acta* (1973),[2646] investigated glucose and insulin response in eight epileptic children treated for three to eight years with PHT (200–300 mg/day). Glucose tolerance was normal in all, but insulin responses were slightly altered: three patients had lowered, and three had delayed insulin peaks.

MENNEAR AND GOSSEL, *Toxicology and Applied Pharmacology* (1973),[1355] studied the effect of PHT (5 mg/kg), administered intraperitoneally, on blood glucose levels in normally fed mice. PHT did not alter resting blood glucose levels, but did reduce glucose tolerance. PHT did not interfere with the hypoglycemic effect of injected insulin, but reversed the hypoglycemic effect of tolbutamide.

ESPOSITO-AVELLA AND MENNEAR, *Proceedings of the Society of Experimental Biology and Medicine* (1973),[1015] studied the protective effect of PHT against alloxan-induced diabetes in mice. The authors found that both PHT (10–45 mg/kg), administered intraperitoneally, and D-glucose administered intravenously afforded complete protection against alloxan. The authors conclude that both D-glucose and PHT exert their protective effects by binding to the pancreatic beta-cell.

SCHIMMEL AND GRAHAM, *Hormone and Metabolic Research* (1974),[1509] studied the protective effect of PHT against streptozotocin-induced diabetes in rats. Intravenous injection of PHT, 20 mg/kg, nineteen minutes prior to or within sixty minutes after administration of streptozotocin, was found to prevent the development of diabetes.

STAMBAUGH AND TUCKER, *Diabetes* (1974),[1583] describe the successful treatment, with PHT, of five patients with functional hypoglycemia previously unresponsive to dietary management.

Clinical reversal of hypoglycemia was observed in all five cases. In addition, laboratory tests confirmed this observation in both six-hour glucose tolerance and insulin level tests, performed before and after PHT therapy. (See p. 11.)

CUDWORTH AND CUNNINGHAM, *Clinical Science and Molecular Medicine* (1974),[924] studied glucose tolerance tests, serum insulin, and growth hormone levels in healthy volunteers before and after receiving PHT, 100 mg every eight hours, for fourteen days. Although the response of insulin to oral glucose was reduced in some individuals, glucose tolerance remained normal. No changes in growth hormone levels were observed.

MADSEN, HANSEN AND DECKERT, *Acta Neurologica Scandanavica* (1974),[1327] investigated intravenous glucose tolerance in eight patients before and during treatment with PHT. They found that neither glucose tolerance nor insulin secretion was affected after a glucose load. In eight additional patients, who had for several years been treated with PHT, the results were comparable.

PETRACK, CZERNIK, ITTERLY, ANSELL AND CHERTOCK, *Diabetes* (1976),[2022] demonstrated that PHT (2.7 µg/ml) suppressed the second-phase release of both insulin and glucagon from isolated perfused rat pancreas. The authors suggest that PHT might therefore suppress glucagon secretion in insulin-dependent juvenile diabetics.

CALLAGHAN, FEELY, O'CALLAGHAN, DUGGAN, McGARRY, CRAMER, WHEELAN AND SELDRUP, *Acta Neurologica Scandinavica* (1977),[1762] demonstrated that non-toxic levels of PHT do not disturb carbohydrate tolerance or insulin levels in epileptic patients.

DRAZNIN, AYALON, HOERER, OBERMAN, HARELL, RAVID AND LAURIAN, *Acta Diabetologica Latina* (1977),[1809] demonstrated that PHT (300 mg/day, for three days) significantly decreased insulin release after glucose ingestion, but did not alter the basal insulin level in obese patients.

Because a secondary hyperinsulinemia has been suggested to play an important role in the pathogenesis of obesity, PHT is proposed as a possible treatment for this condition.

PACE AND LIVINGSTON, *Diabetes* (1979),[2011] studied the effects of PHT on insulin release and metabolism of isolated rat islets of Langerhans. Glucose and veratridine were used to stimulate insulin release by activating the calcium and sodium channels. PHT (100 μM) inhibited glucose-stimulated insulin release (77%) and glycolysis (74%). PHT also inhibited veratridine-stimulated insulin release (60%) and glycolysis (100%). When extracellular calcium was raised from 2.5 to 5.0 mM, PHT's effects were less.

Noting that PHT has been reported to hyperpolarize the beta-cell membrane and to inhibit glucose-induced spike activity, the authors conclude that the inhibitory action of PHT on the pancreatic beta-cell is due to its regulatory effect on sodium and calcium channels.

HERCHUELZ, LEBRUN, SENER AND MALAISSE, *European Journal of Pharmacology* (1981),[2589] investigated the mechanism by which PHT inhibits glucose-stimulated insulin release by studying its effects on calcium and rubidium fluxes in isolated pancreatic islets.

PHT inhibited both basal and glucose-stimulated calcium uptake by islet cells and markedly reduced the secondary rise in calcium efflux normally provoked by glucose. PHT also decreased the calcium exchange evoked by an increase in extracellular calcium concentration. Rubidium uptake was not affected, indicating that PHT's effects on insulin release were not attributable to activation of sodium-potassium-ATPase.

The authors conclude that PHT inhibits glucose-induced insulin release by limiting calcium entry into islet cells.

SIEGEL, JANJIC AND WOLLHEIM, *Diabetes* (1982),[2952] studied the inhibition of insulin release by PHT in rat pancreatic islet culture. PHT (80 μM), added during the second phase of glucose-induced biphasic insulin release, resulted in marked and rapid inhibition. PHT also significantly reduced glucose-induced calcium uptake of islet cells.

The authors suggest that PHT inhibits glucose-stimulated insulin release by regulating voltage-dependent calcium channels.

Lipid Metabolism – HDL

HOUCK, JACOB AND MAENGWYN-DAVIES, *Journal of Clinical Investigation* (1960),[172] showed a decrease in dermal lipids in rats treated with PHT (25 mg/day, for two to sixteen days).

NAKAMURA AND MASUDA, *Archives Internationales de Pharmacodynamie et de Therapie* (1966),[265] demonstrated a marked decrease in dermal lipids (triglycerides, cholesterol and phospholipids) and a decrease in the conversion of [14C]-acetate into these compounds with PHT (50 mg/kg/day) for five weeks.

CHUNG, *Journal of Atherosclerosis Research* (1967),[56] studied the effect of PHT on aortic lipid concentrations. Daily oral administration of PHT (50 mg/day) to rabbits for thirty days resulted in significant reduction of aortic concentrations of cholesterol and phospholipids, and an increase in triglyceride concentration. No significant changes in concentrations of these lipids were noted in liver or plasma. These effects of PHT were not observed when an atherogenic diet was fed to the rabbits.

ARIYOSHI AND REMMER, *Naunyn-Schmiedeberg Archiv fur Pharmakologie* (1968),[529] found that, in rats, PHT (80 mg/kg, for six days) had a protective effect on the fatty infiltration of the liver produced by alcohol or a choline-free diet.

NIKKILA, KASTE, EHNHOLM AND VIIKARI, *Acta Medica Scandinavica* (1978),[2002] measured the serum high-density lipoproteins (HDL) and other lipoprotein and apolipoprotein A levels in twenty-eight epileptic patients who received PHT as their only medication and in forty-four healthy male and forty-nine female controls. The patients treated with PHT had significantly higher HDL levels than the controls.

The authors state that since serum HDL shows an inverse correlation with the risk of coronary heart disease, epileptic patients taking PHT may be protected from this disease.

LUOMA, SOTANIEMI, PELKONEN, AND MYLLYLA, *Scandinavian Journal of Clinical and Laboratory Investigation* (1980),[2740] studied plasma HDL-cholesterol (HDL-C) and hepatic cytochrome P-450 concentrations in eighteen epileptic patients (twelve on PHT alone, five on PHT plus other antiepileptics, and one on carbamazepine alone) who were undergoing diagnostic liver biopsy because of altered hepatic function.

Mean HDL-C levels and cytochrome P-450 concentrations were higher in the PHT-alone group than in controls, but not as high as those in the polytherapy group. Serum

triglyceride level was inversely related to the hepatic cytochrome P-450 content.

The authors conclude that increased plasma HDL-C levels in the treated patients correlate with drug-induced hepatic microsomal enzyme activity.

LUOMA, MYLLYLA, SOTANIEMI, LEHTINEN AND HOKKANEN, *European Neurology* (1980),[2734] compared HDL-C levels in forty-three normal subjects to those in ninety-seven patients on long-term therapy with PHT, carbamazepine and phenobarbital, alone or in combination. Thirty-eight patients on PHT alone and eleven on PHT plus phenobarbital had significantly higher HDL-C levels than controls. HDL-C to total cholesterol ratios were also increased. Patients on carbamazepine alone (twenty) did not show increased HDL-C levels.

NENCINI, *Pharmacological Research Communications* (1982),[2821] reported that PHT (10–100 µM) increased cyclic AMP levels and free fatty acid release under resting conditions, and with isoprenaline treatment, in rat brown adipose tissue. Ouabain, as well as lowered intracellular sodium and potassium, inhibited these effects.

LUOMA, SOTANIEMI AND ARRANTO, *Scandinavian Journal of Clinical Laboratory Investigation* (1983),[2739] utilizing antipyrine kinetics, evaluated the relationship between serum low-density and high-density lipoprotein-cholesterol and liver microsomal enzyme induction in thirty epileptics and thirty normal controls. All patients had been treated with PHT alone or in combination with phenobarbital and/or carbamazepine for at least two years.

The treated patients had higher HDL-C levels and higher HDL-C to total-cholesterol ratios than control subjects. LDL/HDL-C ratio was reduced, indicating a cholesterol transfer from LDL to HDL. Serum total-cholesterol, LDL-C and triglycerides, however, were the same in both groups. The antipyrine clearance rate, which served as a measure of microsomal enzyme induction, was enhanced two-fold in the treated group, as compared to the controls.

CHALMERS AND JOHNSON, *Journal of Neurology, Neurosurgery and Psychiatry* (1983),[2383] found that PHT (500 mg the evening prior to testing) increased exercise-induced free fatty acids, blood glycerol and total ketone concentrations.

The authors suggest that PHT enhances lipid breakdown after exercise.

MAGUIRE, MURTHY AND HALL, *European Journal of Pharmacology* (1985),[2757] reported that, in mice, administration of PHT and other hydantoins (20 mg/kg per day, intraperitoneally), for sixteen days, led to lower serum concentrations of cholesterol and triglycerides. The authors found that PHT and the other agents tested had significant hypolipidemic activity and were more effective than clofibrate in lowering serum cholesterol and triglycerides.

See also Clinical Cardiac section and Refs. 1968, 2282, 2319, 2323, 2652, 2732, 2733, 2741, 2742, 2946.

Pituitary-Adrenal Hormones

BONNYCASTLE AND BRADLEY, *Endocrinology* (1960),[520] found that pretreatment with PHT blocks the adrenal ascorbate depletion which follows unilateral adrenalectomy in rats. PHT also blocked intravenous vasopressin and subcutaneous epinephrine stimulation of adrenocorticotropic hormone (ACTH) release. The authors suggest the hypothalamus or pituitary as possible sites of inhibition of the release of ACTH.

KRIEGER, *Journal of Clinical Endocrinology and Metabolism* (1962),[198] found that

administration of PHT (300 mg/day), for one to two weeks, in eight normal volunteers, affected pituitary-adrenal function by reducing metyrapone-stimulated ACTH release. The effects of injected ACTH were unaffected by PHT.

OLIVER AND TROOP, *Steroids* (1963),[482] found that PHT (15 mg/kg), given to rats orally for twenty days, reduced the rise in plasma corticosterone levels produced by the stress of pentobarbital-induced anesthesia. The authors suggest that PHT diminishes the pituitary-adrenal response to this stress.

WERK, MacGEE AND SHOLITON, *Journal of Clinical Investigation* (1964),[377] in studies in man, found PHT (300–400 mg/day) caused a net increase in excretion of 6-hydroxycortisol and an unconjugated polar metabolite. There was also a relative decrease in conjugated tetrahydro derivatives.

HOUCK AND PATEL, *Nature* (1965),[171] demonstrated that PHT (25 mg/day, for two days) prevented loss of dermal collagen and release of collagenase induced by cortisol administration to young rats.

DILL, *Archives Internationales de Pharmacodynamie et de Therapie* (1966),[76] reported that PHT (100 mg/day) did not inhibit the initial elevation of the plasma level of corticosterone in rats stressed by laparotomy. However, PHT did reduce the duration of the effect.

RINNE, *Medicina et Pharmacologia Experimentalis* (1967),[303] found that patients on PHT released less ACTH in response to metyrapone than controls. The response of these patients to exogenous ACTH was normal and intravenous vasopressin caused normal release of ACTH from the pituitary gland.

The author suggests that PHT alters ACTH release by regulating hypothalamic function.

KUNTZMAN AND SOUTHREN, *Advances in Biochemical Psychopharmacology* (1969),[1240] demonstrated that the metabolism of cortisol in liver microsomes of guinea pigs was markedly increased by pretreatment with PHT (50–100 mg/kg, daily for four to ten days).

CHOI, THRASHER, WERK, SHOLITON AND OLINGER, *Journal of Pharmacology and Experimental Therapeutics* (1971),[896] studied the effect of PHT on the metabolism of injected radiolabeled cortisol in humans. PHT increased cortisol turnover kinetics, but did not affect normal plasma cortisol binding.

WERK, THRASHER, SHOLITON, OLINGER AND CHOI, *Clinical Pharmacology and Therapeutics* (1971),[1679] studied, for up to twenty-four months, cortisol production and metabolism in twenty-one patients with convulsive disorders, with and without PHT therapy.

During PHT therapy there was a positive correlation between cortisol secretion rates, measured by isotope dilution method, and an increase in urine ratio of 6-hydroxycortisol to 17-hydroxycorticosteroids. The cortisol secretion rate was found to increase significantly when the ratio of the hydroxycortisol to corticosteroids increased more than 0.14.

HAQUE, THRASHER, WERK, KNOWLES AND SHOLITON, *Journal of Clinical Endocrinology and Metabolism* (1972),[1128] found that PHT markedly increases the metabolism of dexamethasone in humans.

EVANS, WALKER, PETERS, DYAS, RIAD-FAHMY, THOMAS, RIMMER, TSANACLIS, AND SCANLON, *British Journal of Pharmacology* (1985),[2485] found that morning concentrations of cortisol in saliva and plasma of epileptic patients receiving PHT were the same as those observed in healthy volunteers not receiving PHT. However, cortisol half-life, as determined by an intravenous dexamethasone method, was significantly reduced in the PHT-treated patients. Because there was a correlation between the half-life of cortisol and antipyrine, the authors suggest that the reduced half-life of cortisol may relate to the degree of microsomal enzyme induction in PHT-treated patients.

The authors state that the normal morning levels of cortisol observed in PHT-treated patients, in spite of the reduced half-life, may be explained by increased cortisol secretion, which compensates for increased cortisol metabolism.

See also Refs. 171, 268, 451, 483, 486, 776, 964, 1351, 1480, 1627, 1678, 2382, 3053.

Pituitary-Thyroid Function

OPPENHEIMER, FISHER, NELSON AND JAILER, *Journal of Clinical Endocrinology and Metabolism* (1961),[276] observed lowered serum protein-bound iodine (PBI) levels in thirty-six patients receiving PHT. Despite the lowered PBI levels there was no clinical evidence of hypothyroidism in any of the patients. The authors found no evidence of a direct effect of PHT on the thyroid gland uptake or hormone synthesis. They suggest that PHT lowers serum PBI by interfering with the binding of thyroxine to plasma protein.

CANTU AND SCHWAB, *Archives of Neurology* (1966),[44] found that the administration of PHT (300–400 mg daily) to thirty-nine adult patients for two weeks was associated with reduction in PBI levels, but there was no change in normal thyroid function. Triiodothyronine (T_3) uptake by red blood cells and thyroid ^{131}I uptake were unchanged in the five patients in whom these were measured.

MENDOZA, FLOCK, OWEN AND PARIS (1966),[494] demonstrated that PHT increased metabolism of thyroxine (T_4) in rats. PHT also produced a decrease in concentration of PBI, although it did not alter the uptake of ^{131}I-T_3 from plasma by erythrocytes.

HEYMA, LARKINS, PERRY-KEENE, PETER, ROSS AND SLOMAN, Clinical Endocrinology (1977),[1898] in a randomized controlled trial of the effect of long-term PHT therapy, found that triiodothyronine (T_3) and thyrotropin concentrations were not affected by PHT. Thyroxine (T_4) concentrations were reduced. This appeared to be due to diminished protein binding and enhanced degradation of T_4.

The authors note that an increased rate of conversion of T_4 to T_3 may explain why patients on PHT seldom exhibit clinical features of hypothyroidism, even though T_4 concentrations may be low.

GINSBERG, CHEN AND WALFISH, Annals of Endocrinology (Paris) (1979),[2541] studied the effect of PHT on the rat hypothalamus-pituitary-thyroid system. In intact rats treated with PHT (5 mg/100 g body weight/day), for seven days, serum T_4 was lower and there was no increase in thyroid stimulating hormone (TSH), in response to TRH injection. In thyroidectomized rats receiving T_4 replacement, PHT lowered serum T_4 and T_3, but did not change the T_4/T_3 ratio. There was also no increase in TSH. In another experiment, PHT inhibited the expected rise in TSH in rats subjected to cold, implying inhibition of endogenous TRH activity.

The authors conclude that PHT has multiple sites of action on rat thyroid function.

GAMBERT AND GARTHWAITE, Hormone and Metabolic Research (1980),[2194] found that PHT increased basal levels of thyroid stimulating hormone and prolactin in hypothyroid rats. This effect was not observed in euthyroid animals.

FABER, LUMHOLTZ, KIRKEGAARD AND FRIIS, Annals of Endocrinology (1983),[2486] studied the turnover of ^{125}I- or ^{131}I-labeled T_4, T_3 and reverse T_3 in patients before and after treatment with PHT (350 mg/day) for two weeks. PHT reduced the bioavailability of T_4, increased the T_4 to T_3 conversion rate and increased the nondeiodinative metabolic pathways of T_4.

MANN AND SURKS, Endocrinology (1983),[2761] reported that PHT influenced specific T_3 binding by nuclear T_3 receptors in hepatic tissue from euthyroid and athyreotic rats. PHT (20 mg/100 g body weight) resulted in a 14–24% decrease in specific nuclear binding in nuclei from euthyroid rats and 24% in athyreotic rats compared to control. Similar effects of PHT (10–300 µM) were noted in in vitro studies using solubilized T_3 receptors.

SURKS, ORDENE, MANN AND KUMARA-SIRI, Journal of Clinical Endocrinology and Metabolism (1983),[2994] studied the effect of PHT on thyrotropin releasing hormone (TRH)-induced thyroid stimulating hormone (TSH) secretion in humans and rats.

In four patients, PHT (100 mg t.i.d.), for fourteen days, decreased serum T_4 (22%), free T_4 (31%), and free serum T_3 (6%). Basal TSH levels were unchanged, but the integrated TSH response after TRH injection decreased.

In euthyroid rats, PHT (5 mg/100 g body weight daily, for nine days) caused no change in TRH-induced TSH release. When PHT (5 mg/100 g body weight, every eight hours for 48 hours) was given to athyreotic rats, significant increases in pituitary TSH, but not in plasma TSH, were observed.

PHT (100 μM) caused a 74% decrease in TSH release by cultured anterior pituitary cells in the presence of TRH.

The authors suggest that PHT inhibits TRH-induced TSH release.

FRANKLYN, SHEPPARD AND RAMSDEN, *European Journal of Clinical Pharmacology* (1984),[2507] measured free T_4 and T_3 in thirty-one patients on chronic PHT therapy. They found significant reduction in levels of both hormones and suggest that PHT not only alters thyroid hormone protein binding, but also cellular metabolism of thyroid hormones.

DAVIS, LYNAM, FRANKLYN, DOCHERTY AND SHEPPARD, *European Neuroendocrine Association Abstracts* (1985),[2434] found that both T_3 and PHT (50–150 μM) reduced prolactin messenger RNA levels in cultured rat pituitary cells, supporting the premise that PHT may act as a partial T_3 agonist. The authors suggest that PHT has therapeutically relevant intracellular, as well as cell membrane, effects.

FRANKLYN, DAVIS, RAMSDEN AND SHEPPARD, *Journal of Endocrinology* (1985),[2506] studied the effect of PHT on the binding of T_3 to isolated nuclei from rat anterior pituitary tissue. PHT (50–200 μM) inhibited nuclear binding of T_3 in a dose-dependent fashion. PHT also decreased TRH-stimulated TSH release from rat anterior pituitary cells. The authors conclude that PHT can influence thyroid hormone action at the receptor level.

GINGRICH, SMITH, SHAPIRO AND SURKS, *Endocrinology* (1985),[2540] reported that PHT (100–400 μM) inhibited triiodothyronine (T_3)-stimulated growth rate in a rat

pituitary tumor cell line (GC) that produces growth hormone. PHT also inhibited production of growth hormone messenger RNA and growth hormone itself over the same concentration range. The authors suggest that PHT decreases T_3 effects by inhibiting T_3 nuclear-receptor binding.

See also Refs. 488, 490, 491, 492, 1125, 1479, 2271, 2425, 2644, 2689, 2760, 2917, 2996, 3018, 3042.

Other Pituitary Hormones

TAKAHASHI, KIPNIS AND DAUGHADAY, *Journal of Clinical Investigation* (1968),[487] found, in humans, that growth hormone secretion during sleep was not affected by PHT.

MITTLER AND GLICK, *Abstracts of the Fourth International Congress on Endocrinology* (1972),[1368] studied the effect of PHT (40 μg/ml) on the release of oxytocin from isolated rat pituitary gland. Increasing potassium in the medium increased oxytocin release. Preincubation with PHT reduced this stimulated release of oxytocin by 35%.

GUZEK, RUSSELL AND THORN, *Acta Pharmacologica et Toxicologica* (1974),[1105] demonstrated that PHT (40 μg/ml) inhibits the release of vasopressin from isolated rat neurohypophysis. The effect was observed both during release conditions and after electrical stimulation of the hypophysis.

The authors note that their observations are relevant to the other situations in which PHT has been shown to have a regulatory effect on release of insulin, glucagon and calcitonin.

CHALMERS AND JOHNSON, *Journal of Neurology, Neurosurgery and Psychiatry* (1983),[2383] found that PHT (500 mg the evening prior to testing) increased human growth hormone levels induced by thirty-minute exercise.

Calcitonin and Parathyroid Hormone

PENTO, GLICK AND KAGAN, *Endocrinology* (1973),[1406] studied the effect of intravenous PHT on calcitonin secretion in the pig. Normal basal levels of calcitonin secretion were not significantly changed by PHT. When calcitonin secretion was stimulated by means of glucagon or calcium administration, PHT tended to reduce the level of elevation in plasma calcitonin produced by these two stimuli.

The authors state that these findings are in accord with other demonstrations that PHT does not alter normal basal secretion of pituitary-adrenal hormones; but when unusual stimuli are present, PHT exerts a regulatory influence.

HARRIS, JENKINS AND WILLS, *British Journal of Pharmacology* (1974),[1131] reported that PHT (15 μg/ml) significantly inhibited parathyroid hormone-induced calcium release from mouse brain calvaria in culture. Phenobarbital (5–25 μg/ml) had no effect.

PENTO, *Hormone and Metabolic Research* (1976),[2017] observed that PHT slows the onset and prolongs the duration of pentagastrin-stimulated calcitonin secretion in the pig.

HAHN, SCHARP, RICHARDSON, HALSTEAD, KAHN AND TEITELBAUM, *Journal of Clinical Investigation* (1978),[1878] reported that PHT inhibited basal and hormonally-stimulated bone resorption as measured by calcium and [³H]-hydroxyproline release in cultures of rat forelimb rudiments. PHT's effect was independent of cAMP and synergistic with that of human calcitonin.

LERNER AND HANSTROM, *Acta Pharmacology and Toxicology* (1980),[2708] found that PHT (50 μg/ml) inhibited both bone resorption and release of lysosomal enzymes (β-glucuronidase and β-galactosidase) in mouse calvarial bone in organ culture. The authors suggest that inhibition of lysosomal enzyme release may be one important mechanism by which PHT inhibits bone resorption.

IVIC AND KLISIC, *Stereologi Iugoslavica* (1981),[2613] found that PHT (400 μM) inhibited sodium-potassium-ATPase in thyroid parafollicular cells, while slightly stimulating the same activity in parathyroid cells. The authors suggest that this may be a mechanism by which PHT inhibits calcitonin release.

YI, SEITZ AND COOPER, *Federation Proceedings* (1987),[3095] using a radioimmunoassay, found that PHT (100 μM) inhibited the release of calcitonin induced by high extracellular calcium (2.5 mM) in rat thyroparathyroid complexes *in vitro*. Release of calcitonin in normal calcium (1 mM) was unaffected.

The calcium channel blocker, nitrendipine, also inhibited calcium-stimulated calcitonin release. A calcium channel activator (BAY-K-8644) reversed the inhibitory effects of both PHT and nitrendipine.

The authors suggest that PHT inhibits stimulated calcitonin secretion by interacting with calcium channels in thyroid parafollicular cells.

See also Refs 343, 1104, 1485, 1840, 2088, 2281, 2571, 2574, 2623, 2671, 2672, 2707, 2854, 2855.

Renin

CHURCHILL, McDONALD, CHURCHILL, *Journal of Pharmacology and Experimental*

Therapeutics (1979),[2394] found that PHT (40–320 μM) stimulated renin secretion from rat renal cortical slices. The effect was blocked by incubating the slices in potassium-free medium and by ouabain (1 mM). The authors state that renin secretion is directly dependent on the transmembrane sodium gradient and that PHT stimulates secretion by increasing that gradient.

MIGDAL, SLICK, ABU-HAMDAN AND MC-DONALD, *Journal of Pharmacology and Experimental Therapeutics* (1980),[1985] investigated the effect of PHT on renal hemodynamics and renin release in dogs. Infused into the renal artery (0.18 mg/kg/min.), PHT significantly altered renal hemodynamics, resulting in increased renal blood flow and decreased renal vascular resistance. Renin secretion was increased seven-fold. PHT also increased urine volume, sodium secretion and osmolar clearance.

The authors conclude that PHT is both a natriuretic and a diuretic.

CADNAPAPHORNCHAI, PONTES AND MC-DONALD, *American Journal of Physiology* (1984),[2373] and CADNAPAPHORNCHAI, KELLNER AND MCDONALD, *Federation Proceedings* (1986),[2372] in further studies, reported that PHT's stimulation of renin release is mediated through the renal nerves and by inhibition of alpha adrenoceptors. (See also Ref. 2371.)

Prostaglandins

KARMAZYN, HORROBIN, MORGAN, MANKU, ALLY AND KARMALI, *IRCS Medical Science* (1977),[1921] studied norepinephrine-induced, prostaglandin-dependent vasoconstriction in the rat mesenteric vascular bed. PHT produced a dose-dependent inhibition (50% at 10 μg/ml) of the vasoconstriction response to norepinephrine (10 ng) and potassium chloride (2 mg). In other experiments PHT competitively inhibited the vasoconstrictive effects of prostaglandin E_2.

The authors suggest that PHT's effects on prostaglandins may explain its usefulness in many clinical disorders including cardiovascular and muscle disorders, pain, asthma, and endocrine and neural dysfunctions. (See also Ref. 2660.)

KATSUMATA, GUPTA, BAKER, SUSSDORF AND GOLDMAN, *Science* (1982),[2651] reported that, in mice, both PHT and glucocorticoids, through a common receptor, inhibit formation of 6-ketoprostaglandin F_1 and thromboxane B_2 which are the stable metabolites of prostacyclin and thromboxane A_2. (See also Ref. 2561.)

The following studies demonstrate that PHT has anti-anoxic and anti-ischemic effects in brain, nerve, retina, heart and lung. These protective effects of PHT have been demonstrated in whole animal, isolated organ and tissue culture studies.

Cerebral

EMERSON, *Proceedings of the Society for Experimental Biology and Medicine* (1943),[2177] demonstrated that PHT (100 mg/kg, intraperitoneally) protected mice against the lethal effects of acute anoxia induced in a decompression chamber at atmospheric pressures equivalent to those at more than 10,000 feet. In the PHT-treated animals mortality was three out of thirty, compared to thirteen out of thirty in the untreated control group.

HOFF AND YAHN, *American Journal of Physiology* (1944),[164] studied the effect of PHT on tolerance of rats and mice to severe acute hypoxia induced by reduced atmospheric pressures. Decompression was carried out at the rate of 100 mm Hg per minute. Rats and mice given single doses of PHT tolerated lower pressures or withstood a given low pressure for a longer time than controls. PHT-treated animals could be taken to extraordinarily low pressures and survive. This protective action could be demonstrated within ten minutes and persisted as long as forty-eight hours.

FORDA AND McILWAIN, *British Journal of Pharmacology* (1953),[717] electrically stimulated guinea pig brain slices at 500 and 2,000 Hz, 3.5 V. At this level more oxygen per gm per hour was used. When PHT (100 μM) was added, this increase in the use of oxygen was reduced.

The increase in oxygen use produced by the less intense stimulation of 50 Hz, 1.3 V or 2 V, was not changed by PHT.

GAYET-HALLION, BERTRAND, *Comptes Rendus des Seances de la Societe de Biologie* (1959),[118] found that PHT (80 mg/day) prolonged respiratory activity in rats that were immersed in water at 14–15°C, for periods varying from trial to trial. PHT given intraperitoneally three hours before the test prolonged respiratory activity and increased survival.

NAIMAN AND WILLIAMS, *Journal of Pharmacology and Experimental Therapeutics* (1964),[263] found that PHT (50–120 mg/kg) prolonged the duration of respiratory activity in cats and guinea pigs subjected to nitrogen anoxia as well as in the decapitated guinea pig head.

The anti-anoxic effect of PHT was thought to be due in part to a direct protective effect on the respiratory neurons of the central nervous system.

BALDY-MOULINIER, *European Neurology* (1971–2),[790] found that PHT protected cats against the effects of cerebral ischemia induced by clamping the aorta.

KOGURE, SCHEINBERG, KISCHIKAWA AND BUSTO, *Dynamics of Brain Edema* (1976),[2213] studied the protective effects of several drugs against ischemic brain injury in experimental stroke in rats. PHT (30 mg/kg), administered intraperitoneally ten minutes prior to induction of stroke, increased post-ischemic cerebral blood flow, preserved energy compounds and prevented the ischemia-induced rise in cyclic AMP as well as edema. In addition, PHT was the only drug tested that prevented sodium content changes in tissue.

The authors conclude that these results support the view that PHT protects against ischemia-induced brain damage by decreasing the metabolic rate of the brain and increasing concentrations of brain energy reserve.

VEDERNIKOV, SHINSKAYA AND STRELKOV, *Pathological Physiology and Experimental Therapeutics* (1978),[2263] demonstrated that PHT (25–200 mg/kg) has a remarkably positive effect on the survival rate (80–90% versus 0–10% in controls) of mice exposed to hypoxia in a hypobaric chamber.

ALDRETE, ROMO SALAS, JANKOVSKY AND FRANATOVIC, *Critical Care Medicine* (1979),[1718] studied the effects of pretreatment with PHT (15 mg/kg, intravenously) and thiopental on post-ischemic brain damage in rabbits. The authors conclude that pretreatment with PHT protects against ischemic cerebral lesions, as evidenced by both neurological recovery and microscopic findings. (See also Ref. 2142.)

GOLDMAN, ALDRETE AND SHERRILL, *7th World Congress of Anesthesiologists Abstract* (1980),[1864] demonstrated that PHT (70–85 mg/kg) had a protective effect

against acute hypoxia, without ischemia, in mice.

BREMER, YAMADA AND WEST, *Neurosurgery* (1980),[2157] found that PHT (30 mg/kg, every eight hours), in primates, prevented both edema and infarction in the cerebral ischemia produced by embolization of the internal carotid artery.

ARTRU AND MICHENFELDER, *Stroke* (1980),[1728] found that PHT increased survival time 123% in mice breathing 5% oxgen. In addition, pretreatment with intravenous PHT (12.5–50 mg/kg) decreased the rate of potassium accumulation in cerebrospinal fluid following 20 minutes of anoxia in dogs.

ARTRU AND MICHENFELDER, *Anesthesia and Analgesia* (1981),[2144] compared the cerebral protective effects of pretreatment with intravenous PHT (50 and 150 mg/kg), pentobarbital (33 mg/kg), and hypothermia following experimentally-induced circulatory arrest in anesthetized rabbits. Cerebrospinal fluid (CSF) potassium accumulation, an indication of brain cell injury, was measured ten and twenty minutes following ischemia. PHT (50 mg/kg) significantly reduced CSF potassium accumulation. PHT's effect was greater than that of pentobarbital or hypothermia.

The authors state that their findings support the hypothesis that PHT's cerebral protective effects during ischemia are linked to its reduction of cerebral potassium accumulation. (See also Ref. 2145.)

FUKUDA, TABUSE, FUJII AND KOHAMA, *Epilepsy Abstracts* (1982),[2193] demonstrated that PHT tended to increase cerebral blood flow after recirculation following total cerebral ischemia produced by aortic occlusion in dogs. (See also Ref. 2192.)

NEMOTO, SHIU, NEMMER AND BLEYAERT, *Protection of Tissues Against Hypoxia* (1982),[2820] studied the effects of ten drugs on the liberation of free fatty acids (FFA) during complete global ischemia in rats. Of the drugs tested, PHT was the most effective in attenuating FFA liberation.

The authors state that if their hypothesis that there is a direct cause-and-effect relationship between FFA liberation and the evolution of ischemic brain injury is correct, these findings have important clinical implications.

FUKUDA, TABUSE, IHARA, TANABE, IKEDA AND KOHAMA, *Circulatory Shock* (1983)[2516] studied the protective effects of PHT (15 mg/kg, intravenously), thirty minutes before ischemia, on post-ischemic brain damage in dogs. Cerebral blood flow was significantly increased in the PHT group compared to controls, even in the pre-ischemic period. Post-ischemic EEG recovery was faster and potassium accumulation in the cerebral venous blood after recirculation was less in the PHT group. In addition, PHT stabilized water and electrolyte balance in the cerebral cortex.

OSAWA, *Journal of Tokyo Medical College* (1983),[2844] studied the effect of PHT on brain circulation and brain tissue respiration following experimentally induced cardiac arrest in dogs. Intravenous PHT (20 mg/kg) was administered either thirty minutes prior to cardiac arrest, or immediately following cardiopulmonary resuscitation (CPR). Animals receiving only CPR served as controls. CPR was performed five or ten minutes after cardiac arrest in all groups.

PHT treatment resulted in increases in regional cerebral blood flow, oxygen availability and brain mitochondria respiratory activity, as well as delay in EEG flattening. These protective effects were most significant in the animals pretreated with PHT.

URAM, NEMOTO AND WINTER, *Anesthesiology* (1983),[3039] showed that the cerebral protective drugs, PHT and thiopental, had markedly different effects on the surface tension and pressure of monolayers of bovine brain phosphotidylinositol than ketamine and halothane, which do not have cerebral protective effects. The authors suggest that these effects on the cell membrane relate to the differential blockade of ionic channels and the inhibition of enzyme systems, which are critical to the cerebral protective effects of PHT and thiopental.

IMAIZUMI, SUZUKI, KINOUCHI AND YOSHIMOTO, *Brain Nerve* (1986),[2609] evaluated a series of drugs for their ability to prolong survival time in mice subjected to hypoxia (4% oxygen, 96% nitrogen).

None of the animals in the control group survived more than eight minutes, mean survival time three minutes. PHT (100 mg/kg) was the most effective of the drugs tested. In the PHT-treated group, 70% survived for an hour or more compared to 45% in the suloctidil-treated group, 23.5% in the vitamin E-treated group, none in the phenobarbital-treated group, and none for any of the other drugs tested.

The authors conclude that PHT is markedly effective as a protective agent in hypoxia.

ABIKO, SUZUKI, MIZOI, OBA AND YOSHIMOTO, *Noshinkei* (1986),[2272] based on their observation of PHT's protective effect on brain during hypoxic states in mice,[2609] studied the effects of PHT in a canine ischemia model in which blood flow could be precisely regulated.

Five animals served as control. Fifteen were treated in groups of five, receiving either 7, 10, or 30 mg/kg PHT intravenously. Five others received a combination of PHT (10 mg/kg), mannitol (2 g/kg) and vitamin E (30 mg/kg). Mannitol and vitamin E were given as free-radical scavengers. All drugs were given twenty minutes prior to the induction of ischemia (blood flow reduced to one-tenth normal). The ischemic state was maintained for one hour before circulation was restored.

Brain electrical activity was monitored throughout the procedure. Time to flat EEG was recorded, as was the activity for three hours after restoration of circulation. In the untreated group the EEG became flat in 6.8 ±3.1 minutes, and only one of the five animals showed recovery of activity after circulation was restored. PHT prolonged the time to loss of EEG activity (29.6 to 42 minutes), shortened time to initial recovery of low-voltage activity, and improved degree of recovery, in a dose-dependent pattern (see below).

Animals per group (5)	Time to flat EEG (min.)	EEG recovery (min.)*	Recovery ** microvolts (no. animals)
Control	6.8	***	≥ 30 (1)
PHT 7mg/kg	29.6	8.2	50–100 (2) 100–200 (3)
PHT 10mg/kg	32.0	8.5	100–200 (5)
PHT 30mg/kg	42.0	6.3	100–200 (3) ≥200 (2)
PHT 10mg/kg, plus mannitol and vitamin E	36.0	1.4	≥200 (5)

* Time to initial appearance of low-voltage slow wave activity, when circulation restored after one hour of ischemia.
** Measured three hours after circulation restored.
*** One of the five control animals showed some EEG recovery—time not given.

Brain swelling (observed by craniotomy) was not seen in any of the animals during ischemia, but appeared gradually one hour after circulation was reestablished in the untreated animals. Treatment with PHT significantly prevented brain swelling. Correlated with this effect, and indicative of a reduction in blood-brain barrier damage, was decreased extravasation of Evans blue dye into brain tissue. PHT (30 mg/kg) alone, and the combination treatment had the greatest protective effects.

LEE, SANCESARIO, TETZLAFF AND KREUTZBERG, *Society for Neuroscience Abstracts* (1986),[2698] found that PHT (25–100 mg/kg), phenobarbital (20–50 mg/kg) and clonazepam (0.2–0.5 mg/kg) protected against hippocampal CA1 pyramidal cell loss in gerbils subjected to ten minutes of hypoxia produced by carotid clamping. The drugs were administered fifteen minutes following removal of the carotid clamps and then once or twice per day for three days.

Cardiac

GUPTA, UNAL, BASHOUR AND WEBB, *Diseases of the Chest* (1967),[496] were the first to demonstrate that PHT (20 mg/kg, intravenously) increases coronary blood flow in dogs.

NAYLER, MCINNES, SWANN, RACE, CARSON AND LOWE, *American Heart Journal* (1968),[402] demonstrated, in dogs, that PHT (3.5 mg/kg) increases coronary blood flow and reduces myocardial oxygen consumption, without altering the work capacity of the left ventricle.

ZEFT, REMBERT, CURRY AND GREENFIELD, *Cardiovascular Research* (1973), [1711] in a study examining coronary blood flow, found that in intact conscious dogs, with the heart rate uncontrolled, PHT (5 mg/kg) produced a mean increase of 61% in coronary blood flow. With the heart rate controlled by ventricular pacing, a similar dose of PHT produced a mean increase in coronary blood flow of 57%. There was no significant change in either aortic blood flow or peripheral vascular resistance.

ZEFT, WHALEN, RATLIFF, DAVENPORT AND McINTOSH, *The Journal of Pharmacology and Experimental Therapeutics* (1968),[392] conducted a study to evaluate the hypothesis that PHT, 20 mg/kg initially, followed by 5 mg/kg every eight hours for seventy-two hours, would be effective in preventing death from ventricular arrhythmias resulting from experimental myocardial infarction. The left anterior descending coronary artery of forty farm pigs was gradually occluded. The farm pig was chosen because its coronary artery pattern is relatively constant and similar to that of man.

Almost twice as many control animals (eleven of twenty) expired as PHT-treated animals (six of twenty). Although the sample was not large enough to be conclusive, the authors state that there is an indication that PHT, used prophylactically, increases the chance of survival in experimental myocardial infarction in pigs.

As a result of this experiment the authors suggest that consideration should be given to the use of PHT on a regular basis to prevent fatalities originating from coronary artery disorders.

RAINES AND NINER, *Neuropharmacology* (1975),[2032] studied the response to bilateral carotid occlusion in cats before and after administration of PHT. Occlusion produced the expected increases in diastolic blood pressure, heart rate and occasional cardiac arrhythmias. PHT (5 mg/kg) reduced the reflex-induced tachycardia. Higher doses (10 mg/kg) reduced the hypertensive responses as well as the tachycardia.

ALDRETE AND CUBILLOS, *Sixth European Congress of Anaesthesiology* (1982),[2279] compared the protective effects of PHT and thiopentone to placebo in rabbits subjected to anoxia under anesthesia. Intravenous PHT (15 mg/kg) significantly delayed the onset of change in heart rate and ventricular fibrillation, compared to thiopentone and placebo. Beneficial blood pressure changes were also observed in the PHT-treated animals.

Pulmonary

GORDON, GOLDSMITH AND CHARIPPER, *Proceedings of the Society for Experimental Biology and Medicine* (1944),[2200] demonstrated that PHT (15 mg), administered intraperitoneally ninety minutes prior to injury, prolonged the survival time and reduced the extent of lung hemorrhage in rats subjected to reduced barometric pressures (equivalent to an altitude of 39,000–49,000 feet).

MOSS, *Bulletin of the New York Academy of Medicine* (1973),[1374] demonstrated, in dogs, that PHT pretreatment provided protection against lung damage under conditions of hypoxia induced by hemorrhagic trauma.

Six untreated dogs evidenced pulmonary edema, hemorrhage, congestion and atelectasis typical of shock lung.

None of eight dogs pretreated with PHT (5 mg/kg, intramuscularly) one hour prior to the hemorrhage regimen showed evidence of shock lung. Their lungs appeared normal both grossly and microscopically.

STEIN AND MOSS, *Surgical Forum* (1973),[1591] in a controlled study, found that pretreatment with PHT (5 mg/kg), two hours prior to hemorrhage, afforded statistically significant protection against "shock lung" in rats and dogs.

MENTZER, ALEGRE AND NOLAN, *Surgical Forum* (1975),[1981] studied the effects of PHT (1 mg/kg) on pulmonary vascular resistance and pulmonary vascular caliber in dogs.

The authors conclude that PHT is a pulmonary vasodilator, that its effects are independent of myocardial performance or changes in systemic resistance, and that its mechanism of action is not mediated through adrenergic receptor sites. The authors suggest that PHT may have a beneficial effect in patients with alveolar hypoxia and pulmonary hypertension by reducing pulmonary vascular resistance.

DAS, AYROMLOOI, TOBIAS, DESIDERIO AND STEINBERG, *Pediatric Research* (1980),[1791] studied the effects of PHT on fetal rabbit lung ischemia *in vivo*. Normal levels of coenzyme A (CoA), acetyl CoA, and long-chain acetyl CoA were restored after treatment with PHT (7 mg/kg). NADH/NAD ratio was increased in hypoxic, untreated lung and restored to normal after treatment with PHT.

FLICK, HOEFFEL AND WEBSTER, *Federation Proceedings* (1982),[2185] demonstrated that PHT (10 mg/kg) counteracts the increased vascular permeability which results from air emboli in sheep. Increases in leakage of lung lymph fluid and protein during emboli were 90% greater without PHT.

AMY, LEGRAND, LEVITZKY, WELCH AND SCHECHTER, *Journal of Trauma* (1981),[2291] demonstrated PHT's effects in preventing the development of shock lung in anemic animals following hemorrhagic shock. Untreated animals had grossly hemorrhagic lungs with diffuse interstitial and alveolar congestion, hemorrhage and edema. None of the animals receiving intravenous PHT (5 mg/kg), either one hour before or fifteen minutes after hemorrhage, had gross or histopathologic evidence of shock lung.

The authors state that their findings suggest that PHT may be efficacious in preventing adult respiratory distress syndrome when administered as soon as possible to patients with major traumatic blood loss.

WOHNS AND KERSTEIN, *Critical Care Medicine* 1982),[2269] reported that PHT (5 mg/kg) protected dogs against the development of pulmonary edema during isolated cerebral hypoxia, but not during noncerebral systemic hypotension. They evaluated both pulmonary histology and gaseous exchange.

The authors hypothesize that, because the development of neurogenic pulmonary edema is hypothalamically mediated, PHT may prevent cerebral hypoxia from triggering neurogenic pulmonary edema by stabilizing the hypothalamus.

Nerve, Purkinje Fibers, Retina

PINCUS, GROVE, MARINO AND GLASER, *Presented at the International Society of Neurochemistry* (1969),[1419] observed that PHT (100 μM) reduced the abnormal accumulation of intracellular sodium in hypoxic nerves. In normally functioning, oxygenated nerves, PHT did not affect intracellular sodium.

The authors state that PHT has been shown to have a stabilizing influence on virtually all excitable membranes. They note that these effects have been seen in a wide variety of vertebrate and invertebrate species. (See also Refs. 285, 293.)

BASSETT, BIGGER AND HOFFMAN, *The Journal of Pharmacology and Experimental Therapeutics* (1970),[804] found that PHT protected canine Purkinje fibers during hypoxia.

To determine the effect of PHT, a Purkinje fiber preparation of the isolated heart was stimulated electrically at a constant rate, and the electrical responses were measured until optimal performance was established. Then, hypoxia was induced by perfusion with a nitrogen-carbon dioxide mixture. This hypoxia caused a fall in resting and action potential amplitude, phase zero max rate of rise (V_{max}), and conduction velocity. PHT (.01–.1 μM) significantly delayed these hypoxia-induced effects, especially the fall in phase zero V_{max}. In another set of experiments, PHT, given after hypoxia-induced depression of the Purkinje fibers, transiently improved action potential amplitude, conduction velocity and V_{max}.

The authors conclude that PHT's effectiveness in abolishing arrhythmias arising from coronary artery occlusion may be due, in part, to its ability to maintain and/or improve Purkinje fiber V_{max} and conduction.

HONDA, PODOS AND BECKER, *Investigative Ophthalmology* (1973),[1160] observed the protective effect of PHT (100 μM) against oxygen deprivation in the retina of rabbits as registered on one of the two major peaks of the electroretinogram.

Preservation of Energy Compounds

WOODBURY, TIMIRAS AND VERNADAKIS, *Hormones, Brain Function, and Behavior* (1957),[483] reported that PHT increased glycogen in rat brain.

BERNSOHN, POSSLEY AND CUSTOD, *Pharmacologist* (1960),[17] demonstrated that PHT (25 mg/kg), two hours prior to measurement, more than doubled creatinine phosphate levels in rat brain. With control values of 3.30 μM/gm of brain, creatinine phosphate values were 1.30 for chlordiazepoxide, 4.40 for chlorpromazine, and 7.38 for PHT.

BRODDLE AND NELSON, *Federation Proceedings* (1968),[37] found that PHT (50 mg/kg) can decrease brain metabolic rate 40 to 60%, as well as increase the concentrations of brain energy compounds measured, i.e.,

phosphocreatine, serum and brain glucose and glycogen.

HUTCHINS AND ROGERS, *British Journal of Pharmacology* (1970),[739] found that PHT (20 mg/kg, intraperitoneally) increased the concentration of brain glycogen in mouse brain by 7% at 30 minutes and by 11% at 120 minutes.

GILBERT, GRAY AND HEATON, *Biochemical Pharmacology* (1971),[1071] demonstrated that brain glucose levels were increased in mice who received PHT (20 mg/kg). The authors also found that PHT significantly increased the uptake of xylose by brain slices, without affecting glucose utilization by cerebral cortex slices.

The authors concluded that PHT stimulates glucose transport into the brain. They considered the possibility that, with PHT, the extra glucose may play a role independent of its more obvious one as a substrate in oxidative metabolism, such as stabilization of water molecules in the cell membrane, with a consequent stabilizing effect on neuronal excitability.

KOGURE, SCHEINBERG, KISHIKAWA AND BUSTO, *Dynamics of Brain Edema* (1976),[2213] using a rat stroke model to study focal cerebral infarction, demonstrated that PHT (30 mg/kg, intraperitoneally), thirty minutes prior to stroke, preserved energy compounds and prevented the ischemia-induced rise of cyclic AMP in brain.

McCANDLESS, FEUSNER, LUST AND PASSONNEAU, *Journal of Neurochemistry* (1979),[2229] demonstrated that PHT (25 mg/kg, intraperitoneally) counteracted the maximal electroshock-induced decreases in phosphocreatine, ATP, glucose and glycogen in mouse cerebellum.

MUSCLE BASIC MECHANISMS

Skeletal Muscle

PARISI AND RAINES, *Federation Proceedings* (1963),[1400] studied the effect of PHT on the soleus nerve of the cat, and on neuromuscular transmission via this nerve.

Repeated nerve volleys caused post-tetanic repetitive discharge of the motor nerve terminals which, in turn, caused a contractile post-tetanic potentiation in the muscle. The authors found that intravenous PHT (20 mg/kg) abolished this abnormal muscle post-tetanic potentiation. When a normal muscle was given a single volley, PHT did not affect normal twitch.

The authors placed emphasis on this selective action of PHT, which enables it to counteract post-tetanic repetitive activity without interfering with normal transmission or contraction.

JURNA AND LANZER, *Naunyn-Schmiedebergs Archives of Pharmacology* (1969), [2636] reported the inhibitory effects of intravenous PHT on reserpine-induced rigidity, as evidenced by increased alpha and decreased gamma motor activity. PHT (50 mg/kg) consistently normalized alpha and gamma reflex activity. The authors suggest that PHT's effects result from its inhibition of facilitatory processes that follow repetitive activation. (See also Refs. 182, 183.)

KUHN, DOUWES AND KERN, *Klinische Wochenschrift* (1969),[2216] found that PHT abolished the myotonia induced with 2, 4-dichlorophenoxyacetate in rat diaphragm.

BAKER, OKAMOTO AND RIKER, *Pharmacologist* (1971),[789] found that, in a cat soleus nerve-muscle preparation, pretreatment with PHT counteracted abnormal excitability produced by exogenous acetylcholine. The authors note that PHT selectively suppresses the post-tetanic potentiation of motor nerve terminals without impairing single-impulse transmission.

RUTLEDGE, SOHN AND SARDINAS, *Pharmacologist* (1971),[1494] studied the effect of PHT on hyperexcitability in a cat soleus nerve-muscle preparation. PHT (20–40 mg/kg) counteracted succinylcholine-induced muscle fasciculation and twitch potentiation, but did not impair normal neuromuscular transmission.

GRUENER AND STERN, *Nature, New Biology* (1972),[1103] studied the effects of PHT on muscle fibers from steroid-treated mice.

Myopathy was induced in twelve adult mice by the daily intraperitoneal injection of dexamethasone over eight to twelve weeks. Six of these mice then received injections of PHT (25 mg/kg) at 48, 24, 4 and 2 hours prior to measurement of the electrophysiological properties of the extensor digitorum longus muscle. Six mice were untreated.

In PHT-treated animals with steroid-induced myopathy, the abnormally low resting potentials, threshold potentials, and excitability were restored to normal levels.

PHT was also given to six of twelve normal mice (not treated with steroids), using the same schedule of administration. PHT had no effect on the normal muscle properties in these animals.

The authors conclude that PHT reverses the membrane effects produced by chronic administration of corticosteroids in mice by correcting the abnormal ion distribution or permeabilities.

SU AND FELDMAN, *Archives of Neurology* (1973),[1602] in a microelectrode study of *in vivo* rat neuromuscular transmission, found that intravenous PHT (10–40 mg/kg) had no effect on normal muscle resting potential or miniature endplate potential (mepp) frequency or amplitude. However, when the neuromuscular junction was abnormally stimulated by depolarization with high potassium (35 mM), PHT increased the resting potential of the muscle membrane by 15% and decreased mepp frequency by 60%. The onset of PHT's effect was rapid, occurring within ten minutes.

The authors conclude that PHT stabilizes both the motor-nerve ending and the muscle membrane. They suggest that this stabilizing effect could be a factor in the success of PHT in the treatment of generalized myokymia and myotonia.

ROSES, BUTTERFIELD, APPEL AND CHESTNUT, *Archives of Neurology* (1975),[2057] demonstrated that PHT corrects the membrane defect in red blood cells of patients with myotonic muscular dystrophy, as revealed by electron spin resonance spectroscopy.

In myotonic red cell membrane there was increased membrane fluidity and decreased polarity. PHT normalized fluidity differences in spectra derived from myotonic erythrocytes, but had no significant effect on normal erythrocyte spectra.

HERZBERG, CHALLBERG, HESS AND HOWLAND, *Biochemical and Biophysical Research Communications* (1975),[1897] observed that when dystrophic mice are treated with both PHT and lithium chloride, the abnormally elevated potassium efflux, characteristic of dystrophic diaphragm, returns to within normal limits.

The authors note that treatment of normal animals with PHT and lithium chloride does not produce significant inhibition of efflux of potassium, so that the effect appears to be specific for the dystrophic state.

YAARI, RAHAMIMOFF AND PINCUS, *Israel Journal of Medical Science* (1976),[2131] demonstrated that PHT (100–200 μM) either increases or decreases the evoked endplate potential at frog neuromuscular junction, depending on whether the calcium in the medium was high or low. (See also Ref. 2130.)

ANDERSON AND RAINES, *Neurology* (1976),[1722] demonstrated that a combination of PHT and chlorpromazine markedly reduced decerebrate rigidity in cats. Since this treatment did not impair neuromuscular transmission or motor coordination, the authors suggest it may be of value for treating the muscle rigidity in some upper motor neuron lesions. (See also Ref. 2031.)

HULCE, *Society for Neuroscience Abstracts* (1977),[1903] examining the basis for the beneficial effect of PHT and chlorpromazine in reducing decerebrate rigidity, demonstrated separate effects of the two agents. PHT (40 mg/kg) reduces the total time of extensor rigidity seen after vestibular stimulation, while chlorpromazine reduces the peak force.

ENTRIKIN, SWANSON, WEIDOFF, PATTERSON AND WILSON, *Science* (1977),[1824] found that PHT (20 mg/kg) injected daily for forty days after hatching markedly improved the righting ability of dystrophic chicks. The characteristically high activity of acetylcholinesterase in dystrophic posterior latissimus dorsi muscles was simultaneously reduced to normal levels. (See also Refs. 2164, 2165.)

ENTRIKIN AND BRYANT, *Epilepsy Abstracts* (1978),[2178] in studying the mechanism by which the righting ability of dystrophic chickens was improved by PHT, examined posterior latissimus dorsi muscles *in vitro* by microelectrode stimulation and recording.

The authors conclude that PHT effects an improvement by decreasing the abnormal tendency for the muscle to fire repetitively. (See also Ref. 2179.)

HERSHKOWITZ, MAHANY, BAIZER AND RAINES, *Neuroscience Abstracts* (1978),[2591] studied the effects of PHT on extensor muscle tone and gamma motoneuron activity in decerebrate cats. PHT reduced extensor tone by 25% at 10 mg/kg and by 50% at 20 mg/kg.

The authors state that these effects provide a rationale for the use of PHT in the treatment of abnormally increased muscle tone.

KWIECINSKI, *Neurology* (1978),[2682] studied the effects of PHT, procainamide, ajmaline, isoptin, hydrocortisone and glucose on clofibrate-induced myotonia in rats and in isolated denervated muscle. PHT was the only drug tested that significantly reduced the intensity of the myotonic discharges. PHT also lessened the decline of the myotonic muscle response during continued direct stimulation.

SILVERMAN, ATWOOD AND BLOOM, *Experimental Neurology* (1978),[2081] found that PHT improved motor control of hind limbs in dystrophic mice. Electromyographic assay demonstrated PHT's ability to reduce the dystrophic myotonic activity within fifteen minutes of a single injection.

FURMAN AND BARCHI, *Annals of Neurology* (1978),[1842] demonstrated that PHT, in concentrations clinically effective in controlling hereditary myotonia in humans, inhibited the myotonia induced by aromatic monocarboxylic acids in rats.

OZAWA, KOMATSU AND SATO, *Journal of the Pharmaceutical Society of Japan* (1978),[2010] demonstrated that PHT (25 mg/kg), administered intraperitoneally for nine to eleven days to dystrophic mice, restored the resting membrane potential of skeletal muscle. Comparable studies in normal mice demonstrated that PHT did not affect normal skeletal muscle.

GAGE, LONERGAN AND TORDA, *British Journal of Pharmacology* (1980),[1843] reported that PHT (10 µg/ml) has both pre- and postsynaptic effects at the mouse sternomastoid and diaphragm neuromuscular junction. PHT reduced the amplitude of the muscle endplate potentials by decreasing the average number of quanta of acetylcholine released in response to an action potential and by decreasing the amplitude of the voltage response to each quantum of acetylcholine. Reduction in spontaneous miniature endplate potential amplitude was due to a decrease in the time constant of decay of the miniature endplate currents (i.e., decreased average open time of endplate channels).

IONASESCU, IONASESCU, WITTE, FELD, CANCILLA, KAEDING, KRAUS AND STERN, *Journal of the Neurological Sciences* (1980),[1905] studied altered protein synthesis in breast muscle cell cultures from dystrophic chick embryos. PHT (20 µg/ml) significantly increased total protein and myosin synthesis and creatine kinase in cells, while decreasing creatine kinase in the medium. The effects were specific since neither turnover for total protein and myosin nor noncollagen protein content were changed.

PINCUS, YAARI AND ARGOV, *Antiepileptic Drugs: Mechanisms of Action* (1980),[2023] evaluating the effects of PHT on calcium flux at the frog neuromuscular junction, found that PHT (200 µM), in normal calcium medium, reduced quantal content and endplate potential amplitude. In low calcium medium, however, PHT increased quantal content and endplate potential amplitude. PHT increased miniature endplate potential frequency irrespective of calcium concentration. The authors also found that PHT had a frequency-dependent effect on synaptic transmission: the higher the frequency of stimulation, the greater PHT's inhibitory effect.

ENTRIKIN, PATTERSON AND WILSON, *Experimental Neurology* (1981),[2180] in a blind study including twenty-five, thirty and ninety-day trials, found that PHT (in gradually increasing doses of 10–60 mg/kg, intraperitoneally, twice a day) improved righting ability in dystrophic chickens as early as the tenth day of treatment. Improvement, compared to the untreated chickens, was still present at ninety days, although the disease had progressed in all animals.

PHT also reduced plasma creatine kinase and plasma and fast-twitch muscle acetylcholinesterase activity.

HUDECKI, POLLINA, HEFFNER AND BHARGAVA, *Experimental Neurology* (1981),[2207] found that PHT (40 mg/kg, daily) significantly improved the righting ability of dystrophic chickens during a ninety-day trial.

KWIECINSKI, *European Journal of Clinical Investigation* (1984),[2683] showed that PHT (30 μg/ml) inhibited experimentally induced myotonia and completely suppressed the self-sustaining repetitive activity in human myotonic intercostal muscle fibers. Latencies at rheobase were decreased and the number of spikes during a current pulse was markedly diminished. During tetanic isometric contraction, the abnormal myotonic relaxation and the electromyographic after-activity were completely abolished by PHT.

The author suggests that PHT inhibits myotonic activity by decreasing voltage-dependent sodium conductance.

AICHELE, PAIK AND HELLER, *Experimental Neurology* (1985),[2278] studied the efficacy of PHT, procainamide and tocainide in murine genetic myotonia. All three drugs were initially effective against myotonia; however, the duration of the effect was longest for PHT, 89% of its maximum effect still present three hours after injection, compared with 25% for tocainide, and no effect for procainamide. The authors note that the effectiveness of the drugs correlated with their potency in blocking isolated sodium currents.

SELZER, DAVID AND YAARI, *Brain Research* (1984),[2944] found that PHT (100–300 μM) strongly suppressed the tetanic and post-tetanic potentiation of muscle endplate potentials induced by stimulation (30 Hz), but had only slight effects at low frequencies (0.5 Hz). The authors suggest that PHT's frequency-dependent suppression of excitatory synaptic transmission may also be important in its regulation of hyperexcitability in the CNS.

DAVID, SELZER AND YAARI, *Brain Research* (1985),[2429] demonstrated that PHT (100–300 μM) suppressed aminopyridine-induced presynaptic afterdischarges and repetitive muscle-fiber activation in a frog nerve-muscle preparation. At the presynaptic terminal, PHT suppressed abnormal afterdischarges, while the primary action potential was never abolished.

The authors note that PHT's actions on afterdischarge generation are compatible with its known stabilization of hyperexcitable membranes.

McKINNEY, *Neuroscience Letters* (1985),[2781] using intracellular recording techniques, found that PHT (100 μM) reversed veratridine-induced membrane depolarization in frog skeletal muscle by approximately one-third. PHT also inhibited veratridine-induced sodium influx in a dose-dependent manner. The author notes that these findings are consistent with PHT's effects in neurons.

RAINES, MAHANY, BAIZER, SWOPE AND HERSHKOWITZ, *Journal of Pharmacology and Experimental Therapeutics* (1985),[2889] evaluated PHT's ability to reduce motor manifestations of decerebrate rigidity in cats. PHT diminished the force necessary to collapse hyperextended limbs, reduced gamma motoneuron discharges, and markedly depressed mechanical and electromyographic responses evoked by stretch from both forelimb and hindlimb extensor muscles.

The authors conclude that PHT has both central and peripheral muscle relaxing effects, consistent with its usefulness in the treatment of spasticity.

YAARI, SELZER AND DAVID, *Brain Research* (1985),[3092] studied the effects of PHT (100–300 μM) in frog nerve-muscle preparations using intracellular recordings from muscle endplates and extracellular recordings from motor nerve terminals and their parent axons. With PHT, the number of impulses transmitted across the synapse decreased in a dose-dependent manner. Fewer impulses were transmitted at higher rates of stimulation (100–200 Hz). However, even at lower stimulation frequencies (30–50 Hz), PHT markedly inhibited the buildup of endplate potential amplitude after repetitive nerve stimulation (tetanic potentiation).

HARTMAN, FIAMENGO AND RIKER, *Anesthesiology* (1986),[2576] found that pretreatment with intravenous PHT (30 mg/kg) suppressed succinylcholine-induced motor nerve terminal repetitive firing and post-tetanic potentiation, as well as muscle fasciculations, in an *in situ* cat soleus neuromuscular preparation. PHT was found to be more effective than d-tubocurarine in suppressing the fasciculations. In addition, PHT enhanced succinylcholine's desired blocking effect, while d-tubocurarine reduced it.

The authors comment that succinylcholine, a depolarizing neuromuscular blocker used in anesthesia, has a number of undesirable side effects which can be reduced by suppressing fasciculations. They suggest that PHT may be clinically useful as a preventative when succinycholine is used.

Smooth Muscle

DRUCKMAN AND MOORE, *Proceedings of the Society for Experimental Biology and Medicine* (1955),[465] studied the effect of PHT on isolated rabbit intestine smooth muscle contractions. PHT (60–80 μg/ml) decreased the amplitude of contractions.

The authors state that this direct effect of PHT on intestinal smooth muscle, in addition to its stabilizing effect on the central nervous system, is relevant to its use in the treatment of clinical conditions of intestinal hypermotility and spasticity.

KHAN AND McEWEN, *Proceedings of the Canadian Federation of Biological Societies* (1967),[192] studied the effect of PHT and 5,5-diphenyl-2-thiohydantoin (DTH) on the activity of isolated uterine tissue from the albino rat. PHT and DTH decreased the rate and amplitude of contractions. To attain complete relaxation PHT was required in a concentration of 33 μg/ml, and for DTH, 17 μg/ml was required.

WOODBURY AND KEMP, *Psychiatria, Neurologia, Neurochirurgia* (1971),[1696] showed that PHT tended to reduce toward normal the amplitude of contraction of the smooth muscle of rat ileum when it had been rendered hyperexcitable by barium ions.

Other work from their laboratory showed that small amounts of PHT increased the release of acetylcholine from parasympathetic nerve endings in the wall of rat ileum and also from intramural ganglia, thus stimulating contraction of the ileum. However, when contraction of the ileum was made excessive by the addition of acetylcholine, PHT inhibited the excessive contractions. The authors refer to this selective action of PHT as a biphasic effect.

CHOU, KUIPER AND HSIEH, *Gastroenterology* (1972),[899] noting that PHT has been used in the treatment of spastic colon, studied the effects of PHT on phasic motor activity and contractile state of an *in situ* segment of the ascending colon and terminal ileum of dog.

PHT decreased the contractile state of both ileum and colon, making them more distensible, and also decreased the phasic activity of the colon.

FERRARI AND FURLANUT, *Archives Internationales de Pharmacodynamie et de Therapie* (1973),[1021] studied the effect of PHT on the mechanical and electrical activity of the isolated guinea pig ileum preparations.

PHT enhanced muscular relaxation and regulated the response of smooth muscle to acetylcholine stimulation. The authors note that these effects are consonant with PHT's stabilization of excitable membranes.

VANASIN, BASS, MENDELOFF AND SCHUSTER, *American Journal of Digestive Diseases* (1973),[1644] studied the direct effect of PHT on isolated strips of smooth muscle of colon from fourteen humans and twenty-four dogs. Whether stimulated with acetylcholine, 5-hydroxytryptamine, or electrically, PHT significantly increased relaxation time and decreased contraction time, compared to controls.

The authors conclude that PHT can act directly on smooth muscle, as well as on neuromuscular junctions, and that their observations suggest a basis for the therapeutic use of PHT in the treatment of spastic colon syndrome. (See also Refs. 2380, 2437.)

MELACINI, FURLANUT, FERRARI AND VOLTA, *Archives Internationales de Pharmacodynamie et de Therapie* (1975),[1978] demonstrated that PHT counteracts repetitive discharge under sustained depolarization of guinea pig taenia coli, yet does not affect normal membrane resistance.

KHAN, *Archives Internationales de Pharmacodynamie et de Therapie* (1982),[2660] found that PHT (7.5–120 μM) and diphenylthiohydantoin inhibited spontaneous motility of rat uterus in a dose-dependent manner. PHT reduced the stimulatory effects of ouabain, acetylcholine, oxytocin, ATP and prostaglandins I_2 and E_2 and increased the inhibitory effects of theophylline and nitroglycerin.

CALIXTO AND DE-LIMA, *Brazilian Journal of Medical and Biological Research* (1983),[2375] reported that PHT caused a dose-dependent, noncompetitive inhibition of the contractions induced by norepinephrine, acetylcholine and serotonin in isolated rat vas deferens. PHT also antagonized calcium-induced contractions of the depolarized vas deferens in a competitive manner. The authors suggest that PHT achieves its therapeutic effect, at least in part, by reducing calcium influx in excitable membranes.

CARDIOVASCULAR BASIC MECHANISMS

Cardiac Arrhythmias

HARRIS AND KOKERNOT, *American Journal of Physiology* (1950), [141] found that PHT prevented ectopic contractions in dogs subjected to operative coronary occlusion.

By using a method of gradual coronary occlusion, cardiac ischemia was produced causing ventricular arrhythmias. PHT was found to suppress the ectopic discharges in these hearts. Confidence in the interpretation of the results was gained by the observation of quick diminution of frequency of ectopic complexes almost immediately after injection of PHT. Without PHT, these ectopic complexes returned.

The authors found that in their experiments it was possible to control all ventricular tachycardias by adequate amounts of PHT.

MOSEY AND TYLER, *Circulation* (1954), [260] showed that intravenous PHT (10–30 mg/kg) reversed ouabain-induced ventricular tachycardia in dogs.

SCHERF, BLUMENFELD, TANER AND YILDIZ, *American Heart Journal* (1960), [410] found that PHT (5 mg/kg) reversed aconitine- and delphinine-induced ventricular and atrial arrhythmias in dogs.

LANG, BAZIKI, PAPPELBAUM, GOLD, BERNSTEIN, HERROLD AND CORDAY, *American Journal of Cardiology* (1965), [2218] demonstrated that intravenous PHT (6–15 mg/kg) reversed aconitine-induced atrial and ventricular arrhythmias, digitalis-induced ar-

rhythmias and cerebral venous shunt-induced arrhythmias in dogs.

The use of auto-transplanted heart-lung and cerebral venous shunt preparations permitted the authors to conclude that PHT exerted its beneficial action directly on the myocardium.

COX, PITT, BROWN AND MOLARO, *Canadian Medical Association Journal* (1966), [64] using microelectrodes, found that PHT promptly abolished acetylcholine-induced arrhythmias in isolated atrial tissue.

GUPTA, VOLLMER, BASHOUR AND WEBB, *Federation Proceedings* (1967), [2204] studied the effects of PHT in dog myocardium made ischemic by anterior coronary artery ligation. PHT (10 mg/kg) restored the refractory periods in the ischemic zones to normal and doubled the diastolic threshold. PHT had no effect on refractory period or diastolic threshold of the normal myocardium.

HOCKMAN, MAUCK AND CHU, *American Heart Journal* (1967), [163] using electrical stimulation of diencephalic and mesencephalic loci in dogs and cats induced a spectrum of ventricular arrhythmias which frequently persisted for five minutes or longer after stimulation. Intravenous PHT (10 mg/kg) not only abolished the ectopic ventricular rhythms, but also prevented their induction by a subsequent stimulus for periods varying from thirty minutes to seven hours.

The authors suggest that PHT's therapeutic effects on the heart may at least in part be due to its central nervous system action.

ROSATI, ALEXANDER, SCHAAL AND WALLACE, *Circulation Research* (1967),[308] studied the effects of intravenous PHT (10 mg/kg) in canine hearts using intraventricularly implanted electrodes. In spontaneously beating hearts and external pacemaker-controlled hearts, PHT increased sinus rate, decreased atrioventricular conduction time, and had little or no effect on Purkinje conduction or total ventricular activation time. PHT raised the threshold of atrial and ventricular muscle, with no change in refractory periods.

In chronic heart block, PHT produced no change in ventricular pacemaker activity; but, when ventricular tachycardia was induced by toxic doses of deslanoside, PHT abolished the ectopic arrhythmia and restored the control rhythm. (See also Ref. 519.)

STEIN AND KLEINFELD, *Circulation* (1967),[2982] studied the effect of PHT on the sinoatrial node of rabbit heart. Sinoatrial pacemaker action potentials were recorded using intracellular microelectrodes during constant perfusion of varying concentrations of PHT (1–100 μM). PHT slowed the heart rate by decreasing the slope of diastolic depolarization of the action potential.

The authors note that the ability of PHT to depress automaticity of sinoatrial cells by reducing or eliminating diastolic depolarization suggests that PHT may have a similar effect on ectopic foci, which may explain its antiarrhythmic actions.

BIGGER, BASSETT AND HOFFMAN, *Circulation Research* (1968),[19] studied the effects of PHT (.01–100 μM) on isolated, perfused canine Purkinje fibers.

In stimulated fibers which were partially depolarized or had a low rate of rise of the action potential despite a normal resting potential, PHT increased the phase zero rate of rise of the action potential. PHT also protected such fibers from further decreases in action potential rate of rise caused by high-frequency stimulation.

In spontaneously firing Purkinje fibers which showed generalized diastolic depolarization and decreased maximum diastolic potential, PHT decreased excessive depolarization and increased resting potential. PHT also protected the fibers from the abnormal automaticity induced by ouabain and isoproterenol, without interfering with the latter's therapeutic effects.

The authors emphasize that, unlike quinidine, PHT protects against frequency-dependent decreases in depolarization rate and does not depress conduction velocity or stimulation threshold.

HELFANT, RICCIUTTI, SCHERLAG AND DAMATO, *American Journal of Physiology* (1968),[157] studied the effects of digitalis and PHT on myocardial ion fluxes in dogs. Toxic doses of digitalis caused myocardial potassium loss and arrhythmias, both of which were promptly reversed by PHT (5 mg/kg).

HILMI AND REGAN, *American Heart Journal* (1968),[404] compared the effectiveness of procainamide, lidocaine, propranolol and PHT in digitalis-induced ventricular tachycardia in dogs. PHT and lidocaine were the most successful in conversion of ventricular tachycardia to normal sinus rhythm.

PHT restored and maintained normal sinus rhythm in six of seven animals.

LESBRE, CATHALA, SALVADOR, FLORIO, LESCURE AND MERIEL, *Archives des Maladies du coeur et des Vaisseaux* (1969),[1264] studied the cardiac effects of PHT in ten digitalis-intoxicated dogs. In the first experiment they found that PHT (10 mg/kg) did not lengthen the P-R interval in seven animals and actually shortened it in three.

In another experiment in the same animals, a ligature was placed on both branches of the left coronary artery, creating ventricular dysrhythmias and atrial extrasystoles. In nine of ten cases the arrhythmia and extrasystoles disappeared either during or immediately after injection of PHT. For a thirty-minute period, following intravenous PHT, it was difficult to induce new ventricular arrhythmias by clamping the artery.

The authors note that PHT corrects disturbances of both atrial and ventricular excitability without impairing atrioventricular conduction, ventricular contractility or systemic blood pressure.

SPERELAKIS AND HENN, *American Journal of Physiology* (1970),[1580] studied the effect of PHT (.01–18 μM) on membrane potentials of individual chick heart cells in tissue culture.

PHT was found to prevent hyperexcitability caused by both strontium and electrical stimulation. While PHT protected against these insults, it did not affect the normal function of heart cells as measured by resting potentials and the maximum rate of rise or duration of the action potential.

SINGH, SINHA, RASTOGI, DUA AND KOHLI, *Japanese Journal of Pharmacology* (1971),[1557] studied the antiarrhythmic properties of PHT in dogs. Arrhythmias were induced by means of aconitine (injected into the cerebral ventricle or intravenously), ether-epinephrine and coronary ligation. PHT was effective against all types of arrhythmias, irrespective of their central nervous system or peripheral origin.

CURTIS, *University of Michigan Doctoral Thesis* (1971),[927] reported that PHT (100 μM) was effective in terminating ex-perimentally-induced atrial fibrillation in dogs.

GILLIS, McCLELLAN, SAUER AND STANDAERT, *Journal of Pharmacology and Experimental Therapeutics* (1971),[2197] in a study of cardiac sympathetic nerve activity, demonstrated that intravenous PHT (up to 20 mg/kg/min) counteracted deslanoside-induced sympathetic nerve firing and simultaneously converted deslanoside-induced ventricular tachycardia to sinus rhythm.

LOH, *Federation Proceedings* (1974),[2224] demonstrated in isolated atrial trabeculae of the frog that PHT produced a net gain of tissue potassium and reduction of potassium efflux with an accompanying prolongation of action potential duration and an elevation of resting potential.

The author suggests that PHT's effects on transmembrane potentials are due to its membrane stabilizing actions.

LISANDER, JAJU AND WANG, *European Journal of Pharmacology* (1975),[2720] demonstrated the rapid (one- to three-minute) effectiveness of PHT in treating cardiac arrhythmias resulting from electrical stimulation of the perifornical region of cat hypothalamus. The mean effective dose of PHT required to prevent arrhythmias via the intravenous route was 11.9 mg/kg, and via the vertebral artery route and the fourth ventricular route, less than 2 mg/kg.

The authors conclude that, in addition to its direct actions on the heart, PHT has a strong antiarrhythmic effect via the central nervous system.

CHAI, LEE AND WANG, *Archives Internationales de Pharmacodynamie et de Therapie* (1976),[1768] studied the effect of PHT on arrhythmias induced by occlusion of the common carotid arteries in cats. Intravenous, intravertebral artery, intracarotid artery, intracerebroventricular and intrahypothalamic routes of administration of PHT were all effective at different doses.

The authors conclude that PHT exerts potent antiarrhythmic effects through its action on the central nervous sytem.

CORR AND GILLIS, *Federation Proceedings* (1976),[1783] demonstrated, in cats, that pretreatment with PHT significantly reduced premature ventricular contractions following anterior descending coronary artery occlusion. None of the seven treated animals developed ventricular fibrillation.

The authors conclude that PHT can suppress premature ventricular contractions and ventricular fibrillation during the early stages of myocardial infarction.

HONDEGHEM, *Journal of Electrocardiology* (1976),[1900] demonstrated that intravenous PHT (5 mg/kg) markedly increased the stimulation threshold of ischemic canine myocardium, but had no effect on normal myocardium.

EHRING AND HONDEGHEM, *Proceedings of the Western Pharmacological Society* (1978),[1815] studied the effects of PHT on isolated guinea pig heart papillary muscle. PHT (60–100 μM) decreased action potential V_{max} only when stimulus frequency was high or when the cells were depolarized. PHT's effects were less when the cells were hyperpolarized.

Based on this evidence, the authors suggest that PHT achieves its antiarrhythmic effects by binding to open sodium channels, thus regulating sodium influx.

ALMOTREFI AND BAKER, *British Journal of Pharmacology* (1980),[2143] demonstrated that PHT (3.6–18 μM) produces significant dose-dependent increases in electrical stimulation threshold and ventricular fibril-

lation threshold as measured in the Langendorff perfused rabbit heart.

GRENADER, PONAMAREVA, ZURABISHVILI AND VASIEV, *Biofizika* (1982),[2557] reported that PHT (2–8 μg/ml) decreased the fast inward sodium current in strips of rabbit atrium and ventricle. Consistent with this, refractoriness of the cardiac tissue also increased, more in atrial than ventricular tissue.

The authors suggest that these effects are important in PHT's antiarrhythmic actions and note that they are selective for damaged myocardium. Normal myocardium is not affected by PHT.

QUEST, BREED AND GILLIS, *Journal of Cardiovascular Pharmacology* (1982),[2887] studied the effects of PHT on cardiac slowing produced by peripheral vagus nerve stimulation (1–10 Hz) and by direct injection of acetylcholine. To avoid autonomic reflex mechanisms, vagotomized animals with transected spinal cords were used.

Intravenous PHT (0.5 to 1 mg/kg/min) significantly reduced the bradycardia produced by the higher frequencies of vagal nerve stimulation (3, 5 and 10 Hz). This inhibitory effect appeared immediately after the start of intravenous PHT.

Bradycardia produced by high concentrations of acetylcholine was also significantly inhibited by PHT, and this inhibition persisted from 90 to 120 minutes after cessation of PHT.

SANCHEZ-CHAPULA AND JOSEPHSON, *Journal of Molecular Cell Cardiology* (1983),[2922] reported that PHT (20 μM) inhibited sodium currents in rat ventricular cells in a voltage- and use-dependent manner.

The authors state that PHT's depression of the cardiac sodium current may be an important mechanism of its antiarrhythmic effects. The authors suggest that PHT binds preferentially to inactivated sodium channels and prolongs their recovery.

WATANABE AND BAILEY, *Annals of the New York Academy of Sciences* (1984),[3063] reviewed the regulation of cardiac function by the autonomic nervous system as it relates to various antiarrhythmic drugs, including PHT.

The authors note that, in addition to its direct effect on cardiac tissues, PHT modifies sympathetic nerve activity. They cite several animal studies in which PHT has been shown to decrease activity of cardiac sympathetic nerves with resultant reduction in contractile force, blood pressure and heart rate. PHT has also been shown to reduce the excessive cardiac sympathetic nerve stimulation produced by cardiac glycosides. Pretreatment with PHT has been shown to prevent the increase in sympathetic nerve activity and subsequent cardiac arrhythmias induced by posterior hypothalamic electrical stimulation.

HASHIMOTO, ISHII, KOMORI AND MITSU-HASHI, *Heart and Vessels* (1985),[2577] studied the effects of PHT, as well as other antiarrhythmic drugs, on ventricular arrhythmias induced by digitalis, adrenaline, and two-stage coronary ligation. PHT (9.8–12.1 μg/ml) was effective in controlling the arrhythmias produced by all three methods.

Protection Against Digitalis Toxicity

HELFANT, SCHERLAG AND DAMATO, *Circulation* (1967),[155] and *Clinical Research* (1967),[685] demonstrated that intravenous PHT (5 mg/kg), given prophylactically to dogs, protected against digitalis toxicity. With PHT, 72 to 224% more digitalis was required to produce toxic arrhythmias. The authors state that PHT's effect on the toxic-

therapeutic ratio of digitalis has important clinical implications.

LÜLLMANN AND WEBER, *Arztliche Forschung* (1968)[233] and *Naunyn-Schmiedebergs Archiv fur Pharmakologie* (1968),[403] found that PHT (20–80 mg/kg) given intravenously to guinea pigs almost doubled the amount of intravenous digoxin necessary to produce death. The normalization of rhythm by PHT occurred without interfering with the beneficial effects of digitalis.

SCHERLAG, HELFANT, RICCIUTTI AND DA-MATO, *American Journal of Physiology* (1968),[1507] observed that, in dogs, PHT (5 mg/kg, intravenously) consistently converted digitalis-induced ventricular tachycardia to sinus rhythm with a corresponding reversal of the digitalis-induced potassium efflux. Improvement in myocardial contractility with digitalis was not altered by PHT.

With PHT pretreatment, the toxicity of digitalis was markedly delayed and the rate of myocardial potassium efflux slowed.

BASKIN, DUTTA AND MARKS, *British Journal of Pharmacology* (1973),[801] in a study of the guinea pig heart, showed that PHT (30–100 μM) and potassium significantly prevent ouabain intoxication without interfering with its inotropic benefits.

WATSON AND WOODBURY, *Archives Internationales de Pharmacodynamie et de Therapie* (1973),[1663] studying ouabain intoxication in guinea pigs, observed that PHT prevented ouabain-induced electrolyte changes and arrhythmias. Under some conditions, pretreatment with PHT (80 mg/kg) reduced the lethality of ouabain from 90% to 34%.

The authors found that PHT normalized plasma potassium, as well as intracellular concentrations of sodium, potassium and chloride, in cardiac muscle. They suggest that the antiarrhythmic effect of PHT is due to an action on active transport of electrolytes across cell membrane.

HANSEN AND WAGENER, *Zeitschrift fur Kardiologie und Angiologie* (1974),[1122] by using both isolated atrium and barbiturate-damaged heart-lung preparations of guinea pigs, showed that the toxic arrhythmogenic side effects of digoxin are prevented by PHT (3–5 μg/ml), without affecting its inotropic benefits.

The authors suggest that by the addition of PHT, glycoside dosages can be beneficially increased in patients with cardiac failure.

TAKEYA, HOTTA AND YAJIMA, *Journal of Aichi Medical University Association* (1980),[3001] reported that PHT (30–50 μM) inhibited both chronotropic and inotropic effects of grayanotoxin, and chronotropic effects of G-strophanthin on spontaneous pacemaker activity in isolated guinea-pig right atrial preparations. The authors conclude that PHT reduced grayanotoxin and G-strophanthin induced sodium influx.

GARAN, RUSKIN AND POWELL, *American Journal of Physiology* (1981),[2525] in a study evaluating the role of PHT's central nervous system effects in its control of cardiac arrhythmias, found that PHT (10 mg) administered directly into the cerebrospinal fluid (cisterna magna) protected against digoxin-induced arrhythmias in ten anesthetized dogs.

Time to onset of ventricular arrhythmias was significantly longer in the PHT-treated animals (50 minutes compared to 19 minutes in controls). Five of the PHT-treated dogs remained free of ventricular fibrillation for the entire three-hour observation period, compared to one of ten in the control group. PHT, administered by an intravenous route, had a similar, but slightly less, protective effect.

The protective action of PHT was less under conditions of bilateral vagectomy, confirming PHT's regulatory effect on the heart via the nervous system.

RHEE, *Fourth International Symposium on Calcium-Binding Proteins in Health and Disease* (1983),[2904] studied the effects of PHT, as well as dimethylpropanolol (DMP) and quinidine, on radioisotopic rubidium and calcium uptake in specialized canine cardiac tissues including sinoatrial node, Purkinje fibers, left ventricular muscle and aorta.

An arrhythmogenic dose of ouabain significantly reduced rubidium uptake in all tissue types. Both PHT and DMP, at doses sufficient to control the ouabain-induced arrhythmias, significantly increased rubidium uptake in the left ventricle and Purkinje fiber samples. In the sinoatrial node PHT decreased rubidium uptake, while DMP had no effect. Neither drug affected uptake in aortic tissue.

In a second series of experiments, PHT, DMP and quinidine were found to reduce calcium uptake by membrane vesicles prepared from the left ventricle.

The author concludes that PHT's effects on monovalent cation flux, and its antiarrhythmic actions, are due to its regulation of calcium channels or binding.

Cardiac Conduction

HELFANT, SCHERLAG AND DAMATO, *Circulation* (1967),[154] in studies on dogs concluded that PHT (5 mg/kg) consistently reversed the atrioventricular conduction (AVC) prolongations induced by procainamide.

SCHERLAG, HELFANT AND DAMATO, *American Heart Journal* (1968),[327] compared the effects of PHT and procainamide on AVC in digitalis-intoxicated and normal canine heart. PHT consistently converted more acetylstrophanthidin-induced ventricular tachycardia to sinus rhythm than did procainamide and completely restored AVC to control values. In contrast, procainamide, in doses necessary to counteract digitalis-induced ventricular tachycardia, exacerbated the AVC prolongation produced by the glycoside.

The authors state that the effect of PHT on AVC makes this a unique drug since it abolishes both the ventricular ectopia and AVC abnormalities produced by the glycoside.

BIGGER, STRAUSS AND HOFFMAN, *Federation Proceedings* (1968),[22] studied the effects of PHT on the conducting system in anesthetized dogs with electrodes chronically implanted at selected sites, and in isolated rabbit hearts by means of intracellular microelectrodes. In dogs, PHT (5–10 mg/kg) accelerated AVC by 20% under control conditions and in the presence of incomplete atrioventricular (AV) block and atrial flutter.

In rabbit heart, PHT increased AVC in the presence of partial AV block. PHT also improved impaired AVC caused by acetylcholine (ACh) without altering the ACh-induced sinus bradycardia.

WAX, WEBB AND ECKER, *Surgical Forum* (1969),[1668] observed the effect of PHT on the resting potential and action potential of ventricular heart muscle of the rat. With intravenous PHT (5 mg/kg) the resting potential plateau phase and the recovery period were both lengthened.

The authors note that these actions of PHT stabilized the heart, making it less susceptible to early reentry from circus mechanisms or other aberrant stimuli.

KLEINFELD AND STEIN, *Circulation* (1968),[1221] electrically stimulated isolated canine Purkinje and ventricular fibers and studied the action potentials. They found that PHT (.01–100 μM) decreased the effective refractory period of both fibers, with the greater effect being in the Purkinje fiber.

BIGGER, WEINBERG, KOVALIK, HARRIS, CRANEFIELD AND HOFFMAN, *Circulation Research* (1970),[828] examined the effects of PHT on excitability, automaticity and conduction in the canine heart *in situ* and on threshold voltage and action potential duration in isolated Purkinje fibers.

In the *in situ* heart, PHT (10 mg/kg) shortened the refractory period and enhanced conduction in ventricular muscle without changing diastolic threshold and only slightly decreasing automaticity in the specialized ventricular conducting system. It also increased fibrillation thresholds in both the atrium and ventricle. Shortening of the refractory period was accompanied by a decrease in the Q-T interval, consistent with clinical observations in PHT-treated patients.

In the isolated fibers PHT (0.1 μM) decreased action potential duration and the intracellular current pulse required to bring the fibers to firing threshold, while increasing threshold voltage.

The authors comment that PHT's ability to increase membrane responsiveness, thereby enhancing conduction, appears to be an important aspect of its antiarrhythmic actions and adds to its clinical safety.

ROSEN, DANILO, ALONSO AND PIPPENGER, *Journal of Pharmacology and Experimental*

Therapeutics (1976),[2055] demonstrated in isolated Purkinje fibers that the effect of PHT is determined by the initial state of conduction in the fiber which was experimentally altered by stretch, exposure to ouabain or perfusion with a solution in which all sodium ions were replaced by tetraethylammonium.

Depending upon the state of conduction in the fiber, PHT was shown either to enhance or to reduce conduction.

EL-SHERIF AND LAZZARA, *Circulation* (1978),[1822] studied the mechanism of action of PHT on reentrant ventricular arrhythmias in dogs, utilizing direct recordings of the reentrant pathway from the epicardial surface of the infarction zone.

PHT, in therapeutic doses, consistently prolonged refractoriness of potentially reentrant pathways in the infarction zone. On the other hand, PHT had no significant effect on conduction in the normal adjacent zone.

ARNSDORF AND MEHLMAN, *Journal of Pharmacology and Experimental Therapeutics* (1978),[1726] observed in sheep cardiac Purkinje fibers, injured by ischemia or stretch, that PHT (5 μg/ml) can restore impulse propagation by causing normalization of the action potential.

The authors note that clinically PHT can eliminate functional bundle branch block.

WASSERSTROM AND FERRIER, *Journal of Molecular and Cellular Cardiology* (1982),[3062] reported that both PHT (7.9–12 μM) and quinidine (1.6 μM) abolished or reduced acetylstrophanthidin-induced oscillatory afterpotentials and aftercontractions in isolated canine false tendons and Purkinje tissue. PHT hyperpolarized the tissue, but did not alter the threshold;

whereas quinidine raised the threshold. Both drugs partially reversed the inotropic effects of acetylstrophanthidin.

The authors note that PHT is clinically effective against digitalis-induced arrhythmias, but that quinidine is contraindicated because it can depress conduction and thereby precipitate arrhythmias.

SCHEUER AND KASS, *Circulation Research* (1983),[2931] investigated the effects of PHT (5–100 μM) on electrical and mechanical activity of isolated calf and dog Purkinje fibers. In addition to lowering and shortening the plateau phase of the action potential and twitch tension, PHT also reduced voltage-dependent calcium current.

Cardiac Calcification

RETTURA, STAMFORD AND SEIFTER, *Paper presented at Northeast Regional Meeting of American Chemical Society* (1973),[1454] conducted a controlled study of the effect of PHT in mice with predisposition to cardiac calcification. This calcification was enhanced by stress.

The authors found that PHT reversed the calcification process as determined grossly, microscopically and by chemical analysis. The authors suggest that this might be one mechanism by which PHT is effective in the prevention of cardiac arrhythmias.

Cardiac Hypoxia

BASSETT, BIGGER AND HOFFMAN, *The Journal of Pharmacology and Experimental Therapeutics* (1970),[804] reported that PHT protected canine Purkinje fibers during hypoxia.

Purkinje fibers in isolated heart preparations were stimulated electrically at a constant rate, and the electrical responses were measured until optimal performance was established. Then hypoxia was induced by perfusion with a nitrogen-carbon dioxide mixture, resulting in a sharp reduction in electrical response. During hypoxia, PHT improved electrical response, as measured by phase zero V_{max}. PHT also improved electrical response when the Purkinje fibers had already been depressed by hypoxia.

The authors suggest that the protective and therapeutic action of PHT on Purkinje fibers may in part explain its effectiveness in suppressing arrhythmias caused by myocardial ischemia and hypoxia.

ALDRETE AND CUBILLOS, *Anesthesia and Analgesia* (1984),[2280] compared the effects of PHT (15 mg/kg), thiopental (40 mg/kg), and placebo on hemodynamic tolerance and survival after severe hypoxia in rabbits.

PHT significantly delayed the onset of bradycardia and hypotension compared to thiopental and placebo. Survival was highest (eight of twelve) in the PHT-treated group compared to the thiopental group (three of twelve) and the placebo group in which none survived. (See also Ref. 2279.)

See also Anti-anoxic Effects of PHT.

Hypertension

RAINES AND NINER, *Neuropharmacology* (1975), [2032] demonstrated in cats that PHT (10–20 mg/kg) reduced systolic and diastolic blood pressure and heart rate, which had been elevated by carotid occlusion.

LEW, *Proceedings of the Society of Experimental Biology and Medicine* (1975),[1282] found that PHT increased the concentration of norepinephrine in the hypothalamus, cerebellum and brainstem in a strain of naturally hypertensive rats.

The author notes that a deficiency in norepinephrine in the hypothalamus has been reported in hypertension, and that certain treatments effective in reducing high blood pressure produce an increase of norepinephrine in the hypothalamus.

DADKAR, GUPTE AND DOHADWALLA, *Medical Biology* (1979),[1789] studied the effect of PHT on spontaneously hypertensive rats which exhibit many features similar to human essential hypertension.

PHT (5–20 mg/kg), orally for five days, elicited a dose-dependent fall in elevated systolic blood pressure, and increased norepinephrine concentration in the hypothalamus.

PHT did not lower blood pressure in a group of rats with normal blood pressure.

See also Refs. 414, 1480, 1717, 1797, 1892, 2090, 2168, 2316, 2668.

High-Density Lipoproteins— Atherosclerosis

Phenytoin's ability to raise HDL-C levels and to improve the HDL/LDL cholesterol ratio has been well documented, suggesting a role for PHT as a preventive in atherosclerosis (see Clinical—Cardiovascular section). This evidence, taken together with the fact that PHT protects brain, cardiac and other tissues against the damaging effects of hypoxia or ischemia, as in stroke or myocardial infarction, makes this a promising area for PHT's clinical use.

For laboratory studies on the mechanisms by which PHT achieves its effects on HDL-C, see Metabolic and Endocrine Regulatory Effects, p. 123.

OTHER STUDIES

Behavior and Cognitive Function

FINK AND SWINYARD, *Journal of Pharmaceutical Sciences* (1962),[99] compared a group of pharmacological agents in an effort to detect possible tranquilizing effects. One of the tests showed that PHT markedly reduced amphetamine toxicity in aggregated mice. From their studies the authors conclude that PHT possesses tranquilizing properties and should be more fully studied in patients.

TEDESCHI, TEDESCHI, MUCHA, COOK, MATTIS AND FELLOWS, *Journal of Pharmacology and Experimental Therapeutics* (1959),[749] and CHEN, BOHNER AND BRATTON, *Archives Internationales de Pharmacodynamie et de Therapie* (1963),[419] found that PHT suppressed fighting behavior in mice.

CHEN AND BOHNER, *Archives Internationales de Pharmacodynamic et de Therapie* (1960),[740] found, in mice, that PHT significantly inhibited scratching behavior induced by mescaline.

COHEN AND BARONDES, *Science* (1967),[59] found that PHT (35 mg/kg) significantly improved retention of learned behavior in mice given puromycin, a protein-synthesis inhibitor.

GORDON, *Recent Advances in Biological Psychiatry* (1968),[126] found that PHT (15–30 mg/kg) improved the deteriorated performance of older rats in both habituation and conditioned avoidance paradigms, but did not affect normal behavior in young rats.

The author notes that these findings have possible application to aging in humans. He comments that the decrease in memory function and slowing of task performance in aged humans has been postulated to be caused by an abnormal prolongation of electrophysiological activity in brain, akin to static or noise, and that PHT might exert its therapeutic effects by reducing such activity.

GORDON, CALLAGHAN AND DOTY, *Pharmacologist* (1968),[1088] reported that PHT did not appear to affect the performance of normal young adult rats, but that PHT enhanced the learning level and stable memory of aged rats for avoidance paradigms. These beneficial effects were more pronounced the more difficult and novel the task.

In parallel biochemical studies the authors found that PHT increased brain poly-ribosomal protein, rapidly-labeled RNA, and DNAase activity.

DOTY AND DALMAN, *Psychonomic Science* (1969),[702] found PHT (20–60 mg/kg), thirty minutes prior to each training session, facilitated learning on discrimination and avoidance tasks. The enhancement of performance was more prominent among older rats.

BLOCK AND MOORE, *Personal communication*,[670] found that protein-deficient pigs did not perform as well as normal pigs during extinction of a conditioned avoidance response. The performance of these protein-deficient pigs was significantly improved by pretreatment with PHT.

MOURAVIEFF-LESUISSE AND GIURGEA, *Archives Internationales de Pharmacodynamie et de Therapie* (1970),[1376] found that PHT (80 mg/kg) shortened spinal fixation time in normal rats and also in those in which spinal fixation time had been prolonged by electroshock. The authors note that spinal fixation time reflects a form of memory consolidation process within spinal cord reflexes.

BERNSTEIN AND JOHNSON, *Bulletin of Environmental Contamination and Toxicology* (1973),[823] while studying the effects of PHT on estrogen metabolism in pesticide-treated quail, observed that DDT caused excitability and aggressive behavior in the quail and that PHT reduced this excitable and aggressive behavior, without any apparent sedative effect.

GEHRES, RANDALL, RICCIO AND VARDARIS, *Physiology and Behavior* (1973),[1058] found that pretreatment with PHT (20 mg/kg, subcutaneously) markedly reduced the retrograde amnesia produced by lowered body temperature in rats. In addition, electrophysiological data indicated that PHT reduced the paroxysmal electrical activity induced in the hippocampus and amygdala by the lowered body temperature.

GIBBS AND NG, *Brain Research Bulletin* (1976),[1851] found that PHT (100 μM) counteracted amnesia induced by ouabain and cycloheximide in one-day-old chicks. (See also Ref. 2196.)

FILE AND LISTER, *Neuroscience Letters* (1983),[2493] reported that PHT (10 mg/kg, intraperitoneally) reversed the anxiogenic effects of Ro 5-4864, a selective ligand for benzodiazepine micromolar receptors in rats.

PAULE AND KILLAM, *Federation Proceedings* (1984),[2852] studied the effects of PHT (2.5–40 mg/kg/day, for a two-week period) on the performance of incremental repeated acquisition and incremental fixed-ratio tasks in epileptic baboons. At or below doses of PHT necessary for maximal control of induced seizures (20 mg/kg/day, achieving blood levels of 7–8 μg/ml), the animals showed less variability in response rates for the most difficult tasks.

The authors suggest that PHT made the baboons more attentive to the learning task and note that their results are consistent with other reports of PHT's benefits in human cognitive processes. (See Refs. 2473, 2853.)

STUDIES IN HUMANS

These studies deal with normal human beings. For more detailed summaries, see Clinical—Thought, Mood and Behavior section.

HAWARD, *Drugs and Cerebral Function* (1970),[1139] found PHT (150 mg) effective to a significant degree in improving concentration in twelve college students.

SMITH AND LOWREY, *Drugs, Development and Cerebral Function* (1972),[1564] in a double-blind study, found that PHT (100 mg, t.i.d.) improved cognitive performance to a significant level in twenty volunteer hospital employees.

HAWARD, *Revue de Medecine Aeronautique et Spatiale* (1973),[1140] found PHT (150 mg) significantly improved performance in three separate groups of pilots in simulated flying and radar-fixing tasks.

HOUGHTON, LATHAM AND RICHENS, *European Journal of Clinical Pharmacology* (1973),[1168] examined the effect of PHT in six normal volunteers with regard to critical flicker fusion threshold (CFF). No significant change in CFF was observed at 200, 300 and 400 mg of PHT, as tested hourly from one to seven hours after ingestion of PHT.

SMITH AND LOWREY, *Journal of the American Geriatrics Society* (1975),[1565] in a double-blind study, found improvement in cognitive functions in a group of elderly normal subjects given PHT, 100 mg, twice daily.

BARRATT, FAULK, BRANDT AND BRYANT, *Neuropsychobiology* (1986),[2311] used brain mapping techniques to examine the effects of PHT on the N100 sensory visual potential, as well as the late positive complex (LPC), which reflects cognitive processing. The authors emphasize that augmentation of the N100 potential is associated with impulsivity and attentional distraction.

The N100 and LPC potentials were recorded from six normal subjects given the task of counting a series of bright and dim light flashes. Recordings were made before, and one hour after, the subject received either PHT (100 mg) or placebo, depending on the trial.

PHT significantly reduced the intensity response of N100 at the vertex and anterior temporal sites, with a lesser reduction at the frontal pole.* In addition, PHT enhanced the frontal negative portion of the slow wave LPC component, but not the positive portion of the slow wave or P300 LPC components.

The authors comment that their findings are consistent with behavioral evidence that PHT reduces impulsivity and improves concentration.

* Plasma levels of PHT at one hour ranged from 0.6 to 0.8 μg/ml, indicating that plasma levels do not always correlate with PHT's effects.

Sleep

COHEN, DUNCAN AND DEMENT, *Electroencephalography and Clinical Neurophysiology* (1968),[58] studied the effect of PHT (9 mg/kg, daily) on the sleep patterns of cats. PHT decreased rapid eye movement (REM) sleep time significantly. REM periods were both shorter and less frequent. There was no consistent change in any non-REM sleep time.

ZUNG, *Psychophysiology* (1968),[397] studied the effects of PHT on sleep in ten adults, between the ages of twenty and forty-six, using all-night EEG and EOG (electrooculogram) recordings. Comparison between control and drug nights indicated that, with PHT, the time spent in REM sleep was significantly decreased, and non-REM sleep was increased.

WOLF, RODER-WANNER AND BREDE, *Epilepsia* (1984)[3080] studied polygraphic sleep patterns (EEG, EOG, ECG and respiration) in forty epileptic patients who were not on any medication. They compared phenobarbital and PHT in a randomized crossover design. With both phenobarbital and PHT sleep onset came sooner, but with PHT light sleep was decreased and deep sleep increased.

The authors state, "The decrease of light to the benefit of deep sleep, together with the rapid sleep onset, make PHT look like an excellent sleeping medication." In addition, they comment that few patients report sleep hangovers with PHT.

DECLERCK, MARTENS AND WAUQUIER, *Neuropsychobiology* (1985),[2445] studied the effects of one night's sleep deprivation on sleep patterns in normal individuals and in epileptic patients. In the patients taking PHT, the authors found increased non-REM sleep, decreased eye movements during REM sleep and an overall stabilized sleep pattern.

See also Clinical—Thought, Mood and Behavior section, p. 16; and Refs. 2777, 3079.

Pain

STILLE, *Nervenarzt* (1960),[352] in a study of the basis for the beneficial effect of PHT on pain, found that PHT (20 mg/kg) reduces the cortical response to single electrical stimuli or low-frequency series stimulation of the reticular formation in rabbits. The author states that PHT differs from the barbiturates and chlorpromazine in that it does not change the arousal reaction produced by frequent electrical stimulation of the mesencephalic reticular formation, nor the EEG arousal reaction to sensory stimulation.

SEEMAN, CHAU-WONG AND MOYYEN, *Canadian Journal of Physiology and Pharmacology* (1972),[1524] found that anesthetizing membrane concentrations of PHT or morphine in guinea pig brain synaptosomes and human erythrocytes were close to those predicted by the Meyer-Overton rule of anesthesia, indicating that they both have local anesthetic properties. (See also Ref. 2941.)

GRAFOVA, DANILOVA AND KRYZHANOVSKII, *Bulletin of Experimental Biology and Medicine (USSR)* (1979),[2550] studied the effects of PHT on the application of tetanus toxin, strychnine, penicillin, potassium chloride and ouabain to rat dorsal spinal cord. PHT (100 mg/kg, intramuscularly) suppressed the pain syndrome caused by potassium chloride and ouabain, but had only a weak action against that produced by tetanus toxin, strychnine and penicillin. (See also Ref. 2202.)

KENDIG, COURTNEY AND COHEN, *Journal of Pharmacology and Experimental Therapeutics* (1979),[2212] compared the anesthetic molecular properties and frequency-dependent sodium channel blocking actions of PHT, phenobarbital, the local anesthetic benzocaine, and the volatile general anesthetic diethyl ether at the frog node of Ranvier. Some blockage of resting sodium channels was seen with all the agents tested, but frequency-dependent sodium channel-block was produced only by PHT and phenobarbital.

FOONG, SATOH AND TAKAGI, *Journal of Pharmacological Methods* (1982),[2503] reported that PHT (40–120 mg/kg, intraperitoneally) suppressed bradykinin-induced aversive behavior in a rat tooth-pulp pain model.

FROMM, CHATTHA, TERRENCE AND GLASS, *European Journal of Pharmacology* (1982),[2515] studied the effects of PHT and carbamazepine (CBZ) on segmental and periventricular interneurons of the spinal trigeminal nucleus oralis of cats. Therapeutic serum levels of PHT and CBZ facilitated segmental inhibition, but depressed the periventricular inhibition, while also depressing the response of trigeminal nucleus neurons to an unconditioned maxillary nerve stimulus.

The authors note that the depression of neuronal activity by PHT and CBZ is selective, leaving some inhibitory pathways functioning normally, thus greatly enhancing their effectiveness. They suggest that PHT and CBZ may act to control pain in trigeminal neuralgia, and abnormal electrical activity in the nervous system more generally, by a relative facilitation of inhibitory feedback mechanisms. (See also Ref. 1838.)

HITCHCOCK AND TEIXEIRA, *Applied Neurophysiology* (1982),[2597] compared the effects of PHT (1.25–50 mg/kg), sodium valproate and carbamazepine (CBZ) on the neurotransmitter-related enzymatic activity of the rat anterior mesencephalic periaqueductal grey matter, which is an integrative center for pain systems. PHT caused the greatest reduction in glutamate dehydrogenase and GABA, and it was the only drug to increase semi-aldehyde dehydrogenase activity.

The authors hypothesize that PHT and CBZ, but not sodium valproate, may activate central pain-suppressive systems by reducing the inhibitory effect of GABA on the periaqueductal grey pain suppressive pathways.

YAARI AND DEVOR, *Neuroscience Letters* (1985),[3090] reported that intraaortic PHT (1–10 mg) or topically applied PHT in doses as low as 100 μM to exposed desheathed neuromas, in rats, reduced or blocked abnormal spontaneous neuroma discharges. In spite of its marked suppression of this discharge, and in contrast to the action of local anesthetics, PHT did not block conduction of nerve impulses evoked by direct stimulation of the neuroma. PHT's actions were thus selective for the abnormal activity.

The authors note that spontaneous discharges from nerve-end neuromas and from other sites of nerve injury and disease have been implicated as a cause of paresthesias and pain associated with amputation, peripheral nerve trauma and a wide range of other neurological conditions. They suggest that the clinical analgesic action of PHT may, at least in part, result from direct suppression of ectopic impulses generated in the region of nerve damage.

McLEAN, *Society for Neuroscience Abstracts* (1986),[2782] evaluating mechanisms of neuropathic pain relief, used mouse dorsal root ganglion cells and ganglia obtained from patients undergoing surgery for chronic pain. To simulate the rapid burst firing observed in human sensory nerves in association with pain, calcium concentration in the extracellular medium was lowered to 0.1 mM. Both PHT (2 μg/ml) and carbamazepine (2 μg/ml) inhibited the rapid burst firing induced by the low calcium in both mouse and human ganglia. Resting membrane properties were unaffected.

The author notes that the effects of both PHT and CBZ were selective for sustained repetitive activity and occurred at levels corresponding to their free fractions in plasma. The author concludes that this limitation of rapid firing could explain, at least in part, the success of PHT and CBZ in treating neuropathic pain.

Drug Addiction and Withdrawal

FERTZIGER, LYNCH AND STEIN, *Brain Research* (1974),[1026] reported that PHT (15–30 mg/kg, twice daily) decreased the naloxone-induced withdrawal syndrome in morphine-dependent rats. The authors state that abrupt withdrawal of morphine is known to increase neuronal excitability in animals as well as man.

The PHT-treated animals contrasted sharply with controls in some aspects of the abstinence syndrome. Hyperexcitability was remarkably reduced and significantly fewer "wet dog" or body shakes occurred in the PHT-treated groups.

FERTZIGER, STEIN AND LYNCH, *Psychopharmacologia* (1974),[1027] investigated the effects of pretreatment with PHT on the morphine-induced mania response in cats.

The authors note that in the cat, morphine is known to produce a species-specific excitant or manic response. This response includes extreme excitation and agitation, with explosive impulsivity, abrupt jumping and intermittent vocalizing. Pretreatment with PHT (15 mg/kg, twice daily for four to six days) prevented these hypermanic responses to morphine.

The authors suggest that PHT may prove useful in reducing some of the withdrawal symptoms commonly seen in human addicts.

SPRAGUE AND CRAIGMILL, *Research Communications in Chemical Pathology and Pharmacology* (1976),[2977] showed that PHT (10–20 mg/kg) not only reduced the severity of handling-induced convulsions, but also elevated the threshold of the startle reflex, used as a measure of central nervous system excitability, during ethanol withdrawal in mice.

SAAD, OSMAN, MUSTAFA AND HUSSEIN, *IRCS Medical Science* (1977),[2062] found that PHT reduced naloxone-induced withdrawal symptoms in morphine-dependent rats.

COOKSON AND MANN, *Neuroscience Abstracts* (1978),[1781] reported that intravenous PHT (35 mg/kg) reversed the morphine-induced catalepsy in rats within fifteen minutes. PHT also prevented the appearance of catalepsy when given prior to morphine.

The authors suggest that PHT may correct excessive morphine-induced calcium-dependent neurotransmitter release, which causes the cataleptic response.

Healing

SKIN, MUCOUS MEMBRANES AND CONNECTIVE TISSUE

SHAFER, BEATTY AND DAVIS, *Proceedings of the Society of Experimental Biology and Medicine* (1958),[337] found that pretreatment with PHT (25–50 mg/day), for eighteen days prior to making an incision, produced a dramatic increase in tensile strength of healing wounds in rats. (See also Refs. 335, 336.)

HOUCK, JACOB AND MAENGWYN-DAVIES, *Journal of Clinical Investigation* (1960),[172] found that PHT (25 mg/day) decreases dermal water and fat and increases collagen in rat skin. HOUCK AND JACOB[502] showed that PHT diminished the catabolic effect of cortisol which reduces hexosamine, nitrogen and collagen fractions in the skin of young rats.

KELLN AND GORLIN, *Dental Progress* (1961),[189] confirmed the wound healing effects of PHT in rats by showing that two-weeks pretreatment with PHT (50 mg/day) increased tensile strength and fibroblast growth compared with controls at seventy-two hours after abdominal incision.

SHAFER, *Journal of Dental Research* (1965),[336] found that PHT (5–25 μg/ml) stimulated growth and [³H]-thymidine incorporation of normal human gingival fibroblasts in tissue culture.

KOLBERT, *American Journal of Ophthalmology* (1968),[504] reported that oral PHT (50 mg/day), for two days pre-operatively and twice weekly for two weeks post-operatively, increased the tensile strength of corneal wounds in rabbits.

HOUCK, CHENG AND WATERS, *Antiepileptic Drugs* (1972),[1164] reported that treatment with PHT (100 mg/kg/day, for twelve days) increased the amount of insoluble collagen in the connective tissue of rats. In addition, they observed an increase in another protein (insoluble, noncollagenous) which they termed scleroprotein. With this increase of scleroprotein, there was a significant reduction in the amount of triglyceride or neutral fats.

The authors note that these findings in animals are consistent with improved wound healing observed clinically.

BAZIN AND DELAUNAY, *Comptes Rendues Academie Sciences* (1972),[811] demonstrated that in rats treated with PHT for twenty-one days, the collagen content was unchanged in healthy skin, but was increased by 21% in granulomatous tissue. The degree of collagen maturation was increased in both.

EISENBERG, WILLIAMS, STEVENS AND SCHOFIELD, *Journal of International Research Communications* (1974),[2176] demonstrated that PHT (55 μM) inhibits the activity of collagenase and collagen peptidase *in vitro*.

The authors noted that PHT's inhibition of collagenase may be related to its effectiveness in treating epidermolysis bullosa. (See Refs. 1738, 1817, 2153.)

KASAI AND HACHIMINE, *Bulletin of Tokyo Dental College* (1974),[2647] found that PHT (1–5 μg/ml) stimulated collagen synthesis in all four fibroblast lines tested. The response was greatest in the two lines derived from gingival tissue.

STAPLE AND NAKEEB, *Journal of Dental Research* (1978),[2258] demonstrated in rats that, whereas dermal allograft survival was not prolonged, initial union of host and graft epithelium was more rapid in PHT recipients.

BERGENHOLTZ AND HANSTROM, *Biochemical Pharmacology* (1979),[2155] demonstrated that PHT (20 μg/ml) increased incorporation of radioactive collagen into cat palatal mucosa grown in organ culture. PHT also decreased collagen degradation.

HANSTROM AND JONES, *Medical Biology* (1979),[1882] showed that PHT prevented collagen degradation in cat palatal mucosa during organ culture.

GOULTSCHIN AND SHOSHAN, *Biochimica et Biophysica Acta* (1980),[1867] demonstrated inhibition of collagen breakdown in gingival tissue obtained from five PHT-treated patients during periodontal surgery and maintained in culture for four days. DNA content of the tissue was also increased compared to controls.

NISHIKASE, FURUYA AND TAKASE, *IRCS Medical Science* (1980),[2004] reported that PHT lowered the levels of lipid peroxide, as well as granulation tissue and fluid exudate, in carageenin-induced inflammation and granulomas in rats.

The authors conclude that PHT's inhibition of lipid peroxide accounts for its reduction of granuloma tissue and fluid exudate formation, both manifestations of the inflammatory response.

MOY, TAN, HOLNESS AND UITTO, *Clinical Research* (1983),[2811] studied the effects of PHT (25–50 μg/ml) on the metabolism of collagen in human skin fibroblast cultures. Prolyl hydroxylase and collagenase activity was markedly reduced at these PHT concentrations. PHT did not affect thymidine incorporation or hydroxyproline formation.

The authors conclude that PHT affects the post-translational modification of collagen and may reduce its enzymatic degradation, and suggest PHT's usefulness in patients with increased collagenase activity.

MATSUO AND YAJIMA, *Japanese Journal of Oral Biology* (1985),[2773] found that PHT (5–40 µg/ml) stimulated both rat fibroblast proliferation and collagen fibrogenesis in tissue culture.

STRESS ULCERS

REQUENA, FORTE, KNOPF, SCHERRER, KIRSCHNER AND LEVOWITZ, *Surgical Forum* (1972),[2900] studied the protective effects of PHT and vitamin A on the formation of stress ulcers in fasted and restrained rats. Both PHT (50 mg, twice daily, subcutaneously) and vitamin A (50,000 units intramuscularly as a one-time dose) markedly decreased the incidence of stress ulcers compared to controls (p<0.01). When PHT and vitamin A were given together, an even stronger protective effect was noted.

PHT also prevented intracellular potassium depletion. The authors suggest that the protective action of PHT stems from its membrane stabilizing properties which, in turn, prevent intracellular potassium depletion and the consequent deleterious effects of the back diffusion of hydrogen ions.

TASSE, *The Canadian Journal of Surgery* (1982),[3005] found that PHT (50 mg, intramuscularly) significantly reduced the formation of stress ulcers in restrained, fasted rats. Vitamin A had no protective effects. The author notes the need for further studies of PHT's effects at lower doses. (See also Ref. 3028.)

BONE

FRYMOYER, *Journal of Trauma* (1967),[1840] demonstrated a statistically significant in-

creased rate of union of fibula fractures in rats treated with PHT (4 mg/kg/day). Clot organization was greater in the treated animals than in controls at fifteen days. At thirty days, the number of fracture unions, quality of callus, amount of compact bone and total fracture score were all greater in the PHT-treated group.

SKLANS, TAYLOR, SHKLAR, *Journal of Oral Surgery* (1967),[343] demonstrated that treatment with PHT (40 mg/kg/day), starting either prior to fracture or at the time of fracture, accelerated healing of experimentally produced mandibular fractures in rabbits.

Histologically, the PHT-treated animals showed earlier clot organization and increased vascular and connective tissue formation at the site of the healing fracture compared to controls.

GUDMUNDSON AND LIDGREN, *Acta Orthopaedica Scandinavica* (1973),[1104] in a controlled study, found that PHT (50 mg/kg/day) accelerates healing of experimentally-induced tibial fractures in mice. The tensile strength of healing unstable fractures and the breaking strength of healing fractures were significantly greater in the PHT-treated group than in controls. In the PHT-treated animals the fracture callus contained a larger amount of extractable collagen.

The authors conclude that a higher rate of collagen synthesis may contribute to the better rate of healing of fractures observed with PHT.

LIVER

SMITH AND ROBINSON, *Proceedings of the Western Pharmacology Society* (1962),[505] reported that, in rat, intraperitoneal PHT (10 mg/day), prior to and continuing after hepatectomy, significantly stimulated liver regeneration compared to controls, as measured by both wet and dry liver weights. The PHT-treated animals also showed a much greater fibroblastic reaction around the hepatectomy sites.

SHAFER, *Journal of Oral Therapeutics and Pharmacology* (1966),[335] demonstrated, in rats, that PHT (10 mg/day), beginning ten days prior to hepatectomy, stimulated liver regeneration, as measured by wet and dry liver weight. In a second experiment, in mice, they found that PHT increased [³H]-thymidine uptake, indicating a stimulation of nucleic acid synthesis and liver cell proliferation.

REMMER, *8th International Congress of Gastroenterology* (1968),[2248] reported improved liver healing after partial hepatectomy as reflected by increased liver weight and protein in rats treated with PHT (50 mg/kg/day).

KHAN, *Garyounis Medical Journal* (1979),[2659] studied the effects of PHT (100 mg/kg/day, intraperitoneally, daily for nine days) on liver growth in normal rats and on liver regeneration in partially hepatectomized rats. PHT increased liver weight in both groups compared to controls, with no increase in hepatic water. In addition, PHT stimulated an adhesive reaction around the area of partial hepatectomy which was not seen in controls.

The authors conclude that PHT can have a stimulating effect on cells of non-connective tissue origin in both normal and injured livers. However, PHT increases fibroblast proliferation selectively in the injured liver.

SPINAL CORD

GERBER, OLSON AND HARRIS, *Neurosurgery* (1980),[2195] studied functional recovery after spinal cord injury in animals treated

with PHT. Intravenous PHT (20 mg/kg) at time of injury or thirty minutes following injury, and again at six hours, was compared to conventional steroid treatment and no treatment.

At two weeks, recovery in the PHT-treated group was significantly greater: three of eleven could run and five could walk, compared to one of five in the steroid-treated group and none in the control group. At six weeks, nine of the eleven PHT-treated animals were running with little motor deficit, compared to two of five in the steroid-treated group and none in the control group.

The authors conclude that PHT may offer clinical protection from neurological deficits caused by spinal cord injury.

CARIES

ROVIN, SABES, EVERSOLE AND GORDON, *Journal of Dental Research* (1973),[1485] studied the effect of PHT in preventing caries. The authors state that during the course of a previous study on periodontal disease in rats, there had been an unsuccessful attempt to produce gingival hyperplasia with PHT. Although they were unsuccessful in producing gingival hyperplasia, they noticed that the PHT-treated rats did not develop caries.

As a result of this observation, the authors conducted a controlled study of the effect of PHT on the prevention of caries in rats. A ligature of the first mandibular molar was used as the irritant for inducing experimental caries. PHT had a marked effect in retarding caries in these animals. The effect was particularly apparent for five months; at the end of ten months, the effect was less.

The authors conclude that PHT acted as a caries retarder and that there could be clinical application for their findings. (See also Ref. 1724.)

See also Refs. 171, 188, 499, 500, 501, 2107, and Clinical—Healing section.

Temperature Regulation

GAYET-HALLION, *Comptes Rendus de la Societe Biologique* (1959),[2531] reported that PHT (80–100 mg/kg, intraperitoneally) produced a rapid lowering of rat body temperature (approximately 5 degrees). A similar effect was observed in guinea pig.

LOTTI, TORCHIANA AND PORTER, *Archives Internationales de Pharmacodynamie et de Therapie* (1973),[1306] found that PHT (17 mg/kg) offset lowered body temperature and suppression of locomotion induced by reserpine in mice.

KORCZYN, SHAVIT, AND SCHLOSBERG, *European Journal of Pharmacology* (1980),[1932] reported that PHT (5 mg/kg), as well as dantrolene sodium and procaine, reduced mortality from succinylcholine-induced malignant hyperpyrexia in chicks. Mortality in PHT-treated chicks was 27%, compared to 66% in the control group.

The authors suggest that PHT's protective effects are due to its prevention of excessive intracellular calcium accumulation.

See also Clinical—Fever and Temperature Regulation, p. 69.

Acute Radiation Exposure

LAIRD AND FONNER, *U.S. Army Medical Research Lab, Fort Knox, Ky.* (1957),[213] studied the protective effects of PHT in the hyperacute radiation syndrome. Pretreatment with PHT (94 mg/kg) delayed the onset and reduced the severity of convulsive activity and increased the median survival time as much as three- to ten-fold in mice exposed to massive doses of x-radiation (between 55,000 and 150,000 roentgens), compared with controls.

LEVAN, GORDON AND STEFANI, *Journal of Pharmaceutical Sciences* (1970),[1267] compared survival of mice exposed to 750 rads whole-body irradiation, with and without PHT pretreatment. There were 450 animals in each group.

PHT (3 mg/kg, intraperitoneally) significantly prolonged survival of the irradiated mice. By the nineteenth day after irradiation, all of the control animals had died. At thirty days, 55% of the PHT-treated animals were still alive.

CURRAN AND EL-MOFTY, *Journal of Dental Research* (1983),[2420] reported that PHT (20–50 mg/kg) protected normal rat parotid gland from the damaging effects of a single x-ray dose of 2000 rads, in a dose-dependent manner. Damage was assessed histologically and by serum amylase. The authors attribute this protective effect to PHT's calcium-antagonist actions.

Effects on Malignant Cell Growth

LEVAN, GORDON AND STEFANI, *Onocology* (1972),[1268] reported that intraperitoneal PHT (3 mg/kg/day, for three days) prolonged the life span of mice that had been implanted with Ehrlich ascites tumor. On day twenty-two, 43% of the PHT-treated mice were alive compared with no survivors in the control group.

LEVO, *Naunyn-Schmeideberg's Archiv fur Pharmakologie* (1974),[1279] in a controlled study, observed that PHT (0.5 mg/day, for seven days) reduced the incidence of lung adenomas induced by urethane in SWR mice. Fourteen mice were treated with PHT, fifteen were injected with the solvent used to suspend PHT, and fifteen were untreated. The animals were sacrificed after twelve weeks.

The fifteen mice treated with solvent had a total of seventy adenomas. The fifteen untreated mice had a total of sixty-eight adenomas. The fourteen mice treated with PHT had a total of forty-one adenomas. (See also Ref. 1955.)

KORNBLITH, CALLAHAN AND CASWELL, *Neurosurgery* (1978),[1934] reported that PHT inhibited the growth of seven of ten cultured human astrocytoma cell lines. PHT (20–100 µg/ml) produced significant dose-dependent growth reduction. At comparable doses, the growth of normal fibroblasts and astrocytes was unaffected.

KORNBLITH, HARTNETT, ANDERSON, QUINDLEN AND SMITH, *Neurosurgery* (1979),[1933] described significant growth inhibition by PHT of two murine astrocytoma cell lines in tissue culture. When the same tumor cells were implanted subcutaneously or intracranially in rats, the PHT-treated group showed significantly slower rates of tumor growth than the untreated group. Both tumor volume and number of actively dividing tumor cells were less in the PHT-treated group.

ANISIMOV, OSTROUMOVA AND DILMAN, *Bulletin of Experimental Biology and Medicine* (1980),[2294] reported that administration of PHT (7.5 mg/kg/day) for three weeks prior to the induction of rat mammary tumors by 7,12-dimethylbenzanthracene reduced the incidence of such tumors by approximately 25%.

DILMAN AND ANISIMOV, *Gerontology* (1980),[1806] reported that treatment of female C3H/Sn mice with PHT (2 mg/day, five days per week), decreased spontaneous tumor incidence by 2.3 times and prolonged mean life span by 25%, compared to controls. A similar effect was observed with phenformin.

SHIBA AND WEINKAM, *Cancer Chemotherapy and Pharmacology* (1983),[2949] studied the effects of PHT, in combination with the chemotherapy agent procarbazine, on the lifespan of mice implanted with L1210 ascites leukemia cells. Procarbazine by itself increased lifespan by 29–32%. The addition of PHT (60 mg/kg) increased lifespan by a further 24%. Phenobarbital was effective to a lesser degree and methylprednisolone had no effect.

The authors suggest that PHT achieves its beneficial effects on lifespan by inducing cytochrome P-450 enzymes and thus increasing the production of metabolites of procarbazine with antitumor activity.

LEMON, STOHS, HEINICKE, PFEIFFER AND CAMPBELL, *Proceedings of the American Association for Cancer Research* (1984),[2701] noting reports of a lower incidence of breast and genital cancer among epileptic women taking anticonvulsants for more than ten years, evaluated the prophylactic activity of PHT against 7,12-dimethylbenzanthracene (DMBA)-induced mammary tumors in female rats. All control rats (133) developed breast carcinoma within six to nine months of DMBA exposure.

Oral PHT (0.1%, in water), started fifteen days prior to DMBA exposure and continued for the six- to nine-month observation period, protected eleven of fifty-nine rats indefinitely from mammary tumors (p<.01). The combination of PHT and monthly subcutaneous estriol treatment prevented mammary tumors in fifteen of sixteen animals.

The authors found that PHT induced hepatic aryl hydrocarbon hydroxylases and other monooxygenases after one week and suggest that the protective action of PHT is due to its ability to increase DMBA metabolism. (See also Ref. 2587.)

SINGER AND SLESINGER, *Epilepsia* (1985),[2956] studied the effects of PHT, phenobarbital, carbamazepine and valproic acid on the growth and neurochemistry of a neuroblastoma X glioma cell clone (NG 108-15) in culture. All four agents suppressed cell growth, but PHT (12.5–50 μg/ml) and valproic acid had the greatest effect. PHT also decreased activity of choline acetyltransferase and β-galactosidase.

See also Refs. 507, 967, 1205, 1323, 1324, 1475, 1769, 1807, 1935, 1993, 2045, 2093, 2293, 2379, 2381, 2387, 2454, 2455, 2540, 2750, 2754, 3095.

Acquired Immunodeficiency Syndrome

ZIMMER, LEHR, KORNHUBER, BREITAG, MONTAGNIER AND GIETZEN, *Blut* (1986), [3099] exposed lymphocytes from twenty-four normal controls and twenty-four patients treated with PHT (300–450 mg/day for a minimum of ten days) to ^{125}I-labeled human immunodeficiency virus (HIV). After one-hour, cell radioactivity was measured as an index of virus binding.

Virus binding was significantly less in the lymphocytes from the PHT-treated patients. Mean counts per minute were 4,000 (range 2,000–7,000) in the PHT group, compared to 80,000 (range 64,000–92,000) in the control group. Similar differences were observed when an immunofluorescence assay was used.

To determine whether the inhibition of HIV binding was specific to PHT or shared by other drugs, the authors evaluated HIV binding to lymphocytes from twenty additional patients treated with ampicillin, haldoperidol, phenobarbital, flunarizine, or nimodipine. Only PHT inhibited HIV binding.

In another series of experiments, the functional integrity of the lymphocytes from PHT-treated patients was evaluated by performing surface-marker determinations with monoclonal antibodies. The PHT-treated lymphocytes reacted with all of the antibodies tested (OKT3, OKT4, OKT8, OKT11), and the T-cell subpopulations calculated by this means were the same as those of controls.

The authors conclude that PHT inhibits HIV binding to T-lymphocytes and might therefore be useful in the prevention and treatment of AIDS. (See also Ref. 2700.)

ANTI-TOXIC EFFECTS OF PHT

The toxic effects of many substances, both in man and in the laboratory, have been reported to be diminished or counteracted by PHT. The substances listed here are those with particular clinical relevance. Some are poisons; others are therapeutic but can have toxic effects, especially in overdose.

Alcohol withdrawal: (Refs. 383, 571, 2141, 2182; Lab. study: Ref. 2977);

Alloxan induced diabetes: (Lab. studies: Refs. 1015, 1092, 1354);

Amphetamine toxicity: (Ref. 1904; Lab. study: Ref. 99);

Antidepressants (tricyclics, e.g., amitriptyline, imipramine) induced arrhythmias and conduction defects: (Refs. 1382, 1428, 1430, 2257, 2348, 2377, 2565, 2674, 2675, 2764, 2830; Lab. studies: Refs. 2674, 2675, 2778);

Bilirubin toxicity in newborns: (Refs. 1388, 1926, 2465);

Carbamazepine induced water intoxication· (Refs. 2020, 2089, 2640);

Chloral hydrate induced cardiac arrhythmias: (Ref. 1873);

Clofibrate induced myotonic states: (Lab. study: Ref. 2682);

Cyanide toxicity in nerve: (Lab. studies: Refs. 699, 812);

Digitalis and other cardiac glycoside induced arrhythmias. Use of PHT permits more digitalis to be used before toxic effects occur and does not interfere with the inotropic benefits of digitalis in animals and humans: (Refs. 61, 62, 80, 82, 158, 187, 215, 248, 310, 318, 407, 415, 418, 597, 753, 754, 832, 880, 905, 941, 969, 991, 1007, 1052, 1084, 1114, 1121, 1122, 1151, 1170, 1209, 1214, 1264, 1289, 1402, 1434, 1488, 1508, 1515, 1562, 1563, 1590, 1705, 1707, 1889, 2083, 2163, 2331, 2393, 2569, 2620, 2758, 2985; Lab. studies: 19, 149, 150, 151, 153, 154, 155, 233, 249, 260, 308, 327, 328, 403, 404, 405, 514, 519, 685, 699, 714, 799, 800, 802, 805, 812, 860, 963, 978, 1079, 1277, 1507, 1663, 1696, 2224, 2250, 2484, 2577, 2676, 2723, 2769, 2905, 3061);

Gold induced nephropathy: (Lab. study: Ref. 1525);

Heroin withdrawal: (Refs. 290, 1033);

Insecticide toxicity: *DDT:* (Refs. 701, 943, 944, 998, 999, 1253, 1349, 1510, 1666, 2431; Lab. studies: Refs. 823, 914, 921, 1022, 3017). *Dieldrin:* (Ref. 2431). *Organophosphates:* (Lab. studies: Refs. 2349, 2766). *Permethrin:* (Lab. study: Ref. 3017);

Lidocaine induced seizures: (Ref. 2916);

Lithium induced nervous system toxicity: (Ref. 1637);

LSD (lysergic acid diethylamide) toxicity: (Refs. 1616, 1904);

Mephenytoin: (Lab. study: Ref. 567);

Mephobarbital: (Lab. study: Ref. 567);

Methaqualone intoxication: (Lab. study: Ref. 1529);

Metrizamide induced neurotoxicity and seizures in patients undergoing neuroradiological procedures: (Refs. 2709, 2882, 3054);

Misonidazole induced peripheral neuropathy: (Refs. 2114, 2342, 2868, 3060);

Morphine withdrawal and mania: (Lab. studies: Refs. 1026, 1027, 1781, 2062);

Phenothiazine induced neuroleptic malignant syndrome: (Ref. 2822);

Polychlorinated biphenyl (PCB) toxicity (carcinogenesis): (Ref. 2583);

Reserpine induced hyperexcitability, rigidity and hypothermia: (Lab. studies: Refs. 182, 183, 1306, 1643);

Spider and snake venom: (Refs. 1844, 2789);

Steroid induced muscle weakness and skin changes: (Refs. 377, 425, 896, 1128, 1594; Lab. studies: Refs. 171, 451, 482, 483, 504, 1103, 2063);

Streptozotocin induced diabetes: (Lab. study: Ref. 1509);

Strychnine toxicity: (Ref. 625; Lab. studies: Refs. 90, 1208, 2662, 2724, 2774);

Succinylcholine induced muscle fasciculation: (Lab. studies: Refs. 1494, 2576);

Tetanus toxin: (Refs. 2359, 2913).

Trimethadione: (Lab. study: Ref. 567);

CHEMISTRY, METABOLISM AND
DETERMINATION OF PHT

The physicochemical properties and pharmacokinetics of phenytoin have been extensively reviewed. (See, for example, Refs. 1859, 2284, 2364, 2385, 2631, 2930, 3081, 3085.) Only a brief summary is given here.

Chemical Structure of PHT

$$H_5C_6 - C - N(H) - C = O$$

(structure of 5,5-diphenylhydantoin showing H_5C_6 and H_5C_6 groups attached to a central C, linked to an N–H, C=O, NH, and O=C five-membered ring)

Chemistry and Metabolism

Phenytoin (5,5-diphenylhydantoin, 5,5-diphenyl-2,4-imidazolidinedione) is composed of a five-membered hydantoin ring with two phenyl groups at the five position. PHT has a molecular weight of 256.26 in the free acid form, and 274.26 as the sodium salt. It is highly lipophilic and can be solubilized in alkali and many organic solvents but, as the free acid, it is poorly soluble in water with a true dissociation constant (pKa') of 8.31. It is 80% nonionized at physiological pH (7.4). The aqueous solubility of phenytoin at pH 7.5 is 21.9 μg/ml at 25°C and, in plasma, the apparent solubility is 75 μg/ml at 37°C due to high plasma protein binding.

Absorbed predominantly from the duodenum and, to a lesser extent, from the jejunum and ileum, PHT is rapidly and reversibly bound (90% on average) to intravascular proteins, especially albumin (see Refs. 440, 788, 916, 1000, 1126, 1232, 1233, 1288, 1314, 1315, 1316, 1393, 1442, 2355). The plasma half-life shows considerable variation from individual to individual (average eighteen hours; range seven to forty-two hours) and may vary within individuals, depending on physiological conditions, such as stress, injury (i.e., burns), pregnancy, viral infections, surgical procedures, and age (see Refs. 2354, 2417, 2522, 2616, 2704, 2706, 2712, 2719, 2970). Both interethnic and interphenotype differences in ability to metabolize PHT have been described (see Refs. 2292, 2336, 2477, 2779, 3086).

Less than 5% of phenytoin is excreted unchanged in the urine. Metabolism is by hepatic microsomal enzymes and the major metabolite, 5-(4-hydroxyphenyl)-5-phenylhydantoin (HPPH) is not active. Arene oxide and epoxide intermediates have been described. (See Refs. 69, 179, 205, 269, 284, 359, 361, 440, 442, 443, 444, 445, 446, 452, 453, 521, 528, 544, 553, 554, 555, 1044, 1051, 1076, 1247, 1669, 1697, 1859, 2284, 2334, 2335, 2336, 2337, 2364, 2385, 2395, 2587, 2631, 2684, 2779, 2810, 2873, 2930, 3081, 3083.)

At the organ or system level, PHT has been reported to have wide distribution in brain, liver, muscle and fat, as measured in various species. Most of the tissue PHT is in bound form. Free PHT is found in all transcellular fluids including cerebrospinal fluid, saliva, semen, milk, gastrointestinal fluid and bile.

Levels of PHT in the brain are one to three times those of total (free and bound) drug in plasma and six to ten times those of free drug in plasma. In humans, the brain/plasma ratio for PHT averages 1.52, although white matter (at 1.73) contains more than gray matter. (See Refs. 101, 267, 269, 531, 794, 862, 1082, 1215, 1383, 1471, 1539, 1687, 1704, 2310, 2892.) Brain tumor tissue seems to take up even more (see Refs. 400, 2959). The suggestion has been made that depolarized or rapidly firing cells bind more phenytoin.

At cellular and subcellular levels, neurons appear to bind more PHT than glia. Nuclear, mitochondrial and microsomal fractions all bind PHT, apparently nonspecifically. Studies of protein binding indicate that brain tissue binding correlates with protein concentration, cations, temperature and ionic strength, thus fulfilling the criteria for nonspecific binding. However, there is some evidence for specific binding (see Refs. 1863, 2351, 2369, 2797, 2829, 2947).

PHT also binds to lipids. Total brain lipid mixtures have the greatest activity, while those obtained by extraction of subcutaneous fat (chloroform-methanol extraction) show no binding of tritiated PHT (see Refs. 1860, 1861, 1862, 1863, 2547). All of the phospholipids show some degree of PHT binding, while gangliosides, cholesterol, cerebrosides and other natural lipids have no binding activity. Among the phospholipids, dipalmitoyl and dioleoyl lecithins have the greatest binding activity (80%). Since PHT binds to both phospholipids and protein, the potential for lipid-PHT-lipid, protein-PHT-lipid, and protein-PHT-protein binding exists. Consistent with this, PHT-induced alterations in membrane fluidity have been documented.

Determination

The determination of serum phenytoin levels has proven to be useful in seizure patients where steady state total blood levels usually serve as a guide to effective seizure control, and in determining insufficient or excessive doses, or noncompliance. In nonseizure disorders the correlation of blood levels with therapeutic effects varies. For example, in cardiac arrhythmias the effective blood level range has been reported to be similar to that used for seizure control. However, in thought, mood and behavior disorders, therapeutic effects are frequently observed at much lower blood levels. For patients with the disorders for which PHT is effective, routine blood levels are not necessary, especially when doses of 100–300 mg/day are being used and the desired therapeutic effect is being achieved.

Increasing attention is being devoted to the question of whether free, and not just total, PHT levels should be measured (see Refs. 2301, 2315, 2354, 2365, 2488, 2514, 2661, 2679, 2704, 2706, 2713, 2714, 2839, 2860, 2866, 2908, 3011, 3034, 3045).

New assays for the determination of PHT levels are continually being developed. These include gas chromatography and immunological techniques. Miniaturization has been achieved so that salivary samples or even capillary blood from a finger stick may be used (see Refs. 2286, 2299, 2313, 2426, 2580, 2663, 2840, 3038, 3045). A home assay has been introduced (see Refs. 2403, 2404). It is beyond the scope of this bibliography to review all these methods. The reader is referred to the following:

Refs. 2277, 2295, 2303, 2346, 2400, 2403, 2404, 2408, 2433, 2489, 2545, 2566, 2582, 2595, 2596, 2618, 2630, 2632, 2634, 2665, 2677, 2755, 2787, 2796, 2828, 2843, 2871, 2898, 2937, 2973, 3011, 3027, 3033, 3059, 3074.

Appendix

Exchange of Letters Between
Governor Nelson Rockefeller and Secretary of
HEW Elliot Richardson

April 19, 1972

Dear Mr. Secretary:

It has come to my attention that a great many published reports, written over a thirty-year period by physicians and other scientists, have indicated that the substance phenytoin has a broad range of beneficial uses. Further, it is my understanding that physicians are prescribing phenytoin for many purposes other than its original indicated use, in 1938, as an anticonvulsant. In spite of the evidence of phenytoin's broad usefulness, I understand that today, in 1972, its only listed indication is that of an anticonvulsant.

I realize that the Food and Drug Administration is set up essentially to rectify errors of commission. This certainly does not fall into that category. However, I believe a public clarification of the status of phenytoin by the FDA would be most valuable, and timely.

I enclose with this letter a publication, *The Broad Range of Use of Phenytoin —Bibliography and Review*, that extensively deals with this subject.

I hope you will give this your consideration.

With warm regard,

Sincerely,
/s/ Nelson A. Rockefeller

June 22, 1972

Dear Governor Rockefeller:

Please forgive the delay of this response to your April 19 letter concerning the current status of the drug, phenytoin.

Conversations with health officials within the Department have revealed that phenytoin (PHT) was introduced in 1938 as the first essentially nonsedating anticonvulsant drug. The dramatic effect of PHT and its widespread acceptance in the treatment of convulsive disorders may have tended to obscure a broader range of therapeutic uses.

A review of the literature reveals that phenytoin has been reported to be useful in a wide range of disorders. Among its reported therapeutic actions are its stabilizing effect on the nervous system, its antiarrhythmic effect on certain cardiac disorders, and its therapeutic effect on emotional disorders.

The fact that such broad therapeutic effects have been reported by many independent scientists and physicians over a long period of time would seem to indicate that the therapeutic effects of phenytoin are more than that of an anticonvulsant.

The FDA encourages the submission of formal applications which, of course, would include the necessary supporting evidence for the consideration of approval for a wider range of therapeutic uses.

Your interest in encouraging the Department to provide a public clarification of the status of phenytoin is very welcome and I hope that this information is responsive to your concerns.

With warm regard,

> Sincerely,
> /s/ Elliot L. Richardson

Survey of Use of Phenytoin in 1975

There follows a survey by IMS America, Ltd.[1] (year ending March, 1975) of the number of prescriptions of PHT[2] and diagnosis and desired action.

Description of Method of Data Collection—The survey by IMS America, Ltd. is a continuing study of private medical practice in the United States; the study began in 1956. Data are obtained from a representative panel of physicians who report case history information on private patients seen over a given period of time.

Fifteen hundred physicians report four times a year on a forty-eight-hour period of their practice. Each physician fills out a case record form for every private patient treated. Case histories are returned to IMS America, Ltd. for processing. The books are coded and edited by pharmacists. All information is recorded on computer tapes, from which the monthly and quarterly reports are compiled.

Physicians in private practice are selected at random and include representatives of all specialties.

---

[1] Formerly Lea Associates.
[2] This survey is of the prescriptions for the best known trade name of PHT.

Desired Action	No. of Prescriptions in Thousands	Desired Action	No. of Prescriptions in Thousands
Anticonvulsant	3,057	Stimulant	11
Prophylaxis	255	Calming Effect and Tranquilizer	11
Curb Cardiac Arrhythmia	124	Antinauseant	10
Anticoagulant	121	Uterine Sedative	9
Symptomatic	64	Antidepressant	7
Pain Relief	62	Prophylaxis and Sedative-Unspecific	6
Sedative-Unspecific	46	Antispasmodic	5
Control Heart Rate	27	Mood Elevation	5
Relieve Headache	24	Antiallergic and Anticonvulsant	4
Withdrawal Symptoms	19	Prevent Migraine	4
Analgesic	17	Control Vertigo	4
Psychotherapeutic	17	GI Antispasmodic	4
Control Dizziness	17	Antihemorrhagic	3
Antineuritic	16	Relieve Headache and Anticonvulsant	3
Reduce Tension	15	Cardiotonic	3
Relieve Migraine	12	No Reason Given	1,820
Anticonvulsant and Prophylaxis	12		
Sedative Night and Promote Sleep	12	TOTAL	5,827

Diagnosis	No. of Prescriptions in Thousands	Diagnosis	No. of Prescriptions in Thousands
DISEASES OF CNS AND SENSORY ORGANS	2,534	Late Effects of Intracranial Abscess	16
Epilepsy—not otherwise specified	1,052	Subarachnoid Hemorrhage	10
Grand Mal	452	Intracranial Spinal Abscess	10
Cerebral Hemorrhage	178	Other Neuralgia or Neuritis	9
Cerebral Arteriosclerotic Congestion	177	SYMPTOMS AND SENILITY	1,354
Other Diseases of the Brain	176	Convulsions	1,145
Petit Mal	99	Syncope or Collapse	44
Trigeminal Neuralgia	89	Encephalopathy	27
Cerebral Embolism/Thrombosis	80	Jacksonian Epilepsy	26
Cerebral Paralysis/Seizure	48	Headache—not otherwise specified	22
Stroke—not otherwise specified	38	Vertigo	13
Other Cerebral Paralysis	28	Tension Headache	12
Migraine	20	Other Ill Defined Conditions	12
Facial Paralysis	20	MENTAL DISORDERS	656
		Unspecified Alcoholism	118
		Chronic Alcoholism	113

(*continued*)

Diagnosis	No. of Prescriptions in Thousands	Diagnosis	No. of Prescriptions in Thousands
MENTAL DISORDERS (*continued*)		Arteriosclerotic Coronary	
Other Drug Addiction	74	Artery Disease	17
Acute Alcoholism	45	Heart Block	9
Depressive Reaction	44		
Other Mental Deficiency	41	SPECIFIC CONDITIONS WITHOUT	
Primary Childhood Behavior		SICKNESS	386
Disorders	37	Surgical Aftercare	361
Other Schizophrenia	24	Medical Aftercare	25
Alcoholic Psychosis	23		
Presenile Psychosis	21	NEOPLASMS	306
Hysteria—not otherwise		Malignant Neoplasms—Other	
specified	21	Unspecified Sites	103
Psychosis with Organic Brain		Unspecified Neoplasms Brain/	
Disorder	18	Nervous System	60
Neurotic Depressive Reaction	16	Malignant Neoplasms of the	
Other Pathological Personality	15	Brain	41
Epileptic Psychosis	13	Malignant Neoplasms of the	
CIRCULATORY DISORDERS	452	Nervous System—	
Disorders of Heart Rhythm	107	Unspecified	24
Myocardial Infarction	49	Benign Neoplasms of the Brain	
Arteriosclerotic Heart Disease	43	or Other Parts of the	
Essential Benign		Nervous System	22
Hypertension	35	Malignant Neoplasms of the	
Other Hypertensive		Lung—Unspecified	19
Arteriosclerotic Heart		Malignant Neoplasms of	
Disease	33	Thoracic Organs	15
Angina Pectoris	27		
Myocardial Occlusion	26	ACCIDENTS AND POISONING	228
Coronary Artery Disease with		Head Injuries	129
Selected Complications	26	Other Accidents—Poisoning	35
Arteriosclerosis without		Effects of Poisons	28
Gangrene	23	Injury of Nerves of Spinal	
Myocardial Occlusions with		Cord	21
Complications	17	Fractures	16
		ALL OTHERS	212
		TOTAL[1]	6,127

[1] Since occasionally more than one diagnosis is given per prescription, the total for diagnosis is not exactly the same as the total for desired action.

FDA Drug Bulletin, April, 1982

Use of Approved Drugs for Unlabeled Indications

"The appropriateness or the legality of prescribing approved drugs for uses not included in their official labeling is sometimes a cause of concern and confusion among practitioners.

"Under the Federal Food, Drug, and Cosmetic (FD&C) Act, a drug approved for marketing may be labeled, promoted, and advertised by the manufacturer only for those uses for which the drug's safety and effectiveness have been established and which FDA has approved. These are commonly referred to as 'approved uses.' This means that adequate and well-controlled clinical trials have documented these uses, and the results of the trials have been reviewed and approved by FDA.

"The FD&C Act does not, however, limit the manner in which a physician may use an approved drug. Once a product has been approved for marketing, a physician may prescribe it for uses or in treatment regimens or patient populations that are not included in approved labeling. Such "unapproved" or, more precisely, 'unlabeled' uses may be appropriate and rational in certain circumstances, and may, in fact, reflect approaches to drug therapy that have been extensively reported in medical literature.

"The term 'unapproved uses' is, to some extent, misleading. It includes a variety of situations ranging from unstudied to thoroughly investigated drug uses. Valid new uses for drugs already on the market are often first discovered through serendipitous observations and therapeutic innovations, subsequently confirmed by well-planned and executed clinical investigations. Before such advances can be added to the approved labeling, however, data substantiating the effectiveness of a new use or regimen must be submitted by the manufacturer to FDA for evaluation. This may take time and, without the initiative of the drug manufacturer whose product is involved, may never occur. For that reason, accepted medical practice often includes drug use that is not reflected in approved drug labeling.

"With respect to its role in medical practice, the package insert is informational only. FDA tries to assure that prescription drug information in the package insert accurately and fully reflects the data on safety and effectiveness on which drug approval is based."

References

1. Agarwal, S. L. and Bhargava, V., Effect of drugs on brain acetylcholine levels in rats, *Indian J. Med. Res.*, 52: 1179-1182, 1964.

2. Alarcon-Segovia, D., Wakim, K. G., Worthington, J. W., and Ward, L. E., Clinical and experimental studies on the hydralazine syndrome and its relationship to systemic lupus erythematosus, *Medicine*, 46: 1-33, 1967.

3. Alvarez, W. C., Pseudo-ulcer, *Gastroenterology*, 14: 321-323, 1950.

4. Alvarez, W. C., "Why, that's our Jimmy," *Mod. Med.*, 75-76, 1968.

5. Aring, C. D., Management of fits in adults, *Ohio Med. J.*, 37: 225-230, 1941.

6. Aston, R. and Domino, E. F., Differential effects of phenobarbital, pentobarbital and diphenylhydantoin on motor cortical and reticular thresholds in the rhesus monkey, *Psychopharmacologia*, 2: 304-317, 1961.

7. Baer, P. N., Davis, R. K., and Merrit, A. D., Studies on Dilantin hyperplastic gingivitis: the role of magnesium, *J. Dent. Res.*, 44: 1055, 1965.

8. Baldwin, R. W. and Kenny, T. J., Medical treatment of behavior disorders, *Learning Disabilities*, J. Hellmuth, Ed., 2: 313-327, Special Child Publications of The Seattle Seguin School, Inc., Seattle, 1966.

9. Baxi, S. M., Trigeminal neuralgia: treatment with diphenylhydantoin, *Antiseptic*, 58: 329-330, 1961.

10. Becker, R. and Balshüsemann, T., Treatment of facial pain, *Deutsch Med. Wschr.*, 90: 2014-2020, 1965.

11. Putnam, T. J. and Merritt, H. H., Experimental determination of the anticonvulsant properties of some phenyl derivatives, *Science*, 85: 525-526, 1937.

12. Belton, N. R., Etheridge, J. E., Jr., and Millichap, J. G., Effects of convulsions and anticonvulsants on blood sugar in rabbits, *Epilepsia*, 6: 243-249, 1965.

13. Bente, D., Schönhärl, E., and Krump-Erlangen, J., Electroencephalographic findings in stutterers and their application to medical therapy, *Archiv fur Ohren-, Nasen- und Kehlkopfheilkunde*, 169: 513-519, 1956.

14. Bergouignan, M., Fifteen years of therapeutic trials in essential trigeminal neuralgia: the place of diphenylhydantoin and its derivatives, *Rev. Neurol.* (Paris), 98: 414-416, 1958.

15. Bergouignan, M., Successful cures of essential facial neuralgias by sodium diphenylhydantoinate, *Rev. Laryng.* (Bordeaux), 63: 34-41, 1942.

16. Bergouignan, M. and d'Aulnay, N., Effects of sodium diphenylhydantoin in essential trigeminal neuralgia, *Rev. Otoneuroopthal.* (Paris), 23: 427-431, 1951.

17. Bernsohn, J., Possley, L., and Custod, J. T., Alterations in brain adenine nucleotides and creatinine phosphate *in vivo* after the administration of chlorpromazine, JB-516, Dilantin and RO 5-0650 (Librium), *Pharmacologist*, 2: 67, 1960.

18. Bernstein, H., Gold, H., Lang, T. W., Pappelbaum, S., Bazika, V., and Corday, E., Sodium diphenylhydantoin in the treatment of recurrent cardiac arrhythmias, *JAMA*, 191: 695-697, 1965.

19. Bigger, J. T., Jr., Bassett, A. L., and Hoffman, B. F., Electrophysiological effects of diphenylhydantoin on canine Purkinje fibers, *Circ. Res.*, 22: 221-236, 1968.

20. Bigger, J. T., Jr., Harris, P. D., and Weinberg, D. I., Effects of diphenylhydantoin on cardiac conduction and repolarization, *Amer. J. Cardiol.*, 19: 119-120, 1967.

21. Bigger, J. T., Jr., Schmidt, D. H., and Kutt, H., The relationship between the antiarrhythmic effect and the plasma level of diphenylhydantoin sodium (Dilantin), *Bull. N.Y. Acad. Med.*, 42: 1039, 1966.

22. Bigger, J. T., Jr., Strauss, H. C., and Hoffmann, B. F., Effects of diphenylhydantoin on atrioventricular conduction, *Fed. Proc.*, 27: 406, 1968.

23. Blatman, S. and Metcalf, D. R., Abnormal electroencephalograms in asthmatic children, *Amer. J. Dis. Child.*, 102: 531, 1961.

24. Blaw, M. E. and Torres, F., Treatment of pseudoretardation associated with epilepsy, *Mod. Treatm.*, 4: 799-816, 1967.

25. Bodkin, L. G., Oral therapy for pruritus ani, *Amer. J. Dig. Dis.*, 12: 255-257, 1945.

26. Bodkin, L. G., Pruritus ani: a review of oral therapy, *Amer. J. Dig. Dis.*, 14: 109-113, 1947.

27. Boelhouwer, C., Henry, C. E., and Glueck, B. C., Positive spiking: a double blind control study on its significance in behavior disorders, both diagnostically and therapeutically, *Amer. J. Psychiat.*, 125: 473-481, 1968.

28. Bogoch, S., Diphenylhydantoin: therapeutic uses and mechanisms of action, *Dreyfus Medical Foundation*, 1968.

29. Booker, H. E., Matthews, C. G., and Slaby, A., Effects of diphenylhydantoin on physiological and psychological measures in normal adults, *Neurology*, 17: 949-951, 1967.

30. Bose, B. C., Saifi, A. Q., and Sharma, S. K., Studies on anticonvulsant and antifibrillatory drugs, *Arch. Int. Pharmacodyn.*, 146: 106-113, 1963.

31. Braham, J. and Saia, A., Phenytoin in the treatment of trigeminal and other neuralgias, *Lancet*, 2: 892-893, 1960.

32. Braverman, I. M., and Levin, J., Dilantin-induced serum sickness: case report and inquiry into its mechanism, *Amer. J. Med.*, 35: 418-422, 1963.

33. Bray, P. F., Diphenylhydantoin (Dilantin) after 20 years: a review with re-emphasis by treatment of 84 patients, *Pediatrics*, 23: 151-161, 1959.

34. Brennan, R. W., Dehejia, M., Kutt, H., and McDowell, F., Diphenylhydantoin intoxication attendant to slow inactivation of isoniazid, *Neurology*, 18: 183, 1968.

35. Brill, N. Q., and Walker, E. F., Psychopathic behavior with latent epilepsy, *J. Nerv. Ment. Dis.*, 101: 545-549, 1945.

36. Brittingham, T. E., Lutcher, C. L., and Murphy, D. L., Reversible erythroid aplasia induced by diphenylhydantoin, *Arch. Intern. Med.*, 113: 764-768, 1964.

37. Broddle, W. D. and Nelson, S. R., The effect of diphenylhydantoin on energy reserve levels in brain, *Fed. Proc.*, 27: 751, 1968.

38. Brown, W. T. and Solomon, C. I., Delinquency and the electroencephalograph, *Amer. J. Psychiat.*, 98: 499-503, 1942.

39. Buchthal, F. and Svensmark, O., Aspects of the pharmacology of Phenytoin (Dilantin) and phenobarbital relevant to their dosage in the treatment of epilepsy, *Epilepsia*, 1: 373-384, 1959-1960.

40. Burke, E. C. and Peters, G. A., Migraine in childhood: a preliminary report, *A.M.A. J. Dis. Child.*, 92: 330-336, 1956.

41. Byrne, J. E. and Dresel, P. E., A model for evaluating

drugs which prolong post-countershock periods of normal sinus rhythm (NSR), *Pharmacologist,* 10: 220, 1968.

42. Cameron, A. J., Baron, J. H., and Priestley, B. L., Erythema multiforme, drugs, and ulcerative colitis, *Brit. Med. J.,* 2: 1174-1178, 1966.

43. Campbell, E. W., Jr., and Young, J. D., Jr., Enuresis and its relationship to electroencephalographic disturbances, *J. Urol.,* 96: 947-949, 1966.

44. Cantu, R. C. and Schwab, R. S., Ceruloplasmin rise and PBI fall in serum due to diphenylhydantoin, *Arch. Neurol.,* 15: 393-396, 1966.

45. Cantu, R. C., Schwab, R. S., and Timberlake, W. H., Comparison of blood levels with oral and intramuscular diphenylhydantoin, *Neurology,* 18: 782-784, 1968.

46. Case, W. G., Rickels, K., and Bazilian, S., Diphenylhydantoin in neurotic anxiety, *Amer. J. Psychiat.,* 126: 254-255, 1969.

47. Caspers, H. and Wehmeyer, H., The action of diphenylhydantoin on the seizure threshold of the brain, *Z. Ges. Exp. Med.,* 129: 77-86, 1957.

48. Caveness, W., Adams, R. D., Pope, A., and Wegner, W. R., The role of the dorsal root ganglia in the production of the lancinating pains of central nervous system syphilis, *Trans. Amer. Neurol. Assn.,* 60-64, 1949.

49. Chaiken, B. H., Goldberg, B. I., and Segal, J. P., Dilantin sensitivity: report of a case of hepatitis with jaundice, pyrexia and exfoliative dermatitis, *New Eng. J. Med.,* 242: 897-898, 1950.

50. Chang, T. and Glazko, A. J., Quantitative assay of 5,5'-diphenylhydantoin (Dilantin) and 5-(4-hydroxyphenyl)-5'-phenylhydantoin by gas-liquid chromatography, *Clin. Res.,* 16: 339, 1968.

51. Chao, D., Sexton, J. A., and Davis, S. D., Convulsive equivalent syndrome of childhood, *J. Pediat,* 64: 499-508, 1964.

52. Chenoweth, M. B., Clinical uses of metal binding drugs, *Clin. Pharmacol. Ther.,* 9: 365-387, 1968.

53. Childress, R. H., Higgs, L. M., Boyd, D. L., and Williams, J. F., Jr., Effect of diphenylhydantoin on left ventricular function in patients with heart disease, *Circulation,* 33-34: 73, 1966.

54. Chinitz, A., Seelinger, D. F., and Greenhouse, A. H., Anticonvulsant therapy in trigeminal neuralgia, *Amer. J. Med. Sci.,* 252: 62-67, 1966.

55. Christensen, K., On the preparation and stability of Phenytoin solutions for injection, *Dansk Tidsskr. Farm.,* 34: 97-109, 1960.

56. Chung, A. C., The influence of diphenylhydantoin (Dilantin) on the development of atherosclerosis in rabbits, *J. Atheroscler. Res.,* 7: 373-379, 1967.

57. Chung, A. C., Duren, B. Y., and Houck, J. C., Effect of diphenylhydantoin administration upon concentration of liver and aortic lipids, *Proc. Soc. Exp. Biol. Med.,* 110: 788-789, 1962.

58. Cohen, H. B., Duncan, R. F., II, and Dement, W. C., The effect of diphenylhydantoin on sleep in the cat, *Electroenceph. Clin. Neurophysiol.,* 24: 401-408, 1968.

59. Cohen, H. D. and Barondes, S. H., Puromycin effect on memory may be due to occult seizures, *Science,* 157: 333-334, 1967.

60. Cole, J. O. and Davis, J. M., Brief report of papers on diphenylhydantoin in plenary session, American College of Neuropsychopharmacology, fifth annual meeting, *Psychopharm. Bull.* 4: 28-31, 1967.

61. Conn, R. D., Diphenylhydantoin sodium in cardiac arrhythmias, *New Eng. J. Med.,* 272: 277-282, 1965.

62. Conn., R. D., New drugs for old hearts: newer antiarrhythmic and diuretic agents, *Postgrad. Med.* 42: 71-79, 1967.

63. Corday, E., Lang, T. W., Bazika, V., and Pappelbaum, S., Antiarrhythmic acts directly on myocardium, *JAMA,* 193: 28, 1965.

64. Cox, A. R., Pitt, W., Brown, T. C. K., and Molaro, A., Antiarrhythmic action of diphenylhydantoin (Dilantin) studied in isolated cardiac tissue, *Canad. Med. Assn. J.,* 94: 661, 1966.

65. Crawford, S. E. and Jones. C. K., Fatal liver necrosis and diphenylhydantoin sensitivity, *Pediatrics,* 30: 595-600, 1962.

66. Crue, B. L., Jr., Alvarez-Carregal, E., and Todd, E. M., Neuralgia: consideration of central mechanisms, *Bull. Los Angeles Neurol. Soc.,* 29: 107-132, 1964.

67. Crue, B. L., Jr., Todd, E. M., and Duemler, L. P., Pain as sensory epilepsy, *Bull. Los Angeles Neurol. Soc.,* 32: 53, 1967.

68. Crue, B. L., Jr., Todd, E. M., and Loew, A. G., Clinical use of mephenesin carbamate (Tolseram) in trigeminal neuralgia, *Bull. Los Angeles Neurol. Soc.,* 30: 212-215, 1965.

69. Cucinell, S. A., Factors affecting drug metabolism, *Bull. N.Y. Acad. Med.,* 42: 324, 1966.

70. Popek, K., Czechs make anticonvulsants a must for coma victims, *Med. World News,* 33, March 8, 1968.

71. Dahl, J. R., Diphenylhydantoin toxic psychosis with associated hyperglycemia, *Calif. Med.,* 107: 345-347, 1967.

72. Dam, M., Organic changes in Phenytoin intoxicated pigs, *Acta Neurol. Scand.,* 42: 491-494, 1966.

73. Dam, M. and Olesen, V., Intramuscular administration of Phenytoin, *Neurology,* 16: 288-292, 1966.

74. Dayton, P. G., Cucinell, S. A., Weiss, M., and Perel, J. M., Dose dependence of drug plasma level decline in dogs, *J. Pharm. Exp. Ther.,* 158: 305-316, 1967.

75. de la Vega, P., Clinical results of the treatment of Sydenham's chorea with sodium diphenylhydantoin, *Rev. Clin. Esp.* 24: 113-115, 1947.

76. Dill, R. E., Discrepancy of adrenal responses in diphenylhydantoin treated rats, *Arch. Int. Pharmacodyn.,* 160: 363-372, 1966.

77. Dill, W. A., Kazenko, A., Wolf, L. M., and Glazko, A. J., Studies on 5,5'-diphenylhydantoin (Dilantin) in animals and man, *J. Pharm. Exp. Ther.,* 118: 270-279, 1956.

78. Dimsdale, H., Migraine, *Practitioner,* 198: 490-494, 1967.

79. Dixon, R. L., The interaction between various drugs and methotrexate, *Toxic. Appl. Pharmacol.,* 12: 308, 1968.

80. Dorph, M., Coronary care units and the aggressive management of acute myocardial infarction, *Delaware Med. J.* 44-48, February, 1968.

81. Dorsey, J. F., Hayslip, G. W., and Anderson, K., Tic douloureux: treatment with diphenylhydantoin, *Clin. Med.,* 6: 1395-1397, 1959.

82. Dreifus, L. S., Rabbino, M. D., and Watanabe, Y., Newer agents in the treatment of cardiac arrythmias, *Med. Clin. N. Amer.,* 48: 371-387, 1964.

83. Druskin, M. S., Anticonvulsants and anemia, *Clin. Med.,* 71: 1911-1916, 1964.

84. Druskin, M. S., Wallen, M. H., and Bonagura, L., Anticonvulsant associated megaloblastic anemia: response to 25 microgm. of folic acid administered by mouth daily, *New Eng. J. Med.,* 267: 483-485, 1962.

85. Dubois, E. L., Toxic hepatic necrosis associated with taking Dilantin, Tridione and phenobarbital, *Amer. J. Clin. Path.,* 20: 153-158, 1950.

86. Duma, R. J., Hendry, C. N., and Donahoo, J. S., Hypersensitivity to diphenylhydantoin (Dilantin): a case report with toxic hepatitis, *Southern Med. J.,* 59: 168-170, 1966.

87. Dutton, P., Phenytoin toxicity with associated meningeal reaction, *J. Ment. Sci.,* 104: 1165-1166, 1958.

88. Eissner, H., Diphenylhydantoin exanthema in the form of infectious mononucleosis, *Arch. Toxik.,* 18: 282-295, 1960.

89. Endröczi, E. and Fekete, T., Amino acid composition of the Ammon's horn and the effect of anticonvulsant drugs, *Acta Physiol. Acad. Sci. Hung.,* 32: 389-398, 1967.

90. Esplin, D. W., Effects of diphenylhydantoin on synaptic transmission in cat spinal cord and stellate ganglion, *J. Pharm. Exp. Ther.,* 120: 301-323, 1957.

91. Fabrykant, M., Further studies on electrocerebral dysfunction and the use of anticonvulsants in labile diabetes, *Ann. Intern. Med.,* 38: 814-823, 1953.

92. Fabrykant, M. and Pacella, B. L., Labile diabetes: electroencephalographic status and effect of anticonvulsive therapy, *Ann. Intern. Med.*, 29: 860-877, 1948.

93. Ferngren, H. and Paalzow, L., Studies on electrically induced seizures and their antagonism by anticonvulsants during neonatal development in the mouse, *Acta Pharmacol. Toxicol.*, 25: 60, 1967.

94. Festoff, B. W. and Appel, S. H., Effect of diphenylhydantoin on synaptosome sodium-potassium-ATPase, *J. Clin. Invest.*, 47: 2752-2758, 1968.

95. Fetterman, J. L. and Shallenberger, W. D., Further studies in Dilantin sodium therapy of epilepsy, *Dis. Nerv. System*, 2: 383-389, 1941.

96. Fichman, M. P. and Bethune, J. E., The role of adrenocorticoids in the inappropriate antidiuretic hormone syndrome, *Ann. Intern. Med.*, 68: 806-820, 1968.

97. Fichman, M. P., Kleeman, C. R. and Bethune, J. E., Inhibition of antidiuretic hormone secretion by diphenylhydantoin, *Arch. Neurol.*, 22: 45–53, 1970.

98. Finch, E. and Lorber, J., Methaemoglobinaemia in the newborn: probably due to Phenytoin excreted in human milk, *J. Obstet. Gynaec. Brit. Emp.*, 61: 833-834, 1954.

99. Fink, G. B. and Swinyard, E. A., Comparison of anticonvulsant and psychopharmacologic drugs, *J. Pharm. Sci.*, 51: 548-551, 1962.

100. Finkelman, I. and Arieff, A. J., Untoward effects of Phenytoin sodium in epilepsy, *JAMA*, 118: 1209-1212, 1942.

101. Firemark, H., Barlow, C. F., and Roth, L. J., The entry, accumulation and binding of diphenylhydantoin-2-C^{14} in brain: studies on adult, immature and hypercapnic cats, *Int. J. Neuropharmacol.*, 2: 25-38, 1963.

102. Fishbeck, R. and Zucker, G., Phenytoin (5,5-diphenylhydantoin) hypersensitivity presenting a clinical picture of scarlatiniform erythroderma, *Deutsch. Gesundh.*, 21: 1273-1277, 1966.

103. Floyd, F. W., The toxic effects of diphenylhydantoin: a report of 23 cases, *Clin. Proc. Child Hosp., D. C.*, 17: 195-201, 1961.

104. Forshaw, J. W. B., Megaloblastic anemia associated with anticonvulsant therapy, *Postgrad. Med. J.* (London), 33: 242-243, 1957.

105. Fox, V., Treatment of the non-neurologic complications of alcoholism, *Mod. Treatm.*, 3: 502-508, 1966.

106. Frankel, S. I,. Dilantin sodium in the treatment of epilepsy, *JAMA*, 114: 1320-1321, 1940.

107. Frantzen, E., Hansen, J. M., Hansen, O. E., and Kristensen, M., Phenytoin (Dilantin) intoxication, *Acta Neurol. Scand.*, 43: 440-446, 1967.

108. Freed, L. F., The psychopath: a social challenge, *Med. Proc.*, 13: 408-414, 1967.

109. Frey, H. H., Kampmann, E., and Nielsen, C. K., Study on combined treatment with phenobarbital and diphenylhydantoin, *Acta Pharmacol. Toxic.*, 26: 284-292, 1968.

110. Freyhan, F. A., Effectiveness of diphenylhydantoin in management of nonepileptic psychomotor excitement states, *Arch. Neurol. Psychiat.*, 53: 370-374, 1945.

111. Friedman, A. P., The migraine syndrome, *Bull. N.Y. Acad. Med.*, 44: 45-62, 1968.

112. Friedman, A. P. and Merritt, H. H., Treatment of headache, *JAMA*, 163: 1111-1117, 1957.

113. Gabka, J., On the therapy of idiopathic and symptomatic head and facial pains, *Med. Mschr.*, 17: 430-443, 1963.

114. Galindo, A. M. and Ginabreda, J. M. S., Treatment of chorea minor with diphenylhydantoin sodium, *Ann. Med.* (Barcelona), 34: 165-168, 1947.

115. Garouette, J. V., A suggested mechanism of action for the anticonvulsant properties of diphenylhydantoin, *Tulane U. Med. Fac. Bull.*, 24: 319-328, 1965.

116. Gatenby, P. B. B., Anticonvulsants as a factor in megaloblastic anemia in pregnancy, *Lancet*, 2: 1004-1005, 1960.

117. Gautray, J. P. and Natter, S., The significance of EEG and of neuro-sedative therapies in the gynecology clinic, *Ann. Endocr.*, 22: 173-185, 1961.

118. Gayet-Hallion, T. and Bertrand, I., Favorable action of diphenylhydantoin on the resistance of rats to drowning, *Compt. Rend. Soc. Biol.*, 153: 757-759, 1959.

119. Gellerman, G. L. and Martinez, C., Fatal ventricular fibrillation following intravenous sodium diphenylhydantoin therapy, *JAMA*, 200: 337-338, 1967.

120. Gellman, V., A case of diphenylhydantoin (Dilantin) intoxication, *Manitoba Med. Rev.*, 46: 388-390, 1966.

121. Gershbein, L. L., Effect of drugs and catecholamines on rat diaphragm carbohydrate metabolism, *J. Pharm. Sci.*, 55: 846-848, 1966.

122. Gilbert, J. C., Ortiz, W. R., and Millichap, J. G., The effects of anticonvulsant drugs on the permeability of brain cells to D-xylose, *J. Neurochem.*, 13: 247-255, 1966.

123. Golbert, T. M., Sanz, C. J., Rose, H. D., and Leitschuh, T. H., Comparative evaluation of treatments of alcohol withdrawal syndromes, *JAMA*, 201: 99-102, 1967.

124. Goldschlager, A. W. and Karliner, J. S., Ventricular standstill after intravenous diphenylhydantoin, *Amer. Heart J.*, 74: 410-412, 1967.

125. Goldstein, N., Leider, M., and Baer, R. L., Drug eruptions from anticonvulsant drugs, *Arch. Derm.*, 87: 612-617, 1963.

126. Gordon, P., Diphenylhydantoin and procainamide normalization of suboptimal learning behavior, *Recent Advances Biol. Psychiat.*, 10: 121-133, 1968.

127. Goodwin, F. B., Oral therapy in anogenital pruritus, *J. Nat. Proct. Assn.*, 18: 84-87, 1946.

128. Granick, S., The induction *in vitro* of the synthesis of δ-aminolevulinic acid synthetase in chemical porphyria: a response to certain drugs, sex hormones, and foreign chemicals, *J. Biol. Chem.*, 241: 1359-1375, 1966.

129. Green, J. B., Dilantin in the treatment of lightning pains, *Neurology*, 11: 257-258, 1961.

130. Green, J. B., Electroencephalographic findings in a case of acute reaction to Dilantin, *Electroenceph. Clin. Neurophysiol.*, 20: 201-202, 1966.

131. Gretter, T. E., Danner, P. K., Nibbelink, D. W., Green, D., and Sahs, A. L., The effect of diphenylhydantoin (Dilantin) on acute intermittent porphyria, *Trans. Amer. Neurol. Assn.*, 88: 176-178, 1963.

132. Grissom, J. H., Sy, B. G., Duffy, J. P., and Dunea, G., Dangerous consequence from use of Phenytoin in atrial flutter, *Brit. Med. J.*, 4: 34, 1967.

133. Gropper, A. L., Diphenylhydantoin sensitivity: report of fatal case with hepatitis and exfoliative dermatitis, *New Eng. J. Med.*, 254: 522-523, 1956.

134. Grosz, H. J., Dilantin intoxication—with a report of one case, *Amer. Pract. Dig. Treatm.*, 7: 1633-1636, 1956.

135. Gupta, R. C. and Kofoed, J., Toxicological statistics for barbiturates, other sedatives, and tranquilizers in Ontario: a 10-year survey, *Canad. Med. Assn. J.*, 94: 863-865, 1966.

136. Gydell, K., Megaloblastic anemia in patients treated with diphenylhydantoin and primidone, *Acta Haemat.*, 17: 1-15, 1957.

137. Hamfelt, A., Killander, A., Malers, E., and de Verdier, C., Megaloblastic anemia associated with anticonvulsant drugs, *Acta Med. Scand.*, 177: 549-555, 1965.

138. Hansen, J. M., Kristensen, M., Skovsted, L., and Christensen, L. K., Dicoumarol-induced diphenylhydantoin intoxication, *Lancet*, 2: 265-266, 1966.

139. Hansen, H. A., Nordqvist, P., and Sourander, P., Megaloblastic anemia and neurologic disturbances combined with folic acid deficiency: observations on an epileptic patient treated with anticonvulsants, *Acta Med. Scand.*, 176: 243-251, 1964.

140. Harinasuta, U. and Zimmerman, H. J., Diphenylhydantoin sodium hepatitis, *JAMA*, 203: 1015-1018, 1968.

141. Harris, A. S. and Kokernot, R. H., Effects of diphenylhydantoin sodium (Dilantin sodium) and phenobarbital sodium upon ectopic ventricular tachycardia in acute myocardial infarction, *Amer. J. Physiol.*, 163: 505-516, 1950.

142. Harris, J. and Ritchie, K., Anticonvulsant effects on copper uptake by neural tissue, *Fed. Proc.*, 25: 2091, 1966.

143. Harris, P. D., Bigger, J. T., Jr., Weinberg, D., and Malm, J. R., Use of diphenylhydantoin in ventricular arrhythmias following open heart surgery, *Surg. Forum*, 17: 185-188, 1966.

144. Hartmann, J. F., High sodium content of cortical astrocytes: electron microscope evidence, *Arch. Neurol.*, 15: 633-642, 1966.

145. Hatzmann, I., Neuhold, R., and von Rittner, W., Exfoliative dermatitis after hydantoin therapy, *Ann. Pediat.* (Basel), 179: 305-316, 1952.

146. Hausser, E., Bergoz, R. and Croci, D., Megaloblastic anemia provoked by antiepileptic medications, *Nouv. Rev. Franc. Hemat.*, 4: 221-232, 1964.

147. Hawkins, C. F. and Meynell, M. J., Macrocytosis and macrocytic anemia caused by anticonvulsant drugs, *Quart. J. Med.*, 27: 45-63, 1958.

148. Hawkins, C. F. and Meynell, M. J., Megaloblastic anemia due to Phenytoin sodium, *Lancet*, 2: 737-738, 1954.

149. Helfant, R. H., Scherlag, B. J., and Damato, A. N., The comparative electrophysiological effects of diphenylhydantoin and procaine amide in the digitalis intoxicated and nondigitalized heart, *Clin. Res.*, 15: 206, 1967.

150. Helfant, R. H., Scherlag, B. J., and Damato, A. N., The use of diphenylhydantoin in ventricular arrhythmias unresponsive to procaine amide: a dissociation of procaine amide's actions on automaticity and conduction, *Circulation*, 36: 139, 1967.

151. Helfant, R. H., Scherlag, B. J., and Damato, A. N., Diphenylhydantoin prevention of arrhythmias in the digitalis-sensitized dog after direct-current cardioversion, *Circulation*, 37: 424-428, 1968.

152. Helfant, R. H., Scherlag, B. J., and Damato, A. N., Diphenylhydantoin toxicity, *JAMA*, 201: 894, 1967.

153. Helfant, R. H., Scherlag, B. J., and Damato, A. N., Electrophysiological effects of direct current countershock before and after ouabain sensitization and after diphenylhydantoin desensitization in the dog, *Circ. Res.*, 22: 615-623, 1968.

154. Helfant, R. H., Scherlag, B. J., and Damato, A. N., The electrophysiological properties of diphenylhydantoin sodium as compared to procaine amide in the normal and digitalis intoxicated heart, *Circulation*, 36: 108-118, 1967.

155. Helfant, R. H., Scherlag, B. J., and Damato, A. N., Protection from digitalis toxicity with the prophylactic use of diphenylhydantoin sodium: an arrhythmic-inotropic dissociation, *Circulation*, 36: 119-124, 1967.

156. Helfant, R. H., Scherlag, B. J., and Damato, A. N., Use of diphenylhydantoin sodium to dissociate the effects of procaine amide on automaticity and conduction in the normal and arrhythmic heart, *Amer. J. Cardiol.*, 20: 820-825, 1967.

157. Helfant, R. H., Ricciutti, M. A., Scherlag, B. J., and Damato, A. N., Effect of diphenylhydantoin sodium (Dilantin) on myocardial A-V potassium difference, *Amer. J. Physiol.*, 214: 880-884, 1968.

158. Helfant, R. H., Lau, S. H., Cohen, S. I., and Damato, A. N., Effects of diphenylhydantoin on atrioventricular conduction in man, *Circulation*, 36: 686-691, 1967.

159. Herman, C. J. and Bignall, K. E., Effects of diphenylhydantoin on spontaneous and evoked activity in the cat under chloralose anesthesia, *Electroenceph. Clin. Neurophysiol.*, 23: 351-359, 1967.

160. de la Herran, J., Martinez-Lage, J. M., and Molina, P., Treatment of trigeminal neuralgia with diphenylhydantoin and disulphur of pyridoxine, *Medicina Clinica*, 38: 375-378, 1962.

161. Hirschmann, J., On the interval treatment of migraine, *Ther. Umsch.*, 21: 48-51, 1964.

162. Hoaken, P. C. S., and Kane, F. J., Jr., Unusual brain syndrome seen with diphenylhydantoin and pentobarbital, *Amer. J. Psychiat.*, 120: 282-283, 1963.

163. Hockman, C. H., Mauck, H. P., Jr., and Chu, N., ECG changes resulting from cerebral stimulation. III. Action of diphenylhydantoin on arrhythmias, *Amer. Heart J.*, 74: 256-260, 1967.

164. Hoff, E. C. and Yahn, C., The effect of sodium 5,5-diphenylhydantoinate (Dilantin sodium) upon the tolerance of rats and mice to decompression. *Amer. J. Physiol.*, 141: 7-16, 1944.

165. Hofmann, W. W., Cerebellar lesions after parenteral Dilantin administration, *Neurology*, 8: 210-214, 1958.

166. Holecková, R., Some experiences in treatment of cardiac arrhythmias using diphenylhydantoin, *Vnitrni. Lek.*, 13: 1195-1196, 1967.

167. Holland, P. and Mauer, A. M., Diphenylhydantoin-induced hypersensitivity reaction, *J. Pediat.*, 66: 322-332, 1965.

168. Hopf, H. C., On the alteration of transmission function of peripheral motor nerve fibers through diphenylhydantoin, *Deutsch Z. Nervenheilk*, 193: 41-56, 1968.

169. Horsfield, G. I. and Chalmers, J. N. M., Megaloblastic anemia associated with anticonvulsant therapy, *Practitioner*, 191: 316-321, 1963.

170. Horwitz, S. J., Klipstein, F. A., and Lovelace, R. E., Relation of abnormal folate metabolism to neuropathy developing during anticonvulsant drug therapy, *Lancet*, 1: 563-565, 1968.

171. Houck, J. C. and Patel, Y. M., Proposed mode of action of corticosteroids on the connective tissue, *Nature*, 206: 158-160, 1965.

172. Houck, J. C., Jacob, R. A., and Maengwyn-Davies, G. D., The effect of sodium Dilantin administration upon the chemistry of the skin, *J. Clin. Invest.*, 39: 1758-1762, 1960.

173. Huisman, J. W., The estimation of some important anticonvulsant drugs in serum, *Clin. Chim. Acta*, 13: 323-328, 1966.

174. Husby, J., Delayed toxicity and serum concentrations of Phenytoin, *Danish Med., Bull.*, 10: 236-239, 1963.

175. Iannone, A., Baker, A. B., and Morrell, F., Dilantin in the treatment of trigeminal neuralgia, *Neurology*, 8: 126-128, 1958.

176. Isaacs, H., A syndrome of continuous muscle-fibre activity. *J. Neurol. Neuro-surg. Psychiat.*, 24: 319-325, 1961.

177. Isaacs, H., Quantal squander, *S. A. J. Lab. Clin. Med.*, 10: 93-95, 1964.

178. Itil, T. M., Rizzo, A. E., and Shapiro, D. M., Study of behavior and EEG correlation during treatment of disturbed children, *Dis. Nerv. Syst.*, 28: 731-736, 1967.

179. Jensen, B. N. and Grynderup, V., Studies on the metabolism of Phenytoin, *Epilepsia*, 7: 238-245, 1966.

180. Jensen, H. P., The treatment of trigeminal neuralgia with diphenylhydantoin, *Arztl. Wochschr.*, 9: 105-108, 1954.

181. Jonas, A. D., The diagnostic and therapeutic use of diphenylhydantoin in the subictal state and non-epileptic dysphoria, *Int. J. Neuropsychiat.*, 3: S21-S29, 1967.

182. Jurna, I., Depression by antiparkinson drugs of reserpine rigidity, *Naunyn-Schmiedeberg Arch. Pharm.*, 260: 80-88, 1968.

183. Jurna, I. and Regélhy, B., The antagonism between reserpine and some antiparkinson drugs in electroseizure, *Naunyn-Schmiedeberg Arch. Pharm.*, 259: 442-459, 1968.

184. Kabat, H., Drug therapy of cerebellar ataxia and disorders of the basal ganglia, based on cerebellar-striatal antagonism, *Ann. Intern. Med.*, 50: 1438-1448, 1959.

185. Kabat, H. and McLeod, M., Neuromuscular dysfunction and treatment in athetosis, *Conn. Med.*, 23: 710-714, 1959.

186. Kalinowsky, L. B. and Putnam, T. J., Attempts at treatment of schizophrenia and other nonepileptic psychoses with Dilantin, *Arch. Neurol. Psychiat.*, 49: 414-420, 1943.

187. Karliner, J. S., Intravenous diphenylhydantoin sodium (Dilantin) in cardiac arrhythmias, *Dis. Chest*, 51: 256-269, 1967.

188. Kelln, E. E., Further studies of an epilepsy drug, *Dental Prog.*, 3: 271-273, 1963.

189. Kelln, E. E. and Gorlin, R. J., Healing qualities of an epilepsy drug, *Dental Prog.*, 1: 126-129, 1961.

190. Kemp, J. W. and Swinyard, E. A., Diphenylhydantoin inhibition of hexobarbital metabolism by liver microsomes in mice and rats, *Fed. Proc.*, 27: 350, 1968.

191. Kertesz, A., Paroxysmal kinesigenic choreoathetosis: an entity within the paroxysmal choreoathetosis syndrome, *Neurology*, 17: 680-690, 1967.

192. Khan, M. T. and McEwen, H. D., Effect of diphenylhydantoins on rat uterus *in vitro*, *Proc. Can. Fed. Biol. Soc.*, 10: 161, 1967.

193. Kidd, P. and Mollin, D. L., Megaloblastic anemia and vitamin-B_{12} deficiency after anticonvulsant therapy: report of two cases, *Brit. Med. J.*, 2: 974-976, 1957.

194. Kiørboe, E., Phenytoin intoxication during treatment with antabuse (Disulfiram), *Epilepsia*, 7: 246-249, 1966.

195. Kiørboe, E. and Plum, C. M., Megaloblastic anemia developing during treatment of epilepsy, *Acta Med. Scand.*, 179: suppl. 445, 349-357, 1966.

196. Klein, D. F. and Greenberg, I. M., Behavioral effects of diphenylhydantoin in severe psychiatric disorders, *Amer. J. Psychiat.*, 124: 847-849, 1967.

197. Klipstein, F. A., Subnormal serum folate and macrocytosis associated with anticonvulsant drug therapy, *Blood*, 23: 68-86, 1964.

198. Krieger, D. T., Effect of diphenylhydantoin on pituitary-adrenal interrelations, *J. Clin. Endocrinol. Metab.*, 22: 490-493, 1962.

199. Krieger, D. T. and Krieger, H. P., The effect of short-term administration of CNS-acting drugs on the circadian variation of the plasma 17-OHCS in normal subjects, *Neuroendocrinology*, 2: 232-246, 1967.

200. Kristensen, M., Hansen, J. M., Hansen, O. E., and Lund, V., Sources of error in the determination of Phenytoin (Dilantin) by Svensmark and Kristensen's method, *Acta Neurol. Scand.*, 43: 447-450, 1967.

201. Kubanek, J. L. and Rowell, R. C., The use of Dilantin in the treatment of psychotic patients unresponsive to other treatment, *Dis. Nerv. Syst.*, 7: 1-4, 1946.

202. Kugelberg, E. and Lindblom, U., The mechanism of the pain in trigeminal neuralgia. *J. Neurol. Neurosurg. Psychiat.*, 22: 36-43, 1959.

203. Kurtzke, J. F., Leukopenia with diphenylhydantoin, *J. Nerv. Ment. Dis.*, 132: 339-343, 1961.

204. Kutt, H., Intravenous use of diphenylhydantoin sodium, *JAMA*, 201: 210, 1967.

205. Kutt, H., Haynes, J., and McDowell, F., The effect of phenobarbital upon diphenylhydantoin metabolism in man, *Neurology*, 15: 274-275, 1965.

206. Kutt, H., Louis, S., and McDowell, F., Intravenous diphenylhydantoin in experimental seizures: I. Correlation of dose, blood, and tissue level in cats, *Arch. Neurol.*, 18: 465-471, 1968.

207. Kutt, H. and McDowell, F., Management of epilepsy with diphenylhydantoin sodium: dosage regulation for problem patients, *JAMA*, 203: 969-972, 1968.

208. Kutt, H., Winters, W., and McDowell, F., Depression of parahydroxylation of diphenylhydantoin by antituberculosis chemotherapy, *Neurology*, 16: 594-602, 1966.

209. Kutt, H., Winters, W., and McDowell, F., Determination of diphenylhydantoin and phenobarbital metabolites, *Fed. Proc.*, 23: 2346, 1964.

210. Kutt, H., Wolk, M., Scherman, R., and McDowell, F., Insufficient parahydroxylation as cause of Dilantin toxicity, *Neurology*, 13: 356, 1963.

211. Kutt, H., Wolk, M., Scherman, R., and McDowell, F., Insufficient parahydroxylation as a cause of diphenylhydantoin toxicity, *Neurology*, 14: 542-548, 1964.

212. Lach, J. L., Bhansali, K., and Blaug, S. M., The chromatographic separation and determination of diphenylhydantoin and phenobarbital, *J. Amer. Pharm. Assn.*, 47: 48-49, 1958.

213. Laird, R. D. and Fonner, R. L., The protective effect of sodium diphenylhydantoin in the hyperacute radiation syndrome, *U.S. Army Med. Res. Lab., Fort Knox, Kentucky, Report No. 262*, 1957.

214. Lamberts, A. E., Tic douloureux, *J. Mich. State Med. Soc.*, 58: 95-96, 1959.

215. Lang, T. W., Bernstein, H., Barbieri, F. F., Gold, H. and Corday, E., Digitalis toxicity: treatment with diphenylhydantoin, *Arch. Intern. Med.*, 116: 573-580, 1965.

216. Laubscher, F. A., Fatal diphenylhydantoin poisoning: a case report, *JAMA*, 198: 1120-1121, 1966.

217. Lauriault, C. D. and Jim, R. T. S., Diphenylhydantoin toxicity; lymphadenopathy and low platelet count, *Pediatrics*, 37: 341-342, 1966.

218. Lefkowitz, M. M., Effects of diphenylhydantoin on disruptive behavior: study of male delinquents, *Arch. Gen. Psychiat.*, 20: 643-651, 1969.

219. Lee, W. Y., Grummer, H. A., Bronsky, D., and Waldstein, S. S., Acute water loading as a diagnostic test for the inappropriate ADH syndrome, *J. Lab. Clin. Med.*, 58: 937, 1961.

220. Lees, F., Radioactive vitamin B_{12} absorption in the megaloblastic anemia caused by anticonvulsant drugs, *Quart. J. Med.*, 30: 231-248, 1961.

221. Leonard, W. A., Jr., The use of diphenylhydantoin (Dilantin) sodium in the treatment of ventricular tachycardia, *A.M.A. Arch. Intern. Med.*, 101: 714-717, 1958.

222. Levitt, J. M. and Blonstein, M., Toxic amblyopia resulting from sodium diphenyl hydantoinate, *New York J. Med.*, 40: 1538-1539, 1940.

223. Lieberson, A. D., Schumacher, R. R., Childress, R. H., Boyd, D. L., and Williams, J. F., Jr., Effect of diphenylhydantoin on left ventricular function in patients with heart disease, *Circulation*, 36: 692-699, 1967.

224. Lindblom, U., Diphenylhydantoin for trigeminal neuralgia, *Svensk Lakartidn*, 58: 3186-3191, 1961.

225. Lindsley, D. B. and Henry, C. E., The effect of drugs on behavior and the electroencephalograms of children with behavior disorders, *Psychosom. Med.*, 4: 140-149, 1942.

226. Livingston, S., Petersen, D., and Boks, L. L., Hypertrichosis occurring in association with Dilantin therapy, *J. Pediat.*, 47: 351-352, 1955.

227. Livingston, S. and Whitehouse, D., Treatment of headaches in children, *Mod. Treatm.*, 1: 1391-1398, 1964.

228. Livingston, S., Whitehouse, D., and Pauli, L. L., Study of the effects of diphenylhydantoin sodium on the lungs, *New Eng. J. Med.*, 264: 648-651, 1961.

229. Long, M. T., Childress, R. H., and Bond, W. H., Megaloblastic anemia associated with the use of anticonvulsant drugs: report of a case and review of the literature, *Neurology*, 13: 697-702, 1963.

230. Louis, S., Kutt, H., and McDowell, F., The cardiocirculatory changes caused by intravenous Dilantin and its solvent, *Amer. Heart J.*, 74: 523-529, 1967.

231. Louis, S., Kutt, H., and McDowell, F., Intravenous diphenylhydantoin in experimental seizures: II. Effect on penicillin-induced seizures in the cat, *Arch. Neurol.*, 18: 472-477, 1968.

232. Lovelace, R. E. and Horwitz, S. J., Peripheral neuropathy in long-term diphenylhydantoin therapy, *Arch. Neurol.*, 18: 69-77, 1968.

233. Lüllmann, H. and Weber, R., On the action of Phenytoin on digitalis-induced arrhythmia, *Arztliche Forschung*, 22: 49-55, 1968.

234. Lustberg, A., Goldman, D., and Dreskin, O. H., Megaloblastic anemia due to Dilantin therapy, *Ann. Intern. Med.*, 54: 153-158, 1961.

235. McCullagh, W. H. and Ingram, W., Jr., Headaches and hot tempers, *Dis. Nerv. Syst.*, 17: 279-281, 1956.

236. McDonald, D. B., Diphenylhydantoin and multiple system disease, *Grace Hosp. Bull.*, 44: 40-44, 1966.

237. MacIntosh, P. C. and Hutchison, J. L., Megaloblastic anemia due to anticonvulsant therapy: report of a case responding to vitamin B_{12}, *Canad. Med. Assn. J.*, 82: 365-368, 1960.

238. Magee, K. R. and DeJong, R. N., Complications of treatment and side reactions to anticonvulsant drugs, *Mod. Treatm.*, 1: 1138-1149, 1964.

239. Malygina, E. H., Effect of phenobarbital, diphenylhydantoin and trimethadione on the blood sugar level (rabbit), *Farmakol. Toksik.*, 28: 725-727, 1965.

240. Mandelbaum, H. and Kane, L. J., Dilantin sodium poisoning; report of a case with dermatitis exfoliativa, pyrexia and hepatic and splenic enlargement, *Arch. Neurol. Psychiat.*, 45: 769-771, 1941.

241. Manlapaz, J. S., Abducens nerve palsy in Dilantin intoxication, *J. Pediat.*, 55: 73-77, 1959.

242. Mark, V. H., Sweet, W. R., Ervin, F. R., Solomon, P., and Geschwind, N., Brain disease and violent behavior, *Neuroophthalmology*, Chap. 20, 4: 282-287, J. L. Smith, ed., C. V. Mosby, St. Louis, 1968.

243. Marriott, H. J. L., Management of cardiac dysrhythmias complicating acute myocardial infarction, *Geriatrics*, 147-156, Sept., 1968.

244. Martin, C. M., Rubin, M., O'Malley, W. E., Garagusi, V. F., and McCauley, C. E., Comparative physiological availability of brand and generic drugs in man: chloramphenicol, sulfisoxazole, and diphenylhydantoin, *Pharmacologist*, 10: 167, 1968.

245. Massey, K. M., Teratogenic effects of diphenylhydantoin sodium, *J. Oral Ther. Pharmacol.*, 2: 380-385, 1966.

246. Meeuwisse, G., Gamstorp, I., and Tryding, N., Effect of Phenytoin on the tryptophan load test, *Acta Paediat. Scand.*, 57: 115-120, 1968.

247. Melchior, J. C. and Svensmark, O., A case of Phenytoin hypersensitivity, *Acta Paediat. Scand.*, 52: 138-140, 1963.

248. Mercer, E. N. and Osborne, J. A., The current status of diphenylhydantoin in heart disease, *Ann. Intern. Med.*, 67: 1084-1107, 1967.

249. Mercer, E. N., Ziegler, W. G., Wickland, G. F., and Dower, G. E., The effect of diphenylhydantoin upon beating of heart cells grown *in vitro*, *J. Pharm. Exp. Ther.*, 155: 267-270, 1967.

250. Merritt, H. H. and Putnam, T. J., A new series of anticonvulsant drugs tested by experiments on animals, *Arch. Neurol. Psychiat.*, 1: 1003-1015, 1938.

251. Mertens, H. G. and Zschocke, S., Neuromyotonia, *Klin. Wschr.*, 17: 917-925, 1965.

252. Michels, J. G., Wright, G. C., and Gever, G., Synthesis and pharmacological activity of a series of 2-substituted pyridazinones, *J. Med. Chem.*, 9: 612-615, 1966.

253. Middleton, J. W. and Hejtmancik, M. R., Severe leukopenia due to diphenylhydantoin sodium: case report, *Texas State J. Med.*, 46: 520-521, 1950.

254. Millichap. J. G. and Boldrey, E. E., Studies in hyperkinetic behavior: II. Laboratory and clinical evaluations of drug treatments, *Neurology*, 17: 467-472, 1967.

255. Mixter, C. G., Moran, J. M., and Austen, W. G., Cardiac and peripheral vascular effects of diphenylhydantoin sodium, *Amer. J. Cardiol.*, 17: 332-338, 1966.

256. Moore, M. T., Pulmonary changes in hydantoin therapy, *JAMA*, 171: 1328-1333, 1959.

257. Morrell, F., Bradley, W., and Ptashne, M., Effect of diphenylhydantoin on peripheral nerve, *Neurology*, 8: 140-144, 1958.

258. Morrell, F., Bradley, W., and Ptashne, M., Effect of drugs on discharge characteristics of chronic epileptogenic lesions, *Neurology*, 9: 492-498, 1959.

259. Morris, J. V., Fischer, E., and Bergin, J. T., Rare complication of Phenytoin sodium treatment, *Brit. Med. J.*, 2: 1529, 1956.

260. Mosey, L. and Tyler, M. D., The effect of diphenylhydantoin sodium (Dilantin), procaine hydrochloride, procaine amide hydrochloride, and quinidine hydrochloride upon ouabain-induced ventricular tachycardia in unanesthetized dogs, *Circulation*, 10: 65-70, 1954.

261. Mull, J. D. and Mullinax, F., Diphenylhydantoin allergy: clinical and immunological studies, *Arthritis Rheum.*, 9: 525-526, 1966.

262. Munsat, T. L., Therapy of myotonia: a double-blind evaluation of diphenylhydantoin, procainamide, and placebo, *Neurology*, 17: 359-367, 1967.

263. Naiman, J. G. and Williams, H. L., Effects of diphenylhydantoin on the duration of respiratory activity during anoxia, *J. Pharm. Exp. Ther.*, 145: 34-41, 1964.

264. Nakamura, K. and Kurebe, M., Differential effects of antiepileptics on hippocampal and pallidal afterdischarges in cats, *Jap. J. Pharmacol.*, 12: 180-190, 1962.

265. Nakamura, K. and Masuda, Y., Effects of 5,5-diphenylhydantoin and 3-ethoxycarbonyl-5,5-diphenylhydantoin (P-6127) on the dermal and gingival tissues of experimental animals, *Arch. Int. Pharmacodyn.*, 162: 255-264, 1966.

266. Nakamura, K., Masuda, Y., and Nakatsuji, K., Tissue distribution and metabolic fate of 3-ethoxycarbonyl-5,5-diphenylhydantoin (P-6127) and 5,5-diphenylhydantoin in rats, *Arch. Int. Pharmacodyn.*, 165: 103-111, 1967.

267. Nakamura, K., Masuda, Y., Nakatsuji, K., and Hiroka, T., Comparative studies on the distribution and metabolic fate of diphenylhydantoin and 3-ethoxycarbonyl-diphenylhydantoin (P-6127) after chronic administrations to dogs and cats, *Naunyn-Schmiedeberg Arch. Pharm.*, 254: 406-417, 1966.

268. Natelson, S., Walker, A. A., and Pincus, J. B., Chlordiazepoxide and diphenylhydantoin as antagonists to ACTH effect on serum calcium and citrate levels, *Proc. Soc. Exp. Biol. Med.*, 122: 689-692, 1966.

269. Noach, E. L., Woodbury, D. M., and Goodman, L. S., Studies on the absorption, distribution, fate and excretion of $4\text{-}C^{14}$-labeled diphenylhydantoin, *J. Pharm. Exp. Ther.*, 122: 301-314, 1958.

270. Norris, F. H., Jr., Colella, J., and McFarlin, D., Effect of diphenylhydantoin on neuromuscular synapse, *Neurology*, 14: 869-876, 1964.

271. Oberst, B. B., Preventive care of infants and children. VI. School adjustment problems and their relationship to guided growth, *J. Lancet*, 86: 331-334, 1966.

272. Olesen, O. V., Determination of phenobarbital and Phenytoin in serum by ultraviolet spectrophotometry, *Scand. J. Clin. Lab. Invest.*, 20: 63-69, 1967.

273. Olesen, O. V., Disulfiramum (Antabuse) as inhibitor of Phenytoin metabolism, *Acta Pharmacol. Toxicol.*, 24: 317-322, 1966.

274. Olesen, O. V., Determination of 5-(p-hydroxyphenyl)-5-phenylhydantoin (HPPH) in urine by thin layer chromatography, *Acta Pharmacol. Toxicol.*, 26: 222-228, 1968.

275. Olesen, O. V., A simplified method for extracting Phenytoin from serum, and a more sensitive staining reaction for quantitative determination by thin layer chromatography, *Acta Pharmacol. Toxicol.*, 25: 123-126, 1967.

276. Oppenheimer, J. H., Fisher, L. V., Nelson, K. M., and Jailer, J. W., Depression of the serum protein-bound iodine level by diphenylhydantoin, *J. Clin. Endoc. Metab.*, 21: 252-262, 1961.

277. Orth, D. N., Almeida, H., Walsh, F. B., and Honda, M., Ophthalmoplegia resulting from diphenylhydantoin and primidone intoxication, *JAMA*, 201: 485-487, 1967.

278. Parrow, A., Use of anticonvulsive drugs in the treatment of recurrent cardiac arrhythmias, *Acta Med. Scand.*, 180: 413-419, 1966.

279. Patil, K. P., Chitre, R. G., and Sheth, U. K., Anti-folic acid activity of anti-epileptic drugs: Part I. Studies with bacterial cultures, *Indian J. Med. Sci.*, 20: 614-622, 1966.

280. Pennington, G. W. and Smyth, D., Identification reactions of the hydantoin group of drugs, *Arch. Int. Pharmacodyn.*, 152: 285-297, 1964.

281. Penny, J. L., Megaloblastic anemia during anticonvulsant drug therapy, *Arch. Intern. Med.*, 111: 744-749, 1963.

282. Peters, H. A., Eichman, P. L., Price, J. M., Kozelka, F. L., and Reese, H. H., Abnormal copper and tryptophan metabolism and chelation therapy in anti-convulsant drug intolerance, *Dis. Nerv. Syst.*, 27: 97-106, 1966.

283. Petty, C. S., Muelling, R. J., and Sindell, H. W., Accidental, fatal poisoning with diphenylhydantoin (Dilantin), *J. Forensic Sci.*, 2: 279-286, 1957.

284. Petty, W. C. and Karler, R., The influence of aging on the activity of anti-convulsant drugs, *J. Pharm. Exp. Ther.*, 150: 443-448, 1965.

285. Pincus, J. H. and Giarman, N. J., The effect of diphenylhydantoin on sodium-, potassium-, magnesium-stimulated adenosine triphosphatase activity of rat brain, *Biochem. Pharmacol.*, 16: 600-603, 1967.

286. Pincus, J. H. and Glaser, G. H., The syndrome of minimal brain damage in childhood. *New Eng. J. Med.*, 275: 27-35, 1966.

287. Putnam, T. J. and Hood, O. E., Project Illinois: a study of therapy in juvenile behavior problems, *Western Med.*, 231-233, July, 1964.

288. Raines, A. and Levitt, B., The failure of diphenylhydantoin to influence the β-adrenergic receptor of the heart, *Arch. Int. Pharmacodyn.*, 172: 435-441, 1968.

289. Raines, A. and Standaert, F. G., Pre- and postjunctional effects of diphenylhydantoin at the cat soleus neuromuscular junction, *J. Pharm. Exp. Ther.*, 153: 361-366, 1966.

290. Ramirez, E., The use of diphenylhydantoin in the modification of acting-out behavior of post-detoxification addict patients, *Personal communication.* 1967.

291. Rand, B. O., Kelly, W. A., and Ward, A. A., Jr., Electrophysiological studies of the action of intravenous diphenylhydantoin (Dilantin), *Neurology*, 16: 1022-1032, 1966.

292. Rantakallio, P. and Furuhjelm, U., Diphenylhydantoin sensitivity: a case with exfoliative dermatitis and atypical lymphocytes in the peripheral blood, *Ann. Paediat. Fenn.*, 8: 146-151, 1962.

293. Rawson, M. D. and Pincus, J. H., The effect of diphenylhydantoin on sodium, potassium, magnesium-activated adenosine triphosphatase in microsomal fractions of rat and guinea pig brain and on whole homogenates of human brain, *Biochem. Pharmacol.*, 17: 573-579, 1968.

294. Recant, L. and Hartroft, W. S., Lymphoma or drug reaction occurring during hydantoin therapy for epilepsy, *Amer. J. Med.*, 321: 286-291, 1962.

295. Reichelderfer, T. E., Pearson, P. H., and Livingston, S., Thrombocytopenic purpura occurring in association with paradione (paramethadione) and Dilantin sodium (Phenytoin sodium) therapy, *J. Pediat.*, 43: 43-46, 1953.

296. Remmer, H., Estabrook, R. W., Schenkman, J., and Greim, H., Reaction of drugs with microsomal liver hydroxylase: its influence on drug action, *Naunyn-Schmiedeberg Arch. Pharm.*, 259: 98-116, 1968.

297. Resnick, O., The psychoactive properties of diphenylhydantoin: experiences with prisoners and juvenile delinquents, *Int. J. Neuropsychiat.* 3: S30-S48, 1967.

298. Livingston, S., Treatment of epilepsy with diphenylhydantoin sodium (Dilantin sodium), *Post-grad. Med.*, 20: 584-590, 1956.

299. Reynolds, E. H., Effects of folic acid on the mental state and fit-frequency of drug-treated epileptic patients, *Lancet*, 1: 1086-1088, 1967.

300. Reynolds, E. H., Mental effects of anticonvulsants, and folic acid metabolism, *Brain*, 91: 197-214, 1968.

301. Rhind, E. G. and Varadi, S., Megaloblastic anemia due to Phenytoin sodium, *Lancet*, 2: 921, 1954.

302. Rinne, U. K., Effect of diphenylhydantoin treatment on the release of corticotrophin in epileptic patients, *Confin. Neurol.*, 27: 431-440, 1966.

303. Rinne, U. K., Site of the inhibiting action of diphenylhydantoin on the release of corticotrophin in epileptic patients, *Med. Pharmacol. Exp.*, 17: 409-416, 1967.

304. Roberts, H. J., On the etiology, rational treatment and prevention of multiple sclerosis, *Southern Med. J.*, 59: 940-950, 1966.

305. Robinow, M., Diphenylhydantoin hypersensitivity: treatment with 6-mercaptopurine, *Amer. J. Dis. Child.*, 106: 553-557, 1963.

306. Robinson, D. S., MacDonald, M. G., and Hobin, F. P., Sodium diphenylhydantoin reaction with evidence of circulating antibodies, *JAMA*, 192: 171-172, 1965.

307. Robinson, L. J., The gingival changes produced by Dilantin sodium, *Dis. Nerv. Syst.*, 3: 88-94, 1942.

308. Rosati, R. A., Alexander, J. A., Schaal, S. F., and Wallace, A. G., Influence of diphenylhydantoin on electrophysiological properties of the canine heart, *Circ. Res.*, 21: 757-765, 1967.

309. Roseman, E., Dilantin toxicity: a clinical and electroencephalographic study, *Neurology*, 11: 912-921, 1961.

310. Rosen, M., Lisak, R., and Rubin, I. L., Diphenylhydantoin in cardiac arrhythmias, *Amer. J. Cardiol.*, 20: 674-678, 1967.

311. Rosenberg, P. and Bartels, E., Drug effects on the spontaneous electrical activity of the squid giant axon, *J. Pharm. Exp. Ther.*, 155: 532-544, 1967.

312. Rosenfeld, S., Swiller, A. I., Shenoy, Y. M. V., and Morrison, A. N., Syndrome simulating lymphosarcoma induced by diphenylhydantoin sodium, *JAMA*, 176: 491-493, 1961.

313. Ross, A. T. and Jackson, V., Dilantin sodium: its influence on conduct and on psychometric ratings of institutionalized epileptics, *Ann. Intern. Med.*, 14: 770-773, 1940.

314. Rossi, A. O., Psychoneurologically impaired child: community mental health clinic approach, *New York J. Med.*, 67: 902-912, 1967.

315. Rowntree, L. G. and Waggoner, R. W., Prevention of migraine attacks by Dilantin sodium, *Dis. Nerv. Syst.*, 11: 148, 1950.

316. Rudzik, A. D. and Mennear, J. H., Antagonism of anticonvulsants by adrenergic blocking agents, *Proc. Soc. Exp. Biol. Med.*, 122: 278-280, 1966.

317. Rushton, J. G., Medical treatment of trigeminal neuralgia with a note on the results of alcohol injection, *Med. Clin. N. Amer.*, 52: 797-800, 1968.

318. Ruthen, G. C., Antiarrhythmic drugs: Part IV. Diphenylhydantoin in cardiac arrhythmias, *Amer. Heart J.*, 70: 275-278, 1965.

319. Ryan, G. M. S. and Forshaw, J. W. B., Megaloblastic anemia due to Phenytoin sodium, *Brit. Med. J.*, 2: 242-243, 1955.

320. Sack, L. P., The effects of sodium Dilantin on stuttering behavior, *Univ. of Calif., L. A. Doctoral thesis*, 1968.

321. Said, D. M., Fraga, J. R., and Reichelderfer, T. E., Hyperglycemia associated with diphenylhydantoin (Dilantin) intoxication, *Med. Ann. D.C.*, 37: 170-172, 1968.

322. Saltzstein, S. L. and Ackerman, L. V., Lymphadenopathy induced by anti-convulsant drugs and mimicking clinically and pathologically malignant lymphomas, *Cancer*, 12: 164-182, 1959.

323. Sanbar, S. S., Conway, F. J., Zweifler, A. J., and Smet, G., Diabetogenic effect of Dilantin (diphenylhydantoin), *Diabetes*, 16: 533, 1967.

324. Sandberg, D. H., Resnick, G. L., and Bacallao, C. Z., Measurement of serum diphenylhydantoin by gas-liquid chromatography, *Anal. Chem.*, 40: 736-738, 1968.

325. Sasyniuk, B. I. and Dresel, P. E., The effect of diphe-

nylhydantoin on conduction in isolated, blood-perfused dog hearts, *J. Pharm. Exp. Ther.*, 161: 191-196, 1968.

326. Schaaf, M. and Payne, C. A., Effect of diphenylhydantoin and phenobarbital on overt and latent tetany, *New Eng. J. Med.*, 274: 1228-1233, 1966.

327. Scherlag, B. J., Helfant, R. H., and Damato, A. N., The contrasting effects of diphenylhydantoin and procaine amide on A-V conduction in the digitalis-intoxicated and the normal heart, *Amer. Heart J.*, 75: 200-205, 1968.

328. Scherlag, B. J., Helfant, R. H., and Damato, A. N., The relationship between the ionic, inotropic and electrophysiological effects of digitalis, *Circulation*, 36: 230, 1967.

329. Schneider, E., Treatment of dysrhythmic migraine and other forms of cephalalgia with a new combinative preparation (Sanredo), *Schweiz. Med. Wschr.*, 37: 1340-1343, 1963.

330. Schön, A., Treatment with diphenylhydantoin in essential trigeminal neuralgia and in facial spasm, *Gior. Psichiat. Neuropat.*, 92: 1011-1020, 1964.

331. Schönhärl, E., Pharmacotherapeutic experiences in speech and vocal disturbances, *Med. Exp.*, 2: 179-183, 1960.

332. Schulte, C. J. A., and Good, T. A., Acute intoxication due to methsuximide and diphenylhydantoin, *J. Pediat.*, 68: 635-637, 1966.

333. Schwab, R. S., Timberlake, W. H., and Abbott, J. A., Control of side effects of anticonvulsant drugs, *Med. Clin. N. Amer.*, Boston Number, 1139-1150, 1954.

334. Serrate, J. P., Contribution to the treatment of chorea minor by diphenylhydantoin, *Gac. Mèd. Espan.*, 21: 160-161, 1947.

335. Shafer, W. G., The effect of Dilantin sodium on liver DNA and restitution, *J. Oral Ther. Pharm.*, 2: 319-323, 1966.

336. Shafer, W. G., Response of radiated human gingival fibroblast-like cells to Dilantin sodium in tissue culture, *J. Dent. Res.*, 44: 671-677, 1965.

337. Shafer, W. G., Beatty, R. E., and Davis, W. B., Effect of Dilantin sodium on tensile strength of healing wounds, *Proc. Soc. Exp. Biol.*, 98: 348-350, 1958.

338. Shapera, W., Dilantin therapy in certain nervous disorders, *Pittsburgh Med. Bull.*, 29: 732-736, 1940.

339. Shapiro, M., Acceleration of gingival wound healing in non-epileptic patients receiving diphenylhydantoin sodium, *Exp. Med. Surg.*, 16: 41-53, 1958.

340. Shulman, A. and Laycock, G. M., Action of central nervous system stimulant and depressant drugs in the intact animal: Part 3. Dual action of 5-ethyl-5-(1,3-dimethylbutyl) barbiturate, Dilantin and β-methyl-β-n-propylglutarimide, *Europ. J. Pharmacol.*, 2: 17-25, 1967.

341. Shulman, M. H., The use of Dilantin sodium in bronchial asthma: a preliminary report, *New Eng. J. Med.*, 226: 260-264, 1942.

342. Siegel, S. and Berkowitz, J., Diphenylhydantoin (Dilantin) hypersensitivity with infectious mononucleosis-like syndrome and jaundice, *J. Allergy*, 32: 447-451, 1961.

343. Sklans, S., Taylor, R. G., and Shklar, G., Effect of diphenylhydantoin sodium on healing of experimentally produced fractures in rabbit mandibles, *J. Oral Surg.*, 25: 310-319, 1967.

344. Simpson, G. M., Kunz, E., and Slafta, J., Use of sodium diphenylhydantoin in treatment of leg ulcers, *New York J. Med.*, 65: 886-888, 1965.

345. Simpson, W., Severe megaloblastic anemia induced by Phenytoin sodium, *Oral Surg.*, 22: 302-305, 1966.

346. Smith, I. M., Lindell, S. S., Hazard, E. C., and Rabinovich, S., Chemical treatments of staphylococcal infections in mice, *Nature*, 211: 720-722, 1966.

347. Snyder, C. H., Syndrome of gingival hyperplasia, hirsutism, and convulsions: Dilantin intoxication without Dilantin, *J. Pediat.*, 67: 499-502, 1965.

348. Solomon, H. M. and Schrogie, J. J., The effect of phenylramidol on the metabolism of diphenylhydantoin, *Clin. Pharm. Ther.*, 8: 554-556, 1967.

349. Sparberg, M., Diagnostically confusing complications of diphenylhydantoin therapy: a review, *Ann. Intern. Med.*, 59: 914-930, 1963.

350. Standish, S. M. and Clark, P. G., The effect of Dilantin sodium on connective tissue generation in polyvinyl sponge implants, *Transplantation Bull.*, 29: 439-445, 1962.

351. Stevens, H., Paroxysmal choreo-athetosis: a form of reflex epilepsy, *Arch. Neurol.*, 14: 415-420, 1966.

352. Stille, G., On the question of the action of diphenylhydantoin in states of pain: a neurophysiological analysis, *Nervenarzt*, 31: 109-112, 1960.

353. Swan, H. and Sawyer, D. C., Prevention of ventricular fibrillation during experimental hypothermia: failure of sodium diphenylhydantoin, *Arch. Surg.*, 95: 23-26, 1967.

354. Swerdlow, B., Acute brain syndrome associated with sodium diphenylhydantoin intoxication, *Amer. J. Psychiat.*, 122: 100-101, 1965.

355. Tec, L., Efficacy of diphenylhydantoin in childhood psychiatric disorders, *Amer. J. Psychiat.*, 124: 156-157, 1968.

356. Theopold, W., On the use of hydantoin derivatives in chorea minor, *Zschr. Kinderh.*, 69: 305-310, 1951.

357. Tichner, J. B. and Enselberg, C. D., Suicidal Dilantin (sodium diphenylhydantoin) poisoning, *New Eng. J. Med.*, 245: 723-725, 1951.

358. Toman, J. E. P., Neuropharmacologic considerations in psychic seizures, *Neurology*, 1: 444-460, 1951.

359. Toman, J. E. P., Drugs effective in convulsive disorders, *The Pharmacological Basis of Therapeutics*, 3rd Ed., 215-224, Goodman, L. S., Gilman, A., Eds., Macmillan, New York, 1965.

360. Tompsett, S. L., Note on the detection of hexoestrol, stilboestrol, dienoestrol and the p-hydroxy metabolites of phenobarbitone and Phenytoin in urine, *J. Pharm. Pharmacol.*, 16: 207-208, 1964.

361. Triedman, H. M., Fishman, R. A., and Yahr, M. D., Determination of plasma and cerebrospinal fluid levels of Dilantin in the human, *Trans. Amer. Neurol. Assn.*, 85: 166-170, 1960.

362. Turner, W. J., Anticonvulsive agents in the treatment of aggression, *Proc. Symp. Aggressive Behavior, Milan, May 1968*, 353–362, S. Garattini and E. B. Sigg, Eds., Excerpta Medica, Amsterdam, 1969.

363. Turner, W. J., Therapeutic use of diphenylhydantoin in neuroses, *Int. J. Neuropsychiat.*, 3: 94-105, 1967.

364. Turner, W. J., The usefulness of diphenylhydantoin in treatment of non-epileptic emotional disorders, *Int. J. Neuropsychiat.*, 3: suppl. 2, S8-S20, 1967.

365. Tuttle, R. S., and Preston, J. B., The effects of diphenylhydantoin (Dilantin) on segmental and suprasegmental facilitation and inhibition of segmental motoneurons in the cat, *J. Pharm. Exp. Ther.*, 141: 84-91, 1963.

366. Ungar, B. and Cowling, D. C., Megaloblastic anemia associated with anticonvulsant drug therapy, *Med. J. Aust.*, 2: 461-462, 1960.

367. Unger, A. H. and Sklaroff, H. J., Fatalities following intravenous use of sodium diphenylhydantoin for cardiac arrhythmias: report of two cases, *JAMA*, 200: 335-336, 1967.

368. van Wyk, J. J. and Hoffmann, C. R., Periarteritis nodosa: a case of fatal exfoliative dermatitis resulting from "Dilantin sodium" sensitization, *Arch. Intern. Med.*, 81: 605-611, 1948.

369. Vasko, J. S., Elkins, R. C., Fogarty, T. J., and Morrow, A. G., Effects of diphenylhydantoin on cardiac performance and peripheral vascular resistance, *Surg. Forum*, 17: 189-190, 1966.

370. Vastola, E. F. and Rosen, A., Suppression by anticonvulsants of focal electrical seizures in the neocortex, *Electroenceph. Clin. Neurophysiol.*, 12: 327-332, 1960.

371. Vernadakis, A. and Woodbury, D. M., Effects of cortisol and diphenylhydantoin on spinal cord convulsions in developing rats, *J. Pharm. Exp. Ther.*, 144: 316-320, 1964.

372. Vincent, M. C. and Blake, M. I., A note on the analysis of diphenylhydantoin sodium by an ion exchange procedure, *Drug Standards*, 26: 206-207, 1958.

373. Walker, C. F. and Kirkpatrick, B. B., Dilantin treatment for behavior problem children with abnormal electroencephalograms, *Amer. J. Psychiat.*, 103: 484-492, 1947.

374. Wallace, J., Biggs, J., and Dahl, E. V., Determination of diphenylhydantoin by ultraviolet spectrophotometry, *Anal. Chem.*, 37: 410-413, 1965.

375. Walsh, P. J. F., Prophylaxis in alcoholics in the withdrawal period, *Amer. J. Psychiat.*, 119: 262-263, 1962.

376. Weintraub, R. M., Pechet, L., and Alexander, B., Rapid diagnosis of drug-induced thrombocytopenic purpura, *JAMA*, 180: 528-532, 1962.

377. Werk, E. E., Jr., MacGee, J., and Sholiton, L. J., Effect of diphenylhydantoin on cortisol metabolism in man, *J. Clin. Invest.*, 43: 1824-1835, 1964.

378. Werk, E. E., Jr., Thrasher, K., Choi, Y., and Sholiton, L. J., Failure of metyrapone to inhibit 11-hydroxylation of 11-deoxycortisol during drug therapy, *J. Clin. Endoc. Metab.*, 27: 1358-1360, 1967.

379. Westerink, D., Chromatographic separation and microdetermination of phenobarbital, methylphenobarbital, butobarbital and Phenytoin, *Pharm. Weekbl.*, 97: 849-856, 1962.

380. Weidemann, D. H., New viewpoints on migraine therapy, *Med. Mschr.*, 20: 28-30, 1966.

381. Wilske, K. R., Shalit, I. E., Willkens, R. F., and Decker, J. L., Findings suggestive of systemic lupus erythematosus in subjects on chronic anticonvulsant therapy, *Arthritis Rheum.*, 8: 260-266, 1965.

382. Wilson, D. R., Electroencephalographic studies in diabetes mellitus, *Canad. Med. Assn., J.*, 65: 462-465, 1951.

383. Wilhoit, W. M. C., The broader treatment of acute alcoholism and delirium tremens, *J. Florida Med. Assn.*, 52: 254-255, 1965.

384. Winiker-Blanck, E., On the diphenylhydantoin therapy of trigeminal neuralgia, *Deutsch Stomat.*, 5: 321-322, 1955.

385. Ichikawa, J., Kimura, I., Terui, H., Wada, T., Sakurada, T., and Sakurada, S., Biochemical studies on antiepileptic drugs. I. Effect on glucose metabolism in guinea pig brain slices, *Seishin Shinkeigaku Zasshi*, 69: 1089-1100, 1967.

386. Wolnisty, C., Polyneuritis of pregnancy effectively managed with Dilantin: report of a case, *Obstet. Gynec.*, 23: 802-803, 1964.

387. Woodbury, D. M., Effect of diphenylhydantoin on electrolytes and radiosodium turnover in brain and other tissues of normal, hyponatremic and postictal rats, *J. Pharm. Exp. Ther.*, 115: 74-95, 1955.

388. Woodbury, D. M., Effect of diphenylhydantoin on pentylene tetrazol-induced seizures in developing rats, *Pharmacologist*, 8: 176, 1966.

389. Woodbury, D. M. and Esplin, D. W., Neuropharmacology and neurochemistry of anticonvulsant drugs, *Proc. Assn. Res. Nerv. Ment. Dis.*, 37: 24-57, 1959.

390. Yunis, A. A., Arimura, G. K., Lutcher, C. L., and Blasquez, J., Reversible erythroid aplasia induced by Dilantin: mechanism of action of Dilantin, *J. Lab. Clin. Med.*, 64: 1021, 1964.

391. Yunis, A. A., Arimura, G. K., Lutcher, C. L., Blasquez, J., and Halloran, M., Biochemical lesion in Dilantin-induced erythroid aplasia, *Blood*, 30: 587-600, 1967.

392. Zeft, H. J., Whalen, R. E., Ratliff, N. B., Jr., Davenport, R. D., Jr., and McIntosh, H. D., Diphenylhydantoin therapy in experimental myocardial infarction, *J. Pharm. Exp. Ther.*, 162: 80-84, 1968.

393. de Zeeuw, R. A. and Feitsma, M. T., Separation and identification of some barbiturates, bromoureides, Phenytoin and glutethimide by means of two-dimensional thin-layer chromatography, *Pharm. Weekbl.*, 101: 957-976, 1966.

394. Zetler, G., The harmine tremor and its antagonists, *Arch. Exper. Path. U. Pharmakol.*, 231: 34-54, 1957.

395. Zimmerman, F. T., Explosive behavior anomalies in children on an epileptic basis, *New York J. Med.*, 56: 2537-2543, 1956.

396. Zipes, D. P. and Orgain, E. S., Refractory paroxysmal ventricular tachycardia, *Ann. Intern. Med.*, 67: 1251-1257, 1967.

397. Zung, W. W. K., Effect of diphenylhydantoin on the sleep-dream cycle: an EEG study in normal adults, *Psychophysiology*, 5: 206, 1968.

398. Agarwal, S. P. and Blake, M. I., Determination of the pKa' value for 5,5-diphenylhydantoin, *J. Pharm. Sci.*, 57: 1434-1435, 1968.

399. Alvarez, W. C., Why patients avoid telling what is wrong, *Mod. Med.*, 53-54, Nov. 18, 1968.

400. Rosenblum, I. and Stein, A. A., Preferential distribution of diphenylhydantoin in primary human brain tumors, *Biochem. Pharmacol.*, 12: 1453-1454, 1963.

401. Sayar, B. and Polvan, O., Epilepsy and bronchial asthma, *Lancet*, 1: 1038, 1968.

402. Nayler, W. G., McInnes, I., Swann, J. B., Race, D., Carson, V., and Lowe, T. E., Some effects of diphenylhydantoin and propranolol on the cardiovascular system, *Amer. Heart J.*, 75: 83-96, 1968.

403. Lüllman, H. and Weber, R., Inhibition of cardiac glycoside-induced arrhythmia by Phenytoin, *Naunyn-Schmiedeberg Arch. Pharm.*, 259: 182-183, 1968.

404. Hilmi, K. I. and Regan, T. J., Relative effectiveness of antiarrhythmic drugs in treatment of digitalis-induced ventricular tachycardia, *Amer. Heart J.*, 76: 365-369, 1968.

405. Mierzwiak, D. S., Mitchell, J. H., and Shapiro, W., The effect of diphenylhydantoin (Dilantin) and quinidine on left ventricular function in dogs, *Amer. Heart J.*, 74: 780-791, 1967.

406. Mierzwiak, D. S., Shapiro, W., McNalley, M. C., and Mitchell, J. H., Cardiac effects of diphenylhydantoin (Dilantin) in man, *Amer. J. Cardiol.*, 21: 20-22, 1968.

407. Wehrmacher, W. H., Dilantin in the management of cardiac arrhythmias, *Curr. Med. Dig.*, 36: 45-49, 1969.

408. Shine, K. I., Kastor, J. A., and Yurchak, P. M., Multifocal atrial tachycardia: clinical and electrocardiographic features in 32 patients, *New Eng. J. Med.*, 279: 344-349, 1968.

409. Seuffert, G. W., Helfant, R. H., Dana, J. F., and Urbach, K. F., Use of diphenylhydantoin in prevention and treatment of cardiac arrhythmias during general anesthesia. *Anesth. Analg.*, 47: 334-339, 1968.

410. Scherf, D., Blumenfeld, S., Taner, D., and Yildiz, M., The effect of diphenylhydantoin (Dilantin) sodium on atrial flutter and fibrillation provoked by focal application of aconitine or delphinine, *Amer. Heart J.*, 60: 936-947, 1960.

411. Carlson, E. E., Viral myocarditis, *Minn. Med.*, 51: 829-836, 1968.

412. Lawrie, D. M., Higgins, M. R., Godman, M. J., Oliver, M. F., Julian, D. G., and Donald, K. W., Ventricular fibrillation complicating acute myocardial infarction, *Lancet*, 2: 523-528, 1968.

413. Blachly, P. H., Diphenylhydantoin and arrhythmias, *JAMA*, 202: 173, 1967.

414. Editor, Hypertension in a young man, *JAMA*, 143: 939, 1954.

415. Conn, R. D., Newer drugs in the treatment of cardiac arrhythmia, *Med. Clin. N. Amer.*, 51: 1223-1240, 1967.

416. Criscitiello, M. G., Therapy of atrioventricular block, *New Eng. J. Med.*, 279: 808-810, 1968.

417. Schattenberg, T. T., Echocardiographic diagnosis of left atrial myxoma, *Mayo Clin. Proc.*, 43: 620–627, 1968.

418. Bashour, F. A., Edmondson, R. E., Gupta, D. N., and Prati, R., Treatment of digitalis toxicity by diphenylhydantoin (Dilantin), *Dis. Chest*, 53: 263-270, 1968.

419. Chen, G., Bohner, B., and Bratton, A. C., Jr., The influ-

ence of certain central depressants on fighting behavior of mice, *Arch. Int. Pharmacodyn.*, 142: 30-34, 1963.

420. Editor, Childhood migraine, *New Eng. J. Med.*, 276: 56-57, 1967.

421. Ginabreda, J. M. S., Treatment of chorea with diphenylhydantoin sodium, *Rev. Espan. Pediat.*, 266-272, Mar.-Apr., 1945.

422. Roberts, H. J., Migraine and related vascular headaches due to diabetogenic hyperinsulinism, *Headache*, 7: 41-62, 1967.

423. Gribetz, D., Mizrachi, A., and London, R. B., Neonatal hypocalcemia, Correspondence, *New Eng. J. Med.*, 279: 327, 1968.

424. O'Malley, B. W. and Kohler, P. O., Hypoparathyroidism, *Postgrad. Med.*, 44: 182-186, 1968.

425. Werk, E. E., Sholiton, L. J., and Olinger, C. P., Enzyme inducer, *New Eng. J. Med.*, 276: 877, 1967.

426. Gilbert, J. C., Ortiz, W. R., and Millichap, J. G., The effects of anticonvulsant drugs on the permeability of brain cells to sugars, *Proc. Inst. Med. Chicago*, 25: May, 1965.

427. Werk, E. E., Jr., Sholiton, L. J., and Olinger, C. P., Amelioration of non-tumorous Cushing's syndrome by diphenylhydantoin, *Proc. 2nd Int. Cong. Hormonal Steroids, Excerpta Medica, No. 111*, Milan, 1966.

428. Bodkin, L. G., Pruritus ani, *Amer. Prac.*, 2: 580-581, 1948.

429. Roberts, H. J., The syndrome of narcolepsy and diabetogenic ("functional") hyperinsulinism, with special reference to obesity, diabetes, idiopathic edema, cerebral dysrhythmias and multiple sclerosis (200 patients), *J. Amer. Geriat. Soc.*, 12: 926-976, 1964.

430. Fabrykant, M., Pseudohypoglycemic reactions in insulin-treated diabetics: etiology, laboratory aids and therapy, *J. Amer. Geriat. Soc.*, 12: 221-238, 1964.

431. Ellenberg, M., Treatment of diabetic neuropathy with diphenylhydantoin, *New York J. Med.*, 68: 2653-2655, 1968.

432. Jonas, A. D., *Ictal and subictal neurosis*, C. C. Thomas, Springfield, Ill., 1965.

433. Kong, Y., Chen, J. T. T., Zeft, H. J., Whalen, R. E., and McIntosh, H. D., Natural history of experimental coronary occlusion in pigs: a serial cineangeographic study, *Amer. Heart J.*, 77: 45-54, 1969.

434. Klinefelter, H. F., Greene, C. A., Pauli, L. L. and Livingston, S., Precordial pain in an epileptic relieved by Dilantin, *Johns Hopkins Med. J.*, 124: 25-27, 1969.

435. Bjorge, I., Presthus, J., and Stoa, K. F., A spectrophotometric study on 5,5-diphenylhydantoin, *Norsk Farmaceutisk Selskap*, 19: 17-22, 1957.

436. Koster, R., Mechanism of chlorcyclizine block of diphenylhydantoin in mice, *Pharmacologist*, 6: 187, 1964.

437. Svensmark, O. and Kristensen, P., Determination of diphenylhydantoin and phenobarbital in small amounts of serum, *J. Lab. Clin. Med.*, 61: 501-507, 1963.

438. Wallace, J. E. and Dahl, E. V., New laboratory method for determining Dilantin, *Air Force Systems Command Research and Technology Briefs*, 3: 18-21, Sept., 1965.

439. Panalaks, T., A method for evaluation of physiological availability of diphenylhydantoin by urinary analysis, *Clin. Chim. Acta*, 8: 968-970, 1963.

440. Loeser, E. W., Jr., Studies on the metabolism of diphenylhydantoin (Dilantin), *Neurology*, 11: 424-429, 1961.

441. Schiller, P. J. and Buchthal, F., Diphenylhydantoin and phenobarbital in serum in patients with epilepsy, *Danish Med. Bull.*, 5: 161-163, 1958.

442. Burns, J. J. and Conney, A. H., Enzyme stimulation and inhibition in the metabolism of drugs, *Proc. Roy. Soc. Med.*, 58: 955-960, 1965.

443. Butler, T. C., The metabolic conversion of 5,5-diphenylhydantoin to 5-(p-hydroxyphenyl)-5-phenylhydantoin, *J. Pharm. Exp. Ther.*, 119: 1-11, 1957.

444. Maynert, E. W., The metabolic fate of diphenylhydantoin in the dog, rat and man, *J. Pharm. Exp. Ther.*, 130: 275-284, 1960.

445. Chang, T., Baukema, J., Dill, W. A., Buchanan, R. A., Goulet, J. R., and Glazko, A. J., Metabolic disposition of diphenylhydantoin (DPH) in human subjects following intravenous administration, *Clin. Res.*, 16: 464, 1968.

446. Svensmark, O., Schiller, P. J., and Buchthal, F., 5,5-diphenylhydantoin (Dilantin) blood levels after oral or intravenous dosage in man, *Acta Pharmacol. (Kobenhavn)*, 16: 331-346, 1960.

447. Toman, J. E. P. and Taylor, J. D., Mechanism of action and metabolism of anticonvulsants, *Epilepsia*, Third Series, 1: 31-48, 1952.

448. Rudzik, A. D. and Mennear, J. H., The mechanism of action of anticonvulsants. I. Diphenylhydantoin, *Life Sci.*, 4: 2373-2382, 1965.

449. Morpurgo, C., Aggressive behavior induced by large doses of 2-(2,6-dichlorphenylamino)-2-imidazoline hydrochloride (ST-155) in mice, *Europ. J. Pharmacol.*, 3: 374-377, 1968.

450. Sholiton, L. J., Werk, E. E., and MacGee, J., The effect of diphenylhydantoin *in vitro* on the metabolism of testosterone by rat liver slices, *Acta Endocr.*, 56: 490-498, 1967.

451. Sholiton, L., Werk, E. E., Jr., and MacGee, J., The *in vitro* effect of 5,5'-diphenylhydantoin on the catabolism of cortisol by rat liver, *Metabolism*, 13: 1382-1392, 1964.

452. Kutt, H., Verebely, K., and McDowell, F., Inhibition of diphenylhydantoin metabolism in rat liver microsomes by antituberculosis drugs, *Neurology*, 17: 318-319, 1967.

453. Kutt, H., Verebely, K., and McDowell, F., Inhibition of diphenylhydantoin metabolism in rats and in rat liver microsomes by antitubercular drugs, *Neurology*, 18: 706-710, 1968.

454. Verster, F. de B., Garoutte, J., Ichinosa, H., and Guerrero-Figueroa, R., Mode of action of diphenylhydantoin, *Fed. Proc.*, 24: 390, 1965.

455. Elliott, K. A. C. and van Gelder, N. M., The state of factor I in rat brain: the effects of metabolic conditions and drugs, *J. Physiol.*, 153: 423-432, 1960.

456. Shohl, J., Effects of oral administration of Dilantin sodium on abnormal behavior in the rat, *J. Comp. Psychol.*, 37: 243-250, 1944.

457. Weissman, A., Effect of anticonvulsant drugs on electroconvulsive shock-induced retrograde amnesia, *Arch. Int. Pharmacodyn.*, 154: 122-130, 1965.

458. Toman, J. E. P., The neuropharmacology of antiepileptics, *Electroenceph. Clin. Neurophysiol.*, 1: 33-44, 1949.

459. Ensor, C. R., Bohner, B., and Chen, G., Anticonvulsant effect of Dilantin sodium by intravenous administration in mice, *Proc. Soc. Exp. Med. Biol.*, 100: 133-135, 1959.

460. Hofmann, W. W., Koenig, G., Shumway, N. E., and Hanbery, J. W., Observations of the depressant effects of parenterally administered Dilantin on the cardiovascular system and cerebral cortex, *Stanford Med. Bull.*, 17: 193-197, 1959.

461. Riehl, J. and McIntyre, H. B., A quantitative study of the acute effects of diphenylhydantoin on the electroencephalogram of epileptic patients: Theoretical considerations for its use in the treatment of status epilepticus, *Neurology*, 18: 1107-1112, 1968.

462. Schallek, W. and Kuehn, A., Effects of trimethadione, diphenylhydantoin and chlordiazepoxide on after-discharges in brain of cat, *Proc. Soc. Exp. Biol. Med.*, 112: 813-816, 1963.

463. Chen, G. and Ensor, C. R., Antagonism studies on reserpine and certain CNS depressants, *Proc. Soc. Exp. Biol. Med.*, 87: 602-608, 1954.

464. Lu, F. C., Mazurkiewicz, I. M., Grewal, R. S., Allmark, M. G., and Boivin, P., The effect of sodium fluoride on responses to various central nervous system agents in rats, *Toxic. Appl. Pharmacol.*, 3: 31-38, 1961.

465. Druckman, R. and Moore, F. J., Effects of sodium di-

phenylhydantoinate upon isolated small intestine of the rabbit, *Proc. Soc. Exp. Biol. Med.*, 90: 173-176, 1955.

466. Van Harreveld, A. and Feigen, G. A., Effect of some drugs on the polarization state of spinal cord elements, *Amer. J. Physiol.*, 160: 451-461, 1950.

467. Raines, A. and Standaert, F. G., An effect of diphenylhydantoin on post-tetanic hyperpolarization of intramedullary nerve terminals, *J. Pharm. Exp. Ther.*, 156: 591-597, 1967.

468. Raines, A., Diphenylhydantoin suppression of post-tetanic hyperpolarization in nerve terminals of dorsal root fibers, *Pharmacologist*, 7: 142, 1965.

469. Brumlik, J. and Moretti, L., The effect of diphenylhydantoin on nerve conduction velocity, *Neurology*, 16: 1217-1218, 1966.

470. Hopf, H. C., Effect of diphenylhydantoin on peripheral nerves in man, *Electroenceph. Clin. Neurophysiol.*, 25: 411, 1968.

471. Orozco, A. and Sabelli, H. C., Effect of antiepileptic drugs on calcium-induced hyperexcitability in earthworm ventral cords, *Pharmacologist*, 10: 161, 1968.

472. Korey, S. R., Effect of Dilantin and Mesantoin on the giant axon of the squid, *Proc. Soc. Exp. Biol. Med.*, 76: 297-299, 1951.

473. Kivalo, E., Tyrkkö, J., and Marjanen, P., The response to diphenylhydantoin of the neurosecretory substance in the mouse, *Ann. Med. Intern. Fenn.*, 47: 169-173, 1958.

474. Buchthal, F., Svensmark, O., and Schiller, P. J., Clinical and electroencephalographic correlations with serum levels of diphenylhydantoin, *Arch. Neurol.*, 2: 624-630, 1960.

475. Cohn, R., A neuropathological study of a case of petit mal epilepsy, *Electroenceph. Clin. Neurophysiol.*, 24: 282, 1968.

476. Haury, V. G. and Drake, M. E., The effect of intravenous injections of sodium diphenylhydantoinate (Dilantin) on respiration, blood pressure, and the vagus nerve, *J. Pharm. Exp. Ther.*, 68: 36-40, 1940.

477. Hrbek, J., Komenda, S., Dostalova, K., Siroka, A., Beran, I., and Szarowski, E., The acute effect of some drugs on the higher nervous activity in man. VII. Pyridoxine and diphenylhydantoin, *Acta Univ. Palacki Olomuc., Fac. Med.*, 47: 625-638, 1967.

478. Takahashi, M., Effects of antiepileptic drugs on end plate region. Facilitation of acetazolamide, *Hirosaki Med. J.*, 19: 597, 1967.

479. Van Harreveld, A., Foster, R. J., and Fasman, G. D., Effect of diphenylhydantoin on ether and pentobarbital narcosis, *Amer. J. Physiol.*, 166: 718-722, 1951.

480. Toman, J. E. P., Neuropharmacology of diphenylhydantoin, *Int. J. Neuropsychiat.*, 3: S57-S62, 1967.

481. Woodbury, D. M., Effects of chronic administration of anticonvulsant drugs, alone and in combination with desoxycorticosterone, on electroshock seizure threshold and tissue electrolytes, *J. Pharm. Exp. Ther.*, 105: 46-57, 1952.

482. Oliver, J. T. and Troop, R. C., Plasma corticosterone levels in stressed rats following the administration of pentobarbital, morphine and diphenylhydantoin, *Steroids*, 1: 670-677, 1963.

483. Woodbury, D. M., Timiras, P. S., and Vernadakis, A., Modification of adrenocortical function by centrally acting drugs and the influence of such modification on the central response to these drugs, *Hormones, Brain Function, and Behavior*, 38-50, H. Hoagland, Ed., Academic Press, New York, 1957.

484. Staple, P. H., The effects of continued administration of 5:5-diphenylhydantoin (Dilantin) sodium on the adrenal glands in mice, *J. Roy. Micr. Soc.*, 74: 10-21, 1954.

485. Quinn, D. L., Influence of diphenylhydantoin on spontaneous release of ovulating hormone in the adult rat, *Proc. Soc. Exp. Biol. Med.*, 119: 982-985, 1965.

486. Christy, N. P. and Hofmann, A. D., The apparent lack of effect of diphenylhydantoin (Dilantin) upon adrenal cortical response to ACTH in man, *Clin. Res.*, 6: 258-259, 1958.

487. Takahashi, Y., Kipnis, D. M., and Daughaday, W. H.,

Growth hormone secretion during sleep, *J. Clin. Invest.*, 47: 2079-2090, 1968.

488. Levy, R. P. and Marshall, J. S., Short-term drug effects on thyroid function tests, *Arch. Intern. Med.*, 114: 413-416, 1964.

489. Zaninovich, A. A., Farach, H., Ezrin, C., and Volpé, R., Lack of significant binding of L-triiodothyronine by thyroxine binding globulin *in vivo* as demonstrated by acute disappearance of 131-I-labeled triiodothyronine, *J. Clin. Invest.*, 45: 1290-1301, 1966.

490. Oppenheimer, J. H. and Tavernetti, R. R., Studies on the thyroxin-diphenylhydantoin interaction: effect of 5,5'-diphenylhydantoin on the displacement of L-thyroxine from thyroxine-binding globulin (TBG), *Endocrinology*, 71: 496-504, 1962.

491. Oppenheimer, J. H. and Tavernetti, R. R., Displacement of thyroxine from human thyroxine-binding globulin by analogues of hydantoin. Steric aspects of the thyroxine binding site, *J. Clin. Invest.*, 41: 2213-2220, 1962.

492. Oppenheimer, J. H., Role of plasma proteins in the binding, distribution and metabolism of the thyroid hormones, *New Eng. J. Med.*, 278: 1153-1162, 1968.

493. Chin, W. and Schussler, G. C., Decreased serum free thyroxine concentration in patients treated with diphenylhydantoin, *J. Clin. Endocrinol.*, 28: 181-186, 1968.

494. Mendoza, D. M., Flock, E. V., Owen, C. A., Jr., and Paris, J., Effect of 5,5'-diphenylhydantoin on the metabolism of L-thyroxine-^{131}I in the rat. *Endocrinology*, 79: 106-118, 1966.

495. Merritt, H. H. and Foster, A., Vitamin C in epilepsy. Dilantin sodium not a cause of vitamin C deficiency, *Amer. J. Med. Sci.*, 200: 541-544, 1940.

496. Gupta, D. N., Unal, M. O., Bashour, F. A., and Webb, W. R., Effects of diphenylhydantoin (Dilantin) on peripheral and coronary circulation and myocardial contractility in the experimental animal, *Dis. Chest*, 51: 248-255, 1967.

497. Roberts, H. J., Spontaneous leg cramps and "restless legs" due to diabetogenic hyperinsulinism: observations on 131 patients, *J. Amer. Geriat. Soc.*, 13: 602-638, 1965.

498. Bhussry, B. R., and Rao, S., Effect of sodium diphenylhydantoinate on oral mucosa of rats, *Proc. Soc. Exp. Biol. Med.*, 113: 595-599, 1963.

499. Houck, J. C., The resorption of sodium Dilantin produced dermal collagen, *J. Clin. Invest.* 41: 179-184, 1962.

500. Houck, J. C., Dermal chemical response to analogues of Dilantin, *J. Invest. Derm.*, 40: 89-93, 1963.

501. Houck, J. C., Effect of cortisol and age upon the dermal chemical response to Dilantin, *J. Invest. Derm.*, 40: 125-126, 1963.

502. Houck, J. C. and Jacob, R. A., Connective tissue. VII. Factors inhibiting the dermal chemical response to cortisol, *Proc. Soc. Exp. Biol. Med.*, 113: 692-694, 1963.

503. Forscher, B. K. and Cecil, H. C., Biochemical studies on acute inflammation. II. The effect of Dilantin, *J. Dent. Res.*, 36: 927-931, 1957.

504. Kolbert, G. S., Oral diphenylhydantoin in corneal wound healing in the rabbit, *Amer. J. Ophthal.*, 66: 736-738, 1968.

505. Smith, D. L. and Robinson, W. A., The effect of diphenylhydantoin sodium on liver restitution in the rat following hepatectomy, *Proc. West. Pharmacol. Soc.*, 5: 9-12, 1962.

506. Shafer, W. G., Effect of Dilantin sodium analogues on cell proliferation in tissue culture, *Proc. Soc. Exp. Biol. Med.*, 106: 205-207, 1961.

507. Shafer, W. G., Effect of Dilantin sodium on various cell lines in tissue culture, *Proc. Soc. Exp. Biol. Med.*, 108: 694-696, 1961.

508. Shafer, W. G., Effect of Dilantin sodium on growth of human fibroblast-like cell cultures, *Proc. Soc. Exp. Biol. Med.*, 104: 198-201, 1960.

509. Chalmers, J. N. M. and Boheimer, K., Megaloblastic anaemia and anticonvulsant therapy, *Lancet*, 2: 920-921, 1954.

510. P'an, S. Y., Funderburk, W. H., and Finger, K. F., Anti-

convulsant effect of nialamide and diphenylhydantoin, *Proc. Soc. Exp. Biol. Med.*, 108, 680-683, 1961.

511. Conn, R. D., Kennedy, J. W., and Blackmon, J. R., The hemodynamic effects of diphenylhydantoin, *Amer. Heart J.*, 73: 500-505, 1967.

512. Rowe, G. G., McKenna, D. H., Sialer, S., and Corliss, R. J., Systemic and coronary hemodynamic effects of diphenylhydantoin, *Amer. J. Med. Sci.*, 254: 534-541, 1967.

513. Hockman. C. H., Mauck, H. P., Jr., and Hoff, E. C., Experimental neurogenic arrhythmias, *Bull. N.Y. Acad. Med.*, 43: 1097-1105, 1967.

514. Raines, A., Levitt, B., and Standaert, F. G., Factors influencing diphenylhydantoin antagonism of ouabain-induced ventricular arrhythmia in the cat, *Pharmacologist*, 9: 237, 1967.

515. Roberts, J., Levitt, B., and Standaert, F. G., Autonomic nervous system and control of cardiac rhythm, *Nature*, 214: 912-913, 1967.

516. Stannard, M., Sloman, G., and Sangster, L., The haemodynamic effects of Phenytoin sodium (Dilantin) in acute myocardial infarction, *Med. J. Aust.*, 1: 335-337, 1968.

517. Lugo, V. and Sanabria, A., Treatment of extrasystole in chronic Chagasic cardiopathy with diphenylhydantoin, *Acta Medica Venezolana*, 148-151, Mar.-Apr., 1966.

518. Jensen, H. P., The treatment of trigeminal neuralgia with diphenylhydantoin, *Therapiewoche*, 5: 345, 1955.

519. Rosati, R. and Wallace, A. G., Electrophysiologic effects of diphenylhydantoin (Dilantin) on the heart of awake dogs, *Amer. J. Cardiol.*, 19: 147, 1967.

520. Bonnycastle, D. D. and Bradley, A. J., Diphenylhydantoin and the release of adrenocorticotropic hormone in the albino rat, *Endocrinology*, 66: 355-360, 1960.

521. Porter, I. H., The genetics of drug susceptibility, *Dis. Nerv. Syst.*, 27: 25-36, 1966.

522. Bhattacharya, S. S., Kishor, K., Saxena, P. N., and Bhargava, K. P., A neuropharmacological study of gamma-aminobutyric acid (GABA), *Arch. Int. Pharmacodyn.*, 150: 295-305, 1964.

523. de Ropp, R. S., and Snedeker, E. H., Effect of drugs on amino acid levels in brain: excitants and depressants, *Proc. Soc. Exp. Biol. Med.*, 106: 696-700, 1960.

524. Thomas, H. F. and Stone, C. P., Maze performance of albino rats under influence of Dilantin sodium while subjected to electroshock, *J. Psychol.*, 33: 127-132, 1952.

525. Blum, B., A differential action of diphenylhydantoin on the motor cortex of the cat, *Arch. Int. Pharmacodyn.*, 149: 45-55, 1964.

526. Bianchi, C., Anticonvulsant action of some antiepileptic drugs in mice pretreated with rauwolfia alkaloids, *Brit. J. Pharmacol.*, 11: 141-146, 1956.

527. Haward, L. R. C., A study of physiological responses of neurotic patients to diphenylhydantoin, *Int. J. Neuropsychiat.*, 3: S49-S56, 1967.

528. Gerber, N. and Arnold, K., The effect of diphenyl-piperazine compounds and other agents on diphenylhydantoin, zoxazolamine and hexabarbital metabolism, *J. Pharm. Exp. Ther.*, 164: 232-238, 1968.

529. Ariyoshi, V. T. and Remmer, H., The action of phenobarbital and diphenylhydantoin on various fat fractions of liver, *Naunyn-Schmiedeberg Arch. Pharm.*, 260: 90-91, 1968.

530. Pincus, J. H. and Rawson, M. D., Diphenylhydantoin and intracellular sodium concentration, *Neurology*, 19: 419-422, 1968.

531. Kemp, J. W. and Woodbury, D. M., Intracellular distribution of 4-C^{14} diphenylhydantoin (Dilantin) in rat brain, *Pharmacologist*, 4: 159, 1962.

532. Vernadakis, A. and Woodbury, D. M., Effects of diphenylhydantoin and adrenocortical steroids on free glutamic acid, glutamine, and gamma-aminobutyric acid concentrations of rat cerebral cortex, *Inhibitions of the nervous system and gamma-aminobutyric acid*, 242-248, Pergamon Press, Oxford, 1960.

533. Strauss, H. C., Bigger, J. T., Jr., Bassett, A. L. and Hoffman, B. F., Actions of diphenylhydantoin on the electrical properties of isolated rabbit and canine atria, *Circ. Res.*, 23: 463-477, 1968.

534. Ludmer, R. I. and Toman, J. E. P., Some drug effects on cardiac transmembranal potentials, *Fed. Proc.*, 27: 303, 1968.

535. Kimball, O. P. and Horan, T. N., The use of Dilantin in the treatment of epilepsy, *Ann. Intern. Med.*, 13: 787-793, 1939.

536. Janz, D. and Fuchs, U., Are anti-epileptic drugs harmful when given during pregnancy?, *German Med. Monthly*, 9: 20-22, 1964.

537. Andia, J., Westphal, M., Anthone, R., and Anthone, S., Severe, acute diphenylhydantoin intoxication treated with peritoneal lavage, *New York J. Med.*, 1861-1863, 1968.

538. Ayd, F. J., Jr., New uses for an old drug, *Intern. Drug Ther. Newsletter*, 2: 1-2, Jan., 1967.

539. Bakwin, R. M. and Bakwin, H., Psychologic aspects of pediatrics: epilepsy, *J. Pediat.*, 39: 766-784, 1951.

540. Bergman, H., Dilantin sodium in the control of a convulsive disorder during pregnancy, *Med. Rec.*, 155: 105-106, 1942.

541. Berlyne, N., Levene, M., and McGlashan, A., Megaloblastic anemia following anticonvulsants, *Brit. Med. J.*, 1: 1247-1248, 1955.

542. Benians, R. C. and Hunter, R. A., Megaloblastic anemia occurring during treatment of epilepsy with Phenytoin sodium, primidone and phenobarbitone, *J. Ment. Sci.*, 103: 606-609, 1957.

543. Braham, J., Pain in the face, *Brit. Med. J.*, 3: 316, 1968.

544. Burns, J. J., Cucinell, S. A., Koster, R., and Conney, A. H., Application of drug metabolism to drug toxicity studies, *Ann. N.Y. Acad. Sci.*, 123: 273-286, 1965.

545. Gray, W. D., Rauh, C. E. and Shanahan, R. W., The mechanism of the antagonistic action of reserpine on the anticonvulsant effect of inhibitors of carbonic anhydrase, *J. Pharm. Exp. Ther.*, 139: 350-360, 1963.

546. Eadie, M. J., Sutherland, J. M., and Tyrer, J. H., "Dilantin" overdosage, *Med. J. Aust.*, 2: 515, 1968.

547. Filkova, V., Hyperplastic gingivitis resulting from epilepsy treated with Phenytoin, *Deutsch Stomat.*, 18: 294-298, 1968.

548. Fitzpatrick, T. B., Diphenylhydantoin reaction, *Arch. Derm.*, 93: 766-767, 1966.

549. Hudgins, R. L. and Corbin, K. B., An uncommon seizure disorder: familial paroxysmal choreoathetosis, *Brain*, 89: 199-204, 1966.

550. Jonas, A. D., The emergence of epileptic equivalents in the era of tranquilizers, *Int. J. Neuropsychiat.*, 3: 40-45, 1967.

551. Kellaway, P., Crawley, J. W., and Kagawa, N., Paroxysmal pain and autonomic disturbances of cerebral origin: a specific electro-clinical syndrome, *Epilepsia*, 1: 466-483, 1959-1960.

552. Khoury, N. J., When alcoholics stop drinking, *Postgrad. Med.*, 43: 119-123, 1968.

553. Kutt, H., Haynes, J., and McDowell, F., Some causes of ineffectiveness of diphenylhydantoin, *Arch. Neurol.*, 14: 489-492, 1966.

554. Kutt, H., Winters, W., Scherman, R., and McDowell, F., Diphenylhydantoin and phenobarbital toxicity, *Arch. Neurol.*, 11: 649-656, 1964.

555. Kutt, H., Winters, W., Kokenge, R., and McDowell, F., Diphenylhydantoin metabolism, blood levels, and toxicity, *Arch. Neurol.*, 11: 642-648, 1964.

556. McCartan, W. and Carson, J., The use of sodium diphenylhydantoinate, *J. Ment. Sci.*, 85: 965-971, 1939.

557. Merritt, H. H. and Putnam, T. J., Sodium diphenylhydantoinate in the treatment of convulsive disorders, *JAMA*, 111: 1068-1073, 1938.

558. Nelson, D. A. and Ray, C. D., Respiratory arrest from seizure discharges in limbic system, *Arch. Neurol.*, 19: 199-207, 1968.

559. Olesen, O. V., The influence of disulfiram and calcium carbimide on the serum diphenylhydantoin, *Arch. Neurol.*, 16: 642-644, 1967.

560. Pasamanick, B., Anticonvulsant drug therapy of behavior problem children with abnormal electroencephalograms, *A.M.A. Arch. Neurol. Psychiat.*, 65: 752-766, 1951.

561. Pisciotta, A. V., Penalties of progress—Drug-induced hematologic disease, *Postgrad. Med.*, 43: 213-219, 1968.

562. Rail, L., "Dilantin" overdosage, *Med. J. Aust.*, 2: 339, 1968.

563. Rawson, M. D., Diphenylhydantoin intoxication and cerebrospinal fluid protein. *Neurology*, 18: 1009-1011, 1968.

564. Schubert, H. A. and Malooly, D. A., Convulsive equivalent states, *A.M.A. Arch. Intern. Med.*, 104: 585-588, 1959.

565. Tenckhoff, H., Sherrard, D. J., Hickman, R. O., and Ladda, R. L., Acute diphenylhydantoin intoxication, *Amer. J. Dis. Child.*, 116: 422-425, 1968.

566. Voigt, G. C., Death following intravenous sodium diphenylhydantoin (Dilantin), *Johns Hopkins Med. J.*, 123: 153-157, 1968.

567. Weaver, L. C., Swinyard, E. A., and Goodman, L. S., Anticonvulsant drug combinations: diphenylhydantoin combined with other antiepileptics, *J. Amer. Pharm. Assn.*, 47: 645-648, 1958.

568. Snyder, C. H., Syndrome of Dilantin intoxication without Dilantin, *Southern Med. J.*, 57: 1482, 1964.

569. Roseman, E. and Klein, L. J., Epilepsy—facts and fancy, *GP*, 35: 144-152, 1967.

570. Landy, P. J., Lucas, B. G., and Toakley, J. G., "Dilantin" overdosage, *Med. J. Aust.*, 2: 639-640, 1968.

571. Chafetz, M. E., Alcohol withdrawal and seizures, *JAMA*, 200: 195-196, 1967.

572. Editor, Cardiac arrhythmias and sodium diphenylhydantoin—an appraisal, *JAMA*, 201: 142-143, 1967.

573. Bonnycastle, D. D., Bonnycastle, M. F., and Anderson, E. G., The effect of a number of central depressant drugs upon brain 5-hydroxytryptamine levels in the rat, *J. Pharm. Exp. Ther.*, 135: 17-20, 1962.

574. Garrettson, L. K., Perel, J. M., and Dayton, P. G., Methylphenidate interaction with both anticonvulsants and ethyl biscoumacetate a new action of methylphenidate, *JAMA*, 207: 2053-2056, 1969.

575. Bonnycastle, D. D., Paasonen, M. K., and Giarman, N. J., Diphenylhydantoin and brain-levels of 5-hydroxytryptamine, *Nature*, 178: 990-991, 1956.

576. Lynk, S. M. and Amidon, E., Chemotherapy with delinquents, *Mich. Med.*, 762-766, Oct., 1965.

577. Gangloff, H. and Monnier, M., The action of anticonvulsant drugs tested by electrical stimulation of the cortex, diencephalon and rhinencephalon in the unanesthetized rabbit, *Electroenceph. Clin. Neurophysiol.*, 9: 43-58, 1957.

578. Riley, H. D., Jr., Harris, R. L., and Nunnery, A. W., The pediatric pharmacology unit of the Children's Memorial Hospital: studies in neonatal pharmacology, *Okla. State Med. Assn. J.*, 61: 400-410, 1968.

579. Fromm, G. H. and Landgren, S., Effect of diphenylhydantoin on single cells in the spinal trigeminal nucleus, *Neurology*, 13: 34-37, 1963.

580. Franz, D. N. and Esplin, D. W., Prevention by diphenylhydantoin of post-tetanic enhancement of action potentials in nonmyelinated nerve fibers, *Pharmacologist*, 7: 174, 1965.

581. Fink, G. B. and Swinyard, E. A., Modification of maximal audiogenic and electro-shock seizures in mice by psychopharmacologic drugs, *J. Pharm. Exp. Ther.*, 127: 318-324, 1959.

582. Esplin, D. W., Criteria for assessing effects of depressant drugs on spinal cord synaptic transmission, with examples of drug selectivity, *Arch. Int. Pharmacodyn.*, 143: 479-497, 1963.

583. Kong, Y., Heyman, A., Entman, M. L., and McIntosh, H. D., Glossopharyngeal neuralgia associated with bradycardia, syncope, and seizures, *Circulation*, 30: 109-113, 1964.

584. Fromm, G. H. and Killian, J. M., Effect of some anticonvulsant drugs on the spinal trigeminal nucleus, *Neurology*, 17: 275-280, 1967.

585. Haward, L. R. C., Drugs and concentration: cognitive effect of DPH, *Portsmouth J. Psychol.*, 1: 3-5, 1968.

586. Editor, Spasticity in multiple sclerosis, *Brit. Med. J.*, 3: 174, 1968.

587. Michael, M. I. and Williams, J. M., Migraine in children, *J. Pediat.*, 41: 18-24, 1952.

588. Muniz, F. J., Lynch, J., and Nusyowitz, M. L., Diphenylhydantoin (Dilantin) induced chromosomal abnormalities, *Clin. Res.*, 16: 310, 1968.

589. Perez del Cerro, M. and Snider, R. S., Studies on Dilantin intoxication. I. Ultrastructural analogies with the lipidoses, *Neurology*, 17: 452-466, 1967.

590. Russell, M. A. and Bousvaros, G., Fatal results from diphenylhydantoin administered intravenously, *JAMA*, 206: 2118-2119, 1968.

591. Schwartzman, J., McDonald, D. H., and Perillo, L., Sydenham's chorea, *Arch. Pediat.*, 65: 6-24, 1948.

592. Stein, E. and Kleinfeld, M., Effects of diphenylhydantoin on membrane potentials of Purkinje and ventricular muscle fibers in dog heart, *Bull. N.Y. Acad. Med.*, 45: 110, 1969.

593. Geever, E. F., Seifter, E. and Levenson, S. M., Toxicity of diphenylhydantoin and its effect on wound healing in young guinea pigs, *Toxic. Appl. Pharmacol.*, 11: 272-279, 1967.

594. Bashour, F. A., Petty, L. D., and Stephens, C. R., Value of Dilantin prophylaxis in epinephrine induced ventricular arrhythmias in the anesthetized dog, *Clin. Res.*, 17: 14, 1969.

595. Muniz, F., Houston, E., Schneider, R., and Nusyowitz, M., Chromosomal effects of diphenylhydantoins, *Clin. Res.*, 17: 28, 1969.

596. Nichols, R. E. and Walaszek, E. J., Antagonism of drug induced catatonia, *Fed. Proc.*, 24: 390, 1965.

597. Bigger, T. J., Jr., Schmidt, D. H., and Kutt, H., Relationship between the plasma level of diphenylhydantoin sodium and its cardiac antiarrhythmic effects, *Circulation*, 38: 363-374, 1968.

598. Gydesen, C. S. and Gydesen, F. R., Post micturition syndrome, *Rocky Mountain Med. J.*, 60: 35-36, 1963.

599. McNichol, R. W., Cirksena, W. J., Payne, J. T., and Glasgow, M. C., Management of withdrawal from alcohol (including delirium tremens), *Southern Med. J.*, 60: 7-12, 1967.

600. Pearce, K. I., Drug treatment of emotional disorders in general practice psychiatry, *J. Coll. Gen. Prac. Canad.*, 12: 28-32, 1965.

601. Moss-Herjanic, B., Prolonged unconsciousness following electroconvulsive therapy, *Amer. J. Psychiat.*, 124: 112-114, 1967.

602. Gordon, P. and Scheving, L. E., Covariant 24-hour rhythms for acquisition and retention of avoidance learning and brain protein synthesis in rats, *Fed. Proc.*, 27: 223, 1968.

603. Wilson, W. P. and Wolk, M., The treatment of delirium tremens, *N. Carolina Med. J.*, 26: 552-556, 1965.

604. Swinyard, E. A., Smith, D. L., and Goodman, L. S., Analgesic effects of clinically useful antiepileptics, *J. Amer. Pharm. Assn.*, 43: 212-214, 1954.

605. Ende, M., Diphenylhydantoin in tic douloureux and atypical facial pain, *Virginia Med. Monthly*, 84: 358-359, 1957.

606. Bird, A. V., Anticonvulsant drugs and congenital abnormalities, *Lancet*, 1: 311, 1969.

607. Gertenrich, R. L., Fry, A. E., and Hart, R. W., The effects of Mucoplex therapy and oral hygiene on Dilantin gingival hyperplasia, *Amer. J. Ment. Defic.*, 73: 896-902, 1969.

608. Hauser, H. M. and Brewer, E. J., Death?, *Electroenceph. Clin. Neurophysiol.*, 23: 293, 1967.

609. Sabih, K. and Sabih, K., Chromatographic method for

determination of diphenylhydantoin blood level, *Anal. Chem.*, 41: 1452-1454, 1969.

610. Schwartz, R. S., and Costea, N., Autoimmune hemolytic anemia: clinical correlations and biological implications, *Sem. Hemat.*, 3: 2-26, 1966.

611. Reeve, H. S., Phenytoin in the treatment of trigeminal neuralgia, *Lancet*, 1: 404, 1961.

612. Babcock, J. R., Incidence of gingival hyperplasia associated with Dilantin therapy in a hospital population, *J. Amer. Dent. Assn.*, 71: 1447-1450, 1965.

613. Badenoch, J., The use of labelled vitamin B$_{12}$ and gastric biopsy in the investigation of anemia, *Proc. Roy. Soc. Med.*, 47: 426-431, 1954.

614. Bailey, G., Rosenbaum, J. M., and Anderson, B., Toxic epidermal necrolysis, *JAMA*, 191: 979-982, 1965.

615. Bajoghli, M., Generalized lymphadenopathy and hepatosplenomegaly induced by diphenylhydantoin, *Pediatrics*, 28: 943-945, 1961.

616. Baldi, A., Suicide through poisoning with diphenylhydantoin, *Minerva Medicoleg.*, 74: 161-163, 1954.

617. Bernhardt, H., Fatal granulocytopenia following hydantoins—Mesantoin and Dilantin: report of a case, *J. Med. Assn. Alabama*, 19: 193-197, 1950.

618. Bihler, I., The sodium pump and regulation of sugar transport in skeletal muscle, *Pharmacologist*, 10: 198, 1968.

619. Billen, J. R., Griffin, J. W., and Waldron, C. A., Investigations for pyronin bodies and fluorescent antibodies in 5,5-diphenylhydantoin gingival hyperplasia, *Oral Surg.*, 18: 773-782, 1964.

620. Bonard, E. C., Pseudocollagenosis or malignant pseudolymphoma, *Schweiz. Med. Wschr.*, 94: 57-59, 1964.

621. Burton, R. C., Symptomatology—organic or psychogenic?, *New York J. Med.*, 1304-1309, June 1, 1966.

622. Livingston, S., Seizures in a hypertensive patient, *JAMA*, 204: 412, 1968.

623. Livingston, S., Diphenylhydantoin in emotional disorders, *JAMA*, 204: 549, 1968.

624. Corday, E. and Vyden, J. K., Resuscitation after myocardial infarction, *JAMA*, 200: 781-784, 1967.

625. Cotten, M. S. and Lane, D. H., Massive strychnine poisoning: a successful treatment, *J. Mississippi Med. Assn.*, 7: 466-468, 1966.

626. Cucinell, S. A., Conney, A. H., Sansur, M., and Burns, J. J., Drug interactions in man. 1. Lowering effect of phenobarbital on plasma levels of bishydroxycoumarin (Dicumarol) and diphenylhydantoin (Dilantin), *Clin. Pharmacol. Ther.*, 6: 420-429, 1965.

627. Davis, R. K., Baer, P. N., and Palmer, J. H., A preliminary report on a new therapy for Dilantin gingival hyperplasia, *J. Periodont.*, 34: 17-22, 1963.

628. Ellis, F. A., Reactions to Nirvanol, Phenytoin sodium, and phenobarbital, *Southern Med. J.*, 36: 575-599, 1947.

629. Francis, L. E. and Melville, K. I., Effects of diphenylhydantoin on gingival histamine and serotonin, *J. Canad. Dent. Assn.*, 25: 608-620, 1959.

630. Fulop, M., Widrow, D. R., Colmers, R. A., and Epstein, E. J., Possible diphenylhydantoin-induced arrhythmia in hypothyroidism, *JAMA*, 196: 454-456, 1966.

631. Gabler, W. L., The effect of 5,5-diphenylhydantoin on the rat uterus and its fetuses, *Arch. Int. Pharmacodyn.*, 175: 141-152, 1968.

632. Gams, R. A., Neal, J. A., and Conrad, F. G., Hydantoin-induced pseudo-pseudolymphoma, *Ann. Intern. Med.*, 69: 557-568, 1968.

633. Gardner-Medwin, D. and Walton, J. N., Myokymia with impaired muscular relaxation, *Lancet*, 1: 127-130, 1969.

634. Gianni, E. and Bracchetti, A., Pathogenesis of gingival hypertrophy caused by diphenylhydantoin in experimental animals, *Minèrva Stomat.*, 17: 609-612, 1968.

635. Gibson, J. E. and Becker, B. A., Teratogenic effects of diphenylhydantoin in Swiss-Webster and A/J mice, *Proc. Soc. Exp. Biol. Med.*, 128: 905-909, 1968.

636. Girdwood, R. H., Folic acid, *Practitioner*, 199: 368-376, 1967.

637. Goldstein, L. J. and Verrastro, R., Meniere's disease twenty years later, *Eye, Ear, Nose & Throat Monthly*, 46: 746-752, 1967.

638. Hamfelt, A. and Wilmanns, W., Inhibition studies on folic acid metabolism with drugs suspected to act on the myeloproliferative system, *Clin. Chim. Acta*, 12: 144-154, 1965.

639. Hansen, J. M., Kristensen, M., and Skovsted, L., Sulthiame (Ospolot) as inhibitor of diphenylhydantoin metabolism, *Epilepsia*, 9: 17-22, 1968.

640. Hoffbrand, A. V. and Necheles, T. F., Studies on the mechanism of megaloblastic anemia due to anticonvulsants, *Abs. XII Cong. Int. Soc. Hematol.*, 92, New York, 1968.

641. Hoffbrand, A. V. and Necheles, T. F., Mechanism of folate deficiency in patients receiving Phenytoin, *Lancet*, 2: 528-530, 1968.

642. Hunninghake, D. B. and Azarnoff, D. L., Drug interactions with warfarin, *Arch. Intern. Med.*, 121: 349-352, 1968.

643. Hyman, G. A. and Sommers, S. C., The development of Hodgkin's disease and lymphoma during anticonvulsant therapy, *Blood*, 28: 417-427, 1966.

644. Jubiz, W., Meikle, W., West, C. D., and Tyler, F. H., Failure of dexamethasone suppression in patients on chronic diphenylhydantoin therapy, *Clin. Res.*, 17: 106, 1969.

645. Kemp, J. W. and Woodbury, D. M., The influence of diphenylhydantoin on cerebrospinal fluid electrolytes, *Pharmacologist*, 8: 199, 1966.

646. Kiørboe, E., Antabuse as a source of Phenytoin intoxication, *Ugeskr. Laeg.*, 128: 1531-1532, 1966.

647. Kokenge, R., Kutt, H., and McDowell, F., Neurological sequelae following Dilantin overdose in a patient and in experimental animals, *Neurology*, 15: 823-829, 1965.

648. Kruse, R., Rare, but dangerous, hydantoin side effects, *Mschr. Kinderheilk.*, 115: 289-290, 1967.

649. Malpas, J. S., Spray, G. H., and Witts, L. J., Serum folic-acid and vitamin-B$_{12}$ levels in anticonvulsant therapy, *Brit. Med. J.*, 1: 955-957, 1966.

650. Martin, D. A., The therapeutic and toxic effects of tranquilizing drugs: medical aspects, *N. Carolina Med. J.*, 17: 396-401, 1956.

651. Kanzler, M., Malitz, S., and Higgins, J. C., How effective are antidepressants?, *JAMA*, 204: 34, 1968.

652. Merritt, H. H. and Putnam, T. J., Further experiences with the use of sodium diphenylhydantoinate in the treatment of convulsive disorders, *Amer. J. Psychiat.*, 96: 1023-1027, 1940.

653. O'Quinn, S. E., The use of the indirect basophil degranulation test in the investigation of drug allergy, *Southern Med. J.*, 58: 1147-1151, 1965.

654. Patil, K. P., Chitre, R. G., and Sheth, U. K., Anti-folic acid activity of antiepileptic drugs. Part 2—Experimental studies in rats, *Indian J. Med. Sci.*, 20: 623-627, 1966.

655. Plaa, G. L. and Hine, C. H., Hydantoin and barbiturate blood levels observed in epileptics, *Arch. Int. Pharmacodyn.*, 128: 375-382, 1960.

656. Ritchie, E. B. and Kolb, W., Reaction to sodium diphenylhydantoinate (Dilantin sodium) hemorrhagic erythema multiforme terminating fatally, *Arch. Derm. Syph.*, 46: 856-859, 1942.

657. Rosenberg, I. H., Godwin, H. A., Strieff, R. R., and Castle, W. B., Impairment of intestinal deconjugation of dietary folate: a possible explanation of megaloblastic anemia associated with Phenytoin therapy, *Lancet*, 2: 530-532, 1968.

658. Rümke, C. L., Increased susceptibility of mice to seizures after some anticonvulsant drugs, *Europ. J. Pharmacol.*, 1: 369-377, 1967.

659. Rummel, W., and Wellensiek, H. J., Premedication and

nitrous oxide anesthesia, *Arch. Int. Pharmacodyn.*, 122: 339-349, 1959.

660. Sauter, E. K., Diphenylhydantoin toxicity in children, *Arch. Kinderheilk,,* 146: 64-70, 1953.

661. Scherf, D., Changes in the electrocardiogram after intravenous administration of Phenytoin sodium (Dilantin) in the acute experiment, *Bull. N.Y. Med. Coll.*, 6: 82-89, 1943.

662. Slavin, R. G. and Broun, G. O. Jr., Agranulocytosis after diphenylhydantoin and chlorothiazide therapy, *Arch. Intern. Med.*, 108: 940-944, 1961.

663. Snider, R. S. and del Cerro, M., Membranous cytoplasmic spirals in Dilantin intoxication. *Nature*, 212: 536-537, 1966.

664. Steinberg, S. H., Reaction to diphenylhydantoin sodium: report of a case simulating Rocky Mountain spotted fever and review of literature, *Med. Ann. D.C.*, 22: 600-603, 1953.

665. Svensmark, O. and Buchthal, F., Dosage of Phenytoin and phenobarbital in children, *Danish Med. Bull.*, 10: 234-235, 1963.

666. Svensmark, O. and Buchthal, F., Diphenylhydantoin and phenobarbital: serum levels in children, *Amer. J. Dis. Child.*, 108, 82-87, 1964.

667. Szymanski, F. J., and McGrae, J. D., Jr., Fibrous hyperplasia of the nose, possibly related to diphenylhydantoin sodium (Dilantin) therapy, *Arch. Derm.*, 88: 227-228, 1963.

668. Tanimukai, H., Tsukiyama, H., Yamamoto, M., and Yamada, R., A case with Hodgkin's disease-like syndrome induced by diphenylhydantoin, *Brain Nerve*, 15: 77-83, 1963.

669. Strean, L. P., Treatment of ulcers, *Chem. Abst. Biochem. Sec.*, 65: 11219c, 1966 (Merck & Co., Inc. Application for patent, Belg., May 12, 1965).

670. Block, J. D. and Moore, A. U., Hyperresponsive extinction behavior of protein-deprived pigs reduced by diphenylhydantoin *(in press)*.

671. Turner, P., Granulocytopenia after treatment with Phenytoin sodium, *Brit. Med. J.*, 1: 1790, 1960.

672. DaVanzo, J. P., Daugherty, M., Ruckart, R., and Kang, L., Pharmacological and biochemical studies in isolation-induced fighting mice, *Psychopharmacologia*, 9: 210-219, 1966.

673. Jonas, A. D., More experience with diphenylhydantoin, *Amer. J. Psychiatr.*, 124: 1139, 1968.

674. Vernadakis, A. and Woodbury, D. M., Effects of diphenylhydantoin on electroshock seizure thresholds in developing rats, *J. Pharm. Exp. Ther.*, 148: 144-150, 1965.

675. Waites, L. and Nicklas, T. O., Diphenylhydantoin sodium (Dilantin) intoxication in children, *J. Okla. Med. Assn.*, 54: 95-96, 1961.

676. Wallis, W., Kutt, H., and McDowell, F., Intravenous diphenylhydantoin in treatment of acute repetitive seizures, *Neurology*, 18: 513-525, 1968.

677. Watanabe, S., Hypersensitivity angiitis from diphenylhydantoin, *Acta Derm.*, (Kyoto), 59: 121-129, 1964.

678. Webster, J. M., Megaloblastic anemia due to Phenytoin sodium, *Lancet*, 2: 1017-1018, 1954.

679. Weintraub, M., Neonatal hypocalcemia, Correspondence, *New Eng. J. Med.*, 279: 327, 1968.

680. Welch, B. L., Symposium on aggressive behavior, *BioScience*, 18: 1061-1064, 1968.

681. Wilkinson, T., Megaloblastic anemia during antiepileptic therapy, *Med. J. Aust.*, 2: 894, 1959.

682. Levy, L. L. and Fenichel, G. M., Diphenylhydantoin activated seizures, *Neurology*, 15: 716-722, 1965.

683. Yen, H. C. Y., Silverman, A. J., and Salvatore, A., Iproniazid reinforcement of anticonvulsants, *Fed. Proc.*, 19: 181, 1960.

684. Holland, P. and Mauer, A. M., Drug-induced *in vitro* stimulation of peripheral lymphocytes, *Lancet*, 1: 1368-1369, 1964.

685. Helfant, R., Scherlag, B., and Damato, A. N., Protection from digitalis toxicity with prophylactic Dilantin: an electrophysiological-inotropic dissociation, *Clin. Res.*, 15: 206, 1967.

686. Johnson, J., Anticonvulsants and megaloblastic anemia, *J. Ment. Sci.*, 105: 819-820, 1959.

687. Keeran, M., Cardiac arrest following intravenous administration of diphenylhydantoin, *J. Okla. Med. Assn.*, 60: 334-335, 1967.

688. Klein, J. P., Diphenylhydantoin intoxication associated with hyperglycemia, *J. Pediat.*, 69: 463-465, 1966.

689. Klipstein, F. A., Folate deficiency secondary to disease of the intestinal tract, *Bull. N.Y. Acad. Med.*, 42: 638-653, 1966.

690. Krasznai, G. and Gyory, G., Hydantoin lymphadenopathy, *J. Path. Bact.*, 95: 314-317, 1968.

691. Levine, M. C., Lupus erythematosus and anticonvulsant drugs, *Pediatrics*, 33: 144-145, 1964.

692. Matthews, D. M. and Reynolds, E. H., Gastrointestinal function in anticonvulsant megaloblastic anemia, *Lancet*, 1: 210-211, 1966.

693. Jonas, A. D., The distinction between paroxysmal and non-paroxysmal migraine, *Headache*, 79-84, July, 1967.

694. Lucas, B. G., Dilantin overdosage, *Med. J. Aust.*, 2: 639-640, 1968.

695. Toakley, J. G., Dilantin overdosage, *Med. J. Aust.*, 2: 640, 1968.

696. Arushanyan, E. B. and Belozertsev, Y. A., Effects of diphenylhydantoin on different type of central inhibition of the knee-jerk reflex, *Farmakol. Tosik.*, 29: 12-17, 1966.

697. Haward, L. R. C., Differential modifications of verbal aggression by psychotropic drugs, *Proc. Symp. Aggressive Behavior*, Milan, May, 1968, 317-321, S. Garattini and E. B. Sigg, Eds., *Excerpta Medica*, New York, 1969.

698. Swinyard, E. A., Weaver, L. C., and Goodman, L. S., Effect of liver injury and nephrectomy on the anticonvulsant activity of clinically useful hydantoins, *J. Pharm. Exp. Ther.*, 104: 309-316, 1952.

699. Pincus, J. H., Grove, I., Marino, B. B., and Glaser, G. E., Studies on the mechanism of action of diphenylhydantoin, *Arch. Neurol.*, 22: 566-571, 1970.

700. Stephens, J. H. and Shaffer, J. W., A controlled study of the effects of diphenylhydantoin on anxiety, irritability, and anger in neurotic outpatients, *Psychopharmacologia*, 17: 169-181, 1970.

701. Davies, J. E., Edmundson, W. F., Carter, C. H., and Barquet, A., Effect of anticonvulsant drugs on dicophane (D.D.T.) residues in man, *Lancet*, 2: 7-9, 1969.

702. Doty, B. and Dalman, R., Diphenylhydantoin effects on avoidance conditioning as a function of age and problem difficulty, *Psychos. Sci.*, 14: 109-111, 1969.

703. Goodman, L. S. and Gilman, A., *The Pharmacological Basis of Therapeutics*, 2nd Ed., 181-188, Macmillan, New York, 1955.

704. Resnick, O. and Dreyfus, J. J., Jr., Worcester County Jail study: Beneficial effects of DPH on the nervous systems of nonepileptics (condensed), *Dreyfus Medical Foundation*, 1966.

705. Gottwald, W., An outline of the hydantoins, Synopsis der Hydantoine (German), *Fortschritte der Neurologie, Psychiatrie und ihrer Grenzgebiete*, 37: 573-648, 1969.

706. Baldwin, R. W., Behavior disorders in children, *Maryland Med. J.*, 18: 68-71, 1969.

707. Dreyfus, J. J. Jr., The beneficial effects of diphenylhydantoin on the nervous systems of nonepileptics—as experienced and observed in others by a layman. Presented at the Amer. College of Neuropsychopharmacology, Dec. 7, 1966, *Dreyfus Medical Foundation*, 1966.

708. Rosenblum, J. A. and Shafer, N., Effects of diphenylhydantoin (Dilantin) withdrawal on non-epileptics: preliminary report, *Curr. Ther. Res.*, 12: 31-33, 1970.

709. Haward, L. R. C., The organic integrity test as prognostic index in Phenytoin-facilitated autogenic training, *World J. of Psychosynthesis*, 1: 47-51, 1969.

710. Weintraub, M. I., Megahed, M. S., and Smith, B. H., Myotonic-like syndrome in multiple sclerosis, *New York J. Med.*, 70: 677-679, 1970.

711. Bianchine, J. R., Macaraeg, P. V. J., Jr., Lasagna, L., Azarnoff, D. L., Brunk, S. F., Hvidberg, E. F., and Owen, J. A., Jr., Drugs as etiologic factors in the Stevens-Johnson syndrome, *Amer. J. Med.*, 44: 390-405, 1968.

712. Council on Drugs, American Medical Association Drug Evaluations, *JAMA*, 204, 702-710, 1968.

713. Goldberg, J. and Kurland, A. A., Dilantin treatment of hospitalized cultural-familial retardates, *J. Nerv. Ment. Dis.*, 150: 133-137, 1970.

714. Pincus, J. H., Diphenylhydantoin and sodium influx, *Neurology*, 20: 393, 1970.

715. Silbermann, M., *Personal communication*, 1969.

716. Silverman, D., The electroencephalograph and therapy of criminal psychopaths, *Criminal Psychopathology*, 5: 439-457, 1944.

717. Forda, O. and McIlwain, H., Anticonvulsants on electrically stimulated metabolism of separated mammalian cerebral cortex, *Brit. J. Pharmacol.*, 8: 225-229, 1953.

718. Williams, J. and Stevens, H., Familial paroxysmal chorea-athetosis, *Pediatrics*, 31: 656-659, 1963.

719. Capapas, L., Weiss, M. M., and Leight, L., The use of diphenylhydantoin sodium (Dilantin) in the treatment of cardiac arrhythmias, *J. Kentucky Med. Assn.*, 66: 970-975, 1968.

720. Helfant, R. H., Seuffert, G. W., Patton, R. D., Stein, E., and Damato, A. N., The clinical use of diphenylhydantoin (Dilantin) in the treatment and prevention of cardiac arrhythmias, *Amer. Heart J.*, 77: 315-323, 1969.

721. Gautam, H. P., Phenytoin in post-operative cardiac arrhythmias, *Brit. Heart J.*, 31: 641-644, 1969.

722. Delgado, J. M. R., Electrical stimulation of the brain, *Psychology Today*, 3: 49-53, 1970.

723. Rallison, M. L., Carlisle, J. W., Lee, R. E., Jr., Vernier, R. L., and Good, R. A., Lupus erythematosus and Stevens-Johnson syndrome, *Amer. J. Dis. Child.*, 101: 81-94, 1961.

724. Hess, W. R., Interdisciplinary discussion of selected problems with reference to "The Biology of Mind," *Perspect. Biol. Med.*, 13: 267-293, 1970.

725. Broad range of beneficial effects of diphenylhydantoin: one hundred letters, *Dreyfus Medical Foundation*, 1970.

726. Schmidt, R. P. and Wilder, B. J., *Epilepsy: A clinical textbook*, F. A. Davis Co., Phila., 150-153, 1968.

727. Vanasin, B., Bass, D. D., Mendeloff, A. I., and Schuster, M. M., Effect and site of action of diphenylhydantoin (DPH) on gastrointestinal smooth muscle, *Clin. Res.*, 18: 391, 1970.

728. Crane, P. and Swanson, P. D., Diphenylhydantoin and the cations and phosphates of electrically stimulated brain slices, *Neurology*, 20: 1119-1123, 1970.

729. Sokoloff, L., The action of drugs on the cerebral circulation, *Pharmacol. Rev.*, 11: 1-85, 1959.

730. Taylor, A. S., Behcet's syndrome treated with DPH, *Personal communication*, 1969.

731. Escueta, A. V. and Appel, S. H., The effects of electrically induced seizures on potassium transport within isolated nerve terminals, *Neurology*, 20: 392, 1970.

732. Barasch, K., Baras, I., and Galin, M. A., Early ambulation after cataract surgery, *Personal communication*, 1970.

733. Padis, N., Use of DPH to control low blood sugar, *Personal communication*, 1967.

734. Dreifus, L. S., Use of anti-arrhythmic agents other than digitalis, *J. Iowa Med. Soc.*, 60: 192-195, 1970.

735. Jensen, N. O. and Olesen, V. O., The clinical importance of folic acid in patients treated with anticonvulsant drugs, *Excerpta Medica*, 193: 260, 1969.

736. Anthony, J. J., Malignant lymphoma associated with hydantoin drugs, *Arch. Neurol.*, 22: 450-454, 1970.

737. Meadow, S. R., Congenital abnormalities and anticonvulsant drugs, *Proc. Roy. Soc. Med.*, 63: 12-13, 1970.

738. Eisenberg, H., Campbell, P. C., and Flannery, J. T., *Cancer in Connecticut. Incidence characteristics*, 1935-1962, Conn. State Dept. of Health, Hartford, Conn., 1967.

739. Hutchins, D. A. and Rogers, K. J., Physiological and drug-induced changes in the glycogen content of mouse brain, *Brit. J. Pharmacol.*, 39: 9-25, 1970.

740. Chen, G. and Bohner, B., A study of certain CNS depressants, *Arch. Int. Pharmacodyn.*, 125: 1-20, 1960.

741. Millichap, J. G., Egan, R. W., Hart, Z. H., and Sturgis, L. H., Auditory perceptual deficit correlated with EEG dysrhythmias response to diphenylhydantoin sodium, *Neurology*, 19: 870-872, 1969.

742. Covi, L., Derogatis, L. R., Uhlenhuth, E. H., and Kandel, A., Effect of diphenylhydantoin in violent prisoners, *Proc. 7th Cong. of the Int. College of Neuropsychopharmacol.*, Prague, 1970.

743. Cole, J. O., Psychopharmacology: The picture is not entirely rosy, *Amer. J. Psychiat.*, 127: 224-225, 1970.

744. Chamberlain, W., Use of diphenylhydantoin in surgery, *Personal communication*, 1970.

745. Eccles, J. C., The synapse, *Scientific Am.*, 212: 56-66, 1965.

746. Galin, M. A., Kwitko, M., and Restrepo, N., The use of diphenylhydantoin in the treatment of accommodative esotropia, *Proc. Int. Strabismological Assn.*, In *Proc. Int. Ophthalmological Congress*, Mexico, 1969.

747. Jaffe, N. S., Use of diphenylhydantoin in ophthalmic surgery, *Personal communication*, 1966.

748. Wilson, P. *Medical News-Letter*, *Brit. Migraine Assn.*, Bournemouth, England, August, 1970.

749. Tedeschi, R. E., Tedeschi, D. H., Mucha, A., Cook, L., Mattis, P. A., and Fellows, E. J., Effects of various centrally acting drugs on fighting behavior of mice, *J. Pharmacol. and Exp. Therap.* 125: 28-34, 1959.

750. Alvarez, W. C., Enuresis, *Modern Medicine* (Editorial), 95-96, June, 1969.

751. Adamska-Dyniewska, H., Evaluation of myocardial contractility after hydantoinal and ouabain based polycardiographic methods, *Wiad. Lek.*, 23: 1749-1754, 1970.

752. Adamska-Dyniewska, H., Hydantoinal—New use of an old drug, *Wiad. Lek.*, 23: 1111-1115, 1970.

753. Adamska-Dyniewska, H., The effect of diphenylhydantoin sodium given with cardiac glycosides on the left ventricular systole dynamics, *Pol. Med. J.*, 9: 304-308, 1970.

754. Adamska-Dyniewska, H., The value of diphenylhydantoin for combating the rhythm and conduction disorders induced by cardiac glycosides, *Biul. Wojskowej. Akad. Medy.*, 14: 71-77, 1971.

755. Agarwal, S. P. and Blake, M. I., Differentiating spectrophotometric titration of phenobarbital-diphenylhydantoin combinations in nonaqueous medium, *Anal. Chem.*, 41: 1104-1106, 1969.

756. Alarcon-Segovia, D., Fishbein, E., Reyes, P. A., Dies, H., and Shwadsky, S., Antinuclear antibodies in patients on anticonvulsant therapy, *Clin. Exp. Immunol.*, 12: 39-47, 1972.

757. Alexander, E., Medical management of closed head injuries, *Clin. Neurosurg.*, 19: 240-250, 1972.

758. Alexander, E., Surgical management of head injuries in children in the acute phase, *Clin. Neurosurg.*, 19: 251-262, 1972.

759. Allen, C. D. and Klipstein, F. A., Brain folate concentration in folate-deficient rats receiving diphenylhydantoin, *Neurology*, 20: 403, 1970.

760. Allen, J. D., Kofi Ekue, J. M., Shanks, R. G., and Zaidi, S. A., The effect on experimental cardiac arrhythmias of a new anticonvulsant agent, Ko 1173 and its comparison with phenytoin and procainamide, *Brit. J. Pharmacol.*, 39: 183-184, 1970.

761. Alvarez, W. C., *Nerves in collision*, Pyramid House, New York, 1972.

762. American Medical Association Council on Drugs, *AMA drug evaluations*, 12-13 AMA, Chicago, 1971.

763. American Pharmaceutical Association, *Evaluations of drug interactions*, Washington, 1973.

764. Anderson, D. C., Davis, R. J., Dove, J. T., and Griggs, R. C., Cardiac conduction during treatment of myotonia, *Neurology*, 23: 390, 1973.

765. Anderson, R. J. and Raines, A., Suppression by Diphenylhydantoin of afferent discharges arising in muscle spindles of the triceps surae of the cat, *J. Pharmacol. Exp. Ther.*, 191: 290-299, 1974.

766. Anders, M. W. and Latorre, J. P., High-speed ion exchange chromatography of barbiturates, diphenylhydantoin, and their hydroxylated metabolites, *Anal. Chem.*, 42: 1430-1432, 1970.

767. Andreasen, B., Froland, A., Skovsted, L., Andersen, S. A., and Hauge, M., Diphenylhydantoin half-life in man and its inhibition by phenylbutazone: the role of genetic factors, *Acta Med. Scand.*, 193: 561-564, 1973.

768. Andreasen, P. B., Hansen, J. M., Skovsted, L., and Siersbaek-Nielsen, K., Folic acid and the half-life of diphenylhydantoin in man, *Acta Neurol. Scand.*, 47: 117-119, 1971.

769. Andreasen, P. B., Hansen, J. M., Skovsted, L., and Siersbaek-Nielsen, K., Folic acid and phenytoin metabolism, *Epilepsy Abstracts*, 4: 221, 1971.

770. Andreasen, P. B., Lyngbye, J., and Trolle, E., Tests for abnormalities in liver function during long-term diphenylhydantoin therapy in epileptic out-patients. *Acta Med. Scand.*, 194: 261-264, 1973.

771. Ariyoshi, T. and Takabatake, E., Effect of diphenylhydantoin on the drug metabolism and the fatty acid composition of phospholipids in hepatic microsomes, *Chem. Pharm. Bull.*, 20: 180-184, 1972.

772. Ariyoshi, T., Zange, M., and Remmer, H., Effects of diphenylhydantoin on the liver constituents and the microsomal drug metabolism enzyme systems in the partially hepatectomized rats, *J. Pharm. Soc. Jap.*, 94: 526-530, 1974.

773. Arky, R. A., Diphenylhydantoin and the beta cell, *New Eng. J. Med.*, 286: 371-372, 1972.

774. Arnold, K. and Gerber, N., The rate of decline of diphenylhydantoin in human plasma, *Clin. Pharmacol. Ther.*, 11: 121-134, 1970.

775. Arnold, K., Gerber, N., and Levy, G., Absorption and dissolution studies on sodium diphenylhydantoin capsules, *Canad. J. Pharm. Sci.*, 5: 89-92, 1970.

776. Asfeldt, V. H. and Buhl, J., Inhibitory effect of diphenylhydantoin on the feedback control of corticotrophin release, *Acta Endocrinol.*, 61: 551-560, 1969.

777. Atkinson, A. J., Jr., Clinical use of blood levels of cardiac drugs, *Mod. Conc. Cardiovasc. Dis.*, 42: 1-4, 1973.

778. Atkinson, A. J., Jr., Individualization of anticonvulsant therapy, *Med. Clin. N. Amer.*, 58: 1037-1050, 1974.

779. Atkinson, A. J., Jr., MacGee, J., Strong, J., Garteiz, D., and Gaffney, T. E., Identification of 5-metahydroxyphenyl-5-phenylhydantoin as a metabolite of diphenylhydantoin, *Biochem. Pharmacol.*, 19: 2483-2491, 1970.

780. Atkinson, A. J., Jr. and Davison, R., Diphenylhydantoin as an antiarrhythmic drug, *Ann. Rev. Med.*, 25: 99-113, 1974.

781. Ausman, J. I., New developments in anticonvulsant therapy, *Postgrad. Med.*, 48: 122-127, 1970.

782. Ayala, G. F. and Lin, S., Effect of diphenylhydantoin on an isolated neuron, *Fed. Proc.*, 30: Abstract 67, 1971.

783. Azarnoff, D. L., Clinical implications of drug metabolism —introduction, *Chem. Biol. Interactions*, 3: 241-242, 1971.

784. Azzaro, A. J. and Gutrecht, J. A., The effect of diphenylhydantoin (DPH) on the *in vitro* accumulation and catabolism of H³-l-norepinephrine (H³-NE) in cerebral cortex slices, *Neurology*, 23: 431, 1973.

785. Azzaro, A. J., Gutrecht, J. A., and Smith, D. J., Effect of diphenylhydantoin on the uptake and catabolism of L-(3H) norepinephrine *in vitro* in rat cerebral cortex tissue, *Biochem. Pharmacol.*, 22: 2719-2729, 1973.

786. Babb, R. R. and Eckman, P. B., Abdominal epilepsy, *JAMA*, 222: 65-66, 1972.

787. Bach-Y-Rita, G., Lion, J. R., Climent, C. E., and Ervin, F. R., Episodic dyscontrol: A study of 130 violent patients, *Amer. J. Psychiat.*, 127: 49-54, 1971.

788. Baggot, J. D. and Davis, L. E., Comparative study of plasma protein binding of diphenylhydantoin, *Comp. Gen. Pharmacol.*, 4: 399-404, 1973.

789. Baker, T., Okamoto, M., and Riker, W. F., Diphenylhydantoin (DPH) suppression of motor nerve terminal (MNT) excitation by acetylcholine (ACh), *Pharmacologist*, 13: 265, 1971.

790. Baldy-Moulinier, M., Cerebral blood flow and membrane ionic pump, *Europ. Neurol.*, 6: 107-113, 1971/72.

791. Ballek, R. E., Reidenberg, M. M., and Orr, L., Inhibition of diphenylhydantoin metabolism by chloramphenicol, *Lancet*, 150, 1973.

792. Baratieri, A., Gagliardi, V., and Simonetti, E., Further studies on effect of diphenylhydantoin sodium on oro facial tissues in offspring of female mice, *Epilepsy Abstracts*, 6: 91, 1973.

793. Barbedo, A. S., and Banks, T., Paroxysmal supraventricular tachycardia, *New Eng. J. Med.*, 288: 51, 1973.

794. Barlow, C. F., Diphenylhydantoin-2-C¹⁴ in cat brain, *J. Neuropath. Exp. Neurol.*, 22: 348-349, 1965.

795. Baro, W. Z., The non-convulsive convulsive disorder— its diagnosis and treatment, *Western Med.*, March, 1966.

796. Barsky, P., A clinical variant of tic convulsif, *J. Pediat.*, 71: 417-419, 1967.

797. Bartter, F. C. and Schwartz, W. B., The syndrome of inappropriate secretion of antidiuretic hormone, *Amer. J. Med.*, 42: 790-806, 1967.

798. Bashour, F. A., Coffman, G. K., and Ashby, E. A., Effect of diphenylhydantoin (Dilantin) on oxygen uptake by Sarcina lutea, *Clin. Res.*, 14: 439, 1966.

799. Baskin, S. I. and Dutta, S., Effects of antiarrhythmic drugs and ethacrynic acid on the accumulation of ouabain-H by the isolated guinea pig heart, *Fed. Proc.*, 29: 739, 1970.

800. Baskin, S. I. and Dutta, S., Relationships between prevention of ouabain (O) induced arrhythmia by diphenylhydantoin (DPH) and potassium (K) and their effects on ouabain accumulation and electrolyte composition in the heart, *Fed. Proc.*, 30: 394, 1971.

801. Baskin, S. I., Dutta, S., and Marks, B. H., The effects of diphenylhydantoin and potassium on the biological activity of ouabain in the guinea-pig heart, *Brit. J. Pharmacol.*, 47: 85-96, 1973.

802. Baskin, S. I., Melrose, B. L., Ferguson, R. K., Akera, T., and Brody, T. M., The effect of diphenylhydantoin on ouabain-induced arrhythmia and on the formation and dissociation of the ouabain-enzyme complex, *Personal Communication*, 1973.

803. Bassett, A. L., Bigger, J. T., and Hoffman, B. F., Effect of diphenylhydantoin on cat heart muscle, *Circulation*, 35 & 36: 61, 1967.

804. Bassett, A. L., Bigger, J. T., and Hoffman, B. F., Protective action of DPH on canine Purkinje fibers during hypoxia, *J. Pharmacol. Exp. Ther.*, 173: 336-343, 1970.

805. BasuRay, B. N., Dutta, S. N., and Pradhan, S. N., Central action of ouabain: effects of propranolol and diphenylhydantoin on ouabain-induced arrhythmias, *Fed. Proc.*, 30: Abstract 189, 1971.

806. Baugh, C. M. and Krumdieck, C. L., Effects of phenytoin on folic-acid conjugases in man, *Lancet*, 519-522, 1969.

807. Baughmam, F. A. and Randinitis, E. J., Passage of diphenylhydantoin across the placenta, *JAMA*, 213: 466, 1970.

808. Baxter, M. G., Miller, A. A., and Webster, R. A., Some studies on the convulsant action of folic acid, *Brit. J. Pharmacol.*, 48: 350-351, 1973.

809. Baylis, E. M., Crowley, J. M., Preece, J. M., Sylvester, P. E., and Marks, V., Influence of folic acid on blood-phenytoin levels, *Lancet*, 1: 62-64, 1971.

810. Baylis, E. M., Fry, D. E., and Marks, V., Micro-determi-

nation of serum phenobarbitone and diphenylhydantoin by gas-liquid chromatography, *Clin. Chim. Acta*, 30: 93-103, 1970.

811. Bazin, S. and Delaunay, A., Effect of phenytoin on the maturation of collagen in normal skin and granulomatous tissue, *C. R. Acad. Sci. Ser. D.*, 275: 509-511, 1972.

812. Becker, B. and Podos, S. M., Diphenylhydantoin and its use in optic nerve disease, *Symposium on Ocular Therapy*, Vol. VI, I. H. Leopold, Ed., C. V. Mosby Co., St. Louis, 1973.

813. Becker, B., Stamper, R. L., Asseff, C., and Podos, S. M., Effect of diphenylhydantoin on glaucomatous field loss, *Trans. Amer. Acad. Ophthal. Otolaryng.*, 76: 412-422, 1972.

814. Beernink, D. H. and Miller, J. J., Anticonvulsant induced antinuclear antibodies and lupus like disease in children, *Epilepsy Abstracts*, 6: 210, 1973.

815. Bell, W. E. and McCormick, W. F., Striatopallidonigral degeneration, *Arch. Dis. Child.*, 46: 533-538, 1971.

816. Benaim, R., Chapelle, M., and Chiche, P., Action of di-phenylhydantoin on atrioventricular and intraventricular con-duction in humans, *Ann. Cardiol. Angeiol.*, 21: 379-388, 1972.

817. Bender, F., Modern drug therapy of arrhythmia, *Schweiz. Med. Wschr.*, 103: 272-276, 1973.

818. Bennett, W. M., Singer, I., and Coggins, C. H., Guide to drug usage in adult patients with impaired renal function, *JAMA*, 223: 991-997, 1973.

819. Berger, H., Fever: an unusual manifestation of epilepsy, *Postgrad. Med.*, 40: 479-481, 1966.

820. Bergouignan, M., Antiepileptic drugs in the treatment of trigeminal neuralgia, *Presse Med.*, 78: 1832-1834, 1970.

821. Berlin, A., Agurell, S., Borga, O., Lund, L. and Sjoqvist, F., Micromethod for the determination of diphenylhydantoin in plasma and cerebrospinal fluid, *Scand. J. Clin. Invest.*, 29: 281-287, 1972.

822. Bernoulli, C., Diphenylhydantoin, *Schweiz. Med. Wschr.*, 100: 836, 1970.

823. Bernstein, J. D. and Johnson, S. L., Effects of diphe-nylhydantoin upon estrogen metabolism by liver microsomes of DDT-treated Japanese quail, *Bull. Environ. Contam. Toxicol.*, 10: 309-314, 1973.

824. Berry, D. J. and Grove, J., Emergency toxicological screening for drugs commonly taken in overdose, *J. Chromatogr.*, 80: 205-219, 1973.

825. Bhatt, G., Vijayan, N. and Dreyfus, P. M., Myotonia, *Calif. Med.*, 114: 16-22, 1971.

826. Bigger, J. T., Jr., Steiner, C., and Burris, J. O., The ef-fects of diphenylhydantoin on atrioventricular conduction in man, *Clin. Res.*, 15: 196, 1967.

827. Bigger, J. T., Schmidt, D. H., and Kutt, H., A method for estimation of plasma diphenylhydantoin concentration, *Amer. Heart J.*, 77: 572-573, 1969.

828. Bigger, J. T., Weinberg, D. I., Kovalik, T. W., Harris, P. D., Cranefield, P. C., and Hoffman, B. F., Effects of diphe-nylhydantoin on excitability and automaticity in the canine heart, *Circ. Res.*, 26: 1-15, 1970.

829. Birket-Smith, E. and Krogh, E., Motor nerve conduction velocity during diphenylhydantoin intoxication, *Acta. Neurol. Scand.*, 47: 265-271, 1971.

830. Bissett, J. K., deSoyza, N. D. B., Kane, J. J., and Doherty, J. E., Case studies: effect of diphenylhydantoin on induced aber-rant conduction, *J. Electrocardiol.*, 7: 65-69, 1974.

831. Bissett, J. K., deSoyza, N. D. B., Kane, J. J., and Murphy, M. L., Improved intraventricular conduction of premature beats after diphenylhydantoin, *Amer. J. Cardiol.*, 33: 493-497, 1974.

832. Bissett, J. K., Kane, J. J., deSoyza, N., and Doherty, J., Effect of diphenylhydantoin on bundle branch block in man, *Clin. Res.*, 21: 405, 1973.

833. Bissett, J. K., Kane, J., deSoyza, N., and Doherty, J., Im-proved intraventricular conduction after diphenylhydantoin, *Circulation*, 48: 146, 1973.

834. Bittar, E. E., Chen, S. S., Danielson, B. G., and Tong, E. Y., An investigation of the action of diphenylhydantoin on sodium efflux in barnacle muscle fibres, *Acta Physiol. Scand.*, 89: 30-38, 1973.

835. Bjerk, E. M. and Hornisher, J. J., Narcolepsy: a case re-port and a rebuttal, *Electroenceph. Clin. Neurophysiol.*, 10: 550-552, 1958.

836. Black, J. T., Garcia-Mullin, R., Good, E., and Brown, S., Muscle rigidity in a newborn due to continuous peripheral nerve hyperactivity, *Arch. Neurol.*, 27: 413-425, 1972.

837. Black, N. D., The value of diphenylhydantoinate (Dilan-tin) in psychoses with convulsive disorders, *Psychiatr. Quart.*, 13: 711-720, 1939.

838. Blum, M. R., McGilveray, I., Becker, C. E., and Riegel-man, S., Clinical implications derived from pharmacokinetics of diphenylhydantoin (DPH), *Clin. Res.*, 19: 121, 1971.

839. Blum, M., Riegelman, S., and Becker, C. E., Altered pro-tein binding of diphenylhydantoin in uremic plasma, *New Eng. J. Med.*, 286: 109, 1972.

840. Blumenkrantz, N. and Asboe-Hansen, G., Effect of di-phenylhydantoin on connective tissue, *Acta Neurol. Scand.*, 50: 302-306, 1974.

841. Bochner, F., Hooper, W. D., Sutherland, J. M., Eadie, M. J., and Tyrer, J. H., The renal handling of diphenylhydantoin and 5-(P-Hydroxyphenyl)-5-phenylhydantoin, *Clin. Pharmacol. Ther.*, 14: 791-796, 1973.

842. Bochner, F., Hooper, W. D., Tyrer, J. H., and Eadie, M. J., Effect of a delayed-action phenytoin preparation on blood phenytoin concentration, *J. Neurol. Neurosurg. Psychiat.*, 35: 682-684, 1972.

843. Bochner, F., Hooper, W. D., Sutherland, J. M., Eadie, M. J., and Tyrer, J. H., Diphenylhydantoin concentrations in saliva, *Arch. Neurol.*, 31: 57-59, 1974.

844. Bochner, F., Hooper, W. D., Tyrer, J. H., and Eadie, M. J., Factors involved in an outbreak of phenytoin intoxication, *Epilepsy Abstracts*, 5: 245-246, 1971.

845. Bochner, F., Hooper, W., Tyrer, J., and Eadie, M., Clin-ical implications of certain aspects of diphenylhydantoin metab-olism, *Proc. Aust. Assoc. Neurol.*, 9: 171-178, 1973.

846. Bogoch, S. and Dreyfus, J., The broad range of use of diphenylhydantoin, bibliography and review, *The Dreyfus Medical Foundation*, 1970.

847. Booker, H. E., Serum concentrations of free diphenylhy-dantoin and their relationship to clinical intoxication, *Epilepsia*, 14: 96-97, 1973.

848. Booker, H. E., Tormey, A., and Toussaint, J., Concur-rent administration of phenobarbital and diphenylhydantoin: lack of an interference effect, *Neurology*, 21: 383-385, 1971.

849. Borga, O., et al, Plasma protein binding of tricyclic anti-depressants in man, *Psychopharm. Abs.*, 9: 500, 1970.

850. Borga, O., Garle, M., and Gutova, M., Identification of 5-(3, 4-dihydroxyphenyl)-5-phenylhydantoin as a metabolite of 5, 5-diphenylhydantoin (phenytoin) in rats and man, *Phar-macology*, 7: 129-137, 1972.

851. Borgstedt, A. D., Bryson, M. F., Young, L. W., and Forbes, G. B., Long-term administration of antiepileptic drugs and the development of rickets, *J. Pediat.*, 81: 9-15, 1972. (*cf.* Greenlaw, et al., *Clin. Res.*, 20: 56, 1972.)

852. Borofsky, L. G., Louis, S., and Ku't, H., Diphenylhydan-toin in children, *Neurology*, 23: 967-972, 1973.

853. Borondy, P., Dill, W. A., Chang, T., Buchanan, R. A., and Glazko, A. J., Effect of protein binding on the distribution of 5, 5-diphenylhydantoin between plasma and red cells, *Ann. N.Y. Acad. Sci.*, 226: 82-87, 1973.

854. Bose, B. C., Gupta, S. S., and Sharma, S., Effect of anti-convulsant drugs on the acetylcholine content in rat tissues, *Arch. Int. Pharmacodyn.*, 67: 254-261, 1958.

855. Boshes, B. and Arieff, A. J., Clinical experience in the neurologic substance of pain, *Med. Clin. N. Amer.*, 52: 111-121, 1968.

856. Boston Collaborative Drug Surveillance Program, Diphenylhydantoin side effects and serum albumin levels, *Clin. Pharmacol. Ther.*, 14: 529-532, 1973.

857. Boudin, G., Pepin, B., Decroix, G., and Vernant, J. C., Diphenylhydantoin intoxication triggered by antituberculous treatment (2 cases), *Ann. Med. Intern.*, 122: 855-860, 1971.

858. Bouzarth, W. F., The ABC's of emergency care of serious head injuries in industry, *Industr. Med. Surg.*, 39: 25-29, 1970.

859. Bowe, J. C., Cornish, E. J., and Dawson, M., Evaluation of folic acid supplements in children taking phenytoin, *Develop. Med. Child Neurol.*, 13: 343-354, 1971.

860. Boyd, D. L. and Williams, J. F., The effect of diphenylhydantoin (Dilantin) on the positive inotropic action of ouabain, *Amer. J. Cardiol.*, 23: 712-718, 1969.

861. Boykin, M. E. and Hooshmand, H., CSF and serum folic acid and protein changes with diphenylhydantoin treatment: laboratory and clinical correlations, *Neurology*, 20: 403, 1970.

862. Boykin, M. E., *In vivo* and *in vitro* association of 5, 5-diphenylhydantoin with brain subfractions, *Neurology*, 4: 392-393, 1974.

863. Bozza, G. A., Normalization of intellectual development in the slightly brain-damaged, retarded child, *Paper presented at the 4th Italian National Congress on Child Neuropsychiatry*, Genoa, 1971.

864. Bray, P. F., Ely, R. S., and Kelley, V. C., Studies of 17-hydroxycorticosteroids VIII. Adrenocortical function in patients with convulsive disorders, *A.M.A. Arch. Neurol. Psychiat.*, 72: 583-590, 1954.

865. Bray, P. F., Ely, R. S., Zapata, G., and Kelley, V. C., Adrenocortical function in epilepsy I. The role of cortisol (hydrocortisone) in the mechanism and management of seizures, *Neurology*, 10: 842-846, 1960.

866. Bray, P. F., Kelley, V. C., Zapata, G., and Ely, R. S., Adrenocortical function in epilepsy II. The role of corticosterone in the mechanism and management of epilepsy, *Neurology*, 11: 246-250, 1961.

867. Brena, S. and Bonica, J. J., Nerve blocks for managing pain in the elderly, *Postgrad. Med.*, 47: 215-220, 1970.

868. Brennan, R. W., Dehejia, H., Kutt, H., Verebely, K., and McDowell, F., Diphenylhydantoin intoxication attendant to slow inactivation of isoniazid, *Neurology*, 20: 687-693, 1970.

869. Brien, J. F. and Inaba, T., Determination of low levels of 5,5-diphenylhydantoin in serum by gas liquid chromatography, *Epilepsy Abstracts*, 7: 198, 1974.

870. Bright, N. H., Effect of diphenylhydantoin on proline and hydroxyproline excretion in the rat, *Proc. Soc. Exp. Biol. Med.*, 120: 463-465, 1965.

871. Broddle, W. D., and Nelson, S. R., The effect of diphenylhydantoin on brain P-creatine, *Fed. Proc.*, 28: 1771, 1969.

872. Brodows, R. G. and Campbell, R. G., Control of refractory fasting hypoglycemia in a patient with suspected insulinoma with diphenylhydantoin, *J. Clin. Endocr.*, 38: 159-161, 1974.

873. Brown, G. L., and Wilson, W. P., Salicylate intoxication and the CNS with special reference to EEG findings, *Dis. Nerv. Syst.*, 32: 135-140, 1971.

874. Brown, J. M., Drug-associated lymphadenopathies with special reference to the Reed-Sternberg cell, *Med. J. Aust.*, 375-378, 1971.

875. Buchanan, R. A., and Allen, R. J., Diphenylhydantoin (Dilantin) and phenobarbital blood levels in epileptic children, *Neurology*, 21: 866-871, 1971.

876. Buchanan, R. A., Kinkel, A. W., Goulet, J. R., and Smith, T. C., The metabolism of diphenylhydantoin (Dilantin) following once-daily administration, *Neurology*, 22: 126-130, 1972.

877. Buchanan, R. A., Turner, J. L., Moyer, C. E., and Heffelfinger, J. C., Single daily dose of diphenylhydantoin in children, *J. Pediat.*, 83: 479-483, 1973.

878. Buchthal, F. and Lennox-Buchthal, M. A., Diphenylhydantoin, relation of anticonvulsant effect to concentration in serum, *Antiepileptic Drugs*, 193-209, Woodbury, D. M., Penry, J. K., and Schmidt, R. P., Eds., Raven Press, New York, 1972.

879. Buchthal, F. and Svensmark, O., Serum concentrations of diphenylhydantoin (phenytoin) and phenobarbital and their relation to therapeutic and toxic effects, *Psychiat. Neurol. Neurochir.*, 74: 117-136, 1971.

880. Burckhardt, D. and Sefidpar, M., Digitalis intoxication: contribution to diagnosis and therapy, *Schweiz. Rundschau. Med. (Praxis)*, 60: 1705-1711, 1971.

881. Buscaino, G. A., Labianca, O., Caruso, G., De Giacomo, P., and Ferrannini, E., Electromyographic and muscular histoenzymatic findings in a patient with continuous muscular activity syndrome ("Neuromyotonia"), *Acta Neurol. (Naples)*, 25: 206-224, 1970.

882. Calne, D. B., The drug treatment of epilepsy, *Epilepsy Abstracts*, 6: 177, 1973.

883. Cantor, F. K., Phenytoin treatment of thalamic pain. *Brit. Med. J.*, 4: 590-591, 1972.

884. Caracta, A. R., Damato, A. N., Josephson, M. E., Ricciutti, M. A., Gallagher, J. J., and Lau, S. H., Electrophysiologic properties of diphenylhydantoin, *Circulation*, 47: 1234-1241, 1973.

885. Carnay, L. and Grundfest, S., Excitable membrane stabilization by diphenylhydantoin and calcium, *Neuropharmacology*, 13: 1097-1108, 1974.

886. Caspary, W. F., Inhibition of intestinal calcium transport by diphenylhydantoin in rat duodenum, *Epilepsy Abstracts*, 6: 18, 1973.

887. Castleden, C. M., and Richens, A., Chronic phenytoin therapy and carbohydrate tolerance, *Lancet*, 966-967, 1973.

888. Chang, T. and Glazko, A. J., Diphenylhydantoin biotransformation, *Antiepileptic Drugs*, 149-162, Woodbury, D. M., Penry, J. K., and Schmidt, R. P., Eds., Raven Press, New York, 1972.

889. Chang, T., Okerholm, R. A., and Glazko, A. J., A 3-0-methylated catechol metabolite of diphenylhydantoin (Dilantin) in rat urine, *Res. Communications Chem. Path. Pharmacol.*, 4: 13-23, 1972.

890. Chang, T., Savory, A. and Glazko, A. J., A new metabolite of 5, 5-diphenylhydantoin (Dilantin), *Biochem. Biophys. Res. Commun.*, 38: 444-449, 1970.

891. Cheng, P. T. H. and Staple, P. H., Effect of a dorsal dermal surgical wound on the chemical response of rat abdominal skin to chronic administration of sodium diphenylhydantoin, *J. Dent. Res.*, 51: 131-143, 1972.

892. Cheng, T. O. and Damato, A. N., Dilantin in treatment and prevention of cardiac arrhythmias, *Amer. Heart J.*, 78: 285, 1969.

893. Chetchel, A. P., The influence of diphenine on the gum mucosa, *Epilepsy Abstracts*, 3: 203, 1970.

894. Chikhani, P., The use of "diphenylhydantoin sodium" in the treatment of periodontal disease, *Actualities Odontostomat*, 98: 1-8, 1972.

895. Choi, Y. K. and Kee, C. S., Induction of steroid 6 beta-hydroxylase by administration of diphenylhydantoin, *Chem. Abstracts*, 74: 123576C, 1971.

896. Choi, Y., Thrasher, K., Werk, E. E., Sholiton, L. J., and Olinger, C., Effect of diphenylhydantoin on cortisol kinetics in humans, *J. Pharmacol. Exp. Ther.*, 176: 27-34, 1971.

897. Chokroverty, S. and Rubino, F. A., Motor nerve conduction study in patients on long term diphenylhydantoin therapy: correlation with clinical states and serum levels of diphenylhydantoin, folate and cyanocobalamine, *Epilepsy Abstracts*, 7: 111, 1974.

898. Choovivathanavanich, P., Wallace, E. M., and Scaglione, P. R., Pseudolymphoma induced by diphenylhydantoin, *J. Pediat.*, 76: 621-623, 1970.

899. Chou, C. C., Kuiper, D. H., and Hsieh, C. P., Effects of

diphenylhydantoin on motility and compliance of the canine ileum and colon, *Gastroenterology*, 62: 734, 1972.

900. Chriskie, H. W., du Mesnil de Rochemont, W., Etzrodt, H., Grosser, K. D., Schulten, K. H., and Steinbruck, G., Influence of diphenylhydantoin and lidocaine on hemodynamics in patients with fixed-rate pacemakers, *Verh. Deutsch Ges. Inn. Med.*, 77: 960-963, 1971.

901. Christiansen, C., Rodbro, P., and Lund, M., Effect of vitamin D on bone mineral mass in normal subjects and in epileptic patients on anticonvulsants: a controlled therapeutic trial, *Brit. Med. J.*, 208-209, 1973. (*cf.* Christiansen et al., *Brit. Med. J.*, 3: 738, 1972 and *Brit. Med. J.*, 4: 695, 1973.)

902. Christiansen, J. and Dam, M., Influence of phenobarbital and diphenylhydantoin on plasma carbamazepine levels in patients with epilepsy, *Epilepsy Abstracts*, 7: 137, 1974.

903. Christy, N. P. and Hofmann, A. D., Effects of diphenylhydantoin upon adrenal cortical function in man, *Neurology*, 9: 245-248, 1959.

904. Chrobok, F., Quantitative determination of phenytoin in biological material in the presence of phenobarbital and glutethimide, *Epilepsy Abstracts*, 5: 172, 1972.

905. Chung, E. K., The current status of digitalis therapy, *Modern Treatment*, 8: 643-714, 1971.

906. Clark, R. L., Kuhn, J. P., and Du Jovne, C. A., Absence of rickets after chronic dilantin administration: experimental radiological observations in rats, *Invest. Radiol.*, 6: 152-154, 1971.

907. Coburn, R. F., Enhancement by phenobarbital and diphenylhydantoin of carbon monoxide production in normal man, *New Eng. J. Med.*, 283: 512-515, 1970.

908. Cohen, H., Langendorf, R., and Pick, A., Intermittent parasystole—mechanism of protection, *Circulation*, 48: 761-774, 1973.

909. Cohen, M. S., Bower, R. H., Fidler, S. M., Johnsonbaugh, R. E., and Sode, J., Inhibition of insulin release by diphenylhydantoin and diazoxide in a patient with benign insulinoma, *Lancet*, 40-41, 1973.

910. Cole, P., Efficacy of oral diphenylhydantoin in reduction of premature ventricular contractions, *Clin. Pharmacol. Ther.*, 13: 137, 1972.

911. Collan, R., Boyd, W., and Hathaway, B., Effect of halothane on the liver of rats pretreated with diphenylhydantoin and norethindrone, *Scand. J. Clin. Lab. Invest.*, 25: 74, 1970.

912. Conn, H. L., Jr., Mechanisms of quinidine action. *Mechanisms and Therapy of Cardiac Arrhythmias*, 594-596, Dreifus, L. S. and Likoff, W., Eds., Grune and Stratton, New York, 1966.

913. Conners, C. K., Kramer, R., Rothschild, G. H., Schwartz, L., and Stone, A., Treatment of young delinquent boys with diphenylhydantoin sodium and methyphenidate, *Arch. Gen. Psychiat.*, 24: 156-160, 1971.

914. Conney, A. H. and Burns, J. J., Metabolic interactions among environmental chemicals and drugs, *Science*, 178: 576-586, 1972.

915. Conney, A. H., Jacobson, M., Schneidman, K., and Kuntzman, R., Induction of liver microsomal cortisol 6 β-hydroxylase by diphenylhydantoin or phenobarbital: an explanation for the increased excretion of 6-hydroxycortisol in humans treated with these drugs, *Life Sci.*, 4: 1091-1098, 1965.

916. Conard, G. J., Haavik, C. O., and Finger, K. F., Binding of 5,5-diphenylhydantoin and its major metabolite to human and rat plasma proteins, *J. Pharm. Sci.*, 60: 1642-1646, 1971.

917. Cooper, R. G., Greaves, M. S., and Owen, G., Gas liquid chromatographic isolation, identification, and quantitation of some barbiturates, glutethimide, and diphenylhydantoin in whole blood, *Epilepsy Abstracts*, 6: 184, 1973.

918. Costa, P. J., Glaser, G. H., and Bonnycastle, D. D., Effects of diphenylhydantoin (Dilantin) on adrenal cortical function, *A.M.A. Arch. Neurol. Psychiat.*, 74: 88-91, 1955.

919. Covi, L. and Uhlenhuth, E. H., Methodological problems in the psychopharmacological study of the dangerous anti-social personality, *Proc. Int. Symposium on Aggressive Behavior Biochem. Pharmacol. Psychol. Sociol.*, 326-335, May, 1969.

920. Covino, B. G., Wright, R., and Charleson, D. A., Effectiveness of several antifibrillary drugs in the hypothermic dog, *Amer. J. Physiol.*, 121: 54-58, 1955.

921. Cranmer, M. F., Effect of diphenylhydantoin on storage of DDT in the rat, *Toxic Appl. Pharmacol.*, 17: 315, 1970.

922. Critchley, E. M. R., Clark, D. B., and Wikler, A., An adult form of acanthocytosis, *Trans. Amer. Neurol. Assoc.*, 92: 132-137, 1967.

923. Cuan-Perez, M. C. and Ortiz, A., Comparative study of quinidine, propranolol and diphenylhydantoin for preventing recurrence in post-cardioversion auricular fibrillation, *Arch. Inst. Cardiol. Mex.*, 41: 278-284, 1971.

924. Cudworth, A. G. and Cunningham, J. L., The effect of diphenylhydantoin on insulin response, *Clin. Sci. Molec. Med.*, 46: 131-136, 1974.

925. Cummings, N. P., Rosenbloom, A. L., Kohler, W. C. and Wilder, B. J., Plasma glucose and insulin responses to oral glucose with chronic diphenylhydantoin therapy, *Pediatrics*, 51: 1091-1093, 1973.

926. Cunningham, J. L. and Price Evans, D. A., Urinary D-glucaric acid excretion and acetanilide pharmacokinetics before and during diphenylhydantoin administration, *Europ. J. Clin. Pharmacol.*, 7: 387-391, 1974.

927. Curtis, G. P., Experimental atrial fibrillation, *Univ. of Mich., Ann Arbor, Doctoral Thesis*, 1971.

928. Dack, S., Antiarrhythmic agents in the treatment of ventricular tachycardia, *Mechanisms and Therapy of Cardiac Arrhythmias*, 312-320, Dreifus, L. S. and Likoff, W., Eds., Grune and Stratton, New York, 1966.

929. Dalessio, D. J., Medical treatment of tic douloureux, *J. Chronic Dis.*, 19: 1043-1048, 1966.

930. Dalton, C. and Verebely, K., Hypotriglyceridemic activity of 5,5'-diphenyl-2-thiohydantoin (DPTH), *J. Pharmacol. Exp. Ther.*, 180: 484-491, 1971.

931. Daly, R. F. and Sajor, E. E., Inherited tic douloureux, *Neurology*, 23: 937-939, 1973.

932. Dam, M. and Christiansen, J., Evidence of drug action on serum level of carbamazepine, *Epilepsy Abstracts*, 7: 26, 1974.

933. Dam, M., Diphenylhydantoin, neurologic aspects of toxicity, *Antiepileptic Drugs*, 227-235, Woodbury, D. M., Penry, J. K., and Schmidt, R. P. Eds., Raven Press, New York, 1972.

934. Dam, M., The density and ultrastructure of the Purkinje cells following diphenylhydantoin treatment in animals and man, *Acta Neurol. Scand.*, 48: 1-65, 1972.

935. Damato, A. N., Berkowitz, W. D., Patton, R. D., and Lau, S. H., The effect of diphenylhydantoin on atrioventricular and intraventricular conduction in man, *Amer. Heart J.*, 79: 51-56, 1970.

936. Damato, A. N., Diphenylhydantoin: pharmacological and clinical use, *Progr. Cardiovasc. Dis.*, 12: 1-15, 1969.

937. Danckwardt-Lilliestrom, G., Grevsten, S., and Olerud, S., Investigation of effect of various agents on periosteal bone formation, *Upsala J. Med. Sci.*, 77: 125-128, 1972.

938. Daniel, R., Psychiatric drug use and abuse in the aged, *Geriatrics*, 144-156, January, 1970.

939. Daniels, C., Stein, A. A., and Moss, G., The shock lung syndrome: anemia as a predisposing factor, *Surg. Forum*, 24: 1, 1973.

940. Danielson, B. G., Bittar, E. E., Chen, S. S. and Tong, E. Y., Diphenylhydantoin as a blocking agent of the proton-sensitive component of Na efflux in barnacle muscle fibers, *Life Sci.*, 10: 721-726, 1971.

941. Danzig, R., Treatment of arrhythmias associated with acute myocardial infarction, *Nebraska Med. J.*, 56: 474-475, 1971.

942. Daube, J. R., and Peters, H. A., Hereditary essential myoclonus, *Arch. Neurol.*, 15: 587-594, 1966.

943. Davies, J. E., Edmundson, W. F., Maceo, A., Irvin, G. L.,

Cassady, J., and Barquet, A., Reduction of pesticide residues in human adipose tissue with diphenylhydantoin, *Food Cosmet. Toxic.*, 9: 413-423, 1971.

944. Davies, J. E., Pharmacological depletion of adipose pesticide residues, *Clin. Res.*, 19: 27, 1971.

945. Davies, R. O., Diphenylhydantoin in angina pectoris, *Chest*, 66: 421-422, 1974.

946. Davis, J. N., Diphenylhydantoin for hiccups, *Lancet*, 1: 997, 1974.

947. Dawson, K. P., and Jamieson, A., Value of blood phenytoin estimation in management of childhood epilepsy, *Arch. Dis. Child.*, 46: 386-388, 1971.

948. Dawson, K. P., Severe cutaneous reactions to phenytoin, *Arch. Dis. Child.*, 48: 239-240, 1973.

949. Day, H. W., Control and treatment of arrhythmias, *Cardiovascular Therapy, The Art and The Science*, 289-291, Russek, H. I., and Zohman, B. L., Eds., The Williams & Wilkins Co., Baltimore, 1971.

950. DeCastro, J. H. X., Acosta, M. L., Sica, R. E. P., and Guerico, N., Sensory and motor nerve conduction velocity in long-term diphenylhydantoin therapy, *Arq. Neuropsiquiat.*, 30: 215-220, 1972.

951. DeLuca, K., Masotti, R. E., and Partington, M. W., Altered calcium metabolism due to anticonvulsant drugs, *Develop. Med. Child Neurol.*, 14: 318-321, 1972.

952. Delaire, J., Moutet, H., and Talmant, J. C., Facial peripheric hemispasm and Paget's disease of bone, *Rev. Stomat. (Paris)*, 73: 601-612, 1972.

953. Delgado, J. M. R. and Mihailovic, L., Use of intracerebral electrodes to evaluate drugs that act on the central nervous system, *Ann. N.Y. Acad. Sci.*, 64: 644-666, 1956.

954. Delgado, J. M. R., Mora, F. and Sanguinetti, A. M., Reduction by diphenylhydantoin of after-discharges in the amygdala of stimulated rhesus monkey, *Personal Communication*, 1973.

955. Den Hertog, A., The effect of diphenylhydantoin on the electronic component of the sodium pump in mammalian non-myelinated nerve fibers, *Europ. J. Pharmacol.*, 19: 94-97, 1972.

956. Dent, E., Richens, A., Rowe, D. J. F., and Stamp, T. C. B., Osteomalacia with long-term anticonvulsant therapy in epilepsy, *Brit. Med. J.*, 4: 69-72, 1970.

957. Desjacques, P., Study of the diffusion of phenytoin through the cellophane membrane of the artificial kidney used on a patient suffering from uremia and epilepsy, *Epilepsy Abstracts*, 5: 220, 1972.

958. De Sousa, R. C. and Grosso, A., Effects of diphenylhydantoin on transport processes in frog skin (Rana ridibunda), *Epilepsy Abstracts*, 7: 111, 1974.

959. deWolff, F. A., Drug effects on intestinal epithelium, *Doctoral Thesis*, 1973.

960. Dhar, G. J., Peirach, C. A., Ahamed, P. N., and Howard, R. B., Diphenylhydantoin induced hepatic necrosis, *Postgrad. Med.*, 56: 128-129, 1974.

961. Diamond, B. and Yaryura-Tobias, J. A., The use of diphenylhydantoin in non-epileptic psychotics, *V World Congress of Psychiatry*, 1971.

962. Diamond, W. D. and Buchanan, R. A., A clinical study of the effect of phenobarbital on diphenylhydantoin plasma levels, *J. Clin. Pharmacol.*, 306-311, 1970.

963. Diederich, K. W., Herzog, S. and Tielsen, I., Diphenylhydantoin: A comparative study on normal cats and animals intoxicated with digitalis glycosides, *Basic Research in Cardiology*, 69: 289-308, 1974.

964. Dill, R. E., Adrenal cortical response in rats treated with diphenylhydantoin sodium, *Anat. Rec.*, 148: 366, 1964.

965. Dill, W. A., Baukema, J., Chang, T., and Glazko, A. J., Colorimetric assay of 5,5-diphenylhydantoin (Dilantin) and 5 (p hydroxyphenyl) 5 phenylhydantoin, *Epilepsy Abstracts*, 4: 262, 1971.

966. Dill, W. A., Chucot, L., Chang, T., and Glazko, A. J., Simplified benzophenone procedure for determination of diphenylhydantoin in plasma, *Clin. Chem.*, 17: 1200-1201, 1971.

967. Dilman, V. M., Elivbaeva, G. V., Vishnevskii, A. S., Tsyrilina, E. V., and Bulovskaia, L. N., Justification of the use of diphenine (diphenylhydantoin) in oncologic practice, *Vop. Onkol.*, 17: 70-72, 1971.

968. Doe, W. F., Hoffbrand, A. V., Reed, P. I., and Scott, J. M., Jejunal pH and folic acid, *Brit. Med. J.*, 699-700, 1971.

969. Doherty, J. E., Digitalis glycosides. Pharmacokinetics and their clinical implications, *Ann. Intern. Med.*, 79: 229-238, 1973.

970. Domino, E. F. and Olds, M. E., Effects of d-amphetamine, scopolamine, chlordiazepoxide and diphenylhydantoin on self-stimulation behavior and brain acetylcholine, *Psychopharmacologia (Berlin)*, 23: 1-16, 1972.

971. Domzal, T., Effect of diphenylhydantoin on clinical manifestations and excretion of 5-hydroxyindoleacetic acid in Parkinson's disease, *Neurol. Neurochir. Pol.*, 6: 357-360, 1972.

972. Dreifus, L. S. and Watanabe, Y., Current status of diphenylhydantoin, *Amer. Heart J.*, 80: 709-713, 1970.

973. Dreifus, L. S., de Azevedo, I. M., and Watanabe, Y., Electrolyte and antiarrhythmic drug interaction, *Amer. Heart J.*, 88: 95-101, 1974.

974. Dreifus, L. S., Management of intractable atrial arrhythmias, *Mechanisms and Therapy of Cardiac Arrhythmias*, 205-210, Dreifus, L. S. and Likoff, W., Eds., Grune and Stratton, New York, 1966.

975. Dreifus, L. S., Use of quinidine, procainamide and diphenylhydantoin, *Cardiovascular Therapy, The Art and The Science*, 109-112, Russek, H. I. and Zohman, B. L., Eds., The Williams & Wilkins Co., Baltimore, 1971.

976. Dreifuss, F. E. and Sato, S., Anticonvulsant drugs in clinical practice, *Drug Therapy*, 2: 9-22, 1972.

977. Dreifuss, F. E., Diphenylhydantoin and visceral atony, *Drug Therapy*, 3: 101-102, 1973.

978. Dressler, W. E., Rossi, G. V., and Orzechowski, R. F., Effect of several anticonvulsant drugs and procainamide against ouabain-induced cardiac arrhythmias in rabbits, *J. Pharm. Sci.*, 61: 133-134, 1972.

979. Driessen, O. and Emonds, A., Simultaneous determination of antiepileptic drugs in small samples of blood plasma by gas chromatography. Column technology and extraction procedure. *Epilepsy Abstracts*, 7: 203-204, 1974.

980. Dronamraju, K. R., Epilepsy and cleft lip and palate, *Lancet*, 876-877, 1970.

981. Dry, J. and Pradalier, A., Phenytoin intoxication during treatment combined with disulfiram, *Therapie*, 28: 799-802, 1973.

982. Ducker, T. B., Blaylock, R. L. D., and Perot, P. L., Jr., Emergency care of patients with cerebral injuries, *Postgrad. Med.*, 55: 102-110, 1974.

983. Dudley, W. H. C., Jr., and Williams, J. G., Electroconvulsive therapy in delirium tremens, *Dig. Neurol. Psychiat.*, Series XL: 333, 1972.

984. Dujovne, C. A., Clark, R., and Lasagna, L., Calcium and CNS symptoms, *New Eng. J. Med.*, 281: 271-272, July, 1969.

985. Eadie, M. J., Tyrer, J. H., and Hooper, W. D., Aspects of diphenylhydantoin metabolism, *Proc. Aust. Assoc. Neurol.*, 7: 7-13, 1970.

986. Eastham, R. D. and Jancar, J., Macrocytosis associated with anticonvulsant therapy, *Epilepsia*, 11: 275-280, 1970.

987. Eddy, J. D. and Singh, S. P., Treatment of cardiac arrhythmias with phenytoin, *Brit. Med. J.*, 4: 270-273, 1969.

988. Editor, A guide to selection of a systemic antibacterial agent, *Drugs*, 4: 132-145, 1972.

989. Editor, Anticonvulsant drugs and hypocalcaemia, *Brit. Med. J.*, 4: 351, 1973.

990. Editor, Anticonvulsants or antiepileptics, *Behavioral Neuropsychiatry*, 3: 14-16, 1971.

991. Editor, Diphenylhydantoin for digitalis toxicity, *Postgrad. Med.*, 45: 244-245, 1969.

992. Editor, For tic douloureux, lasting relief, *Medical World News*, 14: 66-67, 1973.

993. Editor, Monitoring drug therapy, *Lancet*, 668, 1974.

994. Editor, Phenytoin and carbamazepine combined, *Brit. Med. J.*, 1: 113, 1974.

995. Editor, Some important interactions with anticonvulsant drugs, *J. International Res. Communication*, 2: 5-7, 1974.

996. Editor, Treatment of trigeminal neuralgia, *Brit. Med. J.*, 2: 583-584, 1972.

997. Editors, Panel discussion: hormones and fetal metabolism, *Clin. Pharmacol. Ther.*, 14: 742-747, 1973.

998. Edmundson, W. F., Davies, J. E., Maceo, A., and Morgade, C., Drug and environmental effects on DDT residues in human blood, *Southern Med. J.*, 63: 1440-1441, 1970.

999. Edmundson, W. F., Frazier, D. E., and Maceo, A., Sequential biochemical tests in persons taking pH phenytoin, *Indust. Med.*, 41: 7-11, 1972.

1000. Ehrnebo, M., Agurell, S., Jalling, B., and Boreus, L. O., Age differences in drug binding by plasma proteins: studies on human fetuses, neonates and adults, *Europ. J. Clin. Pharmacol.*, 3: 189-193, 1971.

1001. Eipe, J., Drugs affecting therapy with anticoagulants, *Med. Clin. N. Amer.*, 56: 255-262, 1972.

1002. Eisen, A. A., Woods, J. F., and Sherwin, A. L., Peripheral nerve function in long-term therapy with diphenylhydantoin, *Neurology*, 24: 411-417, 1974.

1003. Eling, T. E., Harbison, R. D., Becker, B. A., and Fouts, J. R., Diphenylhydantoin effect on neonatal and adult rat hepatic drug metabolism, *J. Pharmacol. Exp. Ther.*, 171: 127-134, 1970.

1004. Eling, T. E., Harbison, R. D., Becker, B. A., and Fouts, J. R., Kinetic changes in microsomal drug metabolism with age and diphenylhydantoin treatment, *Europ. J. Pharmacol.*, 11: 101-108, 1970.

1005. Ellenberger, C., Burde, R. M., and Keltner, J. L., Acute optic neuropathy, *Arch. Ophthal.*, 91: 435-438, 1974.

1006. Elliott, T. H. and Natarajan, P. N., Infrared studies of hydantoin and its derivatives, *J. Pharm. Pharmacol.*, 19: 209-216, 1966.

1007. Ellis, J. G. and Dimond, E. G., Newer concepts of digitalis, *Amer. J. Cardiol.*, 17: 759-767, 1966.

1008. Elshove, J. and Van Eck, J. H. M., Congenital malformations, cleft lip and palate in particular, in children of epileptic women, *Ned. Tijdschr. Geneesk.*, 115: 1371-1375, 1971. (*cf.* Elshove, *Lancet*, 1074, 1969.)

1009. Elwood, J. C., Richert, D. A., and Westerfeld, W. W., A comparison of hypolipidemic drugs in the prevention of an orotic acid fatty liver, *Biochem. Pharmacol.*, 21: 1127-1134, 1972.

1010. Erdey, L., Kaplar, L., Takacs, J. and Dessouky, Y. M., Determination of hydantoins in pharmaceutical preparations by gas chromatography, *J. Chromatogr.*, 45: 63-67, 1969.

1011. Erickson, J. D. and Oakley, G. P., Seizure disorder in mothers of children with orofacial clefts: a case control study, *J. Pediat.*, 84: 244-246, 1974.

1012. Escueta, A. V. and Appel, S. H., Brain synapses—an *in vitro* model for the study of seizures, *Arch. Intern. Med.*, 129: 333-344, 1972.

1013. Escueta, A. V. and Appel, S. H., The effects of electroshock seizures on potassium transport within synaptosomes from rat brain, *Epilepsy Abstracts*, 5: 205, 1972.

1014. Escueta, A. V. and Appel, S. H., Diphenylhydantoin and potassium transport in isolated nerve terminals, *J. Clin. Invest.*, 50: 1977-1984, 1971.

1015. Esposito-Avella, M. and Mennear, J. H., Studies on the protective effect of diphenylhydantoin against alloxan diabetes in mice, *Proc. Soc. Exp. Biol. Med.*, 142: 82-85, 1973.

1016. Evans, D. E. and Gillis, R. A., Effect of diphenylhydantoin (DPH) on centrally induced vagal arrhythmias, *Pharmacologist*, 13: Abstract 188, 1971.

1017. Evenson, M. A., Jones, P., and Darcey, B., Simultaneous measurement of diphenylhydantoin and primidone in serum by gas-liquid chromatography, *Clin. Chem.*, 16: 107-110, 1970.

1018. Fariss, B. L. and Lutcher, C. L., Diphenylhydantoin-induced hyperglycemia and impaired insulin release—effect of dosage, *Diabetes*, 20: 177-181, 1971.

1019. FDA, Anticonvulsant linked with birth defect risk, *FDA Drug Bulletin*, July, 1974.

1020. Fedrick, J., Epilepsy and pregnancy: a report from the Oxford record linkage study, *Brit. Med. J.*, 2: 442-448, 1973.

1021. Ferrari, M. and Furlanut, M., Effects of diphenylhydantoin on smooth muscle, *Arch. Int. Pharmacodyn.*, 203: 101-106, 1973.

1022. Ferry, D. G., Owen, D., and McQueen, E. G., The effect of phenytoin on the binding of pesticides to serum proteins, *Proc. Univ. Otago Med. School*, 50: 8-9, 1972.

1023. Fertziger, A. P. and Dunham, P. B., Diphenylhydantoin stimulation of potassium influx in isolated lobster axons, *Epilepsy Abstracts*, 5: 61, 1972.

1024. Fertziger, A. P., Brain extracellular space: some considerations on the role it plays in brain function, *Cond. Reflex*, 8: 224-232, 1973.

1025. Fertziger, A. P., Liuzzi, S. E., and Dunham, P. B., Diphenylhydantoin (Dilantin): stimulation of potassium influx in lobster axons, *Brain Res.*, 33: 592-596, 1971.

1026. Fertziger, A. P., Lynch, J. J., and Stein, E. A., Modification of the morphine withdrawal syndrome in rats, *Brain Res.*, 78: 331-334, 1974.

1027. Fertziger, A. P., Stein, E. A., and Lynch, J. J., Suppression of morphine-induced mania in cats, *Psychopharmacologia*, 36: 185-187, 1974.

1028. Festoff, B. W. and Appel, S. H., The effect of diphenylhydantoin on synaptosome metabolism, *Neurology*, 19: 300, 1969.

1029. Fica, V., Panaitescu, G., Matrescu, F., and Popescu, E., Indications and limitations of anti-arrhythmic drugs, *Med. Intern.*, 23: 523-536, 1971.

1030. Fincham, R. W., Schottelius, D. D., and Sahs, A. L., The influence of diphenylhydantoin on primidone metabolism, *Arch. Neurol.*, 30: 259-262, 1974.

1031. Finkle, B. S., Foltz, R. L., and Taylor, D. M., A comprehensive GC-MS reference data system for toxiciological and biomedical purposes, *J. Chromatogr. Sci.*, 12: 304-328, 1974.

1032. Fish, B., The "one child, one drug" myth of stimulants in hyperkinesis, *Arch. Gen. Psychiat.*, 25: 193-203, 1971.

1033. Fisher, D. and DiMino, J. M., Case presentation of an alternative therapeutic approach for the borderline psychotic heroin addict: diphenylhydantoin, *Br. J. Addict.*, 70: 51-55, 1975.

1034. Fisher, D. D. and Ungerleider, J. T., Grand mal seizures following ingestion of LSD, *Calif. Med.*, 106: 210-211, 1967.

1035. Formby, B., The *in vivo* and *in vitro* effect of diphenylhydantoin and phenobarbitone on K^+-activated phosphohydrolase and (NA^+,K^+)-activated ATPase in particulate membrane fractions from rat brain, *J. Pharm. Pharmacol.*, 22: 81-85, 1970.

1036. Fouts, J. R. and Kutt, H., Diphenylhydantoin, some studies on the biotransformation and interactions with some other drugs and chemicals, *Antiepileptic Drugs*, 163-168, Woodbury, D. M., Penry, J. K., and Schmidt, R. P., Eds., Raven Press, New York, 1972.

1037. Freiwald, M. J., Prevention of complications of Herpes Zoster ophthalmicus with special reference to steroid therapy, *Eye, Ear, Nose and Throat Monthly*, 46: 444-450, 1967.

1038. Frenkel, E. P., McCall, M. S. and Sheehan, R. G., Cerebrospinal fluid folate, and vitamin B^{12} in anticonvulsant-induced megaloblastosis, *J. Lab. Clin. Med.*, 81: 105-115, 1973.

1039. Friedlander, W. J., Epilepsy—1973, *The Clinical Neurology Information Center*, The University of Nebraska Medical Center, 1-45, 1974.

1040. Friedman, A. P., An overview of chronic recurring headache, *Wisconsin Med. J.*, 71: 110-116, 1972.

1041. Friedman, A. P., Treatment of vascular headache, *International Encyclopedia of Pharmacology and Therapeutics*, Section 33, Vol. I: 225-251. Carpi, A., Ed., Pergamon Press, New York, 1972.

1042. Fromm, G. H., Pharmacological consideration of anticonvulsants, *Epilepsy Abstracts*, 2: 194, 1969.

1043. Frost, J. B., Mesoridazine and chlorpromazine in the treatment of alcohol withdrawal syndrome, *Canad. Psychiat. Assoc. J.*, 18: 385-387, 1973.

1044. Gabler, W. L. and Hubbard, G. L., The metabolism of 5,5-diphenylhydantoin (DPH) in nonpregnant and pregnant Rhesus monkeys, *Arch. Int. Pharmacodyn.*, 203: 72-91, 1973.

1045. Gabreels, F. J. M., The influence of phenythoin on the Purkinje cell of the rat, *Epilepsy Abstracts*, 4:131-132, 1971.

1046. Gallagher, B. B., Baumel, I. P., Mattison, R. H., and Woodbury, S. G., Primidone, diphenylhydantoin and phenobarbital: aspects of acute and chronic toxity, *Neurology*, 23: 145-149, 1973.

1047. Gamstorp, I., Meeuwisse, G., and Tryding, N., Tryptophan loading test in convulsive disorders, *Acta Paediat. Scand.*, 55: 656-657, 1966.

1048. Gardner-Medwin, D., Why should we measure serum levels of anticonvulsant drugs in epilepsy? *Clinical Electroencephalography*, 4: 132-134, 1973.

1049. Gardner, C. R. and Webster, R. A., The effect of some anticonvulsant drugs on leptazol and bicuculline induced acetylcholine efflux from rat cerebral cortex, *Brit. J. Pharmacol.*, 47: 652P, 1973.

1050. Garrettson, L. K. and Curley, A., Dieldrin—studies in a poisoned child, *Arch. Environ. Health*, 19: 814-822, 1969.

1051. Garrettson, L. K., Pharmacology of anticonvulsants, *Pediat. Clin. N. Amer.*, 19: 179-191, 1972.

1052. Gattenlohner, W. and Schneider, K. W., The effect of diphenylhydantoin on hemodynamics, *Munchen Med. Wschr.*, 11: 2561-2566, 1969.

1053. Gauchel, F. D., Lehr, H. J., Gauchel, G., and von Harnack, G. A., Diphenylhydantoin in children, *Deutsch Med. Wschr.*, 98: 1391-1396, 1973.

1054. Gauchel, G., Gauchel, F. D., and Birkofer, L., A micromethod for the determination of phenytoin in blood by high speed liquid chromatography, *Epilepsy Abstracts*, 6: 210, 1973.

1055. Gavrilescu, S., Pop, T., and Goia, E., On a case of supraventricular paroxysmal tachycardia resistant to treatment. Transitory conversion into atrial fibrillation by rapid atrial electric stimulation, *Med. Intern (Bucur)*, 24: 1393-1400, 1972.

1056. Gebauer, D., Prevention and therapy of cardiac rhythm disorders. Experiences with a diphenylhydantoin-meprobamate preparation (Cusitan), *Munchen Med. Wschr.*, 113: 436-440, 1971.

1057. Gegick, C. G., Danowski, T. S., Khurana, R. C., Vidalon, C., Nolan, S., Stephan, T., Chae, S., and Wingard, L., Hyperostosis frontalis interna and hyperphosphatasemia, *Ann. Intern. Med.*, 79: 71-75, 1973.

1058. Gehres, L. D., Randall, C. L., Riccio, D. C., and Vardaris, R. M., Attenuation of hypothermic retrograde amnesia produced by pharmacologic blockage of brain seizures, *Physiol. Behav.*, 10: 1011-1017, 1973.

1059. Gerber, N., Lynn, R., and Oates, J., Acute intoxication with 5,5-diphenylhydantoin associated with impairment of biotransformation, *Ann. Intern. Med.*, 77: 765-771, 1972.

1060. Gerber, N., Seibert, R. A., and Thompson, R. M., Identification of a catechol glucuronide metabolite of 5,5-diphenylhydantoin (DPH) in rat bile by gas chromatography (GC) and mass spectrometry (MS), *Epilepsy Abstracts*, 7: 80, 1974.

1061. Gerber, N., Weller, W. L., Lynn, R., Rangno, R. E., Sweetman, B. J., and Bush, M. T., Study of dose-dependent metabolism of 5,5-diphenylhydantoin in the rat using new methodology for isolation and quantitation of metabolites *in vivo* and *in vitro*, *J. Pharmacol. Exp. Ther.*, 178: 567-579, 1971.

1062. Gerich, J. E., Charles, M. A., Levin, S. R., Forsham, P. H., and Grodsky, G. M., *In vitro* inhibition of pancreatic glucagon secretion by diphenylhydantoin, *J. Clin. Endocr.*, 35: 823-824, 1972.

1063. Gerlings, E. D., and Gilmore, J. P., Some cardiac effects of diphenylhydantoin, *Acta Physiol. Pharmacol. Neerl.*, 15: 461-468, 1969.

1064. German, J., Kowal, A., and Ehlers, K. H., Trimethadione and human teratogenesis, *Teratology*, 3: 349-362, 1970.

1065. Gerson, C. D., Hepner, G. W., Brown, N., Cohen, N., Herbert, V., and Janowitz, H. D., Inhibition by diphenylhydantoin of folic absorption in man, *Gastroenterology*, 63: 246-251, 1972.

1066. Gerz, H. O., Dilantin against "painful touching" (dysthesia), *Physician's Drug Manual*, 3: 144, 1972.

1067. Gettes, L. S., The electrophysiologic effects of antiarrhythmic drugs, *Amer. J. Cardiol.*, 28: 526-535, 1971.

1068. Gharib, H. and Munoz, J. M., Endocrine manifestations of diphenylhydantoin therapy, *Metabolism*, 23: 515-524, 1974.

1069. Gianelly, R. E. and Harrison, D. C., Drugs used in the treatment of cardiac arrhythmias, *Disease-A-Month*, 25-32, January 1969.

1070. Gibson, K. and Harris, P., Diphenylhydantoin and human myocardial microsomal (Na$^+$,K$^+$)-ATPase, *Biochem. Biophys. Res. Commun.*, 35: 75-78, 1969.

1071. Gilbert, J. C., Gray, P., and Heaton, G. M., Anticonvulsant drugs and brain glucose, *Biochem. Pharmacol.*, 20: 240-243, 1971.

1072. Gillis, R. A. and Raines, A., A comparison of the cardiovascular effects of diphenylthiohydantoin and diphenylhydantoin, *Europ. J. Pharmacol.*, 23: 13-18, 1973.

1073. Gimenez-Roldan, S. and Esteban, A., Orbicularis oculi "myotonia" in hypothyroid myopathy, *Europ. Neurol.*, 9: 44-55, 1973.

1074. Ginwalla, T. M. S., Gomes, B. C., and Nayak, R. P., Management of gingival hyperplasia in patients receiving Dilantin therapy, *J. Indian Dent. Assn.*, 39: 124-126, 1967.

1075. Glaser, G. H., Diphenylhydantoin, toxicity, *Antiepileptic Drugs*, 219-226, Woodbury, D. M., Penry, J. K., and Schmidt, R. P. Eds., Raven Press, New York, 1972. (*cf.* Adeloye, et al., *Ghana Med. J.*, 10: 56, 1971, Bosso and Chudzik, *Drug Intel. & Clin. Pharma.*, 7: 336, 1973, Greenberg, et al., *Epilepsy Abstracts*, 4: 151, 1971 and Watts, *Pediatrics*, 30: 592, 1962.)

1076. Glazko, A. J. and Chang, T., Diphenylhydantoin, absorption, distribution and excretion, *Antiepileptic Drugs*, 127-136, Woodbury, D. M., Penry, J. K., and Schmidt, R. P., Eds., Raven Press, New York, 1972.

1077. Glazko, A. J., Diphenylhydantoin, chemistry and methods for determination, *Antiepileptic Drugs*, 103-112, Woodbury, D. M., Penry, J. K., and Schmidt, R. P., Eds., Raven Press, New York, 1972.

1078. Glazko, A. J., Diphenylhydantoin, *Epilepsy Abstracts*, 6: 184, 1973.

1079. Godfraind, T., Lesne, M., and Pousti, A., The action of diphenylhydantoin upon drug binding, ionic effects and inotropic action of ouabain, *Arch. Int. Pharmacodyn.*, 191: 66-73, 1971.

1080. Goebel, R. W., Sodium diphenylhydantoin association with oral healing, *J. Oral Surg.*, 30: 191-195, 1972.

1081. Goldberg, M. A., and Todoroff, T., Binding of diphenylhydantoin to brain protein, *Epilepsy Abstracts*, 7: 112, 1974.

1082. Goldberg, M. A. and Todoroff, T., Diphenylhydantoin binding to brain fractions, *Neurology*, 22: 410, 1972.

1083. Goldberg, M. E. and Ciofalo, V. B., Effect of diphenylhydantoin sodium and chlordiazepoxide alone and in combination on punishment behavior, *Psychopharmacologia (Berlin)*, 14: 233-239, 1969.

1084. Goldstein, F. J., Continuing education via pharmatapes: Digitalis I. A basic pharmacological review, *Amer. J. Pharm.*, 145: 135-141, 1973.

1085. Goldstein, R. E., Penzotti, S. C., Kuehl, K. S., Prindle, K. H., Hall, C. A., Titus, E. O., and Epstein, S. E., Correlation of antiarrhythmic effects of diphenylhydantoin with digoxin-induced changes in myocardial contractility, sodium-potassium adenosine triphosphatase activity, and potassium efflux, *Circ. Res.,* 33: 175-182, 1973.

1086. Gordon, E., Respiratory control after acute head injury, *Lancet,* 483, 1973.

1087. Gordon, P., Aging: a search for drug-modifiable degeneracy in the polyribosomes of brain, *Proc. 8th Int. Cong. Geront.,* 1: 4pp., 1969.

1088. Gordon, P., Callaghan, O., and Doty, B., Diphenylhydantoin effects on nucleic acid biochemistry learning and neoplasm, *Pharmacologist,* 10: 169, 1968.

1089. Gordon, P., Molecular approaches to the drug enhancement of deteriorated functioning in the aged, *Advances Geront. Res.,* 3: 199-248, 1971.

1090. Gordon, P., Rational chemotherapy for aging, *Postgrad. Med.,* 40: 152-155, 1970.

1091. Gordon, P., Tobin, S. S., Doty, B., and Nash, M., Drug effects on behavior in aged animals and man: diphenylhydantoin and procainamide, *J. Geront.,* 23: 434-444, 1968.

1092. Gossel, T. A. and Mennear, J. H., Inhibition of alloxan-induced diabetes by diphenylhydantoin sodium, *Pharmacologist,* 13: 238, 1971.

1093. Gossel, T. A., On the mechanism of diphenylhydantoin protection against alloxan-induced diabetes mellitus in mice, *Dissertation Abstracts,* 33: 2729B, 1972.

1094. Gottschalk, L. A., Covi, L., Uliana, R., and Bates, D. E., Effects of diphenylhydantoin on anxiety and hostility in institutionalized prisoners, *Compr. Psychiat.,* 14: 503-511, 1973.

1095. Goudie, J. H. and Burnett, D., A gas chromatographic method for the simultaneous determination of phenobarbitone, primidone and phenytoin in serum using a nitrogen detector, *Epilepsy Abstracts,* 6: 187, 1973.

1096. Grant, R. H. E. and Stores, O. P. R., Folic acid in folate-deficient patients with epilepsy, *Brit. Med. J.,* 4: 644-648, 1970.

1097. Green, R. S. and Rau, J. H., Treatment of compulsive eating disturbances with anticonvulsant medication, *Amer. J. Psychiat.,* 131: 428-432, 1974.

1098. Greenbaum, D. S., Ferguson, R. K., Kater, L. A., Kuiper, D. H., and Rosen, L. W., A controlled therapeutic study of the irritable-bowel syndrome, *New Eng. J. Med.,* 288: 13-16, 1973.

1099. Greenberg, C. and Papper, E. M., The indications for gasserian ganglion block for trigeminal neuralgia, *Anesthesiology,* 31: 566-573, 1969.

1100. Greenberg, I. M., Cerebral dysfunction in general psychiatric office practice, *Dis. Nerv. Syst.,* 33: 637-644, 1972.

1101. Greengard, O. and McIlwain, H., Anticonvulsants and the metabolism of separated mammalian cerebral tissues, *Biochem. J.,* 61: 61-68, 1955.

1102. Grob, P. J. and Herold, G. E., Immunological abnormalities and hydantoins, *Brit. Med. J.,* 2: 561-563, 1972.

1103. Gruener, R. P. and Stern, L. Z., Diphenylhydantoin reverses membrane effects in steroid myopathy, *Nature New Bio.,* 235: 54-55, 1972.

1104. Gudmundson, C. and Lidgren, L., Does diphenylhydantoin accelerate healing of fractures in mice, *Acta Orthop. Scand.,* 44: 640-649, 1973.

1105. Guzek, J. W., Russell, J. T., and Thorn, N. A., Inhibition by diphenylhydantoin of vasopressin release from isolated rat neurohypophyses, *Acta Pharmacol. et Toxicol.,* 34: 1-4, 1974.

1106. Haan, D., *Diagnosis and therapy of cardiac arrhythmia and acute heart disease,* Medizinisch Literarische Verlagsgesellschaft mbH, Uelzen, Germany, 1973.

1107. Haddad, R. I., Positive EEG spike activity in sleep, *JAMA,* 229: 1282, 1974.

1108. Hadfield, M. G. and Boykin, M. E., Effect of diphenylhydantoin administered *in vivo* on 3H-1-norepinephrine uptake in synaptosomes, *Res. Commun. Chem. Pathol. Pharmacol.,* 7: 209-212, 1974.

1109. Hadfield, M. G., Uptake and binding of catecholamines —effect of diphenylhydantoin and a new mechanism of action, *Arch. Neurol.,* 26: 78-84, 1972.

1110. Haft, J. I., Ricciutti, M. A. and Damato, A. N., Effects of IV diphenylhydantoin (DPH) on coronary blood flow and oxygen utilization of the heart, *Clinical Research,* 15: 204, 1967.

1111. Hagen, H., Treatment of cardiac arrhythmias with diphenylhydantoin, *Deutsch Med. Wschr.,* 96: 380-384, 1971.

1112. Haghshenass, M. and Rao, D. B., Serum folate levels during anticonvulsant therapy with diphenylhydantoin, *J. Amer. Geriat. Soc.,* 21: 275-277, 1973.

1113. Hahn, T. J., Hendin, B. A., Scharp, C. R., and Haddad, J. G., Jr., Effect of chronic anticonvulsant therapy on serum 25-hydroxycalciferol levels in adults, *New Eng. J. Med.,* 287: 900-909, 1972.

1114. Haiat, R., Chapelle, M., Benaim, R., Witchitz, S., and Chiche, P., Disappearance of an intraventricular conduction disorder under diphenylhydantoin, *Sem. Hop. Paris,* 47: 2957-2964, 1971.

1115. Hall, W. B., Prevention of Dilantin hyperplasia: a preliminary report, *Bull. Acad. Gen. Dent.,* 20-25, 1969.

1116. Hallaq, I. Y. and Harris, J. D., The syndrome of post-herpetic neuralgia: complication and an approach to therapy, *J. Amer. Osteopath. Assoc.,* 68: 1265-1267, 1969.

1117. Halpern, L. M. and Julien, R. M., Augmentation of cerebellar Purkinje cell discharge rate after diphenylhydantoin, *Epilepsy Abstracts,* 5: 236-237, 1972.

1118. Hancock, J. C. and Bevilacqua, A. R., Temporal lobe dysrhythmia and impulsive or suicidal behavior, *Southern Med. J.,* 64: 1189-1193, 1971.

1119. Handley, A. J., Phenytoin tolerance tests, *Brit. Med. J.,* 3: 203-204, 1970.

1120. Hansen, H. W. and Wagener, H. H., Sodium diphenylhydantoin for the treatment of cardiac arrhythmias, *Munchen Med. Wschr.,* 111: 417-421, 1969.

1121. Hansen, H. W. and Wagener, H. H., Diphenylhydantoin in the treatment of heart failure, *Deutsch. Med. Wschr.,* 96: 1866-1873, 1971.

1122. Hansen, H. W. and Wagener, H. H., Experimental studies on the influence of diphenylhydantoin glycoside effects on the heart, *Herz Kreislauf Zeitschrift Fur Kardiologie und Angiologie in Klinik und Praxis,* 6: 69-72, 1974.

1123. Hansen, H. W., Marquort, B., and Pelz, W., Indications for phenytoin in cardiac arrhythmias, *Deutsch. Med. Wschr.,* 99: 638-642, 1974.

1124. Hansen, J. M., Siersbaek-Nielsen, K. and Skovsted, L., Effect of diphenylhydantoin on the metabolism of carbamazepine-induced acceleration of dicoumarol in man, *Acta Med. Scand.,* 189: 15-19, 1971.

1125. Hansen, J. M., Skovsted, L., Lauridsen, U. B., Kirkegaard, C., and Siersbaek-Nielsen, K., The effect of diphenylhydantoin on thyroid function, *J. Clin. Endocrinol. Metab.,* 39: 785-786, 1974.

1126. Hansotia, P. and Keran, E., Dilantin binding by red blood cells of normal subjects, *Neurology,* 24: 575-578, 1974.

1127. Hansten, P. D., Diphenylhydantoin drug interactions, *Hosp. Formulary Manage.,* 4: 28-29, 1969.

1128. Haque, N., Thrasher, K., Werk, E. E., Jr., Knowles, H. C., Jr., and Sholiton, L. J., Studies on dexamethasone metabolism in man: effect of diphenylhydantoin, *J. Clin. Endocr.,* 34: 44-50, 1972.

1129. Harbison, R. D. and Becker, B. A., Effect of phenobarbital and SKF 525A pretreatment on diphenylhydantoin teratogenicity in mice, *J. Pharmacol. Exp. Ther.,* 175: 283-288, 1970.

1130. Harbison, R. D., Eling, T. E., and Becker, B. A., Effects of diphenylhydantoin on neonatal rat liver drug metabolizing enzymes, *Fed. Proc.,* 28(2): 1969.

1131. Harris, M., Jenkins, M. V. and Wills, M. R., Phenytoin inhibition of parathyroid hormone induced bone resorption *in vitro, Brit. J. Pharmac.*, 50: 405-408, 1974.

1132. Harrison, D. C., Kerber, R. E., and Alderman, E. L., Pharmacodynamics and clinical use of cardiovascular drugs after cardiac surgery, *Amer. J. Cardiol.*, 26: 385-393, 1970.

1133. Hart, B. L., Feline behavior, *Feline Practice*, 3: 8-10, 1973.

1134. Hartshorn, E. A., Interactions of cardiac drugs, *Drug Intell. Clin. Pharm.*, 4: 272-275, 1970.

1135. Hartshorn, E. A., Pyrazolone derivatives (antipyrine, aminopyrine, phenylbutazone, oxyphenbutazone), *Drug Intelligence Clinical Pharmacy*, 6: 6-10, 1972.

1136. Hasbani, M., Pincus, J. H. and Lee, S. H., Diphenylhydantoin and calcium movement in lobster nerves, *Arch. Neurol.*, 31: 250-254, 1974.

1137. Hatch, R. C. and Fischer, R., Cocaine elicited behavior and toxicity in dogs pretreated with synaptic blocking agents, morphine, or diphenylhydantoin, *Epilepsy Abstracts*, 6: 209, 1973.

1138. Hattwick, M. A. W., Weis, T. T., Stechschulte, C. J., Baer, G. M., and Gregg, M. B., Recovery from rabies: a case report, *Ann. Intern. Med.*, 76: 931-942, 1972.

1139. Haward, L. R. C., Effects of sodium diphenylhydantoinate and pemoline upon concentration: a comparative study, *Drugs and Cerebral Function*, 103-120, Smith, W. L., Ed., Charles C Thomas, 1970.

1140. Haward, L. R. C., Effects of DPH (sodium diphenylhydantoinate) upon concentration in pilots, *Rev. Med. Aeronautique Spatiale*, 12: 372-374, 1973.

1141. Haward, L. R. C., The effect of phenytoin-aided autogenic training on stress threshold, *Int. Congress for Psychosomatic Med. and Hypnosis*, Kyoto, Japan, July 12-14, 1967.

1142. Haward, L. R. C., Effects of sodium diphenylhydantoin upon concentration, *Bulletin Brit. Psychol. Soc.*, 22: 50, 1969.

1143. Hedger, R. W., The conservative management of acute oliguric renal failure, *Med. Clin. N. Amer.*, 55: 121-135, 1971.

1144. Heinemann, U. and Lux, H. D., Effects of diphenylhydantoin on extracellular (K+) in cat cortex, *Electroenceph. Clin. Neurophysiol.*, 34: 735, 1973.

1145. Helfant, R., Scherlag, B., and Damato, A., The interaction of procaine amide and diphenylhydantoin on cardiac conductivity and automaticity, *Clin. Res.*, 15: 206, 1967.

1146. Hendricks, G. L., Jr., Barnes, W. T., and Hood, H. L., Seven-year "cure" of lung cancer with metastasis to the brain, *JAMA*, 220: 127, 1972.

1147. Hepner, G. W., Aledort, L. M., Gerson, C. D., Cohen, N., Herbert, V., and Janowitz, H. D., Inhibition of intestinal ATPase by diphenylhydantoin and acetazolamide, *Clin. Res.*, 18: 382, 1970.

1148. Herbinger, W., Result report of a control by an apparatus of 208 myocardial infarct patients in an intensive care station, *Wien. Med. Wschr.*, 121: 518-522, 1971.

1149. Hermansen, K., Antifibrillatory effect of some beta-adrenergic receptor blocking agents determined by a new test procedure in mice, *Acta Pharmacologica*, 28: 17-27, 1969.

1150. Hinkhouse, A., Craniocerebral trauma, *Amer. J. Nurs.*, 73: 1719-1722, 1973.

1151. Hobson, J. D. and Zettner, A., Digoxin serum half-life following suicidal digoxin poisoning, *JAMA*, 223: 147-149, 1973.

1152. Hodgson, E. R. and Reese, H. H., Clinical experiences with dilantin in epilepsies, *Wis. Med. J.*, 38: 968-971, 1939.

1153. Hoefer, P. F. A., Cohen, S. M., and Greeley, D. McL., Paroxysmal abdominal pain—a form of epilepsy in children, *JAMA*, 147: 1-6, 1951.

1154. Hofeldt, F. D., Dippe, S. E., Levin, S. R., Karam, J. H., Blum, M. R., and Forsham, P. H., Effects of diphenylhydantoin upon glucose-induced insulin secretion in three patients with insulinoma, *Diabetes*, 23: 192-198, 1974.

1155. Hogg, P. S., Three cases of 'restless legs' or 'Ekbom's syndrome' as seen in general practice, *Practitioner*, 209: 82-83, 1972.

1156. Holcomb, R., Lynn, R., Harvey, B., Sweetman, B. J., and Gerber, N., Intoxication with 5,5-diphenylhydantoin (Dilantin), *J. Pediat.*, 80: 627-632, 1972.

1157. Holdaway, P. A., Effects of amino-glutethimide and diphenylhydantoin sodium on the rat adrenal cortex, *Proc. Indiana Acad. Sci.*, 77: 427-433, 1968.

1158. Hommes, O. R. and Obbens, E. A., The epileptogenic action of Na-folate in the rat, *J. Neurol. Sci.*, 16: 271-281, 1972.

1159. Honda, Y., Podos, S. M., and Becker, B., The effect of diphenylhydantoin on the electroretinogram of rabbits. I. Effect of concentration, *Invest. Ophthal.*, 12: 567-572, 1973.

1160. Honda, Y., Podos, S. M., and Becker, B., The effect of diphenylhydantoin on the electroretinogram of rabbits. II. Effects of hypoxia and potassium, *Invest. Ophthal.*, 12: 573-578, 1973.

1161. Hooper, W. D., Sutherland, J. M., Bochner, F. et al., The effect of certain drugs on the plasma protein binding of phenytoin, *Epilepsy Abstracts*, 7: 112, 1974.

1162. Hopf, H. C. and Kauer, H., Effect of phenytoin on the excitable cell membrane, *Epilepsy Abstracts*, 4: 89, 1971.

1163. Houben, P. F. M., Hommes, O. R., and Knaven, P. J. H., Anticonvulsant drugs and folic acid in young mentally retarded epileptic patients, *Epilepsia*, 12: 235-247, 1971.

1164. Houck, J. C., Cheng, R. F., and Waters, M. D., Diphenylhydantoin, effects on connective tissue and wound repair, *Antiepileptic Drugs*, 267-273, Woodbury, D. M., Penry, J. K., and Schmidt, R. P., Eds., Raven Press, New York, 1972.

1165. Houck, J. C., Cheng, R. F., and Waters, M. D., The effect of Dilantin upon fibroblast proliferation, *Proc. Soc. Exp. Biol. Med.*, 139: 969-981, 1972.

1166. Houghton, G. W. and Richens, A., Inhibition of phenytoin metabolism by sulthiame in epileptic patients, *Brit. J. Clin. Pharmacol.*, 1: 59-66, 1974.

1167. Houghton, G. W. and Richens, A., Rate of elimination of tracer doses of phenytoin at different steady state serum phenytoin concentrations in epileptic patients, *Brit. J. Clin. Pharmacol.* 1: 155-161, 1974.

1168. Houghton, G. W., Latham, A. N., and Richens, A., Difference in the central actions of phenytoin and phenobarbitone in man, measured by critical flicker fusion threshold, *Europ. J. Clin. Pharmacol.*, 6: 57-60, 1973.

1169. Huessy, H. R., Study of the prevalence and therapy of the choreatiform syndrome or hyperkinesis in rural Vermont, *Acta Paedopsychiat.*, 34: 130-135, 1967.

1170. Huffman, D. H. and Azarnoff, D. L., The use of digitalis, *Ration. Drug Ther.*, 8: 1-7, 1974.

1171. Hughes, R. C. and Matthews, W. B., Pseudo-myotonia and myokymia, *J. Neurol. Neurosurg. Psychiat.*, 32: 11-14, 1969.

1172. Huisman, J. W., Van Heycop Ten Ham, M. W., and Van Zijl, C. H. W., Influence of ethylphenacemide on serum levels of other anti-epileptic drugs, *Epilepsia*, 11: 207-215, 1970.

1173. Humphries, J. O., New methods for the prevention and treatment of ventricular arrhythmias, *Maryland Med. J.*, 17: 75-76, 1968.

1174. Hunninghake, D. B., Drug interactions, *Postgrad. Med.*, 47: 71-75, 1970.

1175. Hunter, J., Maxwell, J. D., Stewart, D. A., Parsons, V., and Williams, R., Altered calcium metabolism in epileptic children on anticonvulsants, *Brit. Med. J.*, 202-204, 1971. (cf. Hahn, et al., *Clin. Res.*, 21: 626, 1973 and Herman and Pippenger, *Neurology*, 23: 437, 1973.)

1176. Iber, F. L., Prevention of alcohol withdrawal seizures, *JAMA*, 221: 608, 1972.

1177. Ide, C. H. and Webb, R. W., Penetrating transorbital injury with cerebrospinal orbitorrhea, *Amer. J. Ophthal.*, 71: 1037-1039, 1971.

1178. Idestrom, C. M., Schalling, D., Carlquist, U., and

Sjoqvist, F., Acute effects of diphenylhydantoin in relation to plasma levels, *Psychol. Med.*, 2: 111-120, 1972.

1179. Imabayashi, K. and Matsumura, S., Four cases of idiopathic renal hematuria with abnormal electroencephalogram, *Jap. J. Clin. Urol.*, 27: 139-144, 1973.

1180. Inaba, T. and Brien, J. F., Determination of the major urinary metabolite of diphenylhydantoin by high-performance liquid chromatography, *J. Chromatogr.*, 80: 161-165, 1973.

1181. Iosub, S., Bingol, N., and Wasserman, E., The pregnant epileptic and her offspring, *Pediat. Res.*, 7: 420, 1973.

1182. Isaacs, H. and Frere, G., Syndrome of continuous muscle fibre activity. Histochemical, nerve terminal and end-plate study of two cases, *South African Medical Journal*, 48: 1601-7, 1974.

1183. Isaacs, H., Continuous muscle fibre activity in an Indian male with additional evidence of terminal motor fiber abnormality, *J. Neurol. Neurosurg. Psychiat.*, 30: 126-133, 1967.

1184. Janz, D. and Schmidt, D., Comparison of spectrophotometric and gas liquid chromatographic measurements of serum diphenylhydantoin concentrations in epileptic outpatients, *Epilepsy Abstracts*, 7: 268, 1974.

1185. Janz, D. and Schmidt, D., Anti-epileptic drugs and failure of oral contraceptives, *Lancet*, 1113, 1974.

1186. Jenkins, D. and Spector, R. G., The actions of folate and phenytoin on the rat heart *in vivo* and *in vitro*, *Biochem. Pharmacol.*, 22: 1813-1816, 1973.

1187. Jensen, O. N. and Olesen, O. V., Subnormal serum folate due to anticonvulsive therapy, *Arch. Neurol.*, 22: 181-182, 1970.

1188. Jensen, R. A. and Katzung, B. G., Electrophysiological actions of diphenylhydantoin on rabbit atria: dependence on stimulation frequency, potassium and sodium, *Circ. Res.*, 26: 17-27, 1970.

1189. Jonas, A. D., Diphenylhydantoin and the treatment of anxiety, *Amer. J. Psychiat.*, 126: 163, 1969.

1190. Jones, G. L. and Kemp, J. W., Characteristics of the hydrogen bonding interactions of diphenylhydantoin with nucleic acids and their components, *Fed. Proc.*, 31: 570, 1972.

1191. Jovanovic, T., Experiences in the treatment of psychoses occurring concomitantly with epilepsy, *Neuropsihiatrija*, 20: 173-183, 1972.

1192. Joynt, R. J. and Green, D., Tonic seizures as a manifestation of multiple sclerosis, *Arch. Neurol.*, 6: 293-299, 1962.

1193. Jubiz, W. and Rallison, M. L., Diphenylhydantoin treatment of glycogen storage diseases, *Arch. Intern. Med.*, 134: 418-421, 1974.

1194. Jubiz, W., Levinson, R. A., Meikle, A. W., West, C. D., and Tyler, F. H., Absorption and conjugation of metyrapone during diphenylhydantoin therapy: mechanism of the abnormal response to oral metyrapone, *Endocrinology*, 86: 328-331, 1970.

1195. Jubiz, W., Meikle, A. W., Levinson, R. A., Mizutani, S., West, C. D., and Tyler, F. H., Effect of diphenylhydantoin on the metabolism of dexamethasone, *New Eng. J. Med.*, 283: 11-14, 1970.

1196. Julien, R. M. and Halpern, L. M., Cerebellar action of diphenylhydantoin on penicillin-induced cerebral cortical epileptic foci, *Fed. Proc.*, 29: Abstract 784, 1970.

1197. Julien, R. M. and Halpern, L. M., Stabilization of excitable membrane by chronic administration of diphenylhydantoin, *J. Pharmacol. Exp. Ther.*, 175: 206-212, 1970.

1198. Julien, R. M. and Halpern, L. M., Diphenylhydantoin: evidence for a central action, *Life Sci.*, 10: 575-582, 1971.

1199. Julien, R. M. and Halpern, L. M., Effects of diphenylhydantoin and other antiepileptic drugs on epileptiform activity and Purkinje cell discharge rates, *Epilepsia*, 13: 387–400, 1972.

1200. Jung, S. S., Chen, K. M., Brody, J. A., Paroxysmal choreoathetosis: report of Chinese cases, *Neurology*, 23: 749-55, 1973.

1201. Jus, K., Jus, A., Gautier, J., Villeneuve, A., Pires, P.,

Pineau, R., and Villeneuve, R., Studies on the action of certain pharmacological agents on tardive dyskinesia and on the rabbit syndrome, *Int. J. Clin. Pharmacol.*, 9: 138-145, 1974.

1202. Kalman, P., Nanassy, A., and Csapo, G., Diphenylhydantoin treatment of atrial tachycardia with heart block, *Z. Kardiologie*, 62: 75-79, 1972.

1203. Kanzawa, F., Hoshi, A., and Kuretani, K., Relationship between antitumor activity and chemical structure in psychotropic agents, *Gann*, 61: 529-534, 1970.

1204. Kaplan, R., Blume, S., Rosenberg, S., Pitrelli, J., and Turner, W. J., Phenytoin, metronidazole and multivitamins in the treatment of alcoholism, *Quart. J. Stud. Alcohol.*, 33: 97-104, 1972.

1205. Kasai, S. and Yoshizumi, T., Effect of diphenylhydantoin sodium on the proliferation of cultured cells *in vitro*, *Bull. Tokyo Dent. Coll.*, 12: 223-234, 1971.

1206. Kater, R. M. H., Roggin, G., Tobon, F., Zeive, P., and Iber, F. L., Increased rate of clearance of drugs from the circulation of alcoholics, *Amer. J. Med. Sci.*, 258: 35-39, 1969.

1207. Kater, R. M. H., Tobon, F., Zeive, P. D., Roggin, G. M., and Iber, F. L., Heavy drinking accelerates drugs' breakdown in liver, *JAMA*, 206: 1709, 1968.

1208. Kato, R., Chiesara, E., and Vassanelli, P., Increased activity of microsomal strychnine-metabolizing enzyme induced by phenobarbital and other drugs, *Biochem. Pharmacol.*, 11: 913-922, 1962.

1209. Kaufmann, G. and Hauser, K., Experience with diphenylhydantoin (antisacer) in the treatment of cardiac arrhythmias, *Schweiz. Med. Wschr.*, 98: 1223-1226, 1968.

1210. Kaufmann, G. and Weber-Eggenberger, S., Hemodynamic changes due to diphenylhydantoin in digitalized cardiac patients, *Schweiz. Med. Wschr.*, 100: 2164-2168, 1970.

1211. Kazamatsuri, H., Elevated serum alkaline phosphatase levels in epilepsy during diphenylhydantoin therapy, *New Eng. J. Med.*, 283: 1411-1412, 1970.

1212. Kazamatsuri, H., Elevated serum alkaline phosphatase levels in the epileptic patients with diphenylhydantoin, *Folia Psychiat. Neurol. Jap.*, 24: 181-189, 1970.

1213. Keltner, J. L., Becker, B., Gay, A. J., and Podos, S. M., Effect of diphenylhydantoin in ischemic optic neuritis, *Trans. Amer. Ophthal. Soc.*, 70: 113-130, 1972.

1214. Kemp, G. L., Treatment of ventricular ectopic rhythms with diphenylhydantoin, *J. Amer. Geriat. Soc.*, 20: 265-267, 1972.

1215. Kemp, J. W. and Woodbury, D. M., Subcellular distribution of 4-^{14}C-diphenylhydantoin in rat brain, *J. Pharmacol. Exp. Ther.*, 177: 342-349, 1971.

1216. Kennedy, C., Anderson, W., and Sokoloff, L., Cerebral blood flow in epileptic children during the interseizure period, *Neurology*, 8: 100-105, 1958.

1217. Kennedy, C., Grave, G. D., Jehle, J. W., and Kupferberg, H. J., The effect of diphenylhydantoin on local cerebral blood flow, *Neurology*, 22: 451-452, 1972.

1218. Kessler, K. M., Individualization of dosage of antiarrhythmic drugs, *Medical Clinics of North America*, 58: 1019-26, 1974.

1219. Ketel, W. B. and Hughes, J. R., Toxic encephalopathy with seizures secondary to ingestion of composition C-4, *Neurology*, 22: 871-876, 1972.

1220. Kizer, J. S., Vargas-Cordon, M., Brendel, K., and Bressler, R., The *in vitro* inhibition of insulin secretion by diphenylhydantoin, *J. Clin. Invest.*, 49: 1942-1948, 1970.

1221. Kleinfeld, M. and Stein, E., Effects of diphenylhydantoin on action potentials of canine Purkinje and ventricular fibers, *Circulation*, 38: 116, 1968.

1222. Knopp, R. H., Sheinin, J. C., and Freinkel, N., Diphenylhydantoin and an insulin-secreting islet adenoma, *Arch. Intern. Med.*, 130: 904-908, 1972.

1223. Kobayashi, I., Yamashita, Y., and Yamazaki, H., Onset of systemic lupus erythematosus during the long-term administration of diphenylhydantoin, *Nippon Naika Gakkai Zasshi*, 60: 851-854, 1971.

1224. Koch-Weser, J., Antiarrhythmic prophylaxis in ambulatory patients with coronary heart disease, *Arch. Intern. Med.*, 129: 763-772, 1972.

1225. Koch, A., Higgins, R., Sande, M., Tierney, J., and Tulin, R., Enhancement of renal Na⁺ transport by Dilantin, *Physiologist*, 5: 168, 1962.

1226. Koch, H. U., Kraft, D., Von Herrath, D., and Schaefer, K., Influence of diphenylhydantoin and phenobarbital on intestinal calcium transport in the rat, *Epilepsy Abstracts*, 6: 109, 1973.

1227. Kootstra, A. and Woodhouse, S. P., The effect of diphenylhydantoin on the Na⁺-K⁺-stimulated ouabain-inhibited ATPase, *Proceedings of the University of Otago Medical School*, 52: 6-7, 1974.

1228. Koppe, J. G., Bosman, W., Oppers, V. M., Spaans, F., and Kloosterman, G. J., Epilepsy and congenital anomalies, *Ned. T. Geneesk.*, 117: 220-224, 1973. (*cf.* Loughnan, et al., *Lancet*, 70, 1973.)

1229. Kormendy, C. G. and Bender, A. D., Experimental modification of the chemistry and biology of the aging process, *J. Pharm. Sci.*, 60: 167-180, 1971.

1230. Koski, C. L., Rifenberick, D. H., and Max, S. R., Energy metabolism in steroid atrophy, *Neurology*, 4: 352, 1974.

1231. Kostov, K. G., Tachev, A. M. and Nastev, G. T., The problem of pseudomyotonia (Isaac's syndrome), *Zh. Neuropatol. Psikhiatr. Korsakov*, 73: 825-829, 1973.

1232. Krasner, J., Drug-protein interaction, *Pediat. Clin. N. Amer.*, 19: 51-63, 1972.

1233. Krasner, J., Giacoia, G. P., and Yaffe, S. J., Drug protein binding in the newborn infant, *Pediat. Res.*, 7: 317, 1973.

1234. Krell, R. D. and Goldberg, A. M., Effect of diphenylhydantoin and ethanol feeding on the synthesis of rat liver folates from exogenous pteroylglutamate (³H), *Epilepsy Abstracts*, 7: 195, 1974.

1235. Krikler, D. M., A fresh look at cardiac arrhythmias, *Lancet*, 1034-1037, 1974.

1236. Krsiak, M. and Steinberg, H., Psychopharmacological aspects of aggression: a review of the literature and some new experiments, *J. Psychosom. Res.*, 13: 243-252, 1969.

1237. Kruger, G., Effect of Dilantin in mice. 1. Changes in lymphoreticular tissue after acute exposure, *Virshows Arch.* (Path. Anat.), 349: 297-311, 1970. (*cf.* Juhasz, et al., *Acta Morphol. Acad. Sci. Hung.*, 18: 147, 1970.)

1238. Krupin, T., Podos, S. M., and Becker, B., Effect of diphenylhydantoin on dexamethasone suppression of plasma cortisol in primary open-angle glaucoma, *Amer. J. Ophthal.*, 71: 997-1002, 1971.

1239. Kuiper, J. J., Lymphocytic thyroiditis possibly induced by diphenylhydantoin, *JAMA*, 210: 2370-2372, 1969.

1240. Kuntzman, R. and Southern, A. L., The effects of CNS active drugs on the metabolism of steroids in man, *Adv. Biochem. Psychopharmacol.*, 1: 205-217, 1969.

1241. Kupferberg, H. J., Quantitative estimation of diphenylhydantoin, primidone and phenobarbital in plasma by gas-liquid chromatography, *Clin. Chim. Acta*, 29: 283-288, 1970.

1242. Kuroiwa, Y. and Araki, S., Lhermitte's sign and reflex tonic spasm in demyelinating diseases with special reference to their localizing value, *Kyushu J. Med. Sci.*, 14: 29-38, 1963.

1243. Kuroiwa, Y. and Shibasaki, H., Painful tonic seizures in multiple sclerosis—treatment with diphenylhydantoin and carbamazepine, *Folia. Psychiat. Neurol. Jap.*, 22: 107-119, 1968.

1244. Kutt, H. and Fouts, J. R., Diphenylhydantoin metabolism by rat liver microsomes and some of the effects of drug or chemical pretreatment on diphenylhydantoin metabolism by rat liver microsomal preparations, *J. Pharmacol. Exp. Ther.*, 176: 11-26, 1970.

1245. Kutt, H. and Penry, J. K., Usefulness of blood levels of antiepileptic drugs, *Arch. Neurol.*, 31: 283-288, 1974.

1246. Kutt, H. and Verebely, K., Metabolism of diphenylhy-

dantoin by rat liver microsomes, *Biochem. Pharmacol.*, 19: 675-686, 1970.

1247. Kutt, H., Biochemical and genetic factors regulating Dilantin metabolism in man, *Ann. N.Y. Acad. Sci.*, 179: 704-722, 1971.

1248. Kutt, H., Diphenylhydantoin interactions with other drugs in man, *Antiepileptic Drugs*, 169-180, Woodbury, D. M., Penry, J. K., and Schmidt, R. P., Eds., Raven Press, New York, 1972. (*cf.* Evans, et al., *Lancet*, 517, 1970.)

1249. Kutt, H., Diphenylhydantoin relation of plasma levels to clinical control, *Antiepileptic Drugs*, 211-218, Woodbury, D. M., Penry, J. K., and Schmidt, R. P., Eds., Raven Press, New York, 1972.

1250. Kutt, H., Haynes, J., Verebely, K. and McDowell, F., The effect of phenobarbital on plasma diphenylhydantoin level and metabolism in man and rat liver microsomes, *Epilepsy Abstracts*, 3: 4, 1970.

1251. Kutt, H., Waters, L., and Fouts, J. R., Diphenylhydantoin-induced difference spectra with rat-liver microsomes, *Chem. Biol. Interactions*, 2: 195-202, 1970.

1252. Kutt, H., Waters, L., and Fouts, J. R., The effects of some stimulators (inducers) of hepatic microsomal drug-metabolizing enzyme activity on substrate-induced difference spectra in rat liver microsomes, *J. Pharmacol. Exp. Ther.*, 179: 101-113, 1971.

1253. Kwalick, D. S., Anticonvulsants and DDT residues, *JAMA*, 215: 120-121, 1971.

1254. Kyosola, K., Abdominal epilepsy, *Ann. Chir. Gyanaec. Fenn.*, 62: 101-103, 1973.

1255. Lamprecht, F., Epilepsy and schizophrenia: a neurochemical bridge, *Epilepsy Abstracts*, 7: 190, 1974.

1256. Landolt, A. M., Treatment of acute post-operative inappropriate antidiuretic hormone secretion with diphenylhydantoin, *Acta Endocr.*, 76: 625-628, 1974.

1257. Larsen, P. R., Atkinson, A. J., Wellman, H. N., and Goldsmith, R. E., Effect of diphenylhydantoin on thyroxine metabolism in man, *J. Clin. Invest.*, 49: 1266-1279, 1970.

1258. Lascelles, P. T., Kocen, R. S., and Reynolds, E. H., The distribution of plasma phenytoin levels in epileptic patients, *J. Neurol. Neurosurg. Psychiat.*, 33: 501-505, 1970.

1259. Lasser, R. P., Management of arrhythmia, *New York J. Med.*, 73: 1775-1777, 1973.

1260. Latham, A. N., Millbank, L., Richens, A., and Rowe, D. J. F., Liver enzyme induction by anticonvulsant drugs, and its relationship to disturbed calcium and folic acid metabolism, *J. Clin. Pharmacol.*, 13: 337-342, 1973.

1261. Lawrence. T., Antiarrhythmic drugs, *Topics on Medicinal Chemistry*, 3:360-363, Wiley-Interscience, New York, 1970.

1262. Lee, S. I. and Bass, N. H., Microassay of diphenylhydantoin: blood and regional brain concentrations in rats during acute intoxication, *Neurology*, 20: 115-124, 1970.

1263. Lefebvre, E. B., Haining, R. G., and Labbe, R. F., Coarse facies, calvarial thickening and hyperphosphatasia associated with long-term anticonvulsant therapy, *New Eng. J. Med.*, 286: 1301-1302, 1972. (*cf.* Falcone and Davidson, *Lancet*, 2: 1112, 1973, Griscom, *New Eng. J. Med.*, 287: 722, 1972, Lefebvre, et al., Nellhaus and Poskanzer, *ibid.*)

1264. Lesbre, J. P., Cathala, B., Salvador, M., Florio, R. Lescure, F., and Meriel, P., Diphenylhydantoin and digitalis toxicity, *Arch. Mal. Coeur.*, 62: 412-437, 1969.

1265. Lesne, M., Sturbois, X. and Wilmotte, L., Modifications by diphenylhydantoin of the pharmacokinetic of digitoxin in the rat, *J. Pharmacol.*, 5: 75-86, 1974.

1266. Letteri, J. M., Mellk, H., Louis, S., Kutt, H., Durante, P., and Glazko, A., Diphenylhydantoin metabolism in uremia, *New Eng. J. Med.*, 285: 648-652, 1971.

1267. LeVan, H., Gordon, P., and Stefani, S., Enhancement of radioresistance in mice treated with diphenylhydantoin, *J. Pharm. Sci.*, 59: 1178-1179, 1970.

1268. LeVan, H., Gordon, P., and Stefani, S., Effect of diphenylhydantoin on survival and morphology of Ehrlich ascites tumor mice, *Oncology*, 26: 25-32, 1972.

1269. Levin, S. R., Booker, J., Smith, D. F., and Grodsky, G. M., Inhibition of insulin secretion by diphenylhydantoin in the isolated perfused pancreas, *J. Clin. Endocr.*, 300: 400-401, 1970.

1270. Levin, S. R., Charles, M. A., O'Connor, M., and Grodsky, G. M., Use of diphenylhydantoin and diazoxide to investigate insulin secretory mechanisms, *Presented at the 8th Congress of International Diabetes Federation*, Brussels, Belgium, 1973.

1271. Levin, S. R., Charles, M. A., O'Connor, M., Hagura, R., Smith, D., and Grodsky, G. M., Comparative effects of diphenylhydantoin (DPH) and diazoxide (DZ) upon biphasic insulin secretion from the isolated, perfused rat pancreas, with computerized correlation of biologic responses. *Presented at the 8th Congress of International Diabetes Federation*, Brussels, Belgium, 1973.

1272. Levin, S. R., Grodsky, G., Hagura, R., Smith, D., Licko, V., and Forsham, P., Comparison of effects of diphenylhydantoin and diazoxide on insulin secretion in the isolated perfused rat pancreas, using computerized correlation of experimental data, *Clin. Res.*, 19: 375, 1971.

1273. Levin, S. R., Grodsky, G. M., Hagura, R., and Smith, D., Comparison of the inhibitory effects of diphenylhydantoin and diazoxide upon insulin secretion from the isolated perfused pancreas, *Diabetes*, 21: 856-862, 1972. (*cf.* Goldberg, *Diabetes*, 18: 101, 1969.)

1274. Levin, S. R., Reed, J. W., Ching, K. N., Davis, J. W., and Blum, R., Inhibition of insulin secretion after diphenylhydantoin (DPH) in diabetes and in obesity, *Clin. Res.*, 20: 198, 1972.

1275. Levin, S. R., Reed, J. W., Ching, K. N., Davis, J. W., Blum, M. R., and Forsham, P. H., Diphenylhydantion: its use in detecting early insulin secretory defects in patients with mild glucose intolerance, *Diabetes*, 22: 194-201, 1973.

1276. Levine, M. C., Reactions to anticonvulsants, *New Eng. J. Med.*, 286: 1217, 1972.

1277. Levitt, B., Raines, A., Sohn, Y. J., Standaert, F. G., and Hirshfeld, J. W., The nervous system as a site of action for digitalis and antiarrhythmic drugs, *Mt. Sinai Med. J.*, 37: 227-240, 1970.

1278. Levitt, M., Nixon, P. F., Pincus, J. H., and Bertino, J. R., Transport characteristics of folates in cerebrospinal fluid; a study utilizing doubly labeled 5-methyltetrahydrofolate and 5-formyltetrahydrofolate, *J. Clin. Invest.*, 50: 1301-1308, 1971.

1279. Levo, Y., The protective effect of hydantoin treatment on carcinogenesis, *Naunyn-Schmiedeberg's Arch. Pharmacol.*, 285: 29-30, 1974.

1280. Levy, J. A., Wittig, E. O., Ferraz, E. C. F., Scleroderma associated with continuous electro-muscular activity, *Arq. Neuro-Psiquiat.*, 23: 283-287, 1965.

1281. Levy, R. H., and Smith, G. H., Dosage regimens of antiarrhythmics, Part 1: Pharmacokinetic properties, *Amer. J. Hosp. Pharm.*, 30: 398-404, 1973.

1282. Lew, G. M., Increased hypothalamic norepinephrine in genetically hypertensive rats following administration of diphenylhydantoin, *Proc. Soc. Exp. Biol. Med.*, 148: 30-32, 1975.

1283. Lewin, E. and Bleck, V., The effect of diphenylhydantoin administration on sodium-potassium-activated ATPase in cortex, *Neurology*, 21: 647-651, 1971.

1284. Lewin, E. and Bleck, V., The effect of diphenylhydantoin administration on cortex potassium-activated phosphatase, *Neurology*, 21: 417-418, 1971.

1285. Lewin, E., Charles, G., and McCrimmon, A., Discharging cortical lesions produced by freezing—the effect of anticonvulsants on sodium-potassium-activated ATPase, sodium and potassium in cortex, *Neurology*, 19: 565-569, 1969.

1286. Lien, E. J., and Gudauskas, G. A., Structure side-effect sorting of drugs—I: Extrapyramidal syndrome, *J. Pharm. Sci.*, 62: 645-647, 1973.

1287. Lifshitz, F. and Maclaren, N. K., Vitamin D-dependent rickets in institutionalized, mentally retarded children receiving long-term anticonvulsant therapy, *J. Pediat.*, 83: 612-620, 1973.

1288. Lightfoot, R. W., Jr., and Christian, C. L., Serum protein binding of thyroxine and diphenylhydantoin, *J. Clin. Endocr.*, 26: 305-308, 1966.

1289. Linde, L. M., Turner, S. W., and Awa, S., Present status and treatment of paroxysmal supraventricular tachycardia, *Pediatrics*, 50: 127-130, 1972.

1290. Lipicky, R. J., Gilbert, D. L., and Stillman, I. M., The effects of diphenylhydantoin on voltage-dependent currents of the squid axon, *Fed. Proc.*, 30: Abstract 65, 1971.

1291. Lipicky, R. J., Gilbert, D. L., and Stillman, I. M., Diphenylhydantoin inhibition of sodium conductance in squid giant axon, *Proc. Nat. Acad. Sci.*, 69: 1758-1760, 1972.

1292. Lisak, R. P., Lebeau, J., Tucker, S. H, and Rowland, L. P., Hyperkalemic periodic paralysis and cardiac arrhythmia, *Neurology*, 22: 810-815, 1972.

1293. Livingston, S., Abdominal pain as a manifestation of epilepsy (abdominal epilepsy) in children. *J. Pediat.*, 38: 687-695, 1951.

1294. Livingston, S. and Livingston, H. L., Diphenylhydantoin gingival hyperplasia, *Amer. J. Dis. Child.*, 117: 265-270, 1969.

1295. Livingston, S. and Pauli, L. L., Diphenylhydantoin and blood dyscrasias, *JAMA*, 320: 211-212, 1974.

1296. Livingston, S., Berman, W., and Pauli, L. L., Anticonvulsant drugs and vitamin D metabolism, *JAMA*, 224: 1634-1635, 1973.

1297. Livingston, S., Berman, W., and Pauli, L. L., Anticonvulsant drugs and vitamin D metabolism, *JAMA*, 226: 787, 1973.

1298. Livingston, S., Berman, W., and Pauli, L. L., Maternal epilepsy and abnormalities of the fetus and newborn, *Lancet*, 2: 1265, 1973.

1299. Lockman, L. A., Hunninghake, D. B., Krivit, W., and Desnick, R. J., Relief of pain of Fabry's disease by diphenylhydantoin, *Neurology*, 23: 871-875, 1973.

1300. Lockman, L. A., Krivit, W., and Desnick, R. J., Relief of the painful crises of Fabry's disease by diphenylhydantoin, *Neurology*, 21: 423, 1971.

1301. Loeser, J. D., Neuralgia, *Postgrad. Med.*, 53: 207-210, 1973.

1302. Lohrenz, J. G., Levy, L., and Davis, J. F., Schizophrenia or epilepsy? A problem in differential diagnosis, *Compr. Psychiat.*, 3: 54-62, 1962.

1303. Longshaw, R. N., Inhibition of hepatic drug metabolism, *Drug Intelligence and Clinical Pharmacy*, 7: 263-270, 1973.

1304. Looker, A. and Conners, C. K., Diphenylhydantoin in children with severe temper tantrums, *Arch. Gen. Psychiat.*, 23: 80-89, 1970.

1305. Loong, S. C. and Ong, Y. Y., Paroxysmal kinesigenic choreoathetosis, *J. Neurol. Neurosurg. Psychiat.*, 36: 921-924, 1973.

1306. Lotti, V. J., Torchiana, M. L., and Porter, C. C., Investigations on the action and mechanism of action of diphenylhydantoin as an antagonist of tetrabenazine and reserpine, *Arch. Int. Pharmacodyn.*, 203: 107-116, 1973.

1307. Lotto, A., Sanna, G. P., Bossi, M., and Lomanto, B., New therapeutic aspects of ventricular arrhythmias, *Cardiol. Prat.*, 22: 1-15, 1971.

1308. Louis, S., Kutt, H. and McDowell, F., Modification of experimental seizures and anticonvulsant efficacy by peripheral stimulation, *Neurology*, 21: 329-336, 1971.

1309. Lovell, R. R. H., Mitchell. M. E., Prineas, R. J., Sloman, J. G., Vajda, F. J., Pitt, A., Habersberger, P., Rosenbaum, M., Nestel, P. J., Goodman, H. T., and Sowry, G. S. C., Phenytoin after recovery from myocardial infarction—controlled trial in 568 patients, *Lancet*, 1055-1057, 1971.

1310. Lowe, C. R., Congenital malformations among infants

born to epileptic women, *Lancet*, 9-10, 1973. (*cf.* Marsh and Fraser, *Teratology*, 7: A-23, 1973.)

1311. Lown, B., Temte, J. V. and Arter, W. J., Ventricular tachyarrhythmias—clinical aspects, *Circulation*, 47: 1364-1381, 1973.

1312. Lucchesi, B. R., The pharmacology and clinical uses of antiarrhythmic drugs, *U. Michigan Med. Cent. J.*, 37: 61-73, 1971.

1313. Ludtke, A. H., Autenrieth, G., and Dankert, D., On the effects of diphenylhydantoin, potassium-magnesium-asparaginate, insulin and female sex hormones on the hypothermic fibrillation threshold of the guinea-pig heart, *Arzneimittelforschung*, 20: 1554-1557, 1970.

1314. Lund, L., Berlin, A., and Lunde, K. M., Plasma protein binding of diphenylhydantoin in patients with epilepsy, *Clin. Pharmacol. Ther.*, 13: 196-200, 1972.

1315. Lunde, K. M., Plasma protein binding of diphenylhydantoin in man, *Acta Pharmacol.*, 29: 152-155, 1971.

1316. Lunde, K. M., Rane, A., Yaffe, S. J., Lund, L., and Sjoqvist, F., Plasma protein binding of diphenylhydantoin in man, *Clin. Pharmacol. Ther.*, 11: 846-855, 1970.

1317. Lund, L., Lunde, P. K., Rane, A., Borga, O. and Sjoqvist, F., Plasma protein binding, plasma concentrations, and effects of diphenylhydantoin in man, *Ann. N.Y. Acad. Sci.*, 179: 723-728, 1972.

1318. Lussier-Lazaroff, J. and Fletcher, B. D., Rickets and anticonvulsant therapy in children: a roentgenologic investigation, *J. Canad. Assn. Radiol.*, 22: 144-147, 1971.

1319. Lutz, E. G., Add vitamins to DPH, urges doctor, *National Spokesman*, 6: 7, 1973.

1320. Lutz, E. G., On vitamins and anticonvulsants, *Medical World News*, 3, 1973.

1321. Mace, J., and Schneider, S., Diphenylhydantoin and rickets, *Lancet*, 1119, 1973.

1322. MacGee, J., The rapid determination of diphenylhydantoin in blood plasma by gas-liquid chromatography, *Med. Res. Lab., V.A. Hosp. and Dept. Bio. Chem. and Exp. Med.*, Cincinnati, Ohio, 1970.

1323. MacKinney, A. A. and Booker, H. E., Diphenylhydantoin effects on human lymphocytes *in vitro* and *in vivo*, *Arch. Intern. Med.*, 129: 988-992, 1972.

1324. MacKinney, A. A. and Vyas, R., Diphenylhydantoin-induced inhibition of nucleic acid synthesis in cultured human lymphocytes, *Proc. Soc. Exp. Biol. Med.*, 141: 89-92, 1972.

1325. Mackinney, A. A. and Vyas, R., The assay of diphenylhydantoin effects on growing human lymphocytes, *J. Pharmacol. Exp. Ther.*, 186: 37-43, 1973.

1326. Maclaren, N. and Lifshitz, F., Vitamin D-dependency rickets in institutionalized, mentally retarded children on long term anticonvulsant therapy. II. The response to 25-hydroxycholecalciferol and to vitamin D, *Pediat. Res.*, 7: 914-922, 1973.

1327. Madsen, S. N., Hansen, J. M. and Deckert, T., Intravenous glucose tolerance during treatment with phenytoin, *Acta Neurol. Scand.*, 50: 257-260, 1974.

1328. Maletzky, B. M. and Klotter, J., Episodic dyscontrol: A controlled replication, *Dis. Nerv. Syst.*, 35: 175-179, 1974.

1329. Maletzky, B. M., Treatable violence, *Med. Times*, 100: 74-79, 1972.

1330. Malherbe, C., Burrill, K. C., Levin, S. R., Karam, J. H., and Forsham, P. H., Effect of diphenylhydantoin on insulin secretion in man, *New Eng. J. Med.*, 286: 339-342, 1972.

1331. Markkanen, T., Himanen, P., Pajula, R. L., and Molnar, G., Binding of folic acid to serum proteins, *Acta Haemat.*, 50: 284-292, 1973.

1332. Markkanen, T., Peltola, O., Himanen, P. and Riekkinen, P., Metabolites of diphenylhydantoin in human plasma inhibits the pentose phosphate pathway of leukocytes, *Pharmacology*, 6: 216-222, 1971.

1333. Martin, C. M., Reliability in product performance in an innovative environment, The Economics of Drug Innovation,

63-82, Cooper, J. D., Ed., *The Proceedings of the First Seminar of Economics of Pharmaceutical Innovation*, 1969.

1334. Martin, W. and Rickers, J., Cholestatic hepatosis induced by diphenylhydantoin. Case report and review of literature, *Wien. Klin. Wschr.*, 84: 41-45, 1972.

1335. Mason, D. T., Amsterdam, E. A., Massumi, R. A., and Zelis, R., Recent advances in antiarrhythmic drugs: clinical pharmacology and therapeutics, *The Acute Cardiac Emergency—Diagnosis and Management*, 95-123, Eliot, R. S., Ed., Futura Publishing, Mount Kisco, New York, 1972.

1336. Mason, D. T., DeMaria, A. N., Amsterdam, E. A., Zelis, R., and Massumi, R. A., Antiarrhythmic agents. II: Therapeutic consideration, *Drugs*, 5: 292-317, 1973.

1337. Mason, D. T., DeMaria, A. N., Amsterdam, E. A., Zelis, R., and Massumi, R. A., Antiarrhythmic agents. I: Mechanisms of action and clinical pharmacology, *Drugs*, 5: 261-291, 1973.

1338. Mason, D. T., Spann, J. F. Jr., Zelis, R., and Amsterdam, E. A., Evolving concepts in the clinical pharmacology and therapeutic uses of the antiarrhythmic drugs, *Cardiovascular Therapy, The Art and the Science*, 122-137, Russek, H. I. and Zohman, B. L., Eds., The Williams & Wilkins Co, Baltimore, 1971.

1339. Mathur, K. S., Wahal, P. K., Seth, H. C. and Hazra, D. K., Diphenylhydantoin sodium in cardiac arrhythmias, *J. Indian Med. Assoc.*, 57: 256-258, 1971.

1340. Matsuzaki, M. and Killam, K. F., Alterations in conditional behavioral and electrographic responses to interrupted visual stimuli following repeated doses of diphenylhydantoin, *Fed. Proc.*, 30: Abstract 483, 1971.

1341. Mattes, L. M., Spritzer, R. C., Nevins, M. A., Weisenseel, A. C., Donoso, E., and Friedburg, C. K., The cardiovascular effects of diphenylhydantoin in patients with cardiac pacemakers, *Circulation*, 37-38 (Suppl. 6): 135, 1968.

1342. Matthews, W. B., Tonic seizures in disseminated sclerosis, *Brain*, 81: 193-206, 1958.

1343. Matthews, W. D. and Connor, J. D., Effects of diphenylhydantoin on interhippocampal evoked responses, *Pharmacologist*, 16: 228, 1974.

1344. Mattson, R. H., Gallagher, B. B., Reynolds, E. H., and Glass, D., Folate therapy in epilepsy, *Arch. Neurol.*, 29: 78-81, 1973.

1345. McAllister, R. G., Jr., The possible role of antiarrhythmic drugs in the prevention of sudden death, *Heart and Lung*, 2: 857-861, 1973.

1346. McCabe, B. F., Chronic burning tongue syndrome, *Ann. Otol. Rhinol. Laryngol.*, 83: 264, 1974.

1347. McCabe, W. S., and Habovick, J. A., Thorazine as an epileptogenic agent, *Amer. J. Psychiat.*, 120: 595-597, 1963.

1348. McIlvanie, S. K., Phenytoin and depression of immunological function, *Lancet*, 323, February, 1972.

1349. McQueen, E. G., Owen, D., and Ferry, D. G., Effect of phenytoin and other drugs in reducing serum DDT levels, *New Zeal. Med. J.*, 75: 208-211, 1972.

1350. Meadow, S. R., Anticonvulsant drugs and congenital abnormalities, *Lancet*, 2: 1296, 1968.

1351. Meikle, W., Jubiz, W., West, C. D., and Tyler, F. H., Effect of diphenylhydantoin (Dilantin) on the metyrapone test demonstrated by a new assay for plasma metyrapone, *Clin. Res.*, 17: 107, 1969.

1352. Melikian, V., Eddy, J. D., and Paton, A., The stimulant effect of drugs on indocyanine green clearance by the liver, *Gut*, 13: 755-758, 1972.

1353. Mendelson, J. H., Biologic concomitants of alcoholism, *New Eng. J. Med.*, 283: 24-32, 1970.

1354. Mennear, J. H. and Gossel, T. A., Inhibitory effect of diphenylhydantoin on the diabetogenic action of alloxan in the mouse, *Diabetes*, 21: 80-83, 1972.

1355. Mennear, J. H., and Gossel, T. A., Interactions between diphenylhydantoin and tolbutamide in mice, *Toxic. Appl. Pharmacol.*, 24: 309-316, 1973.

1356. Meyer, J. G., The teratological effects of anticonvulsants and the effects on pregnancy and birth, *Europ. Neurol.* 10: 179-190, 1973.

1357. Meyer, J. S., Binns, P. M., Ericsson, A. D., and Vulpe, M., Sphenopalatine ganglionectomy for cluster headache, *Arch. Otolaryng.*, 92: 475-484, 1970.

1358. Michell, A. R., The effect of diphenylhydantoin on sodium appetite in rats, *J. Physiol.*, 237: 53-55, 1973.

1359. Mick, B. A., Diphenylhydantoin and intermittent edema, *JAMA*, 225: 1533, 1973.

1360. Miley, C. E. and Forster, F. M., Paroxysmal signs and symptoms in multiple sclerosis, *Neurology*, 24: 458-461, 1974.

1361. Millichap, J. G., Clinical efficacy and usage of anticonvulsants, *Chemical Modulation of Brain Function*, 199-205, Sabelli, H. C., Ed., Raven Press, New York, 1973.

1362. Millichap, J. G., Drugs in management of minimal brain dysfunction, *Ann. N.Y. Acad. Sci.*, 205: 321-334, 1973.

1363. Millichap, J. G., Efficacy, therapeutic regimens of drugs to control hyperkinesis in children with minimal brain dysfunction reported from trials, *Drug Res. Rep.*, 15: S5-S11, 1972.

1364. Mirkin, B. L. and Wright, F., Drug interactions: effect of methylphenidate on the disposition of diphenylhydantoin in man, *Neurology*, 21: 1123-1128, 1971.

1365. Mirkin, B. L., Diphenylhydantoin: placental transport, fetal localization, neonatal metabolism, and possible teratogenic effects, *J. Pediat.*, 78: 329-337, 1971.

1366. Mirkin, B. L., Maternal and fetal distribution of drugs in pregnancy, *Clin. Pharmacol. Ther.*, 14: 643-647, 1973.

1367. Mirkin, B. L., Placental transfer and neonatal elimination of diphenylhydantoin, *Amer. J. Obstet. Gynec.*, 109: 930-933, 1971.

1368. Mittler, J. C. and Glick, S. M., Radioimmunoassayable oxytocin release from isolated neural lobes: responses to ions and drugs, *Abstracts Fourth Int. Cong. Endocr.*, 47, June, 1972.

1369. Mladinich, E. K., Diphenylhydantoin in the Wallenberg syndrome, *JAMA*, 230: 372-373, 1974.

1370. Monson, R. R., Rosenberg, L., Hartz, S. C., Shapiro, S., Heinonen, O. P., and Slone, D., Diphenylhydantoin and selected congenital malformations, *New Eng. J. Med.*, 289: 1050-1052, 1973.

1371. Morgan, R. J., Scleroderma: treatment with diphenylhydantoin, *Cutis*, 8: 278-282, 1971.

1372. Moss, A. J. and Patton, R. D., Diphenylhydantoin, comparison of antiarrhythmic agents, and management of refractory arrhythmias, *Antiarrhythmic Agents*, 52-58, 101-115, Charles C Thomas, Springfield, Ill., 1973.

1373. Moss, G. and Stein, A. A., Cerebral etiology of the shock lung syndrome: protective effect of diphenylhydantoin, *Personal Communication*, 1972.

1374. Moss, G., Shock, cerebral hypoxia and pulmonary vascular control: the centri-neurogenic etiology of the "respiratory distress syndrome", *Bull. N.Y. Acad. Med.*, 49: 689, 1973.

1375. Mountain, K. R., Hirsh, J., and Gallus, A. S., Neonatal coagulation defect due to anticonvulsant drug treatment in pregnancy, *Lancet*, 1: 265-268, 1970. (*cf.* Davies, *Lancet*, 1: 413, 1970.)

1376. Mouravieff-Lesuisse, F. and Giurgea, C., Influence of electro-convulsive shock on the fixation of an experience at spinal level, *Arch. Int. Pharmacodyn.*, 183: 410-411, 1970.

1377. Nabwangu, J. F., Head injury, *E. Afr. Med. J.*, 49: 624-629, 1972.

1378. Narisawa, K., Honda, Y., and Arakawa, T., Effect of diphenylhydantoin administration on single carbon metabolism in folate deficient rats, *Tohoku, J. Exp. Med.*, 110: 359-365, 1973.

1379. Nasello, A. G., Montini, E. E., and Astrada, C. A., Effect of veratrine, tetraethylammonium and diphenylhydantoin on potassium release by rat hippocampus, *Pharmacology*, 7: 89-95, 1972.

1380. Negri, S., An atypical case of Steinert's disease (myotonia dystrophica) in infancy, *Confin. Neurol.*, 33: 323-333, 1971.

1381. Neville, B. G. R., The origin of infantile spasms: evidence from a case of hydranencephaly, *Epilepsy Abstracts*, 6: 179, 1973.

1382. Newtown, R., Amitriptyline and imipramine poisoning in children, *Brit. Med. J.*, 2: 176, 1974.

1383. Nielsen, T. and Cotman, C., The binding of diphenylhydantoin to brain and subcellular fractions, *Europ. J. Pharmacol.*, 14: 344-350, 1971.

1384. Niswander, J. D. and Wertelecki, W., Congenital malformation among offspring of epileptic women, *Lancet*, 1062, May, 1973.

1385. Noach, E. L., VanRees, H. and DeWolff, F. A., Effects of Diphenylhydantoin (DPH) on absorptive processes in the rat jejunum, *Archives Internationales de Pharmacodynamie et de Therapie*, 206: 392-393, 1973.

1386. Norris, J. W. and Pratt, R. F., A controlled study of folic acid in epilepsy, *Neurology*, 21: 659-664, 1971.

1387. Nuki, K. and Cooper, S. H., The role of inflammation in the pathogenesis of gingival enlargement during the administration of diphenylhydantoin sodium in cats, *J. Periodont. Res.*, 7: 102-110, 1972.

1388. O'Leary, J. A., Feldman, M., and Switzer, H. E., Phenobarbital-Dilantin treatment of the intrauterine patient, *J. Reprod. Med.*, 5: 81-83, 1970.

1389. O'Malley, W. E., Denckla, M. B., and O'Doherty, D. S., Oral absorption of diphenylhydantoin as measured by gas liquid chromatography, *Epilepsy Abstracts*, 3: 230, 1970.

1390. O'Reilly, M. V. and MacDonald, R. T., Efficacy of phenytoin in the management of ventricular arrhythmias induced by hypokalaemia, *Brit. Heart J.*, 35: 631-634, 1973.

1391. Oates, R. K. and Tonge, R. E., Phenytoin and the pseudolymphoma syndrome, *Med. J. Aust.*, 371-373, 1971.

1392. Obbens, E. A., Experimental epilepsy induced by folate derivatives, *Epilepsy Abstracts*, 6: 221-222, 1973.

1393. Odar-Cederlof, I. and Borga, O., Kinetics of diphenylhydantoin in uraemic patients: consequences of decreased plasma protein binding, *Europ. J. Clin. Pharmacol.*, 7: 31-37, 1974.

1394. Oge, V., Drug therapy in alcoholism, *Ill. Med. J.*, 139: 606-610, 1971.

1395. Olds, M. E., Comparative effects of amphetamine, scopolamine, chlordiazepoxide, and diphenylhydantoin on operant and extinction behavior with brain stimulation and food reward, *Neuropharmacology*, 9: 519-532, 1970.

1396. Osorio, C., Jackson, D. J., Gartside, J. M., and Goolden, A. W. G., Effect of carbon dioxide and diphenylhydantoin on the partition of triiodothyronine labelled with iodine-131 between the red cells and plasma proteins, *Nature*, 196: 275-276, 1962.

1397. Overall, J. E., Brown, D., Williams, J. D., and Neill, L. T., Drug treatment of anxiety and depression in detoxified alcoholic patients, *Arch. Gen. Psychiat.*, 29: 218-221, 1973.

1398. Pakszys, W. and Domzal, T., Ceruloplasmin stimulation test, *Epilepsy Abstracts*, 7: 107, 1974.

1399. Pakszys, W., Phenytoin, *Epilepsy Abstracts*, 6: 236, 1973.

1400. Parisi, A. F. and Raines, A., Diphenylhydantoin suppression of repetitive activity generated in nerve endings, *Fed. Proc.*, Abstract 22: 390, 1963.

1401. Pashayan, H., Pruzansky, D., and Pruzansky, S., Are anticonvulsants teratogenic?, *Lancet*, 702-703, 1971.

1402. Patton, R. D., and Helfant, R. H., Atrial flutter with one-to-one conduction, *Dis. Chest*, 55: 250-251, 1969.

1403. Payen, J., A study of changes in the gum during treatment with diphenylhydantoin sodium, *Rev. Odonto-Stomatol.*, 19: 47-53, 1972.

1404. Pelkonen, R. and Taskinen, M. R., Effect of diphenylhydantoin on plasma-insulin in insulinoma, *Lancet*, 604-605, 1973.

1405. Pento, J. T., Glick, S. M., and Kagan, A., Diphenylhydantoin inhibition of glucagon- and calcium-stimulated calcitonin release, *Fed. Proc.*, Abstract 31: 251, 1972.

1406. Pento, J. T., Glick, S. M., and Kagan, A., Diphenylhydantoin inhibition of calcitonin secretion in the pig. *Endocrinology*, 92: 330-333, 1973.

1407. Penttila, O., Neuvonen, P. J., Aho, K. and Lehtovaara, R., Interaction between doxycycline and some antiepileptic drugs, *Brit. Med. J.*, 2: 470-472, 1974.

1408. Persijn, G. G. and Van Zeben, W., Generalized lymphadenopathy caused by phenytoin in a six-year-old child, *Epilepsy Abstracts*, 6: 236, 1973.

1409. Peter, J. B., A (Na$^+$ + K$^+$) ATPase of sarcolemma from skeletal muscle, *Biochem. Biophys. Res. Commun.*, 40: 1362-1367, 1970.

1410. Peters, B. H. and Samaan, N. A., Hyperglycemia with relative hypoinsulinemia in diphenylhydantoin toxicity, *New Eng. J. Med.*, 281: 91-92, 1969.

1411. Petroski, D. and Patel, A. N., Diphenylhydantoin for intractable hiccups, *Lancet*, 1: 739, 1974.

1412. Pezcon, J. D., and Grant, W. M., Sedatives, stimulants, and intraocular pressure in glaucoma, *Arch. Ophthal.*, 72: 177-188, 1964.

1413. Pezzimenti, J. F. and Hahn, A. L., Anicteric hepatitis induced by diphenylhydantoin, *Arch. Intern. Med.*, 125: 118-120, 1970.

1414. Phillips, J. R. and Eldridge. F. L., Respiratory myoclonus (Leeuwenhoek's disease), *New Eng. J. Med.*, 289: 1390-1395. 1973.

1415. Pinto, A., Simopoulos, A. M., Uhlenhuth, E. H. and De Rosa, E. R., Responses of chronic schizophrenic females to a combination of diphenylhydantoin and neuroleptics: a double-blind study, *Comprehensive Psychiatry*, 16(6): 529-536, 1975.

1416. Pincus, J. H. and Lee, S. H., Diphenylhydantoin and norepinephrine release, *Neurology*, 22: 410, 1972.

1417. Pincus, J. H., and Lee, S. H., Diphenylhydantoin and calcium in relation to norepinephrine release from brain slices, *Arch. Neurol.*, 29: 239-244, 1973.

1418. Pincus, J. H., Diphenylhydantoin and ion flux in lobster nerve, *Arch. Neurol.*, 26: 4-10, 1972.

1419. Pincus, J. H., Grove, I., Marino. B. B. and Glaser, G. E., Studies on the mechanism of action of diphenylhydantoin, *Presented at the International Soc. Neurochem.*, September, 1969.

1420. Pinkhas, J., Ben-Bassat, M., and DeVries, A., Death in anticonvulsant-induced megaloblastic anemia, *JAMA*, 224: 246, 1973.

1421. Podos, S. M., Becker, B., Beaty, C., and Cooper, D. G., Diphenylhydantoin and cortisol metabolism in glaucoma, *Amer J. Ophthal.*, 74: 498-500, 1972.

1422. Podos, S. M., Glaucoma, *Invest. Ophthal.*, 12: 3-4, 1973.

1423. Poley, J. R., and Bhatia, M., Recurrent abdominal pain: recurrent controversy, *Pediatrics*, 52: 144-145, 1973.

1424. Pollen, R. H., Cat-scratch encephalitis, *Neurology*, 18: 1031-1033, 1968.

1425. Porciello, P. I. and Zanini, S., Diphenylhydantoin: antiarrhythmic drug, *Fracastoro*, 64: 114-135, 1971.

1426. Porciello, P. I., Zanini, S., and Poppi, A., Comparative considerations on two modern antiarrhythmic drugs: lidocaine and diphenylhydantoin, *G. Ital. Cardiol.* 2: 579-583, 1972.

1427. Poschel, B. P. H., A simple and specific screen for benzodiazepine-like drugs, *Psychopharmacologia*, 19: 193-198, 1971.

1428. Postlethwaite, R. J. and Price, D. A., Amitriptyline and imipramine poisoning in children, *Brit. Med. J.*, 2: 504, 1974.

1429. Preston, T. A., Yates, J. D., and Brymer, J. F., Three therapeutic approaches in tachycardia, *Geriatrics*, 28: 110-116, 1973.

1430. Price, D. A. and Postlethwaite, J. R., Amitriptyline and imipramine poisoning in children, *Brit. Med. J.*, 1: 575, 1974.

1431. Pryles, C. V., Livingston, S. and Ford, F. R., Familial paroxysmal choreoathetosis of Mount and Reback, *Pediatrics*, 9: 44-47, 1952.

1432. Puri, P. S., The effect of diphenylhydantoin sodium (Dilantin) on myocardial contractility and hemodynamics, *Amer. Heart J.*, 82: 62-68, 1971.

1433. Puro, D. .G. and Woodward, D. J., Effects of diphenylhydantoin on activity of rat cerebellar Purkinje cells, *Neuropharmacology*, 12: 433-440, 1973.

1434. Quiret, J. C., Bens, J. L., Duboisset, M., Lesbre, P. and Bernasconi, P., Diphenylhydantoin injectable in cardiology, *Arch. Mal. Coeur.*, 67: 87-96, 1974.

1435. Raines, A. and Standaert, F. G., Effects of anticonvulsant drugs on nerve terminals, *Epilepsia*, 10: 211-227, 1969.

1436. Raines, A., Levitt, B., Standaert, F. G. and Sohn, Y. J., The influence of sympathetic nervous activity on the antiarrhythmic efficacy of diphenylhydantoin, *Europ. J. Pharmacol.*, 11: 293-297, 1970.

1437. Raines, A., Sohn, Y. J., and Levitt, B., Spinal excitatory and depressant effects of sodium diphenylthiohydantoinate, *J. Pharmacol. Exp. Ther.*, 177: 350-359, 1971.

1438. Raines, A., Effects of diphenylhydantoin on post-tetanic alterations in the terminals of dorsal root fibers and motor nerves, *Georgetown University Doctoral Thesis*, June, 1965.

1439. Ralston, A. J., Snaith, R. P., and Hinley, J. B., Effects of folic acid on fit-frequency and behaviour in epileptics on anticonvulsants, *Lancet*, 1: 867-868, 1970.

1440. Ramdohr, Von B., Schuren, K. P., Dennert, J., Macha, H.-N. and Schroder, R., Influence of diphenylhydantoin on hemodynamics in recent myocardial infarct., *Verhandlungen der Deutschen Gesellschaft fur Kreislaufforschung*, 35: 444-50, 1969.

1441. Rane, A., Garle, M., Borga, O., Sjoqvist, F., Plasma disappearance of transplacentally transferred diphenylhydantoin in the newborn studied with mass fragmentography, *Clin. Pharmacol. Ther.* 15: 39-45, 1974.

1442. Rane, A., Lunde, P. K. M., Jalling, B., et al., Plasma protein binding of diphenylhydantoin in normal and hyperbilirubinemic infants, *Epilepsy Abstracts*, 4: 223, 1971.

1443. Rane, A., Urinary excretion of diphenylhydantoin metabolites in newborn infant, *J. Pediat.*, 85: 543-545, 1974.

1444. Raskin, N. H., Levinson, S. A., Pickett, J. B., Hoffman, P. M., and Fields, H. L., Postsympathectomy neuralgia, *Amer. J. Surg.*, 128: 75-78, 1974.

1445. Raskovic, J., Phenomenological aspects of the psychotic epileptic state in terms of therapeutic argument, *Neuropsihialrya*, 20: 161-166, 1972.

1446. Ray, A. K., and Rao, D. B., Calcium metabolism in elderly epileptic patients during anticonvulsant therapy, *Epilepsy Abstracts*, 7: 210, 1974.

1447. Raz, S., Zeigler, M., and Caine, M., The effect of diphenylhydantoin on the urethra, *Invest. Urol.*, 10: 293-294, 1973.

1448. Reidenberg, M. M., Odar-Cederlof, I., Von Bahr, C., Borga, O., and Sjoqvist, F., Protein binding of diphenylhydantoin and desmethylimipramine in plasma from patients with poor renal function, *New Eng. J. Med.*, 285: 264-267, 1971.

1449. Reimann, H. A., Abdominal epilepsy and migraine, *JAMA*, 224: 128, 1973.

1450. Reimann, R., Lemmel, W., and Theisen, K., Efficacy and risks of diphenylhydantoin in cardiac arrhythmias, *Munchen Med. Wschr.*, 113: 893-899, 1971.

1451. Reizenstein, P. and Lund, L., Effect of anticonvulsive drugs on folate absorption and the cerebrospinal folate pump, *Epilepsy Abstracts*, 7: 86, 1974.

1452. Remmer, H., Induction of drug metabolizing enzyme system in the liver, *Eur. J. Clin. Pharmacol.*, 5: 116-136, 1972.

1453. Resnekov, L., Drug therapy before and after the electroversion of cardiac dysrhythmias, *Progr. Cardiovasc. Dis.*, 16: 531-538, 1974.

1454. Rettura, G., Stamford, W. and Seifter, E., Reversal of cardiac calcification by diphenylhydantoin, *Paper presented at N.E. Regional Meeting of the American Chemical Society*, Oct. 1973.

1455. Reynolds, E. H., Anticonvulsant drugs, folic acid metabolism and schizophrenia-like psychoses in epilepsy, *Psychische Sto-*

rungen bei Epilepsie, H. Penin, Ed., F. K. Schattauer Verlag, Stuttgart-New York, 1973.

1456. Reynolds, E. H., Anticonvulsant drugs, folic acid metabolism, fit frequency and psychiatric illness, *Psychiat. Neurol. Neurochir.,* 74: 167-174, 1971.

1457. Reynolds, E. H., Anticonvulsants, folic acid and epilepsy, *Lancet,* 1376-1378, June, 1973.

1458. Reynolds, E. H., Chanarin, I., Milner, G. and Matthews, D. M., Anticonvulsant therapy, folic acid and vitamin B[12] metabolism and mental symptoms, *Epilepsia,* 7: 261-270, 1966.

1459. Reynolds, E. H., Mattson, R., and Gallagher, B., Relationships between serum and cerebrospinal fluid anticonvulsant drug and folic acid concentrations in epileptic patients, *Neurology,* 22: 841-844, 1972.

1460. Reynolds, E. H., Streiff, R. R., Wilder, B. J., and Hammer, R. H., Diphenylhydantoin hematologic aspects of toxicity, *Antiepileptic Drugs,* 247-266, Woodbury, D. M., Penry, J. K., and Schmidt, R. P., Eds., Raven Press, New York, 1972. (*cf.* Bottomley, et al., *J. Mich. Dent. Ass.,* 53: 256, 1971 and Kolodzieczak and Prazanowski, *Epilepsy Abstracts,* 5: 149, 1972.)

1461. Reynolds, J. W. and Mirkin, B. L., Urinary corticosteroid and diphenylhydantoin metabolite patterns in neonates exposed to anticonvulsant drugs in utero, *JAMA,* 227: 577, 1974.

1462. Rhee, R. S., Margolin, M., and Pellock, J., Palatal myoclonus and diphenylhydantoin therapy, *New Eng. J. Med.,* 290: 1088-1089, 1974.

1463. Richens, A. and Houghton, G. W., Phenytoin intoxication caused by sulthiame, *Lancet,* 1442-1443, 1973.

1464. Richens, A. and Rowe, D. J. F., Disturbance of calcium metabolism by anticonvulsant drugs, *Brit. Med. J.,* 4: 73-76, 1970.

1465. Richens, A. and Rowe. D. J. F., Anticonvulsant hypocalcemia, *Epilepsy Abstracts,* 5: 224, 1972.

1466. Riddell, D. and Leonard, B. E., Some properties of a coma producing material obtained from mammalian brain, *Neuropharmacology,* 9: 283-299, 1970.

1467. Riehl, J. L. and McIntyre, H. B., Acute effects of Dilantin on the EEG of epileptic patients: a quantitative study, *Electroenceph. Clin. Neurophysiol.,* 28: 94, 1970.

1468. Rifkind, A. B., Gillette, P. N., Song, C. S., and Kappas, A., Drug stimulation of δ-Aminolevulinic acid synthetase and cytochrome P-450 *in vivo* in chick embryo liver, *J. Pharmacol. Exp. Ther.,* 185: 214-225, 1973.

1469. Riker, W. F., The pharmacology of the neostigmine-like facilitatory drug effect at the mammalian neuromuscular junction, *Jap. J. Pharmacol.,* 22: 1, 1972.

1470. Rish, B. L. and Caveness, W. F., Relation of prophylactic medication to the occurrence of early seizures following craniocerebral trauma, *J. Neurosurg.,* 38: 155-158, 1973.

1471. Rizzo, M., Morselli, P. L. and Garattini, S., Further observations on the interactions between phenobarbital and diphenylhydantoin during chronic treatment in the rat, *Biochem. Pharmacol.,* 21: 449-454, 1972.

1472. Robbins, M. M., Aplastic anemia secondary to anticonvulsants, *Amer. J. Dis. Child.,* 104: 64-74, 1962.

1473. Roberts, E., An hypothesis suggesting that there is a defect in the GABA system in schizophrenia, *Neurosciences Research Program Bulletin,* 10: 468-482, 1972.

1474. Roberts, J., The effect of diphenylhydantoin on the response to accelerator nerve stimulation, *Proc. Soc. Exp. Biol. Med.,* 134: 274-280, 1970.

1475. Robineaux, R., Lorans, G., and Beaure D'Augeres, C., Action of diphenylhydantoin on the growth and respiration of cell in culture, *Rev. Europ. Etudes Clin. Biol.,* 15: 1066-1071, 1970.

1476. Rockliff, B. W., and Davis, E. H., Controlled sequential trials of carbamazepine in trigeminal neuralgia, *Arch. Neurol.,* 15: 129-136, 1966.

1477. Rodman, N. F., McDevitt, N. B., and Almond, J. R.,

Platelet function inhibition by diphenylhydantoin, *Fed. Proc.,* 30: Abstract 513, 1971.

1478. Roman, I. C. and Caratzali, A., Effects of anticonvulsant drugs on chromosomes, *Brit. Med. J.,* 234, 1971.

1479. Romero, E., Maranon, A. and Bobillo, E. R., Antithyroid action of hydantoin derivatives, *Rev. Iber. Endocr.,* 101: 363-375, 1970.

1480. Rose, L. I., Williams, G. H., Jagger, P. I., Lauler, D. P., and Thorn, G. W., The paradoxical dexamethasone response phenomenon, *Metabolism,* 18: 369-375, 1969.

1481. Rosenthal, J. E. and Cohen, L. S., Therapeutic predicament—the unresponsive PVC, *Geriatrics,* 28: 88-92, 1973.

1482. Ross, G. S., A technique to study pain in monkeys; effect of drugs and anatomic lesions, *Henry Ford Hosp. Symposium on Pain,* Chap. 8, 100-101, Knighton, R. S. and Dumke, P. R., Eds., Little, Brown and Co., Boston, 1966.

1483. Ross, G. S., Effect of diphenylhydantoin on experimental pain in the monkey, *Neurology,* 15: 275, 1965.

1484. Ross, L. M., Diphenylhydantoin (DPH) induced cleft palate, *Teratology,* 7: A-26, June, 1973.

1485. Rovin, S., Sabes, W. R., Eversole, L. R., and Gordon, H. A., Dilantin as a caries retarder, *J. Dent. Res.,* 52: 267, 1973.

1486. Rubins, S., Lozano, J., Carrasco, H., Lang, T. W., and Corday, E., Tachyarrhythmias: Differential diagnosis and therapy after acute myocardial infarction, *Geriatrics,* 27: 123-133, 1972.

1487. Rudner, E. J., Diphenylhydantoin therapy, *Arch. Derm.,* 102: 561, 1970.

1488. Rumack, B. H., Wolfe, R. R. and Gilfrich, H., Phenytoin (diphenylhydantoin) treatment of massive digoxin overdose, *Brit. Heart J.,* 36: 405-408, 1974.

1489. Rundle, A. T. and Sudell, B., Leucine aminopeptidase isoenzyme changes after treatment with anticonvulsant drugs, *Clin. Chim. Acta,* 44: 377-384, 1973.

1490. Rushton, J. G., Medical treatment of trigeminal neuralgia, *Med. Clin. N. Amer.,* 52: 797-800, 1968.

1491. Ruskin, H. M., Therapeutic Dilantin levels, *New Eng. J. Med.,* 284: 792, 1971.

1492. Rutkowski, M. M., Cohen, S. N., and Doyle, E. F., Drug therapy of heart disease in pediatric patients. II. The treatment of congestive heart failure in infants and children with digitalis preparations, *Amer. Heart J.,* 86: 270-275, 1973.

1493. Rutkowski, M. M., Doyle, E. F. and Cohen, S. N., Drug therapy of heart disease in pediatric patients III. The therapeutic challenge of supraventricular tachyarrhythmias in infants and children, *Amer. Heart J.,* 86: 562-568, 1973.

1494. Rutledge, R., Sohn, Y. J., and Sardinas, A., Interaction of diphenylhydantoin and succinylcholine at the neuromuscular junction, *Pharmacologist,* 13: 265, 1971.

1495. Saad, S. F., El Masry, A. M., and Scott, P. M., Influence of certain anticonvulsants on the concentration of 8-aminobutyric acid in the cerebral hemispheres of mice, *Communications in Behav. Biol.,* 9: February, 1972.

1496. Sabih, K. and Sabih, K., Combined GLC and high-resolution mass spectroscopic analysis of diphenylhydantoin, *J. Pharm. Sci.,* 60: 1216-1220, 1971.

1497. Sampliner, R., Diphenylhydantoin control of alcohol withdrawal seizures, *JAMA,* 230: 1430-1432, 1974.

1498. Sampson, D., Harasymiv, I. and Hensley, W. J., Gas chromatographic assay of underivatized 5,5-diphenylhydantoin (Dilantin) in plasma extracts, *Clin. Chem.,* 17: 382-385, 1971.

1499. Sano, T., Suzuki, F., Sato, S., and Iida, Y., Mode of action of new anti-arrhythmic agents, *Jap. Heart J.,* 9: 161-168, 1968.

1500. Sataline, L., Cardiac standstill simulating epileptic seizures, *JAMA,* 225: 747, 1973.

1501. Satoyoshi, E. and Yamada, K., Recurrent muscle spasms of central origin. A report of two cases, *Arch. Neurol.,* 16: 254-264, 1967.

1502. Satoyoshi, E., Recurrent muscle spasms of central origin, *Trans. Amer. Neurol. Assoc.*, 92: 153-157, 1967.

1503. Saunders, B. A. and Jenkins, L. C., Cardiac arrhythmias of central nervous system origin: possible mechanism and suppression, *Canad. Anaesth. Soc. J.*, 20: 617-628, 1973.

1504. Savini, E. C., Poitevin, R. and Poitevin, J., New treatment of periodontolysis, *Rev. Franc. Odontostomat.*, 19: 55-61, 1972.

1505. Schade, G. H. and Gofman, H., Abdominal epilepsy in childhood, *Pediatrics*, 25: 151-154, 1960.

1506. Scherlag, B. J. and Helfant, R. H., Effect of diphenylhydantoin on acetyl strophanthidin, *Amer. Heart J.*, 81(4): 577-579, 1971.

1507. Scherlag, B. J., Helfant, R. H., Ricciutti, M. A., Damato, A. N., Dissociation of the effects of digitalis on myocardial potassium flux and contractility, *Am. J. Physiology*, 215: 1288-1291, 1968.

1508. Schick, D. and Scheuer, J., Current concepts of therapy with digitalis glycosides, Part II., *Amer. Heart J.*, 87: 391-396, 1974.

1509. Schimmel, R. J., and Graham, D., Inhibition by diphenylhydantoin of the diabetogenic action of streptozotocin, *Horm. Metab. Res.*, 6: 475-477, 1974.

1510. Schoor, W. P., Effect of anticonvulsant drugs on insecticide residues, *Lancet*, 520-521, 1970.

1511. Schreiber, M. M. and McGregor, J. G., Pseudolymphoma syndrome, *Arch. Derm.*, 97: 297-300, 1968.

1512. Schulten, H. K., Etzrodt, H., du Mesnil de Rochemont, W., Chriske, H. W., Grosser, K. D. and Steinbruck, G., Clinical and electrophysiological observations in DPH therapy of arrhythmia, *Verh. Deutsch Ges. Inn. Med.*, 77: 952-956, 1971.

1513. Schussler, G. C., Diazepam competes for thyroxine binding sites, *Chem. Abstracts*, 75: 74395C, 1971.

1514. Schussler, G. C., Similarity of diazepam to diphenylhydantoin, *JAMA*, 218: 1832, 1971.

1515. Schwender, C. F., Antiarrhythmic agents, *Annual Reports in Medicinal Chemistry, 1970*, 80-87, Cain, C. K., Ed., Academic Press, New York, 1971.

1516. Scientific Review Subpanel on Antiarrhythmia Agents, Quinidine-reserpine, Evaluations of Drug Interactions, *American Pharmaceutical Association*, Washington, D.C., 130-131, 1973.

1517. Scientific Review Subpanel on Anticonvulsants, Diphenylhydantoin-Isoniazid, Evaluations of Drug Interactions, *American Pharmaceutical Association*, Washington, D.C., 51-52, 1973.

1518. Scientific Review Subpanel on Anticonvulsants, Diphenylhydantoin-phenobarbital, Evaluations of Drug Interactions, *American Pharmaceutical Association*, Washington, D.C., 54-56, 1973.

1519. Scientific Review Subpanel on Antidiabetic Agents, Insulin-diphenylhydantoin, Evaluation of Drug Interaction, *American Pharmaceutical Association*, Washington, D.C., 90-91, 1973.

1520. Scientific Review Subpanel on Anticonvulsants, Diphenylhydantoin-methylphenidate, Evaluations of Drug Interactions, *American Pharmaceutical Association*, Washington, D.C. 53-54, 1973.

1521. Scientific Review Subpanel on Steroids, Dexamethasone-diphenylhydantoin, Evaluations of Drug Interactions, *American Pharmaceutical Association*, Washington, D.C., 32-34, 1973.

1522. Scientific Review Subpanel on Anticonvulsants, Anticonvulsant therapy, Evaluations of Drug Interactions, *American Pharmaceutical Association*, Washington, D.C., 252-256, 1973.

1523. Scott, M., Peale, A. R., and Croissant, P. D., Intracranial midline anterior fossae ossifying fibroma invading orbits, paranasal sinuses, and right maxillary antrum, *J. Neurosurg.*, 34: 827-831, 1971.

1524. Seeman, P., Chau-Wong, M., and Moyyen, S., The membrane binding of morphine, diphenylhydantoin, and tetrahydrocannabinol, *Canad. J. Physiol. Pharmacol.*, 50: 1193-1200, 1972.

1525. Selye, H. and Szabo, S., Protection by various steroids against gold nephropathy, *J. Europ. Toxicol.*, 6: 512-516, 1972.

1526. Selye, H. and Tuchweber, B., Effect of various steroids upon the toxicity of bile acids, *Int. Symp. Hepatotoxicity*, 63, 1973.

1527. Selye, H., Szabo, S., and Kourounakis, P., Effect of various steroids and nonsteroidal microsomal enzyme inducers upon propoxyphene intoxication, *Neuroendocrinology*, 9: 316-319, 1972.

1528. Selye, H., Szabo, S. and Kourounakis, P., Protection against phenylisothicyanate by various steroids, phenobarbitone and diphenylhydantoin, *J. Pharm. Pharmacol.*, 24: 333-334, 1972.

1529. Selye, H., Szabo, S., and Kourounakis, P., Protection by catatoxic steroids, phenobarbital and diphenylhydantoin against methaqualone intoxication, *Steroids Lipids Res.*, 3: 156-159, 1972.

1530. Selye, H., Szabo, S., and Mecs, I., Protection by catatoxic steroids against the paralysis caused by combined treatment with thyroxine and methylphenidate, *Neuropharmacology*, 11: 693-696, 1972.

1531. Selye, H., Hormones and resistance, *J. Pharm. Sci.*, 60: 1-28, 1971.

1532. Selye, H., Prevention by catatoxic steroids of lithocholic acid-induced biliary concrements in the rat, *Proc. Soc. Exp. Biol. Med.*, 141: 555-558, 1972.

1533. Selye, H., Protection by glucocorticoids against allopurinol nephropathy, *Acta Endocr.*, 69: 347-354, 1972.

1534. Serrano, E. E., Roe, D. B., Hammer, R. H.,, and Wilder, B. J., Plasma diphenylhydantoin values after oral and intramuscular administration of diphenylhydantoin, *Neurology*, 23: 311-317, 1973.

1535. Shah, J. R., Vora, G., Karkhanis, A. V., and Talwalkar, C. V., The effect of diphenylhydantoin on ventilation tests in airway obstruction, *Indian J. Chest. Dis.*, 12: 10-14, 1970.

1536. Shalsha, K. G., The function of newer antiarrhythmic drugs under special consideration of beta blocking adrenergic agents, *Proc. Virchow Med Soc. (N.Y.).* 27: 201-211, 1969.

1537. Shemano, I., Orzechowski, R., Goldstein, S., and Beiler, J. M., Effects of 3,5-diethylhydantoin on resistance to asphyxia in rats, *Toxic. Appl. Pharmacol.* 25: 250-258, 1973.

1538. Sher, S. P., Drug enzyme induction and drug interactions: literature tabulation, *Toxic. Appl. Pharmacol.*, 18: 780-834, 1971.

1539. Sherwin, A. L., Eisen, A. A. and Sokolowski, C. D., Anticonvulsant drugs in human epileptogenic brain, *Presented at the annual meeting of the American Neurological Association and the Canadian Congress of Neurological Sciences*, Montreal, 1973.

1540. Sherwin, I., Suppressant effects of diphenylhydantoin on the cortical epileptogenic focus, *Neurology*, 23: 274-281, 1973.

1541. Shibasaki, H. and Kuroiwa, Y., Painful tonic seizure in multiple sclerosis, *Arch. Neurol.*, 30: 47-51, 1974.

1542. Shinohara, Y., Ventricular fibrillation threshold (VFRT) in experimental coronary occlusion: comparative studies on the effect of G-I-K solution and some new antiarrhythmic agents, *Jap. Circ. J.*, 32: 1269-1281. 1968.

1543. Shoeman, D. W., Benjamin, D. M., and Azarnoff, D. L., The alteration of plasma proteins in uremia as reflected in the ability to bind diphenylhydantoin, *Ann. N. Y. Acad. Sci.*, 226: 127-130, 1973.

1544. Shoeman, D. W., Kauffman, R. E., Azarnoff, D. L., and Boulos, B. M., Placental transfer of diphenylhydantoin as determined at constant drug concentrations in the maternal blood, *Pharmacologist*, 13: 195, 1971.

1545. Shoeman, D. W., Kauffman, R. E., Azarnoff, D. L., and Boulos, B. M., Placental transfer of diphenylhydantoin in the goat, *Biochem. Pharmacol.*, 21: 1237-1244, 1972.

1546. Sholiton, L. J., Werk, E. E. and MacGee, J., The effect of diphenylhydantoin *in vitro* on the formation of the polar metabolites of testosterone by rat liver, *Acta Endocr.*, 62: 360-366, 1969.

1547. Siegel, G. H. and Goodwin, B. B., Sodium-potassium-activated adenosine triphosphatase of brain microsomes: modification of sodium inhibition by diphenylhydantoins, *J. Clin. Invest.*, 51: 1161-1169, 1972.

1548. Siegel, G. J. and Goodwin, B. B., Effects of 5,5-diphenlhydantoin (DPH) and 5-p-hydroxyphenyl-5-phenylhydantoin (HPPH) on brain Na-K-ATPase, *Neurology*, 21: 417, 1971.

1549. Sigwald, J., Raverdy, P., Fardeau, M., Gremy, F., Mace de Lepinay, A., Bouttier, D., and Danic, Mme., Pseudomyotonia, *Rev. Neurol.*, 115: 1003-1014, 1966.

1550. Simon, G. E., Jatlow, P. I., Seligson, H. T., and Seligson, D., Measurement of 5,5-diphenylhydantoin in blood using thin layer chromatography, *Epilepsy Abstracts*, 4: 136, 1971.

1551. Simopoulos, A. M., Pinto, A., Uhlenhuth, E. H., McGee, J. J., and DeRosa, E. R., Diphenylhydantoin (DPH) effectiveness in the treatment of chronic schizophrenics, *Arch. Gen. Psychiat.*, 30: 106-112, 1974.

1552. Simpson, J. F., Use of diphenylhydantoin, *Ann. Intern. Med.*, 78: 305-306, 1973.

1553. Singh, B. N. and Hauswirth, O., Comparative mechanisms of action of antiarrhythmic drugs, *Amer. Heart J.*, 87: 367-382, 1974.

1554. Singh, B. N. and Vaughan Williams, E. M., Effect of altering potassium concentration on the action of lidocaine and diphenylhydantoin on rabbit atrial and ventricular muscle, *Circ. Res.*, 29: 286-295, 1971.

1555. Singh, B. N., Explanation for the discrepancy in reported cardiac electrophysiological actions of diphenylhydantoin and lignocaine, *Brit. J. Pharmacol.*, 41: 385-386, 1971.

1556. Singh, H. P., Hebert, M. A., and Gualt, M. H., Effect of some drugs on clinical laboratory values as determined by technicon SMA 12/60, *Clin. Chem.*, 18: 137-144, 1972.

1557. Singh, N., Sinha, J. N., Rastogi, S. K., Dua, P. R., and Kohli, R. P., An experimental investigation on the antiarrhythmic activity of antiepileptic agents, *Jap. J. Pharmacol.* 21: 755-761, 1971.

1558. Sisca, T. S., An unusual dual hypersensitivity reaction induced by diphenylhydantoin, *Amer. J. Hosp. Pharm.*, 30: 446-449, 1973.

1559. Skrotsky, Y. A., Complications due to antiepileptic therapy in children and adolescents, *Epilepsy Abstracts*, 7: 138-139, 1974.

1560. Slosberg, P. S., Medical therapy for the cerebrovascular insufficiencies; eight years' experience, *Mt. Sinai Med. J.*, 37: 692-698, 1970.

1561. Smith, J. S., Brierley, H. and Brandon, S., Akinetic mutism with recovery after repeated carbon monoxide poisoning, *Psychol. Med.*, 1: 172-177, 1971.

1562. Smith, T. W. and Haber, E., Digitalis, *New Eng. J. Med.*, 289: 1125-1129, 1973.

1563. Smith, T. W., Digitalis glycosides, *New Eng. J. Med.*, 288: 942-946, 1973.

1564. Smith, W. L. and Lowrey, J. B., The effects of diphenylhydantoin on cognitive functions in man, *Drugs, Development, and Cerebral Function*, Smith, W. L., Ed., Charles C Thomas, 344-351, 1972.

1565. Smith, W. L. and Lowrey, J. B., Effects of diphenylhydantoin on mental abilities in the elderly, *J. Amer. Geriat. Soc.*, 23: 207-211, 1975.

1566. Snider, R. S. and del Cerro, M., Diphenylhydantoin, proliferating membranes in cerebellum resulting from intoxication, *Antiepileptic Drugs*, 237-245, Woodbury, D. M., Penry, J. K., and Schmidt, R. P. Eds., Raven Press, New York, 1972.

1567. Sohn, R. S. and Ferrendelli, J. A., Inhibition of Ca^{++} uptake in rat brain synaptosomes by diphenylhydantoin, *Neurology*, 23: 444, 1973.

1568. Solomon, G. E., Hilgartner, M. W., and Kutt, H., Co-agulation defects caused by diphenylhydantoin, *Neurology*, 22: 1165-1171, 1972.

1569. Solomon, P. and Kleeman, S. T., Medical aspects of violence, *Calif. Med.*, 114: 19-24, 1971.

1570. Solow, E. B. and Green, J. B., The simultaneous determination of multiple anticonvulsant drug levels by gas-liquid chromatography, *Neurology*, 22: 540-550, 1972.

1571. Solow, E. B., Metaxas, J. M. and Summers, T. R., Antiepileptic drugs. A current assessment of simultaneous determination of multiple drug therapy by gas liquid chromatography on column methylation, *J. Chromatographic Sci.*, 12: 256-260, 1974.

1572. Sorrell, T. C., Forbes, I. J., Burness, F. R., and Rischbieth, R. H. C., Depression of immunological function in patients treated with phenytoin sodium (sodium diphenylhydantoin), *Lancet*, 1233-1235, 1971.

1573. Sotaniemi, E. A., Arvela, P., Hakkarainen, H. K., and Huhti, E., The clinical significance of microsomal enzyme induction in the therapy of epileptic patients, *Ann. Clin. Res.*, 2: 223-227, 1970.

1574. Sotaniemi, E. A., Hakkarainen, H. K., Puranen, J. A. and Lahti, R. O., Radiologic bone changes and hypocalcemia with anticonvulsant therapy in epilepsy, *Ann. Intern. Med.*, 77(3): 389-394, 1972.

1575. South, J., Teratogenic effect of anticonvulsants, *Lancet*, 2: 1154, 1972.

1576. Spector, R. G., Effects of formyl tetrahydrofolic acid and noradrenaline on the oxygen consumption of rat brain synaptosome-mitrochondrial preparations, *Brit. J. Pharmacol.*, 44: 279-285, 1972.

1577. Spector, R. G., Influence of folic acid on excitable tissues, *Nature New Biol.*, 240: 247-249, 1972.

1578. Spector, R. G., The influence of anticonvulsant drugs on formyl tetrahydrofolic acid stimulation of rat brain respiration *in vitro*, *Epilepsy Abstracts*, 6: 110, 1973.

1579. Speidel, B. D. and Meadow, S. R., Maternal epilepsy and abnormalities of the fetus and newborn, *Lancet*, 839-843, October, 1972.

1580. Sperelakis, N. and Henn, F. A., Effect of diphenylhydantoin on membrane potentials and Na-K-ATPase of cultured chick heart cells, *Amer. J. Physiol.*, 218: 1224-1227, 1970.

1581. Spina, A., Pyridinolcarbamate in the therapy of hemicrania syndromes, *Acta Neurol.*, 27: 610-617, 1972.

1582. Spray, G. H. and Burns, D. G., Folate deficiency and anticonvulsant drugs, *Brit. Med. J.*, 2: 167-168, April, 1972.

1583. Stambaugh, J. E. and Tucker, D., Effect of diphenylhydantoin on glucose tolerance in patients with hypoglycemia, *Diabetes*, 23: 679-683, 1974.

1584. Stamp, T. C. B., Effects of long-term anticonvulsant therapy on calcium and vitamin D metabolism, *Proc. Roy. Soc. Med.*, 67: 64-68, 1974.

1585. Stamp, T. C. B., Round, J. M., Rowe, D. J. F., and Haddad, J. G., Plasma levels and therapeutic effect of 25-hydroxycholecalciferol in epileptic patients taking anticonvulsant drugs, *Brit. Med. J.*, 4: 9-12, 1972.

1586. Staples, R. E., Teratology, *Antiepileptic Drugs*, 55-62, Woodbury, D. M., Penry, J. K., and Schmidt, R. P. Eds., Raven Press, New York, 1972. (*cf.* Kuenssberg and Knox, *Lancet*, 198, 1973, Millar and Nevin, *Lancet*, 328, 1973 and Stenchever and Jarvis, *Amer. J. Obstet. Gynec.*, 109: 961, 1971.)

1587. Starreveld-Zimmerman, A. A. E., Van Der Kolk, W. J., Meinardi, H., and Elshove, J., Are anticonvulsants teratogenic?, *Lancet*, 48-49, July, 1973.

1588. Staunton, C., Stein, A. A., and Moss, G., The cerebral etiology of the respiratory distress syndrome (RDS): universal response, with prevention by unilateral pulmonary denervation, *Surg. Forum*, 24: 1973.

1589. Stavchansky, S. A., Lubawy, W. C. and Kostenbauder, H. B., Increase of hexobarbital sleeping time and inhibition of drug metabolism by the major metabolite of DPH, *Life Sci.* 14: 1535-1539, 1974.

1590. Stazi, C. and Marasa, G., Arrhythmias due to digitalis and their treatment, *Ann. Med. Nav.* (Roma), 77: 51-80, 1972.

1591. Stein, A. A. and Moss, G., Cerebral etiology of the respiratory distress syndrome: diphenylhydantoin (DPH) prophylaxis, *Surg. Forum*, 24: 433-435, 1973.

1592. Stephens, J. H. and Shaffer, J. W., A controlled replication of the effectiveness of diphenylhydantoin in reducing irritability and anxiety in selected neurotic outpatients, *J. Clin. Pharmacol.*, 13: 351-356, 1973.

1593. Stephens, J. H., Shaffer, J. W., and Brown, C. C., A controlled comparison of the effects of diphenylhydantoin and placebo on mood and psychomotor functioning in normal volunteers, *J. Clin. Pharmacol.*, 14: 543-551, 1974.

1594. Stern, L. Z., Gruener, R., and Amundsen, P., Diphenylhydantoin for steroid-induced muscle weakness, *JAMA*, 223: 1287-1288, 1973.

1595. Stevens, H., Nine neuropathies, *Med. Ann.*, 37: 89-97, 1968.

1596. Stevens, M. W. and Harbison, R. D., Placental transfer of diphenylhydantoin: effects of species, gestational age, and route of administration, *Teratology*, 9: 317-326, 1974.

1597. Stevenson, M. M. and Gilbert, E. F., Anticonvulsants and hemorrhagic diseases of the newborn infant, *J. Pediat.*, 516, 1970.

1598. Stone, N., Klein, M. D., and Lown, B., Diphenylhydantoin in the prevention of recurring ventricular tachycardia, *Circulation*, 43: 420-427, 1971.

1599. Stowell, A., Physiologic mechanisms and treatment of histaminic or petrosal neuralgia, *Headache*, 9: 187-194, 1970.

1600. Strauss, H., Rahm, W. E., and Barrera, S. E., Studies on a group of children with psychiatric disorders. I. Electroencephalographic studies, *Psychosom. Med.*, 2: 34-42, 1940.

1601. Strittmatter, W. J. and Somjen, G. G., Depression of sustained evoked potentials and glial depolarization in the spinal cord by barbiturates and by diphenylhydantoin, *Brain Res.*, 55: 333-342, 1973.

1602. Su, P. C. and Feldman, D. S., Motor nerve terminal and muscle membrane stabilization by diphenylhydantoin administration, *Arch. Neurol.*, 28: 376-379, 1973.

1603. Swaiman, K. F. and Stright, P. L., The effects of anticonvulsants on *in vitro* protein synthesis in immature brain, *Brain Res.*, 58: 515-518, 1973.

1604. Swann, W. P., Effects of Dilantin on the repair of gingival wounds, *Indiana University School of Dentistry Thesis*, 1966.

1605. Sweet, W. H. and Wepsic, J. G., Relation of fiber size in trigeminal posterior root to conduction of impulses for pain and touch; production of analgesia without anesthesia in the effective treatment of trigeminal neuralgia, *Trans. Amer. Neurol. Assoc.*, 95: 134-139, 1970.

1606. Tabachnick, M., Hao, Y. L., and Korcek, L., Effect of oleate, diphenylhydantoin and heparin on the binding of 125 I-thyroxine to purified thyroxine-binding globulin, *J. Clin. Endocr.*, 36: 392-394, 1973.

1607. Taitz, L. S., Mental retardation elevated alkaline phosphatase, convulsive disorder and thickening of calvarium, *Epilepsy Abstracts*, 6: 228, 1973. (*cf.* Kattan, *Amer. J. Roentgen.*, 110: 102, 1970.)

1608. Tappaz, M. and Pacheco, H., Effects of convulsant and anticonvulsant drugs on uptake of 14,-C GABA by rat brain slices, *J. Pharmacol.* (Paris), 4: 295-306, 1973.

1609. Tashima, C. K. and De Los Santos, R., Lymphoma and anticonvulsive therapy, *JAMA*, 228: 286-287, 1974.

1610. Tassinari, C. A. and Fine, R. D., Paroxysmal choreoathetosis, *Proc. Aust. Assoc. Neurol.*, 6: 71-75, 1969.

1611. Taylor, C. R., Double-blind crossover study of diphenylhydantoin in angina pectoris, *Chest*, 66: 422-427, 1974.

1612. Taylor, J. D., Krahn, P. M. and Higgins, T. N., Serum copper levels and diphenylhydantoin, *Amer. J. Clin. Path.*, 61: 577-578, 1974.

1613. Tenser, R. B. and Corbett, J. J., Myokymia and facial contraction in brain stem glioma, *Arch. Neurol.*, 30: 425-427, 1974.

1614. Thompson, C. E., Diphenylhydantoin for myotonia congenita, *New Eng. J. Med.*, 286: 893, 1972.

1615. Thurkow, I., Wesseling, H., and Meijer, D. K. F., Estimation of phenytoin in body fluids in the presence of sulphonyl urea compounds, *Clin. Chim. Acta*, 37: 509-513, 1972.

1616. Thurlow, H. J. and Girvin, J. P., Use of anti-epileptic medication in treating "flashbacks" from hallucinogenic drugs, *Canad. Med. Assoc. J.*, 105: 947-948, 1971.

1617. Tigelaar, R. E., Rapport, R. L., Inman, J. K., and Kupferberg, H. J., A radioimmunoassay for diphenylhydantoin, *Epilepsy Abstracts*, 6: 113, 1973.

1618. Tisman, G., Herbert, V., Go, L. T., and Brenner, L., *In vitro* demonstration of immunosuppression without bone marrow suppression by alcohol and bleomycin, *Clin. Res.*, 19: 730, 1971.

1619. Tobin, T., Dirdjosudjono, S., and Baskin, S. I., Pharmacokinetics and distribution of diphenylhydantoin in kittens, *Amer. J. Vet. Res.*, 34: 951-954, 1973.

1620. Tolman, K. G., Jubiz, W., DeLuca, H. F. and Freston, J. W., Rickets associated with anticonvulsant medications, *Clin. Res.*, 20: 414, 1972.

1621. Toman, J. E. P. and Sabelli, H. C., Comparative neuronal mechanisms, *Epilepsia*, 10: 179-192, 1969.

1622. Torretti, J., Hendler, E., Weinstein, E., Longnecker, R. E., and Epstein, F. H., Functional significance of Na-K-ATPase in the kidney: effects of ouabain inhibition, *Amer. J. Physiol.*, 222: 1398-1405, 1972.

1623. Tovi, D., The use of antifibrinolytic drugs to prevent early recurrent aneurysmal subarachnoid haemorrhage, *Acta Neurol. Scand.*, 49: 163-175, 1973.

1624. Treasure, T. and Toseland, P. A., Hyperglycaemia due to phenytoin toxicity, *Arch. Dis. Child.*, 46: 563-564, 1971.

1625. Tuchweber, B., Szabo, S., Kovacs, K., and Garg, B. D., Hormonal and nonhormonal factors influencing pyrrolizidine alkaloid hepatotoxicity, *Int. Symp. Hepatotoxicity*, 89, 1973.

1626. Turner, W. J., Dilantin effect on emotionally disturbed children, *Drugs and Cerebral Function*, 99-102, Smith, W. L., Ed., Charles C Thomas, 1970.

1627. Tyler, F. H., West, C. D., Jubiz, W., and Meikle, A. W., Dilantin and metyrapone: a clinically significant example of enzyme induction, *Trans. Amer. Clin. Climat. Assoc.*, 81: 213-219, 1970.

1628. Tyrer, J. H., Eadie, M. J., and Sutherland, J. M., Investigation of an outbreak of anticonvulsant intoxication, *Proc. Aust. Assoc. Neurol.*, 7: 15-18, 1970.

1629. Tyrer, J. H., Eadie, M. J., and Hooper, W. D., Further observations on an outbreak of diphenylhydantoin intoxication, *Proc. Aust. Assoc. Neurol.*, 8: 37-41, 1971.

1630. Uhlenhuth, E. H., Stephens, J. H., Dim, B. H., and Covi, L., Diphenylhydantoin and phenobarbital in the relief of psychoneurotic symptoms: a controlled comparison, *Psychopharmacologia* (Berlin), 27: 67-84, 1972.

1631. Uono, M., Treatment of myotonic dystrophy, *Naika*, 25: 664-668, 1970.

1632. Vaisrub, S., Diphenylhydantoin and insulin-secreting tumors, *JAMA*, 223: 553-554, 1973.

1633. Vaisrub, S., Diphenylhydantoin and early diabetes, *JAMA*, 226: 191, 1973.

1634. Vajda, F. J. E., Prineas, R. J., and Lovell, R. R. H., Interaction between phenytoin and the benzodiazepines, *Epilepsy Abstracts*, 4: 263, 1971.

1635. Vajda, F. J. E., Prineas, R. J., Lovell, R. R. H., and Sloman, J. G., The possible effect of long-term high plasma levels of phenytoin on mortality after acute myocardial infarction, *Europ. J. Clin. Pharmacol.*, 5: 138-144, 1973.

1636. van der Kleijn, E., Rijntjes, N. V. M., Guelen, P. J. M., and Wijffels, C. C. G., Systemic and brain distribution of diphenylhydantoin in the squirrel monkey, *Antiepileptic Drugs*, 124, Woodbury, D. M., Penry, J. K., and Schmidt, R. P., Eds., Raven Press, New York, 1972.

1637. Van Der Velde, C. D., Toxicity of lithium carbonate in elderly patients, *Amer. J. Psychiat.*, 127: 1075-1077, 1971.

1638. van Dijk, L., Pharmacotherapy of cardiac arrhythmias in acute myocardial infarction, *Folia Med. Neerl.*, 14: 225-236, 1971.

1639. Van Meter, J. C., Buckmaster, H. S., and Shelley, L. L., Concurrent assay of phenobarbital and diphenylhydantoin in plasma by vapor-phase chromatography, *Clin. Chem.*, 16: 135-138, 1970.

1640. Van Rees, H. and Noach, E. L., The intestinal absorption of diphenylhydantoin from a suspension in rats, *Epilepsy Abstracts*, 7: 197, 1974.

1641. Van Rees, H., DeWolff, F. A., Noach, E. L., The influence of diphenylhydantoin on intestinal glucose absorption in the rat, *European J. Pharmacology*, 28: 310-315, 1974.

1642. Van Rees, H., Woodbury, D. M. and Noach, E. L., Effects of ouabain and diphenylhydantoin on electrolyte and water shifts during intestinal absorption in the rat, *Arch. Int. Pharmacodyn.*, 182: 437, 1969.

1643. Van Riezen, H. and Delver, A., The effect of a number of drugs with different pharmacological properties upon reserpine induced hypothermia in mice, *Arzneimittelforschung.*, 21: 1562-1566, 1971.

1644. Vanasin, B., Bass, D. D., Mendeloff, A. I., and Schuster, M. M., Alteration of electrical and motor activity of human and dog rectum by diphenylhydantoin, *Amer. J. Dig. Dis.*, 18: 403-410, 1973.

1645. Vander Ark, C. R. and Reynolds, E. W., Jr., Cellular basis and clinical evaluation of antiarrhythmic therapy, *Med. Clin. N. Amer.*, 53: 1297-1308, 1969.

1646. Vaughan Williams, E. M., The development of new antidysrhythmic drugs, *Schweiz. Med. Wschr.*, 103: 262-271, 1973.

1647. Vedso, S., Rud, C., and Place, J. F., Determination of phenytoin in serum in the presence of barbiturates sulthiame and ethosuximid by thin-layer chromatography, *Scand. J. Clin. Lab. Invest.*, 23: 175-180, 1969.

1648. Verebel, K., Kutt, H., Sohn, Y. J., Levitt, B., and Raines, A., Uptake and distribution of diphenylthiohydantoin (DPTH), *Europ. J. Pharmacol.*, 10: 106-110, 1970.

1649. Villareale, M., Gould, L. V., Wasserman, R. H., Barr, A., Chiroff, R. T., and Bergstrom, W. H., Diphenylhydantoin: effects on calcium metabolism in the chick, *Science*, 183: 671-673, 1974.

1650. Viukari, N. M. A. and Tammisto, P., Central effects of diphenylhydantoin (Dilantin) in epileptic oligophrenics during phenobarbital-primidone withdrawal, sodium bicarbonate, and ammonium chloride administration, *Behav. Neuropsychiatr.*, 1: 13-16, 1969.

1651. Viukari, N. M. A., Diphenylhydantoin as an anticonvulsant: evaluation of treatment in forty mentally subnormal epileptics, *Epilepsy Abstracts*, 3: 150, 1970.

1652. Vulliamy, D., Unwanted effects of anticonvulsant drugs, *Dev. Med. Child. Neurol.*, 13: 107-109, 1971.

1653. Walker, W. J., Treatment of heart failure, *JAMA*, 228: 1276-1278, 1974.

1654. Wallace, J. E., Microdetermination of diphenylhydantoin in biological specimens by ultraviolet spectrophotometry, *Anal. Chem.*, 40: 978-980, 1968.

1655. Wallace, J. E., Simultaneous spectrophotometric determination of diphenylhydantoin and phenobarbital in biologic specimens, *Clin. Chem.*, 15: 323-330, 1969.

1656. Wallace, J. E., Spectrophotometric determination of diphenylhydantoin, *J. Forensic Sci. Soc.*, 11: 552-559, 1966.

1657. Wallis, W. E. and Plum, F., Continuous fasciculations, myokymia and muscle contraction due to peripheral nerve disease, *Trans. Assoc. Amer. Physicians*, 82: 286-292, 1969.

1658. Wallis, W. E., Van Poznak, A., and Plum, F., Generalized muscular stiffness, fasciculations, and myokymia of peripheral nerve origin, *Arch. Neurol.*, 22: 430-439, 1970.

1659. Walsh, G. O., Masland, W., and Goldensohn, E. S., Relationship between paroxysmal atrial tachycardia and paroxysmal cerebral discharges, *Bull. Los Angeles Neurol. Soc.*, 37: 28-35, 1972.

1660. Ware, E., The chemistry of the hydantoins, *Chem. Rev.*, 46: 403-470, 1950.

1661. Watanabe, Y., A-V conduction disturbance: its pathophysiology and pharmacology, *Singapore Med. J.*, 14(3): 249, 1973.

1662. Watson, E. L. and Woodbury, D. M., Effect of diphenylhydantoin on active sodium transport in frog skin, *J. Pharmacol. Exp. Ther.*, 180: 767-776, 1972.

1663. Watson, E. L. and Woodbury, D. M., The effect of diphenylhydantoin and ouabain, alone and in combination, on the electrocardiogram and on cellular electrolytes of guinea-pig heart and skeletal muscle, *Arch. Int. Pharmacodyn.*. 201: 389-399, 1973.

1664. Watson, E. L. and Woodbury, D. M., Effects of diphenylhydantoin on electrolyte transport in various tissues, *Chemical Modulation of Brain Function*, 187-198, Sabelli, H. C., Ed., Raven Press, New York, 1973.

1665. Watson, J. D. and Spellacy, W. N., Neonatal effects of maternal treatment with the anticonvulsant drug diphenylhydantoin, *Obstet. Gynec.*, 37: 881-885, 1971.

1666. Watson, M., Gabica, J., and Benson, W. W., Serum organochlorine pesticides in mentally retarded patients on differing drug regimens, *Clin. Pharmacol. Ther.*, 13: 186-192, 1972.

1667. Watson, P., Brainwave to save life, *London Times*, 1973.

1668. Wax, S. D., Webb, W. R., and Ecker, R. R., Myocardium stabilization by diphenylhydantoin, *Surg. Forum*, 20: 164-166, 1969.

1669. Weber-Eggenberger, S. and Kaufmann, G., Studies on absorption, elimination and antiarrhythmic serum concentrations of diphenylhydantoin (antisacer) in digitalized heart patients, *Z. Kreislaufforsch.*, 60: 420-432, 1971.

1670. Weckman, N. and Lehtovaara, R., Serum and cerebrospinal fluid folate values in epileptics on anticonvulsant treatment, *Scand. J. Clin. Lab. Invest.*, Supp. 101, 120-121, 1968.

1671. Weckman, N. and Lehtovaara, R., Folic acid and anticonvulsants, *Lancet*, 1: 207-208, 1969.

1672. Weinreich, D. and Clark, L. D., Anticonvulsant drugs and self-stimulation rates in rats, *Arch. Int. Pharmacodyn.*, 185: 269-273, 1970.

1673. Weisse, A. B., Moschos, C. B., Passannante, A. J., and Regan, T. J., Comparative effectiveness of procaine amide, lidocaine, and diphenylhydantoin in treating ventricular arrhythmias during acute myocardial infarction, *Circulation*, 38: VI205, 1968.

1674. Weiss, C. F., Yaffe, S. J., Cann, H. M., Gold, A. P., Kenny, F. M., Riley, H. D., Schafer, I., Stern, L., and Shirkey, H. C., An evaluation of the pharmacologic approaches to learning impediments, *Pediatrics*, 46: 142-144, 1970.

1675. Weisse, A. B., Moschos, C. B., Passannante, A. J., Khan, M. I., and Regan, T. J., Relative effectiveness of three antiarrhythmic agents in the treatment of ventricular arrhythmias in experimental acute myocardial ischemia, *Amer. Heart J.*, 81: 503-510, 1971.

1676. Welch, L. K., Appenzeller, O., and Bicknell, J. M., Peripheral neuropathy with myokymia, sustained muscular contraction, and continuous motor unit activity, *Neurology*, 22: 161-169, 1972.

1677. Wepsic, J. G., Tic douloureux: etiology, refined treatment, *New Eng. J. Med.*, 288: 680-681, 1973.

1678. Werk, E. E., Choi, Y., Sholiton, L., Olinger, C., and Haque, N., Interference in the effect of dexamethasone by diphenylhydantoin, *New Eng. J. Med.*, 281: 32-34, 1969.

1679. Werk, E. E., Thrasher, K., Sholiton, L. J., Olinger, C., and Choi, Y., Cortisol production in epileptic patients treated with diphenylhydantoin, *Clin. Pharmacol. Ther.*, 12: 698-703, 1971.

1680. Wesseling, H. and Thurkow, I., Effect of sulphonylureas (tolazamide, tolbutamide and chlorpropamide) on the metabolism of diphenylhydantoin in the rat, *Biochem. Pharmacol.*, 22: 3033-3040, 1973.

1681. Westmoreland, B. and Bass, N. H., Chronic diphenylhydantoin intoxication in the albino rat during pregnancy, *Neurology*, 20: 411, 1970.

1682. Whelton, A., Snyder, D. S., and Walker, W. G., Acute toxic drug ingestions at the Johns Hopkins Hospital 1963 through 1970, *Johns Hopkins Med. J.*, 132: 157-167, 1973.

1683. White, C. W., Jr., Megirian, R., and Swiss, E. D., The effects of diphenylhydantoin sodium, glucose and β-diethylaminoethyl diphenylpropylacetate hydrochloride on cyclopropane-epinephrine arrhythmias in the dog, *Circ. Res.*, 3: 290-292, 1955.

1684. Wilder, B. J., Buchanan, R. A., and Serrano, E. E., Correlation of acute diphenylhydantoin intoxication with plasma levels and metabolite excretion, *Neurology*, 23: 1329-1332, 1973.

1685. Wilder, B. J., Serrano, E. E. and Ramsay, R. E., Plasma diphenylhydantoin levels after loading and maintenance doses, *Clin. Pharmacol. Ther.*, 14: 797-801, 1973.

1686. Wilder, B. J., Streiff, R. R., and Hammer, R. H., Diphenylhydantoin, absorption, distribution, and excretion: clinical studies, *Antiepileptic Drugs*, 137-148, Woodbury, D. M., Penry, J. K., and Schmidt, R. P., Eds., Raven Press, New York, 1972.

1687. Wilensky, A. J. and Lowden, J. A., Interaction of diphenylhydantoin $4^{14}C$ with subcellular fractions of rat brain, *Epilepsy Abstracts*, 5: 194, 1972.

1688. Wilensky, A. J. and Lowden, J. A., The inhibitory effect of diphenylhydantoin on microsomal ATPases, *Life Sci.*, 11: 319-327, 1972.

1689. Wilensky, A. J. and Lowden, J. A., Inadequate serum levels after intramuscular administration of diphenylhydantoin, *Neurology*, 23: 318-324, 1973.

1690. Wilkinson, H. A., Epileptic pain—an uncommon manifestation with localizing value, *Neurology*, 23: 518-520, 1973.

1691. Wilson, J. T. and Wilkinson, G. R., Delivery of anticonvulsant drug therapy in epileptic patients assessed by plasma level analyses, *Neurology*, 24: 614-623, 1974.

1692. Winter, B., Bilateral carotid body resection for asthma and emphysema, *Int. Surg.*, 57: 458-466, 1972.

1693. Wolff, J., Standaert, M. E., and Rall, J. E., Thyroxine displacement from serum proteins and depression of serum protein-bound iodine by certain drugs, *J. Clin. Invest.*, 40: 1373-1377, 1961.

1694. Wood, R. A., Sinoatrial arrest: an interaction between phenytoin and lignocaine, *Brit. Med. J.*, 1: 645, 1971.

1695. Woodbury, D. M. and Kemp, J. W., Some possible mechanisms of action of anti-epileptic drugs, *Pharmakopsychiatr.*, 3: 201-226, 1970.

1696. Woodbury, D. M. and Kemp, J. W., Pharmacology and mechanisms of action of diphenylhydantoin, *Psychiat. Neurol. Neurochir.*, 74: 91-115, 1971.

1697. Woodbury, D. M. and Swinyard, E. A., Diphenylhydantoin, absorption, distribution, and excretion, *Antiepileptic Drugs*, 113-123, Woodbury, D. M., Penry, J. K., and Schmidt, R. P., Eds., Raven Press, New York, 1972.

1698. Woodbury, D. M., Koch, A., and Vernadakis, A., Relation between excitability and metabolism in brain as elucidated by anticonvulsant drugs, *Neurology*, 8: 113-116, 1958.

1699. Woodbury, D. M., Mechanisms of action of anticonvulsants, *Epilepsy Abstracts*, 3: 248, 1970.

1700. Woodbury, D. M., Penry, J. K. and Schmidt, R. P., Eds., *Antiepileptic Drugs*, Raven Press, New York, 1972.

1701. Yalaz, K. and Baytok, V., Mirror movement, *Turk. J. Pediat.*, 12: 85-88, 1970.

1702. Yanagihara, T. and Hamberger, A., Effect of diphenylhydantoin on protein metabolism in the central nervous system—study of subcellular fractions, *Exp. Neurol.*, 31: 87-99, 1971.

1703. Yanagihara, T. and Hamberger, A., Effect of diphenylhydantoin on protein metabolism in neuron and neuroglial fractions of central nervous tissue, *Exp. Neurol*, 32: 152-162, 1971.

1704. Yanagihara, T., Distribution of diphenylhydantoin in the neuronal and glial fractions, *Antiepileptic Drugs*, 125-126, Woodbury, D. M., Penry, J. K., and Schmidt, R. P., Eds., Raven Press, New York, 1972.

1705. Yang, C. P., Persistent ventricular tachycardia. The use of diphenylhydantoin, *J. Kansas Med. Soc.*, 74: 418-421, 1973.

1706. Yaryura-Tobias, J. A. and Neziroglu, F., Violent behaviour, brain dysrhythmia and glucose dysfunction: a new syndrome, *Amer. J. Psychiat.*, 130: 825, 1973.

1707. Yasky, J., Moretti, O., Carosella, C., Phenytoin treatment of cardiac arrhythmias induced by digitalis, *Revista Argentina de Cardiologia*, 41: 53-61, 1973.

1708. Yoshida, T. and Arakawa, T., Serum histidine clearance in children with diphenylhydantoin administration, *Tohoku J. Exp. Med.*, 112: 257-259, 1974.

1709. Yoshimasu, F., Kurland, L. T., and Elveback, L. R., Tic douloureux in Rochester, Minnesota, 1945-1969, *Neurology*, 22: 952-956, 1972.

1710. Zanini, S. and Rossi, R., Ventricular parasystole: effective treatment with diphenylhydantoin, *G. Ital. Cardiol.*, 2: 575-578, 1972.

1711. Zeft, H. J., Rembert, J. C., Curry, C. L., and Greenfield, J. C., Effects of diphenylhydantoin on coronary and systemic haemodynamics in awake dogs, *Cardiovasc. Res.*, 7: 331-335, 1973.

1712. Zeft, H. J., Whalen, R. E., Morris, J. J., Jr., Rummo, N. J., and McIntoch, H. D., Prophylaxis versus treatment of acetylstrophanthidin intoxication, *Amer. Heart J.*, 77: 237-245, 1969.

1713. Affrime, M. and Reidenberg, M. M., The protein binding of some drugs in plasma from patients with alcoholic liver disease, *Europ. J. Clin. Pharmacol.*, 8: 267–9, 1975.

1714. Agapova, E. N. and Mikhalev, I. D., Effectiveness of the use of diphenine in insuloma, *Ter. Arkh.*, 49(9): 124–5, 1977.

1715. Agnew, D. C. and Goldberg, V. D., A brief trial of phenytoin therapy for thalamic pain, *Bulletin Los Angeles Neurol. Soc.*, 41(1): 9–12, 1976.

1716. Aickin, C. C., Deisz, R. A. and Lux, H. D., The effect of diphenylhydantoin and picrotoxin on post-synaptic inhibition, *J. Physiol.*, 284: 125–6, 1978.

1717. Aldrete, J. A. and Franatovic, Y., Postponement of operations—its prevention in patients found to be mildly hypertensive, *Arch. Surg.*, 115: 1204–6, 1980.

1718. Aldrete, J. A., Romo-Salas, F., Jankovsky, L. and Franatovic, Y., Effect of pretreatment with thiopental and phenytoin on postischemic brain damage in rabbits, *Critical Care Medicine*, 7(10): 466–70, 1979.

1719. Aldrete, J. A., Romo-Salas, F., Mazzia, V. D. B. and Tan, S., Diphenylhydantoin for reversal of neurological injury after cardiac arrest, *Rev. Bras. Anest.*, 30(4): 263–7, 1980.

1720. Ali, I. I. and Dutta, S., Distribution of C^{14}-diphenylhydantoin (DPH) in relation to its antidysrhythmic effect in dogs, *Fed. Proc.* 36: 1012, 1977.

1721. Allen, M. A., Wrenn, J. M., Putney, J. W. and Borzelleca, J. F., A study of the mechanism of transport of diphenylhydantoin in the rat submaxillary gland *in vitro*, *J. Pharmacol. Exp. Ther.*, 197(2): 408–13, 1976.

1722. Anderson, R. J. and Raines, A., Suppression of decerebrate rigidity by phenytoin and chlorpromazine, *Neurol.*, 26: 858–62, 1976.

1723. Appenzeller, O., Feldman, R. G. and Friedman, A. P., Migraine, headache, and related conditions, *Arch. Neurol.*, 36: 784–805, 1979.

1724. Apton, R., Dilantin and its relation to caries incidence, *Dent. Hyg.*, 51: 349–51, 1977.

1725. Arnaout, M. A. and Salti, I., Phenytoin in benign insulinoma, *Lancet*, 861, 1976.

1726. Arnsdorf, M. F. and Mehlman, D. J., Observations on the effects of selected antiarrhythmic drugs on mammalian cardiac Purkinje fibers with two levels of steady-state potential: Influences of lidocaine, phenytoin, propranolol, disopyramide and procainamide on repolarization, action potential shape and conduction, *J. Pharmacol. Exp. Ther.*, 207(3): 983–91, 1978.

1727. Artru, A. A. and Michenfelder, J. D., Cerebral potassium release reduced by diphenylhydantoin: mechanism of cerebral protection, *Ann. Neurol.*, 6(2): 151, 1979.

1728. Artru, A. A. and Michenfelder, J. D., Cerebral protective, metabolic, and vascular effects of phenytoin, *Stroke*, 11(4): 377–82, 1980.

1729. Asboe-Hansen, G., Treatment of generalized scleroderma: updated results, *Acta Derm. Venereol.*, 59(5): 465–7, 1979.

1730. Ayala, G. F. and Johnston, D., Phenytoin: electrophysiological studies in simple neuronal systems, *Antiepileptic Drugs: Mechanisms of Action*, 339–51, Glaser, G. H., Penry, J. K. and Woodbury, D. M., Eds., Raven Press, New York, 1980.

1731. Ayala, G. F. and Johnston, D., The influences of phenytoin on the fundamental electrical properties of simple neural systems, *Epilepsia*, 18(3): 299–307, 1977.

1732. Ayala, G. F., Johnson, D., Lin, S., and Dichter, H. N., The mechanism of action of diphenylhydantoin on invertebrate neurons: II. Effects on synaptic mechanisms, *Brain Res.*, 121: 259–70, 1977.

1733. Ayala, G. F., Lin, S. and Johnston, D., The mechanism of action of diphenylhydantoin on invertebrate neurons: I. Effects on basic membrane properties, *Brain Res.*, 121: 245–58, 1977.

1734. Baselt, R. C. and Cravey, R. H., A compendium of therapeutic and toxic concentrations of toxicologically significant drugs in human biofluids, *J. Anal. Toxicol.*, 1: 81–103, 1977.

1735. Baskin, S. I., Leibman, A. J., DeWitt, W. S., Orr, P. L., Tarzy, N. T., Levy, P., Krusz, J. C., Dhopesh, V. P. and Schraeder, P. L., Mechanism of the anticonvulsant action of phenytoin: regulation of central nervous system taurine levels, *Neurology*, 28(4): 331–2, 1978.

1736. Baskin, S. I. and Melrose, B. L., The effect of diphenylhydantoin on the formation and dissociation of the cardiac glycoside—(Na^+ + K^+)-ATPase complex, *Clin. Res.*, 23: 172A, April 1975.

1737. Baratz, R. and Mesulam, M. M., Adult-onset stuttering treated with anticonvulsants, *Arch. Neurol.*, 38: 132, 1981.

1738. Bauer, E. A., Cooper, T. W., Tucker, D. R. and Esterly, N. B., Phenytoin therapy of recessive dystrophic epidermolysis bullosa: clinical trial and proposed mechanism of action on collagenase, *New Eng. J. Med.*, 303(14): 776–81, 1980.

1739. Bayer, R., Kaufmann, R. and Gudjons, M., The effects of diphenylhydantoin on mechanical and electrical properties of isolated cat myocardium, *Naunyn-Schmied. Arch. Pharmacol.*, 298: 273–82, 1977.

1740. Bechtel, P., Delafin, C. and Bechtel, Y., Induction of hepatic cytochrome P-450 and b5 in mice by phenytoin during chronic hypoxia, *C. R. Soc. Biol. (Paris)*, 170(2): 325–30, 1976.

1741. Beckner, T. F. and Idsvoog, P., Drug use and distribution in a pain rehabilitation center, *Am. J. Hosp. Pharm.*, 32: 285–9, 1975.

1742. Benowitz, N. L., Rosenberg, J. and Becker, C. E., Cardiopulmonary catastrophes in drug-overdosed patients, *Med. Clin. North Am.*, 63(10): 267–96, 1979.

1743. Berger, M. and Berchtold, P., Side effects of antiepileptic agents, *Dtsch. Med. Wschr.*, 100: 2552, 1975.

1744. Berger, M., Berchtold, P., Cuppers, H. J., Wiegelmann, W., Drost, H., Sailer, R., Borchard, F. and Zimmermann, H., Suppressibility of serum insulin in patients with insulinoma by somatostatin, diazoxide and diphenylhydantoin, *Presented at 4th International Danube Symposium on Diabetes Mellitus, Dubrovnik*, 1975.

1745. Bianchi, C. P., Cell calcium and malignant hyperthermia, *International Symposium on Malignant Hyperthermia*, 147–51, Gordon, R. A., Britt, B. A. and Kalow, W., Eds., Charles C Thomas, Illinois, 1973.

1746. Bianchi, C., Beani, L. and Bertelli, A., Effects of some antiepileptic drugs on brain acetylcholine, *Epilepsy Abstracts*, 8(9): 231, 1975.

1747. Biberdorf, R. I. and Spurbeck, G. H., Phenytoin in IV fluids: results endorsed, *Drug Intell. Clin. Pharm.*, 12: 300–1, 1978.

1748. Bigger, J. T., Antiarrhythmic drugs in ischemic heart disease, *Hosp. Pract.*, 7: 69–80, 1972.

1749. Bigger, J. T., Heissenbuttel, R. H. and Lovejoy, W. P., Management of cardiac problems in the intensive care unit, *Med. Clin. N. Am.*, 55: 1183–1205, 1971.

1750. Bihler, I. and Sawh, P. C., Effects of Diphenylhydantoin on the transport of Na^+ and K^+ and the regulation of sugar transport in muscle *in vitro*, *Biochim. Biophys. Acta*, 249: 240–51, 1971.

1751. Binnion, P. F. and DasGupta, R. Tritiated digoxin metabolism after prior treatment with propranolol or diphenylhydantoin sodium, *Int. J. Clin. Pharmacol.*, 12: 96–101, 1975.

1752. Biryukov, V. B., The treatment of patients with different forms of myotonia with diphenine and novocainamide, *Zh. Nevropatol, Psikhiatr.*, 76: 1333–5, 1976.

1753. Boller, F., Wright, D. G., Cavalieri, R. and Mitsumoto, H., Paroxysmal "nightmares," *Neurology*, 55: 1026–28, 1975.

1754. Boon, W. H., Benign myoclonus in infants and children, *J. Singapore Paediat. Soc.*, 20(2): 60–8, 1978.

1755. Bowdle, T. A., Neal, G. D., Levy, R. H. and Heimbach, D. M., Phenytoin pharmacokinetics in burned rats and plasma protein binding of phenytoin in burned patients, *J. Pharmacol. Exp. Ther.*, 213(1): 97–9, 1980.

1756. Bricaire, H., Luton, J. P., Wechsler, B., Messing, B. and Halaby, G., Inappropriate secretion of insulin by an islet cell adenoma. Trial treatment with diphenylhydantoin, *Ann. Med. Intern.*, 127(5): 403–7, 1976.

1757. British Medical Journal, Editor, Treatment of tinnitus, *Br. Med. J.*, 1445–6, 1979.

1758. Broser, F., Ditzen, G. and Friedrich, K., Complementary electro-physiological findings in a case of neuromyotonia, *Nervenarzt*, 46: 100–4, 1975.

1759. Buda, F. B. and Joyce, R. P., Successful treatment of atypical migraine of childhood with anticonvulsants, *Mil. Med.*, 144(8): 521–3, 1979.

1760. Bustamante, L., Lueders, H., Pippenger, C. and Goldensohn, E. S., The effects of phenytoin on the penicillin-induced spike focus, *Electroencephalogr. Clin. Neurophysiol.*, 48: 90–7, 1980.

1761. Caillard, C., Menu, A., Plotkine, M. and Rossignol, P., Do anticonvulsant drugs exert protective effect against hypoxia?, *Life Sci.*, 16: 1607–12, 1975.

1762. Callaghan, N., Feely, M., O'Callaghan, M., Duggan, B., McGarry, J., Cramer, B., Wheelan, J. and Seldrup, J., The effects of toxic and non-toxic serum phenytoin levels on carbohydrate tolerance and insulin levels, *Acta Neurol. Scand.*, 56: 563–71, 1977.

1763. Caplan, L. R., Weiner, H., Weintraub, R. M. and Austen, W. G., "Migrainous" neurologic dysfunction in patients with prosthetic cardiac valves, *Headache*, 16: 218–21, 1976.

1764. Carney, J. M., Rosecrans, J. A. and Vasko, M. R., Barbitone-induced tolerance to the effects of sedative hypnotics and related compounds on operant behavior in the rat, *Br. J. Pharmac.*, 65: 183–92, 1979.

1765. Carson, I. W., Lyons, S. M. and Shanks, R. G., Anti-arrhythmic drugs, *Br. J. Anaesth.*, 51: 659–70, 1979.

1766. Celis, G. R., Kula, R. W., Somasundaram, M., Sher, J. H. and Schutta, H. S., Myokymia of segmental spinal cord origin, *Ann. Neurol.*, 8(1): 95, 1980.

1767. Chadda, V. S. and Mathur, M. S., Double blind study of the effects of diphenylhydantoin sodium on diabetic neuropathy, *J. Assoc. Phys. Ind.*, 26: 403–6, 1978.

1768. Chai, C. Y., Lee, T. M. and Wang, S. C., Effects of diphenylhydantoin on cardiac arrhythmias induced by carotid occlusion in the cat, *Arch. Int. Pharmacodyn.*, 219: 180–92, 1976.

1769. Chalfie, M. and Perlman, R. L., Inhibition of catechol-amine synthesis and tyrosine 3-monooxygenase activation in pheochromocytoma cells by diphenylhydantoin, *Neurochem.*, 29: 757–9, 1977.

1770. Chapa-Alvarez, J. R., Francisco-Mendiola, J., Espejo-Plascencia, I. and Rodriguez-Noriega, E., Results obtained in the treatment of burns with sodium diphenylhydantoin, *Personal Communication*, 1981.

1771. Chapman, J. H., Schrank, J. P. and Crampton, R. S., Idiopathic ventricular tachycardia—an intracardiac electrical hemodynamic and angiographic assessment of six patients, *Am. J. Med.*, 59: 470–80, 1975.

1772. Cisson, C. M., Entrikin, R. K. and Wilson, B. W., Actions of phenytoin on acetylcholinesterase (ACHE), creatine kinase (CK) and protein of cultured chick embryo muscle, *Fed. Proc.*, 36: 498, March, 1977.

1773. Clemmesen, J., Incidence of neoplasms in a population on anti-convulsant drugs, *Anti-convulsant Drugs and Enzyme Induction, Study Group 9 of the Institute for Research into Mental and Multiple Handicap*, 123–30, Richens, A. and Woodford, F. P., Eds., Associated Scientific Publication, Amsterdam, 1976.

1774. Cloyd, J. C., Bosch, D. E. and Sawchuk, R. J., Concentration-time profile of phenytoin after admixture with small volumes of intravenous fluids, *Am. J. Hosp. Pharm.*, 35: 45–8, 1978.

1775. Cobbs, B. W. and Kings, S. B., Ventricular buckling: A factor in the abnormal ventriculogram and peculiar hemodynamics associated with mitral valve prolapse, *Am. Heart J.*, 93(6): 741–58, 1977.

1776. Cochran, P. T., Linnebur, A. C., Wright, W. and Matsumoto, S., Electrophysiologic studies in patients with long Q-T syndrome, *Clin. Res.*, 25(2): 88A, Feb. 1977.

1777. Cohan, S. L., Anderson, R. J. and Raines, A., Diphenylhydantoin and chlorpromazine in the treatment of spasticity, *Neurology*, 367, April, 1976.

1778. Cohan, S. L., Raines, A., Panagakos, J. and Armitage, P., Phenytoin and chlorpromazine in the treatment of spasticity, *Arch. Neurol.*, 37: 360–4, 1980.

1779. Cohen, L. S., Diphenylhydantoin sodium (Dilantin), *Current Cardiovascular Topics, Vol. I., Drugs in Cardiology, Part I*, 49–79, Donoso, E., Ed., Stratton Intercontinental Medical Book Corp., New York, 1975.

1780. Connors, B. W., Pentobarbital and diphenylhydantoin effects on the excitability and GABA sensitivity of rat dorsal root ganglion cells, *Society for Neuroscience, 9th Annual Meeting*, Nov. 2–6, 1979.

1781. Cookson, S. L. and Mann, J. D., Reversal and prevention of acute morphine induced catalepsy by phenytoin in naive rats, *Neurosci. Abstr.*, 4: 488, 1978.

1782. Cordone, G., Iester, A., Venzano, V. and Minetti, C., A case of Thomsen's disease associated with hypoparathyroidism, *Minerva Pediatrica.*, 30: 1629–34, 1979.

1783. Corr, P. B. and Gillis, R. A., Beneficial cardiac rhythm effects produced by diphenylhydantoin in experimental myocardial infarction, *Fed. Proc.*, 35: 222, 1976.

1784. Cotler, H. M. and Christensen, H. D., Tissue distribution of diphenylhydantoin, *Fed. Proc.*, 35: 664, 1976.

1785. Counsell, R. E., Ranada, V. V., Kline, W., Hong, B. H. and Buswink, A. A., Potential organ or tumor imaging agents XV: radioiodinated phenytoin derivatives, *J. of Pharmac. Sci.*, 65(2): 285–7, 1976.

1786. Crampton, R. S., Another link between the left stellate ganglion and the long Q-T syndrome, *Am. Heart J.*, 96(1): 130–2, 1978.

1787. Cudworth, A. G. and Barber, H. E., The effect of hydrocortisone phosphate, methylprednisolone and phenytoin on pancreatic insulin release and hepatic glutathione-insulin transhydrogenase activity in the rat, *Eur. J. Pharmacol.*, 31: 23–8, 1975.

1788. Cullen, J. P., Aldrete, J. A., Jankovsky, L. and Romo-Salas, F., Protective action of phenytoin in cerebral ischemia, *Anesth. Analg.*, 58: 165–9, 1979.

1789. Dadkar, M. K., Gupte, R. D. and Dohadwalla, A. M., Effect of diphenylhydantoin on blood pressure of spontaneously hypertensive rats, *Med. Biol.*, 57: 398–401, 1979.

1790. Dalessio, D. J., Medical treatment of trigeminal neuralgia, *Clin. Neurosurg.*, 24: 579–83, 1976.

1791. Das, D., Ayromlooi, J., Tobias, M., Desiderio, D. and Steinberg, H., Effect of Dilantin (D) on hypoxic fetal rabbit lung, *Pediatr. Res.*, 14: 640, 1980.

1792. Data, J. L., Wilkinson, G. R. and Nies, A. S., Interaction of quinidine with anticonvulsant drugs, *New Eng. J. Med.*, 294(13): 699–702, 1976.

1793. Dawson, G. W., Brown, H. W. and Clark, B. G., Serum phenytoin after ethosuximide, *Neurology*, 4(6): 583–4, 1978.

1794. Deisz, R. A. and Lux, H. D., Diphenylhydantoin prolongs post-synaptic inhibition and iontophoretic GABA action in the crayfish stretch receptor, *Neuroscience Letters*, 5: 199–203, 1977.

1795. Deisz, R. A. and Lux, H. D., Postsynaptic inhibition of the crayfish stretch receptor: prolongation by diphenylhydantoin, *Pflugers Arch. Ges. Physiol.*, Suppl. 368: R33, 1977.

1796. Dekeban, A. S. and Lehman, E. J. B., Effects of different dosages of anticonvulsant drugs on mental performance in patients with chronic epilepsy, *Acta Neurol. Scand.*, 52: 319–30, 1975.

1797. de la Torre, R., Murgia-Suarez, J. J. and Aldrete, J. A., Comparison of phenytoin and conventional drug therapy in the treatment of mild hypertension, *Clin. Ther.*, 3(4): 117–24, 1980.

1798. Delgado-Escueta, A. V. and Horan, M. P., Phenytoin: biochemical membrane studies, *Antiepileptic Drugs: Mechanisms of Action*, 377–98, Glaser, G. H., Penry, J. K. and Woodbury, D. M., Eds., Raven Press, New York, 1980.

1799. DeLorenzo, R. J., Phenytoin: calcium- and calmodulin-dependent protein phosphorylation and neurotransmitter release, *Antiepileptic Drugs: Mechanisms of Action*, 399–414, Glaser, G. H., Penry, J. K. and Woodbury, D. M., Eds., Raven Press, New York, 1980.

1800. DeLorenzo, R. J. and Freedman, S. D., Phenytoin inhibition of neurotransmitter release and protein phosphorylation, *Neurology*, 28(4): 367–68, 1978.

1801. DesRosiers, M., Grave, G. D., Kupferberg, H. J. and Kennedy, C., Effects of diphenylhydantoin on local cerebral blood flow, *Pharmacology and Anesthesia*, 339–42, Springer-Verlag, New York, 1975.

1802. Deupree, J. D. and Weaver, J. A., Inhibition of rat brain phosphodiesterases and adenylate cyclase by phenytoin, *Fed. Proc.* 38(3): 754, March, 1979.

1803. De Weer, P., Phenytoin: blockage of resting sodium channels, *Antiepileptic Drugs: Mechanisms of Action*, 353–61, Glaser, G. H., Penry, J. K. and Woodbury, D. M., Eds., Raven Press, New York, 1980.

1804. Dhatt, M. S., Akhtar, M., Reddy, C. P., Gomes, J. A. C., Lau, S. H., Caracta, A. R. and Damato, A. N., Modification and abolition of re-entry within the His-Purkinje system in man by diphenylhydantoin, *Circulation*, 56(5): 720–26, 1977.

1805. Dhatt, M. S., Gomes, J. A. C., Reddy, C. P., Akhtar, M., Caracta, A. R., Lau, S. H. and Damato, A. N., Effects of phenytoin on refractoriness and conduction in the human heart, *J. Cardiovasc. Surg.*, 1: 3–18, 1979.

1806. Dilman, V. M. and Anisimov, V. N., Effect of treatment with phenformin, diphenylhydantoin or L-dopa on life span and tumour incidence in C3H/Sn mice, *Gerontology*, 26: 241–6, 1980.

1807. Dilman, V. M., Bershtein, L. M., Tsyrlina, E. V., Bobrov, Y. F., Kovaleva, I. G., Vasileva, I. A. and Kryloya, N. V., The correction of endocrinous metabolic disturbances in oncological patients. The effect of biguanides (phenformin and adebit), miskleron, and diphenine, *Vopr. Onkol.*, 21(11): 33–9, 1975.

1808. Dodrill, C. B., Diphenylhydantoin serum levels, toxicity, and neuropsychological performance in patients with epilepsy, *Epilepsia*, 16: 593–600, 1975.

1809. Drazin, B., Ayalon, D., Hoerer, E., Oberman, Z., Harell, A., Ravid, R. and Laurian, L., Effect of diphenylhydantoin on patterns of insulin secretion in obese subjects, *Acta Diabetol. Lat.*, 14: 51–61, Jan/Apr 1977.

1810. Dreifus, L. S. and Morganroth, J., Antiarrhythmic agents and their use in therapy, *Pharmacol. Ther.*, 9: 75–106, 1980.

1811. Dretchen, K. L., Standaert, F. G. and Raines, A., Effects of phenytoin on the cyclic nucleotide system in the motor nerve terminal, *Epilepsia*, 18(3): 337–48, 1977.

1812. Duckrow, R. B. and Taub, A., The effect of diphenylhydantoin on self mutilation in rats produced by unilateral multiple dorsal rhizotomy, *Epilepsy Abstracts*, 11(1): 27, 1977.

1813. Duperrat, B., Puissant, A., Saurat, J. H., Delanoe, J., Doyard, P. A. and Grunfels, J. P., Fabry's disease neonatal angiokeratomas. Effect of diphenylhydantoin on acute pain episodes, *Ann. Derm. Syph.* (Paris), 102(4): 392–3, 1975.

1814. Eadie, M. J., The management of vertigo, *Med. J. Aust.*, 135–6, July 26, 1975.

1815. Ehring, G. R. and Hondeghem, L. M., Rate, rhythm and voltage dependent effects of phenytoin: a test of a model of the mechanisms of action of antiarrhythmic drugs, *Proc. West. Pharmacol. Soc.*, 21: 63–5, 1978.

1816. Ehrnebo, M. and Odar-Cederlof, I., Binding of amobarbital, pentobarbital and diphenylhydantoin to blood cells and plasma proteins in healthy volunteers and uraemic patients, *Europ. J. Clin. Pharmacol.*, 8: 445–53, 1975.

1817. Eisenberg, M., Stevens, L. H. and Schofield, P. J., Epidermolysis bullosa—new therapeutic approaches, *Aust. J. Derm.*, 19: 1–8, 1978.

1818. Elfstrom, J., Plasma protein binding of phenytoin after cholecystectomy and neurosurgical operations, *Acta Neurol. Scand.*, 55: 455–64, 1977.

1819. Ellenberg, M., Unremitting painful diabetic neuropathy, *JAMA*, 237(18): 1986, 1977.

1820. Elliott, P. N. C., Jenner, P., Chadwick, D., Reynolds, E. and Marsden, C. D., The effect of diphenylhydantoin on central catecholamine containing neuronal systems, *J. Pharm. Pharmac.*, 29: 41–3, 1977.

1821. Ellis, J. M. and Lee, S. I., Acute prolonged confusion in later life as an ictal state, *Epilepsia*, 19: 119–28, 1978.

1822. El-Sherif, N. and Lazzara, R., Re-entrant ventricular arrhythmias in the late myocardial infarction period, 5. Mechanism of action of diphenylhydantoin, *Circulation*, 57(3): 465–73, 1978.

1823. Entrikin, R. K., Patterson, G. T., Weidoff, P. M. and Wilson, B. W., Righting ability and skeletal muscle properties of phenytoin-treated dystrophic chickens, *Exp. Neurol.*, 61: 650–63, 1978.

1824. Entrikin, R. K., Swanson, K. L., Weidoff, P. M., Patterson, G. T. and Wilson, B. W., Avian muscular dystrophy: functional and bio-chemical improvement with diphenylhydantoin. *Science*, 195: 873–5, 1977.

1825. Esparza-Ahumada, S., Chapa-Alvarez, R., Andrade-Perez, J. S. and Rodriguez-Noriega, E., The improvement of chronic vascular leg ulcers while on treatment with diphenylhydantoin sodium, *Personal Communication*, 1981.

1826. Eviatar, L. and Eviatar, A., Vertigo in children: differential diagnosis and treatment, *Pediatrics*, 59: 833–8, 1977.

1827. Faugier-Grimaud, S., Action of anticonvulsants on pentylenetetrazol-induced epileptiform activity on invertebrate neurones (Helix aspersa), *Epilepsy Abstracts*, 12(11): 489, 1979.

1828. Ferrendelli, J. A., Phenytoin: cyclic nucleotide regulation in the brain, *Antiepileptic Drugs: Mechanisms of Action*, 429–33, Glaser, G. H., Penry, J. K. and Woodbury, D. M., Eds., Raven Press, New York, 1980.

1829. Ferrendelli, J. A. and Kinscherf, D. A., Inhibitory effects of anticonvulsant drugs on cyclic nucleotide accumulation in brain, *Ann. Neurol.*, 5: 533–8, 1979.

1830. Ferrendelli, J. A. and Kinscherf, D. A., Phenytoin: effects on calcium flux and cyclic nucleotides, *Epilepsia*, 18(3): 331–6, 1977.

1831. Ferrendelli, J. A. and Kinscherf, D. A., Similar effects of phenytoin and tetrodotoxin on cyclic nucleotide regulation in depolarized brain tissue, *J. Pharm. Exp. Ther.*, 207(3): 787–93, 1978.

1832. Fincham, R. W. and Schottelius, D. D., Decreased phenytoin levels in antineoplastic therapy, *Ther. Drug Monitoring*, 1: 277–83, 1979.

1833. Finelli, P. F., Phenytoin and methadone tolerance, *New Eng. J. Med.*, 294(4): 227, 1976.

1834. Fisher, J. D., Cohen, H. L., Mehra, R., Altschuler, H., Escher, D. J. W. and Furman, S., Cardiac pacing and pacemakers II. Serial electro-physiologic-pharmacologic testing for control of recurrent tachyarrhythmias, *Am. Heart J.*, 93(5): 658–68, 1977.

1835. Fleming, K., Japanese encephalitis in an Australian soldier returned from Vietnam, *Med. J. Aust.*, 2: 19–23, 1975.

1836. Friis, M. L., Epilepsy among parents of children with facial clefts, *Epilepsia*, 20: 69–76, 1979.

1837. Fromm, G. H., Glass, J. D., Chattha, A. S. and Martinez, A. J., Effect of anticonvulsant drugs on inhibitory and excitatory pathways, *Epilepsia*, 22: 65–73, 1981.

1838. Fromm, G. H., Glass, J. D., Chattha, A. S. and Terrence, C. F., Role of inhibitory mechanisms in trigeminal neuralgia, *Neurology*, 30: 417, 1980.

1839. Fry, B. and Ciarlone, A. E., Phenytoin increases norepinephrine (NE) and serotonin (5-HT) in mouse cerebellum, *Pharmacologist*, 21(3): 183, 1979.

1840. Frymoyer, J. W., Fracture healing in rats treated with diphenylhydantoin (Dilantin), *J. Trauma*, 16(5): 368–70, 1976.

1841. Fukuyama, Y., Ochiai, Y., Hayakawa, T. and Miyagawa, F., Overnight sleep EEG and cerebrospinal fluid monoamines in seizures induced by movement, *Neuropadiatrie*, 10(2): 138–49, 1979.

1842. Furman, R. E. and Barchi, R. L., The pathophysiology of myotonia produced by aromatic carboxylic acids, *Ann. Neurol.*, 4(4): 357–65, 1978.

1843. Gage, P. W., Lonergan, M. and Torda, T. A., Presynaptic and postsynaptic depressant effects of phenytoin sodium at the neuromuscular junction, *Br. J. Pharmac.*, 69: 119–21, 1980.

1844. Gage, P. W. and Spence, I., The origin of the muscle fasciculation caused by funnel-web spider venom, *Epilepsy Abstracts*, 11(9): 364, 1978.

1845. Gallaghan, J. T., Kinetic inhibition studies of microsomal phenytoin (DPH), *Fed. Proc.*, 35(3): 408, 1976.

1846. Gangji, D., Schwade, J. G. and Strong, J. M., Phenytoin-misonidazole: possible metabolic interaction, *Cancer Treat. Rep.*, 64(1): 155–6, 1980.

1847. Garson, A., Kugler, J. D., Gillette, P. C., Simonelli, A. and McNamara, D. G., Control of late postoperative ventricular arrhythmias with phenytoin in young patients, *Am. J. Cardiol.*, 46(2): 290–4, 1980.

1848. Gautray, J. P., Jolivet, A., Goldenberg, F., Tajchner, G., and Eberhard, A., Clinical investigation of the menstrual cycle. II Neuroendocrine investigation and therapy of the inadequate luteal phase, *Fertility and Sterility*, 29(3): 275–281, 1978.

1849. Gelehrter, T. D., Enzyme induction (second of three parts), *New Eng. J. Med.*, 294(11): 589–95, 1976.

1850. Gibberd, F. B. and Webley, M., Studies in man of phenytoin absorption and its implication, *Epilepsy Abstracts*, 9(2): 78, 1976.

1851. Gibbs, M. E. and Ng, K. T., Diphenylhydantoin facilitation of labile, protein-independent memory, *Brain Research Bulletin*, 1: 203–8, 1976.

1852. Gibbs, M. E. and Ng, K. T., Psychobiology of memory: towards a model of memory formation, *Biobehavioral Reviews*, 1: 113–36, 1977.

1853. Gilbert, J. C., Diseases of the cardiovascular system—drugs affecting the cardiovascular system: pharmacological basis of treatment, *Br. Med. J.*, 31–3, 1976.

1854. Gilbert, J. C. and Wyllie, M. G., Effects of anticonvulsant and convulsant drugs on the ATPase activities of synaptosomes and their components, *Br. J. Pharmac.*, 56: 49–57, 1976.

1855. Gilbert, J. C. and Wyllie, M. G., The relationship between nerve terminal adenosine triphosphatases and neurotransmitter release: as determined by the use of antidepressant and other CNS-active drugs, *Br. J. Pharmac.*, 69: 215–25, 1980.

1856. Gill, M. A., Miscia, V. F. and Gourley, D. R., The treatment of common cardiac arrhythmias, *J. Amer. Pharm. Assn.*, NS16(1): 20–9, Jan. 1976.

1857. Gillette, P. C. and Garson, A., Electrophysiologic and pharmacologic characteristics of automatic ectopic atrial tachycardia, *Circulation*, 56: 571–5, 1977.

1858. Glaser, G. H., Penry, J. K. and Woodbury, D. M., Eds., *Antiepileptic Drugs: Mechanisms of Action*, Raven Press, New York, 1980.

1859. Goldberg, M. A., Phenytoin: binding, *Antiepileptic Drugs: Mechanisms of Action*, 323–37, Glaser, G. H., Penry, J. K. and Woodbury, D. M., Eds., Raven Press, New York, 1980.

1860. Goldberg, M. A., Phenytoin, phospholipids and calcium, *Neurology*, 27: 827–33, 1977.

1861. Goldberg, M. A. and Crandall, P. H., Human brain binding of phenytoin, *Neurology*, 28: 881–5, 1978.

1862. Goldberg, M. A. and Todoroff, T., Phenytoin binding to brain phospholipids, *Neurology*, 26: 386, 1976.

1863. Goldberg, M. A., Todoroff, T. and Crandall, P., Phenytoin binding to human brain, *Neurology*, 27(4): 374, 1977.

1864. Goldman, E., Aldrete, J. A. and Sherrill, D., Phenytoin brain protection in acute reversible hypoxia, *7th World Congress of Anaesthesiologists*, Hamburg, 215–6, Sept. 1980.

1865. Goldsmith, S. and From, A. H. L., Arsenic-induced atypical ventricular tachycardia, *New Eng. J. Med.*, 303(19): 1096–8, 1980.

1866. Goodenough, D. J., Fariello, R. G., Annis, B. L. and Chun, R. W. M., Familial and acquired paroxysmal dyskinesias, *Arch. Neurol.*, 35: 827–31, 1978.

1867. Goultschin, J. and Shoshan, S., Inhibition of collagen breakdown by diphenylhydantoin, *Biochim. Biophys. Acta*, 631: 188–91, 1980.

1868. Grafova, V. N., Danilova, E. I. and Kryzhanovskii, G. N., Analgesic effects of antiepileptic drugs in a pain syndrome of spinal origin, *Bull. Exp. Biol. Med.*, 88(8): 837–40, 1979.

1869. Green, R. S. and Rau, J. H., The use of diphenylhydantoin in compulsive eating disorders; further studies, *Anorexia Nervosa*, 377–82, Vigersky, R. A., Ed., Raven Press, New York, 1977.

1870. Greenblatt, D. J., Allen, M. D., Koch-Weser, J. and Shader, R. I., Accidental poisoning with psychotropic drugs in children, *Am. J. Dis. Child*, 130: 507–11, 1976.

1871. Greenblatt, D. J. and Shader, R. I., Intravenous phenytoin, *New Eng. J. Med.*, 1078, 1976.

1872. Griggs, R. C., Moxley, R. T., Riggs, J. E. and Engel, W. K., Effects of acetazolamide on myotonia, *Ann. Neurol.*, 3: 531–7, 1978.

1873. Gustafson, A., Svensson, S. E. and Ugander, L., Cardiac arrhythmias in chloral hydrate poisoning, *Acta Med. Scand.*, 201: 227–30, 1977.

1874. Hadfield, M. G. and Rigby, W. F. C., Dopamine: Adaptive uptake changes in striatal synaptosomes after 30 seconds of intense fighting, *Biochem. Pharmacol.*, 25: 2752–4, 1976.

1875. Hadfield, M. G. and Weber, N. E., Effect of fighting and diphenylhydantoin on the uptake of 3H-1-norepinephrine *in vitro* in synaptosomes isolated from retired male breeding mice. *Biochem. Pharmacol.*, 24: 1538–40, 1975.

1876. Haffner, Z. and Hovarth, E., Pseudomyotonia (Isaacs-syndroma), *Orvosi Hetilap*, 116(49): 2895–7, 1975.

1877. Hahn, T. J., Dibartelo, T. F. and Halstead, L. R., Comparative effects of diphenylhydantoin (DPH) and ouabain (Ou) ^{45}Ca release from cultured fetal rat forelimb rudiments, *Clin. Res.*, 26(5): 681A, 1978.

1878. Hahn, T. J., Scharp, C. R., Richardson, C. A., Halstead, L. R., Kahn, A. J. and Teitelbaum, S. L., Interaction of diphenylhydantoin (phenytoin) and phenobarbital with hormonal mediation of fetal rat bone resorption *in vitro*, *J. Clin. Invest.*, 62: 406–14, 1978.

1879. Hamed, M. A., Abdel-Aal, H. M., Abdel-Aziz, T. M., Nassar, S. K., Sweify, S. M., Atta, S. M., El-Awady, S. M., El-Aref, M., El-Garf, A. R., A trial of diphenylhydantoin in periodic disease (familial Mediterranean fever) in Egyptian children, *J. Egypt. Med. Assoc.*, 58(¾): 205–15, 1975.

1880. Hamer, J., Diseases of the cardiovascular system—cardiac failure, *Br. Med. J.*, 220–4, 1976.

1881. Hansotia, P., Mazza, J. J. and Gatlin, P., Diphenylhydantoin and fragility of erythrocytes in normal subjects and in patients with hereditary spherocytic anemia. *Amer. J. Clin. Path.*, 64(1): 75–9, 1975.

1882. Hanstom, L. and Jones, I. L., The effect of diphenylhydantoin upon degradation of sulphated macromolecules in cat palatal mucosa *in vitro*, *Med. Biol.*, 57: 177–81, 1979.

1883. Hardie, R. A. and Savin, J. A., Drug-induced skin diseases, *Br. Med. J.*, 935–7, 1979.

1884. Haruda, F., Phenytoin hypersensitivity, *Neurology*, 29: 1480–5, 1979.

1885. Harvey, S. C., The effects of ouabain and phenytoin on myocardial noradrenaline, *Arch. Int. Pharmacodyn.*, 213(2): 222–36, 1975.

1886. Hatangdi, V. S., Boas, R. A. and Richards, E. G., Postherpetic neuralgia: management with antiepileptic and tricyclic drugs, *Advances in Pain Research and Therapy*, Vol. 1, 583–587, Bonica, J. J. and Albe-Fessard, D., Eds., Raven Press, New York, 1976.

1887. Haward, L. R. C., Augmentation of autogenic training by sodium diphenylhydantoinate, *World J. Psychosynthesis*, 8: 26–29, 1976.

1888. Haward, L. R. C., Impairment of flying efficiency in anancastic pilots, *Aviation, Space & Environmental Medicine*, 156–161, 1977.

1889. Heesen, H. and Lahrtz, H., Treatment of severe digitalis intoxication in suicidal attempt, *Med. Klin.*, 70: 812–6, 1975.

1890. Hegarty, B. A., Treatment of severe self-imposed overdose of phencyclidine hydrochloride, *Bulletin Sinai Hosp.*, Detroit, 23(3): 147–51, 1975.

1891. Heinonen, O. P., Slone, D. and Shapiro, S., Birth defects and drugs in pregnancy, *Lancet* (Review) 1086, 1977.

1892. Helfant, R. H., Effectiveness of diphenylhydantoin as an antihypertensive, *Personal Communication*, 1975.

1893. Henry, D. A., Bell, G. D. and Glithero, P., Plasma high-density lipoproteins, *New Eng. J. Med.*, 300(14): 798, 1979.

1894. Herishanu, Y., Eylath, U. and Ilan, R., 'In vitro' studies on the fate of diphenylhydantoin in uremia, *Neurosci. Lett.*, 2: 97–101, 1976.

1895. Herishanu, Y., Eylath, U. and Ilan, R., Effects of calcium content of diet on absorption of diphenylhydantoin, *Israel J. Med. Sci.*, 12(12): 1453–6, 1976.

1896. Hertz, L., Drug-induced alterations of ion distribution at the cellular level of the central nervous system, *Pharmacol. Rev.*, 29(1): 35–65, 1977.

1897. Herzberg, G. R., Challberg, M. D., Hess, B. C. and Howland, J. L., Elevated potassium efflux from dystrophic diaphragm: influence of diphenylhydantoin and lithium, *Biochem. Biophys. Res. Commun.*, 63(4): 858–63, 1975.

1898. Heyma, P., Larkins, R. G., Perry-Keene, D., Peter, C. T., Ross, D. and Sloman, J. G., Thyroid hormone levels and protein binding in patients on long-term diphenylhydantoin treatment, *Clin. Endocrin.*, 6: 369–76, 1977.

1899. Homan, R. W., Vasko, M. R. and Blaw, M., Phenytoin plasma concentrations in paroxysmal kinesigenic choreoathetosis, *Neurology*, 30: 673–76, 1980.

1900. Hondeghem, L. M., Effects of lidocaine, phenytoin and quinidine on the ischemic canine myocardium, *J. Electrocardiol.*, 9(3): 203–9, 1976.

1901. Hondeghem, L. M., Effects of quinidine, lidocaine and phenytoin on the excitability of the ischemic rabbit heart, *Proc. West. Pharmacol. Soc.*, 19: 320–22, 1976.

1902. Hufnagl, H. D. and Sen, S., Phenytoin infusions in medical intensive care, *Fortschr. Med.*, 96: 415–24, 1978.

1903. Hulce, V. D., The action of chlorpromazine and phenytoin on muscle rigidity due to cerebellar lesions, *Society for Neuroscience*, III: 372, 7th Annual Meeting, Nov. 7–10, 1977.

1904. Ifabumuyi, O. I. and Jeffries, J. J., Treatment of drug-induced psychosis with diphenylhydantoin, *Can. Psychiatr. Assoc. J.*, 21: 565–9, 1976.

1905. Ionasescu, V., Ionasescu, R., Witte, D., Feld, R., Cancilla, P., Kaeding, L., Kraus, L. and Stern, L., Altered protein synthesis and creatine kinase in breast muscle cell cultures from dystrophic chick embryos, *J. Neurol. Sci.*, 46: 157–68, 1980.

1906. Ionasescu, V., Stern, L. Z., Ionasescu, R. and Rubenstein, P., Stimulatory effects of drugs for protein synthesis on muscle cell cultures in Duchenne dystrophy, *Ann. Neurol*, 5: 107–10, 1979.

1907. Irani, P. F., Purohit, A. V., and Wadia, N. H., The syndrome of continuous muscle fiber activity, *Acta Neurol. Scand.*, 55: 273–88, 1977.

1908. Ishibashi, F., Hamasaki, A., Shibata, Y., Naitoh, Y. and Kawate, R., Protection against alloxan inhibition of insulin release by glucose, cytochalasin B and diphenylhydantoin, *Hiroshima J. Med. Sci.*, 25(4): 199–202, 1976.

1909. Itil, T. M. and Seaman, P., Drug treatment of human aggression, *Prog. Neuro-Psychopharmacol.*, 2: 659–69, 1978.

1910. Jackson, D. L., Satya-Murti, S., Davis, L. and Drachman, D. B., Isaacs syndrome with laryngeal involvement: an unusual presentation of myokymia, *Neurology*, 29: 1612–5, 1979.

1911. JAMA, Questions and Answers, Recurrent transient motor aphasia in 39-year-old woman, *JAMA*, 238(23): 2541–2, 1977.

1912. JAMA, Questions and Answers, Anticonvulsant therapy and athletic performance, *JAMA*, 240(1): 59–60, 1978.

1913. Jannetta, P. J., Glossopharyngeal neuralgia, *JAMA*, 239(20): 2173, 1978.

1914. Jennett, W. B., *An Introduction to Neurosurgery*, 109, C. V. Mosby, St. Louis, 1970.

1915. Johanson, C. E. and Smith, Q. R., Phenytoin-induced stimulation of the Na-K pump in the choroid plexus cerebrospinal fluid system, *Society for Neuroscience*, III: 316, 7th Annual Meeting, Nov. 7–10, 1977.

1916. Johnson, R. N., Englander, R. N., Quint, S. R., Hanna, G. R., Control of excitability and threshold in the thalamocortical motor system of the cat by cerebellar stimulation, *Epilepsy Abstracts*, 9(9): 277, 1976.

1917. Johnston, D. and Ayala, G. F., Diphenylhydantoin: action of a common anticonvulsant on bursting pacemaker cells in aplysia, *Science*, 189: 1009–11, 1975.

1918. Jonas, A. D., When a subclinical psychomotor seizure poses as a neurosis, *Medical Bulletin of the U.S. Army, Europe*, 32(5): 174–76, 1975.

1919. Kamio, M. and Sugita, T., Syncopal attacks with loss of consciousness and abnormal EEG in childhood, *Epilepsy Abstracts*, 10(6): 180, 1977.

1920. Kannan, K., Dash, R. J. and Rastogi, G. K., Evaluation of treatment of painful diabetic neuropathy with diphenylhydantoin, *J. Diabetic Assoc. India*, 18: 199-202, 1978.

1921. Karmazyn, M., Horrobin, D. F., Morgan, R. O., Manku, M. S., Ally, A. I. and Karmali, R. A., Diphenylhydantoin: a prostaglandin antagonist in the rat mesenteric vasculature, *IRCS Medical Science*, 5: 332, 1977.

1922. Kerstein, M. D., and Firestone, L., The role of Dilantin (DPH) in the prevention of the pulmonary lesions associated with CNS hypoxia, *Clin. Res.*, 25(3): 419A, April, 1977.

1923. Keith, D. A., Side effects of diphenylhydantoin: a review, *J. Oral Surg.*, 36: 206–10, 1978.

1924. Kinscherf, D. A. and Ferrendelli, J. A., Tetrodotoxin-like effect of phenytoin on cyclic nucleotide regulation in brain, *Fed. Proc.*, 37(3): 341, 1978.

1925. Kloppel, G., Functional pathomorphology of the pancreatic β cell system—Ultrastructural and calcium-cytochemical studies on insulin biosynthesis and secretion, *Veroeff Pathol.*, 108: 54–8, 1977.

1926. Koch, K. M., Lorenzini, I., Freddara, U., Jezequel, A. M. and Orlandi, F., Type 2 Crigler-Najjar syndrome. Quantitation of ultrastructural data and evolution under therapy with phenytoin, *Gastroenterol. Clin. Biol.*, 2: 831–42, 1978.

1927. Koch-Weser, J., The serum level approach to individualization of drug dosage, *Eur. J. Clin. Pharmacol.*, 9: 1–8, 1975.

1928. Koch-Weser, J. and Sellers, E. M., Binding of drugs to serum albumin (First of two parts), *New Eng. J. Med.*, 294(6): 311–9, 1976.

1929. Koch-Weser, J. and Sellers, E. M., Binding of drugs to serum albumin (Second of two parts), *New Eng. J. Med.*, 294(10): 526–31, 1976.

1930. Komatsu, K. and Sato, M., A comparison between ouabain treated and genetically dystrophic mice with reference to the effect of phenytoin on the membrane potential of their skeletal muscles, *Yakugaku Zasshi*, 99(8): 855–8, 1979.

1931. Kontani, H., Kudo, Y. and Fukuda, H., Effect of drugs affecting sodium permeability on the muscle spindle of the frog, *Folia Pharmacol. Japan*, 72: 325–30, 1976.

1932. Korczyn, A. D., Shavit, S. and Schlosberg, I., The chick as a model for malignant hyperpyrexia, *Eur. J. Pharmacol.*, 61: 187–9, 1980.

1933. Kornblith, P. L., Hartnett, L. C., Anderson, L. P., Quindlen, E. A., and Smith, B. H., Growth-inhibitory effect of diphenylhydantoin on murine astrocytomas, *Neurosurgery*, 5(2): 259–63, 1979.

1934. Kornblith, P. L., Callahan, L. V. and Caswell, P. A., Growth-inhibitory effects of diphenylhydantoin on human brain tumor cells in culture, *Neurosurgery*, 2(2): 122–7, 1978.

1935. Kornblith, P. L., Caswell, P. A., Bogoch, S., Callahan, L. V. and Dreyfus, J., Effects of diphenylhydantoin on cultured human glial cells, *In Vitro*, 324, April, 1976.

1936. Kramer, M. S., Menstrual epileptoid psychosis in an adolescent girl, *Amer. J. Dis. Child.*, 131: 316–7, 1977.

1937. Krumdieck, C. L., Fukushima, K., Fukushima, T., Shiota, T. and Butterworth, C. E., A long-term study of the excretion of folate and pterins in a human subject after ingestion of ^{14}C folic acid, with observations on the effect of diphenylhydantoin administration, *Am. J. Clin. Nutr.*, 31: 88–93, 1978.

1938. Kupferberg, H. J., Lust, W. D., Yonekawa, W., Passonneau, J. V. and Penry, J. K., Effect of phenytoin (Diphenylhydantoin) on electrically-induced changes in the brain levels of cyclic nucleotides and GABA, *Fed. Proc.*, 35: 583, March, 1976.

1939. Kurihara, T., Tawara, S., Araki, S., Okamoto, S. and Shirabe, T., The therapeutic effects of diphenylhydantoin for myotonia and electron microscopic studies of Thomsen's disease, *Clin. Neurol. (Tokyo)*, 16: 661–8, 1976.

1940. Kutt, H. and Solomon, G. E., Phenytoin: relevant side effects, *Antiepileptic Drugs: Mechanisms of Action*, 435–45, Glaser, G. H., Penry, J. K. and Woodbury, D. M., Eds., Raven Press, New York, 1980.

1941. Lala, V. R., Juan, C. S., and AvRuskin, T. W., Effect of diphenylhydantoin (DPH) on arginine-induced glucagon (IRC) secretion in juvenile diabetes mellitus (JDM), *Pediatr. Res.*, 11: 517, April 1977.

1942. LaManna, J., Lothman, E., Rosenthal, M., Somjen, G. and Younts, W., Phenytoin, electric, ionic and metabolic responses in cortex and spinal cord, *Epilepsia*, 18(3): 317–29, 1977.

1943. Lance, J. W., Burke, D. and Pollard, J., Hyperexcitability of motor and sensory neurons in neuromyotonia, *Ann. Neurol.*, 5: 523–32, 1979.

1944. Lancet, Editor, Liquid-protein diets and ventricular tachycardia, *Lancet*, 976, 1978.

1945. Lancet, Editor, Tinnitus, *Lancet*, 1124, 1979.

1946. Lappas, D. G., Powell, W. M. J. and Daggett, W. M., Cardiac dysfunction in the perioperative period, *Anesthesiology*, 47: 117–37, 1977.

1947. Laxer, K. D., Robertson, L. T., Julien, R. M. and Dow, R. S., Phenytoin: relationship between cerebellar function and epileptic discharges, *Antiepileptic Drugs: Mechanisms of Action*, 415–27, Glaser, G. H., Penry, J. K. and Woodbury, D. M., Eds., Raven Press, New York, 1980.

1948. Lechin, F. and van der Dijs, B., Effects of diphenylhydantoin (DPH) on distal colon motility, *Acta Gastroenterol. Latinoam.*, 9(3): 145–52, 1979.

1949. Lee, Y. T., Lee, T. K. and Tsai, H. C., Glossopharyngeal neuralgia as the cause of cardiac syncope, *J. Formosan Med. Assoc.*, 74: 103–7, 1975.

1950. Leon-Sotomayor, L., A new technique in the treatment of thromboembolic stroke, *Angiology*, 31(11): 729–43, 1980.

1951. Levin, S. R., Charles, M. A., O'Connor, M., Grodsky, G. M., Use of diphenylhydantoin and diazoxide to investigate insulin secretory mechanisms, *Amer. J. Physiol.*, 229(1): 49–54, July, 1975.

1952. Levin, S. R., Driessen, J. and Kasson, B., Adenosinetriphosphatases of pancreatic islets: comparison with those of kidney, *Endocr. Soc. Program*, 59: 75 (Abstract 38), 1977.

1953. Levin, S. R., Kasson, B. G. and Driessen, J. F., Adenosine triphosphatases of rat pancreatic islets—comparison with those of rat kidney, *J. Clin. Invest.*, 62: 692–701, 1978.

1954. Levinson, S., Canalis, R. F. and Kaplan, H. J., Laryngeal spasm complicating pseudomyotonia, *Arch. Otolaryngol.*, 102: 185–7, 1976.

1955. Levo, Y., Markowitz, O. and Trainin, N., Hydantoin immunosuppression and carcinogenesis, *Clin. Exp. Immun.*, 19: 521–7, March 1975.

1956. Levy, R. H., Phenytoin: biopharmacology, *Antiepileptic Drugs: Mechanisms of Action*, 315–21, Glaser, G. H., Penry, J. K. and Woodbury, D. M., Eds., Raven Press, New York, 1980.

1957. Lewin, E., Effects of phenytoin on the release of ^{14}C-Adenine derivatives, *Epilepsia*, 18(3): 349–55, 1977.

1958. Lewin, E. and Bleck, V., Cyclic AMP accumulation in cerebral cortical slices: effect of carbamazepine, phenobarbital and phenytoin, *Epilepsia*, 18(2): 237–42, 1977.

1959. Lewis, D. V., Zbiez, K. I. and Wilson, W. A., Diphenylhydantoin depresses firing in the aplysia giant neuron by blocking a slow inward current, *Soc. for Neuroscience*, 251, 9th Annual Meeting, Nov. 2–6, 1979.

1960. Lewis, J. S., Gilbert, B. and Garry, P. J., Glutathione reductase activity coefficients of children on anticonvulsant

drugs and their normal siblings, *Fed. Proc.*, 37 (Abstract 2412): 671, March 1978.

1961. Linden, V., Brevik, J. I., and Hansen, T., Phenytoin, phenobarbitone and serum cholesterol, *Scand. J. Soc. Med.*, 5: 123–5, 1977.

1962. Livingston, S., Phenytoin and serum cholesterol, *Epilepsy Abstracts*, 9(10): 329, 1976.

1963. Loeser, J. D., The management of tic douloureux, *Pain*, 3: 155–62, 1977.

1964. Loeser, J. D., What to do about tic douloureux, *JAMA*, 239(12): 1153–5, 1978.

1965. Loh, C. K., Katz, A. M. and Pierce, E. C., Interactions of diphenylhydantoin and cardiac glycosides on atrial potassium, *Am. J. Physiol.*, 230(4): 965–69, 1976.

1966. Lown, B., Temte, J. V., Reich, P., Gaughan, C., Regestein, Q. and Hai, H., Basis for recurring ventricular fibrillation in the absence of coronary heart disease and its management, *New Eng. J. Med.*, 294(12): 623–29, 1976.

1967. Lublin, F. D., Tsairis, P., Streletz, L. J., Chambers, R. A., Riker, W. F., Van Poznak, A. and Duckett, S. W., Myokymia and impaired muscular relaxation with continuous motor unit activity, *J. Neurol. Neurosurg. Psychiatry*, 42: 557–62, 1979.

1968. Luoma, P. V., Myllyla, V. V., Sotaniemi, E. A. and Hokkanen, T. E. J., Plasma HDL cholesterol in epileptics with elevated triglyceride and cholesterol, *Acta Neurol. Scand.*, 60: 56–63, 1979.

1969. Lust, W. D., Kupferberg, H. J., Yonekawa, W. D., Penry, J. K., Passonneau, J. V. and Wheaton, A. B., Changes in brain metabolites induced by convulsants or electroshock: Effects of anticonvulsant agents, *Molec. Pharmacol.*, 14: 347–56, 1978.

1970. Lutschg, J., Jerusalem, F., Ludin, H. P., Vassella, F. and Mumenthaler, M., The syndrome of 'continuous muscle fiber activity,' *Arch. Neurol.*, 35: 198–205, 1978.

1971. Maisov, N. I., Tolmacheva, N. S. and Raevsky, K. S., Liberation of ^{3}H-gamma-aminobutyric acid (^{3}H-GABA) from isolated nerve endings of the rat's brain under the effect of psychotropic substances, *Farmakol. Toksik.*, 39: 517–20, 1976.

1972. Mathews, E. C., Blount, A. W. and Townsend, J. I., Q-T prolongation and ventricular arrhythmias, with and without deafness, in the same family, *Am. J. Cardiol.*, 29: 702–11, 1972.

1973. Matthews, E. K. and Sakamoto, Y., Pancreatic islet cells: electrogenic and electrodiffusional control of membrane potential, *J. Physiol.*, 246: 439–57, 1975.

1974. Matthews, W. D. and Connor, J. D., Actions of iontophoretic phenytoin and medazepam on hippocampal neurons, *J. Pharmacol. Exp. Ther.*, 201(3): 613–21, 1977.

1975. Matthews, W. D. and Connor, J. D., Effects of diphenylhydantoin and diazepam on hippocampal evoked responses, *Neuropharmacol.*, 15: 181–6, 1976.

1976. Medical Letter on Drugs and Therapeutics, Treatment of cardiac arrhythmias, 20(26): 113–20, 1978.

1977. Medical World News, Editor, New clues to averting liquid-protein deaths, *Medical World News*, 61, 1978.

1978. Melacini, P., Furlanut, M., Ferrari, M. and Volta, S. D., Effects of quinidine and diphenylhydantoin on membrane resistance in smooth muscle, *Arch. Int. Pharmacodyn.*, 213(1): 17–21, 1975.

1979. Melding, P. S. and Goodey, R. J., The treatment of tinnitus with oral anticonvulsants, *J. Laryng.*, 93: 111–22, 1979.

1980. Melikian, A. P., Straughn, A. B., Slywka, G. W. A., Whyatt, P. L. and Meyer, M. C., Bioavailability of 11 phenytoin products, *J. Pharmacokinet. Biopharm.*, 5(2): 133–46, 1977.

1981. Mentzer, R. M., Alegre, C. and Nolan, S. P., Effects of diphenylhydantoin (Dilantin) on the pulmonary circulation, *Surgical Forum*, 26: 217–9, 1975.

1982. Merck Manual of Diagnosis and Therapy, 13th Edition, Merck Sharp & Dohme Research Laboratories, Rahway, New Jersey, 1977.

1983. Mesulam, M. M., Dissociative states with abnormal temporal lobe EEG-multiple personality and the illusion of possession, *Arch. Neurol.*, 38: 176–81, 1981.

1984. Migdal, S. D., Slick, G. L. and McDonald, F. D., Diphenylhydantoin (DPH) renal vasodilator, *Clin. Res.*, 25(3): 273A, 1977.

1985. Migdal, S. D., Slick, G. L., Abu-Hamdan, D. and McDonald, F. D., Phenytoin, renal function and renin release, *J. Pharmacol. Exp. Ther.*, 215(2): 304–8, 1980.

1986. Migdal, S. D., Slick, G. L. and McDonald, F. D., Phenytoin (DPH) renal function and renin secretion (RSR), *Clin. Res.*, 26(3): 471, 1978.

1987. Millichap, J. G., Recurrent headaches in 100 children, *Child's Brain*, 4: 95–105, 1978.

1988. Mohan, K. J., Salo, M. W. and Nagaswami, S., A case of limbic system dysfunction with hypersexuality and fugue state, *Dis. Nerv. Syst.*, 36: 621–4, 1975.

1989. Moore, S. J., Digitalis toxicity and treatment with phenytoin: neurologic mechanism of action, *Heart & Lung*, 6(6): 1035–40, 1977.

1990. Morgan, P. H. and Mathison, I. W., Arrhythmias and antiarrhythmic drugs: mechanism of action and structure-activity relations, *J. Pharm. Sci.*, 65: 467–81, 1976.

1991. Moss, G., The role of the central nervous system in shock: the centroneurogenic etiology of the respiratory distress syndrome, *Critical Care Medicine*, 2(4): 181–5, 1974.

1992. Muller, D. and Leuschner, U., Clinical and neurophysiological findings in blood-level controlled diphenylhydantoin application—considerations on the therapy of myotonic dystrophy, *Psychiatr. Neurol. Med. Psychol.*, 32(8): 464–8, 1980.

1993. Muller, N. R., Tsyrlina, E. V., Ostroumova, M. N. and Shemerovskaya, T. G., The effect of diphenine on the growth and metastasis of experimental malignant tumors, *Vopr. Onkol.*, 21(7): 86–90, 1975.

1994. Neldner, H. K., Treatment of localized linear scleroderma with phenytoin, *Cutis*, 22: 569–72, 1978.

1995. Nelson, E. W., Cerda, J. J., Wilder, B. J. and Streiff, R. R., Effect of diphenylhydantoin on the bioavailability of citris folate, *Am. J. Clin. Nutr.*, 31: 82–7, 1978.

1996. Neuman, R. S. and Frank, G. B., Effects of diphenylhydantoin and phenobarbital on voltage-clamped myelinated nerve, *Can. J. Physiol. Pharmacol.*, 55(1): 42–8, 1977.

1997. Neuvonen, P. J., Penttila, O., Lehtovaara, R. and Aho, K., Effect of antiepileptic drugs on the elimination of various tetracycline derivatives, *Europ. J. Clin. Pharmacol.*, 9: 147–54, 1975.

1998. Nevsimal, O., Suta, M. and Tuhacek, M., The stiffman syndrome, *Cesk. Neurol.*, 30(2): 133–8, 1967.

1999. Newell, I. M., Trigeminal neuralgia: induced remission without surgery, and observations on its aetiology, *Med. J. Aust.*, 1: 605–7, 1976.

2000. Newsom, J. A., Withdrawal seizures in an in-patient alcoholism program, *Currents in Alcoholism*, vol. 6, 11–14, Galanter, M., Ed., Grune and Stratton, New York, 1979.

2001. Nies, A. S., Cardiovascular disorders, I. Alteration of arterial pressure and regional blood flow, *Clinical Pharmacology, Basic Principles in Therapeutics*, K. L. Melmon and H. F. Morrelli, Eds., Macmillan, New York, 1972.

2002. Nikkila, E. A., Kaste, M., Ehnholm, C. and Viikari, J., Elevation of high-density lipoprotein in epileptic patients treated with phenytoin, *Acta Med. Scand*, 204: 517–20, 1978.

2003. Nishida, T., The effects of diphenylhydantoin sodium on the *in vivo* electroretinogram of rabbits, *Epilepsy Abstracts*, 9(2): 47, 1976.

2004. Nishikaze, O., Furuya, E. and Takase, T., Diphenylhydantoin inhibits the production of lipid peroxide in carrageenin induced inflammation in rats, *IRCS Med. Sci.*, 8: 552, 1980.

2005. Ochiai, Y., Hayakawa, T., Fukuyama, Y. and Miragawa, F., Analysis of overnight sleep EEG and cerebrospinal fluid monoamine metabolites in seizures induced by movement, *Epilepsy Abstracts*, 11(8): 297, 1978.

2006. O'Donnell, J. M., Kovacs, T. and Szabo, B., Influence of the membrane stabilizer diphenylhydantoin on potassium and sodium movements in skeletal muscle, *Pflugers Arch*, 358: 275–88, 1975.

2007. Oettinger, L., Interaction of methylphenidate and diphenylhydantoin, *Drug Therapy*, 5: 107–8, 1975.

2008. Opie, L. H., Drugs and the heart—IV antiarrhythmic agents, *Lancet*, 861–8, 1980.

2009. Otto, G., Ludewig, R. and Kotzschke, H. J., Specific action of local phenytoin application on periodontal disease, *Stomatol. DDR*, 27: 262–8, 1977.

2010. Ozawa, H., Komatsu, K. and Sato, M., Reversal by phenytoin (diphenylhydantoin) of the resting membrane potential of skeletal muscle from genetically dystrophic mice, *J. Pharm. Soc. Japan*, 98(3): 386–9, 1978.

2011. Pace, C. S. and Livingston, E., Ionic basis of phenytoin sodium inhibition of insulin secretion in pancreatic islets, *Diabetes*, 28: 1077–82, 1979.

2012. Palmer, G. C., Jones, D. J., Medina, M. A., Palmer, S. J. and Stavinoha, W. B., Anticonvulsants: action on central adenylate cyclase systems, *Pharmacologist*, 20: 231, 1978.

2013. Palmer, G. C., Jones, D. J., Medina, M. A. and Stavinoha, W. B., Anticonvulsant drug actions on *in vitro* and *in vivo* levels of cyclic AMP in the mouse brain, *Epilepsia*, 20: 95–104, 1979.

2014. Pedley, T. A. and Guilleminault, C., Episodic nocturnal wanderings responsive to anticonvulsant drug therapy, *Ann. Neurol*, 2(1): 30–5, 1977.

2015. Pelkonen, R., Fogelholm, R. and Nikkila, E. A., Increase in serum cholesterol during phenytoin treatment, *Br. Med. J.*, 85, 1975.

2016. Pendefunda, G., Oprisan, C., Ciobanu, M. and Cozma, V., Clinico-electromyographic considerations on a case of neuromyotonia, *Rev. Roum. Med. (Neurol. Psychiatr.)*, 13(4): 237–45, 1975.

2017. Pento, J. T., Diphenylhydantoin inhibitions of pentagastrin-stimulated calcitonin secretion in the pig, *Horm. Metab. Res.*, 8: 399–401, 1976.

2018. Peppercorn, M. A., Herzog, A. G., Dichter, M. A. and Mayman, C. I., Abdominal epilepsy—a cause of abdominal pain in adults, *JAMA*, 240(22): 2450–51, 1978.

2019. Peraino, C., Fry, R. J. M., Staffeldt, E. and Christopher, J. P., Comparative enhancing effects of phenobarbital, amobarbital, diphenylhydantoin, and dichlorodiphenyltrichloroethane on 2-acetylaminofluorene-induced hepatic tumorigenesis in the rat, *Cancer Res.*, 35: 2884–90, Oct. 1975.

2020. Perucca, E. and Richens, A., Water intoxication produced by carbamazepine and its reversal by phenytoin, *Br. J. Clin. Pharmacol.*, 9: 302–4P, 1980.

2021. Perry, J. G., McKinney, L. and DeWeer, P., The cellular mode of action of the anti-epileptic drug 5,5-diphenylhydantoin, *Nature*, 272: 271–3, 1978.

2022. Petrack, B., Czernik, A. J., Itterly, W., Ansell, J. and Chertock, H., On the suppression of insulin and glucagon released by diphenylhydantoin, *Diabetes*, 25, Suppl. 1: 380, 1976.

2023. Pincus, J. H., Yaari, Y. and Argov, Z., Phenytoin: electrophysiological effects at the neuromuscular junction, *Antiepileptic Drugs: Mechanisms of Action*, 363–76, Glaser, G. H., Penry, J. K. and Woodbury, D. M., Eds., Raven Press, New York, 1980.

2024. Pollen, D. A., Responses of single neurons to electrical stimulation of the surface of the visual cortex, *Brain Behav. Evol.*, 14: 67–86, 1977.

2025. Porras, C., Barboza, J. J., Fuenzalida, E., Adaros, H. L., de Diaz, A. M. O. and Furst, J., Recovery from rabies in man, *Ann. Int. Med.*, 85: 44–48, 1976.

2026. Prchal, V. and Smythies, J. R., Temporal-lobe epilepsy presenting as fugue state, *Lancet*, 1034, 1977.

2027. Pull, I. and McIlwain, H., Centrally-acting drugs and related compounds examined for action on output of adenine derivatives from superfused tissues of the brain, *Biochem. Pharmacol.*, 25: 293–7, 1976.

2028. Pulsinelli, W. A. and Rottenberg, D. A., Painful tic convulsif, *J. Neurol. Neurosurg. and Psychiat.*, 40(2): 192–5, 1977.

2029. Racy, A., Osborn, M. A., Vern, B. A. and Molinari, G. F., Epileptic aphasia, *Arch. Neurol.*, 37: 419–22, 1980.

2030. Raines, A., Phenytoin revisited, *Epilepsia*, 18(3): 297–8, 1977.

2031. Raines, A., Cohan, S. L., Panagakos, J. and Armitage, P., Utility of chlorpromazine (CPZ) and phenytoin (PH) in spasticity, *Pharmacologist*, 21(3): 183, 1979.

2032. Raines, A. and Niner, J. M., Blockade of a sympathetic nervous system reflex by diphenylhydantoin, *Neuropharmacology*, 14: 61–66, 1975.

2033. Ramsay, R. E., Wilder, B. J., Willmore, L. J. and Perchalski, R. J., Central nervous system penetration of anticonvulsant drugs, *Abstract of Amer. Epilepsy Soc. Ann. Meeting*, 1976.

2034. Rapport, R. L. and Ojemann, G. A., Prophylactically administered phenytoin, *Arch. Neurol.*, 32(8): 539–48, 1975.

2035. Rapport, R. L. and Penry, J. K., A survey of attitudes toward the pharmacological prophylaxis of posttraumatic epilepsy, *J. Neurosurg.*, 38: 159–166, 1973.

2036. Raskin, N. H. and Fishman, R. A., Neurologic disorders in renal failure, *New England Journal of Medicine*, 294(3): 143–8, 1976.

2037. Rau, J. H. and Green, R. S., Compulsive eating: a neuropsychologic approach to certain eating disorders, *Compr. Psychiat.*, 16: 223–31, 1975.

2038. Rau, J. H. and Green, R. S., Soft neurological correlates of compulsive eaters, *J. Nerv. Ment. Dis.*, 166(6): 435–7, 1978.

2039. Ravindran, M., Focal cerebral dysrhythmia—presenting as headache: report of a case, *Clin. Electroencephalogr.*, 9(1): 29–31, 1978.

2040. Reeback, J., Benton, S., Swash, M. and Schwartz, M. S., Penicillamine-induced neuromyotonia, *Br. Med. J.*, 1464–5, 1979.

2041. Reidenberg, M. M., Drug metabolism in uremia, *Clin. Nephrol.*, 4(3): 83–5, 1975.

2042. Reith, H., Availability of phenytoin infusion concentrate, *Drug Intell. Clin. Pharm*, 13(12): 783, 1979.

2043. Reynolds, E. H., Chronic antiepileptic toxicity: a review, *Epilepsia*, 16: 319–52, 1975.

2044. Reynolds, F., Ziroyanis, P. M., Jones, N. F. and Smith, S. E., Salivary phenytoin concentrations in epilepsy and in chronic renal failure, *Lancet*, 384–6, 1976.

2045. Richelson, E. and Tuttle, J. B., Diphenylhydantoin inhibits ionic excitation of mouse neuroblastoma cells, *Brain Res.*, 99: 209–12, 1975.

2046. Riddle, T. G., Mandel, L. J., Goldner, M. M., Dilantincalcium interaction and active Na transport in frog skin, *Europ. J. Pharmacol.*, 33: 189–92, 1975.

2047. Riley, T. L. and Massey, E. W., The syndrome of aphasia, headaches, and left temporal spikes, *Headache*, 20(2): 90–2, 1980.

2048. Roberts, J. and Goldberg, P. B., Changes in responsiveness of the heart to drugs during aging, *Fed. Proc.*, 38(5): 1927–32, 1979.

2049. Robertson, S., Gibbs, M. E. and Ng, K. T., Sodium pump activity, amino acid transport and long-term memory, *Brain Res. Bull.*, 3(1): 53–8, 1978.

2050. Rogers, H. J., Haslam, R. A., Longstreth, J. and Lietman, P. S., Phenytoin intoxication during concurrent diazepam therapy, *J. Neurol. Neurosurg. Psychiatry*, 40: 890–5, 1977.

2051. Rootwelt, K., Ganes, T. and Johannessen, S. I., Effect of carbamazepine, phenytoin and phenobarbitone on serum levels of thyroid hormones and thyrotropin in humans, *Scand. J. Clin. Lab. Invest.*, 38: 731–6, 1978.

2052. Rose, J. Q., Choi, H. K., Schentag, J. J., Krinkel, W. R. and Jusko, W. J., Intoxication caused by interaction of chloramphenicol and phenytoin, *JAMA*, 237(24): 2630–1, 1977.

2053. Rose, M. and Johnson, I., Reinterpretation of the haematological effects of anticonvulsant treatment, *Lancet*, 1349–50, 1978.

2054. Rosen, M., Danilo, P., Alonso, M. and Pippenger, C., Effects of diphenylhydantoin on the electrophysiologic properties of blood-superfused Purkinje fibers, *Fed. Proc.*, 34: 755 (Abstr. 3154), March 1975.

2055. Rosen, M. R., Danilo, P., Alonso, M. and Pippenger, C. E., Effects of therapeutic concentrations of diphenylhydantoin on transmembrane potentials of normal and depressed Purkinje fibers, *J. Pharmacol. Exp. Ther.*, 197(3): 594–604, 1976.

2056. Rosenblatt, S., Schaeffer, D. and Rosenthal, J. S., Effects of diphenylhydantoin on child-abusing parents, *Curr. Ther. Res.*, 19(3): 332–6, 1976.

2057. Roses, A. D., Butterfield, D. A., Appel, S. H. and Chestnut, D. B., Phenytoin and membrane fluidity in myotonic dystrophy, *Arch. Neurol.*, 32 (8): 535–38, 1975.

2058. Rotmensch, H. H., Graff, E., Ayzenberg, O., Amir, C. and Laniado, S., Self-poisoning with digitalis glycosides—successful treatment of three cases, *Israel J. Med. Sci.*, 13: 1109–13, 1977.

2059. Rowell, F. J. and Paxton, J. W., Conformational and chemical requirements for antibody recognition of diphenylhydantoin derivatives, *Immunochem.*, 13: 891–4, 1976.

2060. Runge, M. and Rehpenning, W., Behaviour of salivary electrolytes potassium and calcium in digitalized patients after administration of diphenylhydantoin, *Arzneim-Forsch.*, 24(10): 1696–9, 1974.

2061. Ruskin, J. N., Garan, H., Silver, T. S. and Powell, W. J., CNS-mediated effect of phenytoin in delaying the onset of digoxin-induced ventricular arrhythmias, *Clin. Res.*, 26(3): 267, April 1975.

2062. Saad, S. F., Osman, O. H., Mustafa, A. and Hussein, K. E., Possible involvement of gamma-aminobutyric acid in morphine abstinence in rats, *IRCS Med. Sci.*, 5(7): 317, 1977.

2063. Sabai, Y., Kobayashi, K. and Iwata, M., Effects of an anabolic steroid and vitamin B complex upon myopathy induced by corticosteroids, *European J. Pharmacol.*, 52: 353–9, 1978.

2064. Sansom, L. N., O'Reilly, W. J., Wiseman, C. W., et al., Plasma phenytoin levels produced by various phenytoin preparations, *Epilepsy Abstracts*, 97: 249, 1976.

2065. Sastry, B. S. R. and Phillis, J. W., Antagonism of glutamate and acetylcholine excitation of rat cerebral cortical neurones by diphenylhydantoin, *Gen. Pharmac.*, 7: 411–13, 1976.

2066. Sawaya, M. C. B., Horton, R. W. and Meldrum, B. S., Effects of anticonvulsant drugs on the cerebral enzymes metabolizing GABA, *Epilepsia*, 16: 649–55, 1975.

2067. Schlosser, W., Franco, S. and Sigg, E. B., Differential attenuation of somatovisceral and viscerosomatic reflexes by diazepam, phenobarbital and diphenylhydantoin, *Neuropharmacol.*, 14: 525–31, 1975.

2068. Schmitz, I., Janzik, H. H. and Mayer, K., The personality structure and sexual behavior of patients with epilepsy on long-term therapy with diphenylhydantoin, *Epilepsia*, 16: 412–3, 1975.

2069. Schneider, R. R., Bahler, A., Pincus, J. and Stimmel, B., Asymptomatic idiopathic syndrome of prolonged Q-T interval in a 45-year-old woman, *Chest*, 71: 210–3, 1977.

2070. Schwartz, P. A., Rhodes, C. T. and Cooper, J. W., Solubility and ionization characteristics of phenytoin, *J. Pharm. Sci.*, 66(7): 994–7, 1977.

2071. Schwartz, P. J., Periti, M. and Malliani, A., The long Q-T syndrome, *Am. Heart J.*, 89(3): 378–90, 1975.

2072. Schwarz, J. R. and Vogel, W., Diphenylhydantoin: excitability reducing action in single myelinated nerve fibres, *European J. Pharmacol.*, 44: 241–9, 1977.

2073. Selzer, M. E., The action of phenytoin on a composite electrical-chemical synapse in the lamprey spinal cord, *Ann. Neurol.*, 3(3): 202–6, 1978.

2074. Selzer, M. E., The effect of phenytoin on the action potential of a vertebrate spinal neuron, *Brain Research*, 171: 511–21, 1979.

2075. Selzer, M. E., Phenytoin blocks post-tetanic potentiation at a vertebrate CNS synapse, *Trans. Am. Neurological Assoc.*, 102: 118–20, 1977.

2076. Shah, U. H., Jindal, M. N. and Patel, V. K., Beta-adrenoceptor blockade with diphenylhydantoin (DPH), *Arzneim-Forsch*, 27: 2316–8, 1977.

2077. Shealy, C. N., Drug use in a pain rehabilitation center, *Am. J. Hosp. Pharm.*, 32: 1083, 1975.

2078. Sherwin, A. L., Harvey, C. D., Leppik, I. E. and Gonda, A., Correlation between red cell and free plasma phenytoin levels in renal disease, *Neurol.*, 26: 874–8, 1976.

2079. Sheth, K. J. and Bernhard, G. C., The arthropathy of Fabry disease, *Arthritis Rheum.*, 22(7): 781–3, 1979.

2080. Shintomi, K., Effects of psychotropic drugs on methamphetamine-induced behavioral excitation in grouped mice, *Europ. J. Pharmacol.*, 31: 195–206, 1975.

2081. Silverman, H., Atwood, H. L. and Bloom, J. W., Phenytoin application in murine muscular dystrophy; behavioral improvement with no change in the abnormal intracellular Na : K ratio in skeletal muscles, *Exp. Neurol.*, 62: 618–27, 1978.

2082. Singh, B. N., Gaarder, T. D., Kanegae, T., Goldstein, M., Montgomerie, J. Z. and Mills, H., Liquid protein diets and *torsade de pointes*, *JAMA*, 240(2): 115–9, 1978.

2083. Sirohiya, M. K., Bhatnagar, H. N. S., Shah, D. R. and Narang, N. K., Phenytoin sodium in cardiac arrhythmias, *J. Indian Med. Assoc.*, 64(12): 329–34, 1975.

2084. Smith, I. M. and Burmeister, L. F., Biochemically assisted antibiotic treatment of lethal murine staphylococcus aureus septic shock, *Am. J. Clin. Nutr.*, 30: 1364–8, 1977.

2085. Sneer, A., Colev, V., Dughir, E. and Sneer, I., The protective effect of diphenylhydantoin on the diabetogenic action of alloxan, *Epilepsy Abstracts*, 12(9): 421, 1979.

2086. Snider, S. R. and Snider, R. S., Phenytoin and cerebellar lesions: similar effects on cerebellar catecholamine metabolism, *Arch. Neurol.*, 34: 162–7, 1977.

2087. Sohn, R. S. and Ferrendelli, J. A., Anticonvulsant drug mechanisms, phenytoin, phenobarbital, and ethosuximide and calcium flux in isolated presynaptic endings, *Arch. Neurol.*, 33: 626–9, 1976.

2088. Somerman, M. J., Au, W. Y. W. and Rifkin, B. R., Phenytoin inhibition of bone resorption in organ culture, *J. Dent. Res.*, 56 (Special Issue B) Abstr. 579, 1977.

2089. Sordillo, P., Sagransky, D. M., Mercado, R. and Michelis, M. F., Carbamazepine-induced syndrome of inappropriate antidiuretic hormone secretion—reversal by concomitant phenytoin therapy, *Arch. Intern. Med.*, 138: 299–301, 1978.

2090. Starkova, N. T., Marova, E. I., Lemesheva, S. N., Goncharova, V. N., Atamanova, T. M. and Sedykh, L. P., The effect of diphenin on functional condition of the adrenal cortex in patients with Itsenko-Cushing disease, *Problemy Endokrinologii*, 18: 35–8, Nov/Dec, 1972.

2091. Stavchansky, S. A., Tilbury, R. S., McDonald, J. M., Ting, C. T. and Kostenbauder, H. B., *In vivo* distribution of carbon-11 phenytoin and its major metabolite, and their use in scintigraphic imaging, *J. Nucl. Med.*, 19(8): 936–41, 1978.

2092. St. Louis, E. L., McLoughlin, M. J. and Wortzman, G., Chronic damage to medium and large arteries following irradiation, *J. Canad. Assoc. Radiol.*, 25: 94–104, 1974.

2093. Study, R. E., Phenytoin inhibition of cyclic guanosine 3′:5′-monophosphate (cGMP) accumulation in neuroblastoma cells by calcium channel blockade, *J. Pharmacol. Exp. Ther.*, 215(3): 575–81, 1980.

2094. Suratt, P. M., Crampton, R. S. and Carpenter, M. A., Benign familial biventricular dysrhythmias with syncope limited to late childhood, adolescence and early youth, *Circulation*, 48 (Suppl. IV): 222, 1973.

2095. Swann, W. P., Swenson, H. M. and Shafer, W. G., Effects of Dilantin on the repair of gingival wounds, *J. Periodont.*, 46(5): 302–5, 1975.

2096. Swanson, J. W. and Vick, N. A., Basilar artery migraine, *Neurology*, 28: 782–6, 1978.

2097. Swerdlow, M., The treatment of 'shooting' pain, *Postgrad. Med. J.*, 56: 159–61, 1980.

2098. Swanson, P. D. and Crane, P. O., Diphenylhydantoin and movement of radioactive sodium into electrically stimulated cerebral slices. *Biochem. Pharmacol.*, 21: 2899–905, 1972.

2099. Swift, T. R., Gross, J. A., Ward, L. C. and Flicek, B. O., Electrophysiologic study of patients receiving anticonvulsant drugs, *Neurology*, 29: 581, 1979.

2100. Szyper, M. S. and Mann, J. D., Anorexia nervosa as an interictal symptom of partial complex seizures, *Neurology*, 28(4): 335, 1978.

2101. Tanay, A., Yust, I., Peresecenschi, G., Abramov, A. L. and Aviram, A., Long-term treatment of the syndrome of inappropriate antidiuretic hormone secretion with phenytoin, *Ann. Intern. Med.*, 90: 50–2, 1979.

2102. Taylor, P. H., Gray, K., Bicknell, P. G. and Rees, J. R., Glossopharyngeal neuralgia with syncope, *J. Laryngol. Otol.*, 91: 859–68, 1977.

2103. Thampi, N. S., Mader, M. M. and Earley, R. J., Effect of diphenylhydantoin on levels of cyclic AMP and cyclic GMP in rat brain synaptasomes, *Pharmacologist*, 16: Abstr. 551, Fall, 1974.

2104. Tuttle, J. B., Intracellular recordings from a clonal, tissue-cultured neuron: bioelectric differentiation of anti-metabolite survivors and the action of diphenylhydantoin, *Dissertation Abstracts International*, Section B,38: 91B–92B, 1977.

2105. Tuttle, J. B. and Richelson, E., Phenytoin action on the excitable membrane of mouse neuroblastoma, *J. Pharmacol. Exp. Ther.*, 2(3): 632–7, 1979.

2106. Tyler, G. S., McNeely, H. E. and Dick, M. L., Vascular headache treatment update, *Arizona Med.*, 36: 117–8, 1979.

2107. Vernillo, A. T. and Schwartz, N. B., Collagen and proteoglycan synthesis in 5,5 diphenylhydantoin (Dilantin) treated chondrocytes, *J. Cell. Biol.*, 83(pt. 2): 116a, 1979.

2108. Vincent, T. S., When to use Dilantin in alcoholism, *Resident and Staff Physician*, 22: 50–1, 1976.

2109. von Albert, H. H., Treatment of acute trigeminal neuralgia with intravenous infusions of phenytoin, *Munch. Med. Wsch.*, 120(15): 529–30, 1978.

2110. Wadell, M. C. and Chambers, D. A., Effect of diphenylhydantoin on the cell cycle of a serum free mouse symphocyte system, *Fed. Proc.*, 35(3): 749, March, 1976.

2111. Waller, D. A., Paroxysmal kinesigenic choreoathetosis or hysteria? *Am. J. Psychiat.*, 134(12): 1439–40, 1977.

2112. Walson, P., Trinca, C. and Bressler, R., New uses for phenytoin, *JAMA*, 233(13): 1385–9, 1975.

2113. Walton, J. N., Muscular dystrophies and their management, *Br. Med. J.*, 3(671): 639–42, 1969.

2114. Wasserman, T. H., Phillips, T. L., Van Raalte, G., Urtasun, R., Partington, J., Koziol, D., Schwade, J. G., Gangji, D. and Strong, J. M., The neurotoxicity of misonidazole: potential modifying role by phenytoin sodium and dexamethasone, *Br. J. Radiol.*, 53: 172–3, 1980.

2115. Weinberger, J., Nicklas, W. J. and Berl, S., Mechanism of action of anticonvulsants, *Neurology* 26: 162–166, 1976.

2116. Weiss, T. and Levitz, M., Diphenylhydantoin treatment of bulimia, *Am. J. Psychiatry*, 133(9): 1093, 1976.

2117. Wermuth, B. M., Davis, L. K., Hollister, L. E. and Stunkard, A. J., Phenytoin treatment of the binge-eating syndrome, *Am. J. Psychiat.*, 134(11): 1249–53, 1977.

2118. Wilson, J. T., Huff, J. G. and Kilroy, A. W., Brief clinical and laboratory observations, *J. Pediatr.*, 95(1): 135–8, 1979.

2119. White, R. A. S. and Workman, P., Phenytoin sodium-induced alterations in the pharmacokinetics of misonidazole in the dog, *Cancer Treat. Rep.*, 64: 360–1, 1980.

2120. Wit, A. L., Rosen, M. R. and Hoffman, B. F., Electrophysiology and pharmacology of cardiac arrhythmias, VIII. Cardiac effects of diphenylhydantoin Part A., *Am. Heart J.*, 90(3): 265–72, 1975.

2121. Wit, A. L., Rosen, M. R. and Hoffman, B. F., Electrophysiology and pharmacology of cardiac arrhythmias, VIII. Cardiac effects of diphenylhydantoin Part B., *Am. Heart J.*, 90(3): 397–404, 1975.

2122. Wohns, R. N. W. and Wyler, A. R., Prophylactic phenytoin in severe head injuries, *J. Neurosurg.*, 51: 507–8, 1979.

2123. Wolfe, G. W. and Schnell, R. C., Protection against alloxan-induced alterations in hepatic drug metabolism and plasma glucose levels in the male rat, *Toxicol. App. Pharmacol.*, 48(Pt 2): A69, 1979.

2124. Wolter, M. and Brauer, D., Neuromyotonia syndrome, *Fortschr. Neurol. Psychiat.*, 45: 98–105, 1977.

2125. Woo, E. and Greenblatt, D. J., Choosing the right phenytoin dosage, *Drug Therapy (Hospital Edition)*, 2: 35–41, Oct. 1977.

2126. Woodbury, D. M., Phenytoin: introduction and history, *Antiepileptic Drugs: Mechanisms of Action*, 305–13, Glaser, G. H., Penry, J. K. and Woodbury, D. M., Eds., Raven Press, New York, 1980.

2127. Woodbury, D. M., Phenytoin: Proposed mechanisms of anticonvulsant action, *Antiepileptic Drugs: Mechanisms of Action*, 447–71, Glaser, G. H., Penry, J. K. and Woodbury, D. M., Eds., Raven Press, New York, 1980.

2128. Workman, P., Effects of pretreatment with phenobarbitone and phenytoin on the pharmacokinetics and toxicity of misonidazole in mice, *Br. J. Cancer*, 40: 335–53, 1979.

2129. Workman, P., Bleehen, N. M. and Wiltshire, C. R., Phenytoin shortens the half-life of the hypoxic cell radiosensitizer misonidazole in man: implications for possible reduced toxicity, *Br. J. Cancer*, 41: 302–4, 1980.

2130. Yaari, Y., Pincus, J. H., Argov, Z., Phenytoin and transmitter release at the neuromuscular junction of the frog, *Brain Res.*, 160: 479–87, 1979.

2131. Yaari, Y., Rahamimoff, H. and Pincus, J. H., Action of diphenylhydantoin at the frog neuromuscular junction, *Israel J. Med. Sci.*, 12(2): 171-2, 1976.

2132. York, G. K., Gabor, A. J. and Dreyfus, P. M., Paroxysmal genital pain: an unusual manifestation of epilepsy, *Neurology*, 29: 516–9, 1979.

2133. Yeh, J. Z., Quandt, F. N. and Kirsch, G. E., Comparative studies of phenytoin action on ionic channels in excitable membranes, *Fed. Proc.*, 40(3): 240, 1981.

2134. Young, B., Rapp, R., Brooks, W. H., Madauss, W. and Norton, J. A., Posttraumatic epilepsy prophylaxis, *Epilepsia*, 20: 671–81, 1979.

2135. Young, R. F., Facial pain, *The Practitioner*, 219: 731–7, 1977.

2136. Zapadnyuk, V. I., Zaika, M. U., The therapeutic efficacy of diphenine, *Klin. Med.*, 1: 128–31, 1975.

2137. Zenteno Vacheron, J. S., Carrasco Zanini, J. and Ramos Ramirez, R., Paroxysmal dystonic choreoathetosis. A form of reflex epilepsy (two sporadic cases), *Epilepsy Abstracts*, 10(3): 84, 1977.

2138. Zhiping, Q., Chuanzhen, L., Iiyun, Y., Hanbai, C. and Yue, D., Limb-pain epilepsy—report of 9 cases, *Chin. Med. J.*, 93(4): 265–8, 1980.

2139. Ziegler, B., Hahn, H. J., Ziegler, M. and Fiedler, H., Successful cultivation of isolated islets of Langerhans without attachment: relationship between glucose- and theophylline-induced insulin release and insulin content in rat islets after cultivation, *Endocrinologie*, 69(1): 103–11, 1977.

2140. Zweibel, P. C., Insulinoma: review of seven cases at the Mount Sinai Hospital in light of the current literature, *Mount Sinai J. Med.*, 43(5): 637–56, 1976.

2141. Adams, H.P., Diphenylhydantoin in the treatment of alcohol withdrawal, *JAMA*, 218(4): 598, 1971.

2142. Aldrete, J.A., Romo-Salas, F., Mazzia, V.D.B. and Tan, S.L., Phenytoin for brain resuscitation after cardiac arrest, *Critical Care Medicine*, 9(6): 474-7, 1981.

2143. Almotrefi, A. A. and Baker, J. B. E., Investigation of the antifibrillatory activity of some anticonvulsant γ-aminobutyric acid-transaminase inhibitors in the rabbit isolated heart: comparison with phenytoin and mexiletine, *Br. J. Pharmac.*, 71(2): 635-9, 1980.

2144. Artru, A.A. and Michenfelder, J.D., Anoxic cerebral potassium accumulation reduced by phenytoin: mechanism of cerebral protection?, *Anesth. Analg.*, 60: 41-5, 1981.

2145. Artru, A.A. and Michenfelder, J.D., Influence of hypothermia or hyperthermia alone or in combination with pentobarbital and phenytoin on survival time in hypoxic mice, *Anesth. Analg.*, 60: 867-70, 1981.

2146. Ashizawa, T., Butler, I.J., Harati, Y. and Marshall, R.N. Autosomal dominant form of continuous motor neuron discharge, *Neurology*, 31(2): 59, 1981.

2147. Askanas, V., Engel, W.K., Berginer, V.M., Odenwald, W.F. and Galdi, A., Lysosomal abnormalities in cultured Schwann cells from a patient with peripheral neuropathy and continuous muscle fiber activity, *Ann. Neurol.*, 10: 238-42, 1981.

2148. Austin, G., Ed., *The Spinal Cord: Basic Aspects and Considerations*, Charles C. Thomas, Illinois, 1972.

2149. AvRuskin, T.W., Tio, S.L. and Juan, C.S., Modulating effects of acute and chronic Dilantin administration on the hyperglucagonemia of type-1 diabetes mellitus, *Clin. Res.*, 27(4): 625A, 1979.

2150. Bashour, F.A., Jones, E. and Edmonson, R., Cardiac arrhythmias in acute myocardial infarction: II. Incidence of the common arrhythmias with special reference to ventricular tachycardia, *Dis. Chest*, 51: 520-9, 1967.

2151. Bashour, F.A., Lehmann, J. and Prati, R., Prophylactic use of Dilantin in acute myocardial infarction, *J. Lab. Clin. Med.*, 70(5): 893, 1967.

2152. Baskin, S.I. and Finney, C.M., *The Effects of Taurine on Excitable Tissues*, 405-18, Spectrum Publications, 1981.

2153. Bauer, E.A. and Cooper, T.W., Therapeutic considerations in recessive dystrophic epidermolysis bullosa, *Arch. Dermatol.*, 117: 529, 1981.

2154. Behrens, J.M., Postmotor status epilepticus masking as a stroke, *Postgrad. Med.*, 68(5): 223-6, 1980.

2155. Bergenholtz, A. and Hanstrom, L., The effect of diphenylhydantoin upon the biosynthesis and degradation of collagen in cat palatal mucosa in organ culture, *Biochem. Pharmacol.*, 28: 2653-9, 1979.

2156. Blank, H., Treatment of pachyonychia congenita with phenytoin, *Br. J. Dermatol.*, 106(1): 123, 1982.

2157. Bremer, A.M., Yamada, K. and West, C.R., Ischemic cerebral edema in primates: effects of acetazolamide, phenytoin, sorbitol, dexamethasone, and methylprednisolone on brain water and electrolytes, *Neurosurgery*, 6(2): 149-54, 1980.

2158. Bücking, P.H. and Regli, F., The short periodicity of paroxysmal complex waves in electroencephalographic and clinical course of Creutzfeldt-Jakob disease, *Z. EEG-EMG.*, 10: 80-7, 1979.

2159. Cadnapaphornchai, P., Pontes, C. and McDonald, F.D., Mechanism of effect of phenytoin sodium on renin release, *Fed. Proc.*, 41(4): 1232, 1982.

2160. Cahill, D.W., Knipp, H. and Mosser, J., Intracranial hemorrhage with amphetamine abuse, *Neurology*, 31: 1058-9, 1981.

2161. Chase, T.N., Katz, R.I. and Kopin, I.J., Effect of anticonvulsants on brain serotonin, *Trans. Am. Neurol. Assoc.*, 94: 236-8, 1969.

2162. Check, W.A., 'A remarkable medicine' raises HDL levels, *JAMA*, 247(12): 1686-7, 1982.

2163. Chung, D.C., Anaesthetic problems associated with the treatment of cardiovascular disease: I. Digitalis toxicity, *Can. Anaesth. Soc. J.*, 28(1): 6-16, 1981.

2164. Cisson, C.M., Entrikin, R.K. and Wilson, B.W., Actions of phenytoin on AChE synthesis in cultured chick embryo muscle treated with paraoxon, *Soc. Neurosci. Abstr.*, 310: 986, 1977.

2165. Cisson, C.M., Entrikin, R.K. and Wilson, B.W., Effects of phenytoin on acetylcholinesterase activity and cell protein in cultured chick embryonic skeletal muscle, *Can. J. Physiol. Pharmacol.*, 56(2): 287-93, 1978.

2166. Clark, R.W. and Malarkey, W.B., Seizures and sleep-associated ventilatory dysfunction findings and treatment in 18 cases, *Neurology*, 31(2): 113, 1981.

2167. Craviso, G.L. and Musacchio, J.M., Penytoin (diphenylhydantoin) enhances the binding of dextromethorphan to guinea pig brain, *Fed. Proc.*, 40(3): 324, 1981.

2168. Delini-Stula, A., Radeke, E., Schlicht, G. and Hedwall, P.R., Detection of CNS-depressant properties of antihypertensives: validity of various methods in rodents and estimation of therapeutic margin in hypertensive rats, *Pharmac. Ther.*, 5: 431-44, 1979.

2169. DeLorenzo, R.J., Emple, G.P., and Glaser, G.H., Regulation of the level of endogenous phosphorylation of specific brain proteins by diphenylhydantoin, *J. Neurochem.*, 28: 21-30, 1977.

2170. DeSousa, R.C. and Grosso, A., Interactions of diphenylhydantoin with norepinephrine, theophylline and cyclic AMP in frog skin, *Experientia*, 29: 748-9, 1973.

2171. Deupree, J.D., The role or non-role of ATPase activation by phenytoin in the stabilization of excitable membranes, *Epilepsia*, 18(3): 309-15, 1977.

2172. Dinner, D.S., Lueders, H., Lederman, R. and Gretter, T.E., Aphasic status epilepticus: a case report, *Neurology*, 31: 888-91, 1981.

2173. Donoff, R.B., The effect of diphenylhydantoin on open wound healing in guinea pigs, *J. Surg. Res.*, 24: 41-4, 1978.

2174. Drachman, D.A. and Kapen, S., Sleep disturbance, *JAMA*, 246(2): 163-4, 1981.

2175. Dungan, W.T., Garson, Jr., A. and Gillette, P.C., Arrhythmogenic right ventricular dysplasia: a cause of ventricular tachycardia in children with apparently normal hearts, *Am. Heart J.*, 745-50, 1981.

2176. Eisenberg, M., Williams, J.F., Stevens, L. and Schofield, P.J., Mammalian collagenase and peptidase estimation in normal skin and in the skin of patients suffering from epidermolysis bullosa, *IRCS*, 2: 1732, 1974.

2177. Emerson, G.A., Drug prophylaxis against lethal effects of severe anoxia: VI. Neostigmine bromide and diphenylhydantoin, *Proc. Soc. Exp. Biol. Med.*, 54: 252-4, 1943.

2178. Entrikin, R.K. and Bryant, S.H., Membrane electrical effects of phenytoin on skeletal muscle of dystrophic chickens, *Epilepsy Abstracts*, 11(7): 277, 1978.

2179. Entrikin, R.K. and Bryant, S.H., Suppression of myotonia in dystrophic chicken muscle by phenytoin, *Am. J. Physiol.*, 237(3): C13-6, 1979.

2180. Entrikin, R.K., Patterson, G.T. and Wilson, B.W., Phenytoin, methysergide, and penicillamine in hereditary muscular dystrophy of the chicken, *Exper. Neurol.*, 72: 82-90, 1981.

2181. Ferro, J.M. and Castro-Caldas, A., Palatal myoclonus and carbamazepine, *Ann. Neurol.*, 10(4): 402, 1981.

2182. Finer, M.J., Diphenylhydantoin for treatment of alcohol withdrawal syndromes, *JAMA*, 215(1): 119, 1971.

2183. Flacke, W., Mulke, G. and Schulz, R., Contribution to the effect of drugs on negative-pressure tolerance, *Arch. Exper. Path. u. Pharmakol.*, 220: 469-76, 1953.

2184. Fleckman, A., Erlichman, J., Schubart, U.K. and Fleischer, N., Effect of trifluoperazine, D600, and phenytoin on depolarization and thyrotropin-releasing hormone-induced thyrotropin release from rat pituitary tissue, *Endocrinology*, 108: 2072-7, 1981.

2185. Flick, M.F., Hoeffel, J. and Webster, R.O., Phenytoin attenuates increased lung microvascular permeability in sheep, *Fed. Proc.*, 41(5): 1500, 1982.

2186. Foley, K.M. and Rogers, A., *The Rational Use of Analgesics in the Management of Cancer Pain*—Vol. II, Roche Laboratories, Nutley, NJ, 1981.

2187. Frank-Piskorska, A., Bogoniowska, Z., Baranska, H. and Donicowa, K., Insulin secretion in obese patients treated with diphenylhydantoin (DPH), *Pol. Tyg. Lek.*, 33(2): 41-3, 1978.

2188. Epilepsy drug decreases blistering due to a genetic disease, *NIH Research Resources Reporter*, V(12): 1981.

2189. Friis, M.L., Broeng-Nielson, B., Sindrup, E.H., Lund, M., Fogh-Anderson, P. and Hauge, M., Facial clefts among epileptic patients, *Arch. Neurol.*, 38: 227-9, 1981.

2190. Fromm, G.H., Terrence, C.F., Chattha, A.S. and Glass, J.D., Baclofen in trigeminal neuralgia: a pilot study, *Arch. Neurol.*, 37: 768-71, 1980.

2191. Fry, B.W. and Ciarlone, A.E., Effects of phenytoin on mouse cerebellar 5-hydroxytryptamine and norepinephrine, *Neuropharmacology*, 20: 623-5, 1981.

2192. Fukuda, A., Tabuse, H., Fujii, C. and Kohama, A., Experimental studies on total cerebral ischemia in dogs: II. The effect of phenytoin on electrocorticogram, *Epilepsy Abstracts*, 15(3): 98, 1982.

2193. Fukuda, A., Tabuse, H., Fujii, C. and Kohama, A., Experimental studies on total cerebral ischemia in dogs: I. The effect of phenytoin on regional cerebral blood flow, *Epilepsy Abstracts*, 15(3): 108, 1982.

2194. Gambert, S. R. and Garthwaite, T. L., The effect of diphenylhydantoin on basal and stimulated thyroid stimulating hormone (TSH) and prolactin secretion in euthyroid and hypothyroid rats, *Horm. Metab. Res.*, 12:636-7, 1980.

2195. Gerber, A.M., Olson, W.L. and Harris, J.H., Effect of phenytoin on functional recovery after experimental spinal cord injury in dogs, *Neurosurgery*, 7(5): 472-6, 1980.

2196. Gibbs, M.E. and Ng, K.T., Counteractive effects of norepinephrine and amphetamine on ouabain-induced amnesia, *Pharmac. Biochem. Behav.*, 6(5): 533-7, 1977.

2197. Gillis, R.A., McClellan, J.R., Sauer, T.S. and Standaert, F.G., Depression of cardiac sympathetic nerve activity by diphenylhydantoin, *J. Pharmacol. Exp. Ther.*, 179: 599-600, 1971.

2198. Gilmore, R.L. and Heilman, K.M., Speech arrest in partial seizures: evidence of an associated language disorder, *Neurology*, 31: 1016-9, 1981.

2199. Goncharov, N.P., The effect of substances stimulating and depressing the central nervous system on the quantity and quality of corticosteroids in the blood of dogs and guinea pigs, *Biull. Eksp. Biol. Med.*, 52: 1295-7, 1962.

2200. Gordon, A. S., Goldsmith, E. D. and Charipper, H. A., Effects of thiouracil and sodium 5,5-diphenylhydantoinate (Dilantin sodium) on resistance to lowered barometric pressures, *Proc. Soc. Exp. Biol. Med.*, 56: 202–3, 1944.

2201. Gordon, A.S., Milfay, D. and Diamond, I., Phosphorylation of the membrane-bound acetylcholine receptor: inhibition by diphenylhydantoin, *Ann. Neurol.*, 5(2): 201-3, 1979.

2202. Grafova, V. N. and Danilova, E. I., Action of antiepileptic drugs on myoclonia of spinal origin, *Bull. Exp. Biol. Med.*, 90(11): 1503–6, 1980.

2203. Greene, C.A., Rao, V.S., Maragos, G.D. and Mitchell, J.R., On the relationship migraine—epilepsy, *Nebraska Med. J.*, 56(4): 136-8, 1971.

2204. Gupta, D.N., Vollmer, V., Bashour, F.A. and Webb, W.R., Effect of Dilantin on the excitability of the experimentally infarcted heart, *Fed. Proc.*, 26: 381, 1967.

2205. Hanstrom, L., Lerner, U. and Gustafson, G.T., The effect of diphenylhydantoin upon enzyme release in relation to collagen degradation in cat palatal mucosa during organ culture, *Med. Biol.*, 57: 171-6, 1979.

2206. Holmes, G. L., McKeever, M. and Saunders, Z., Epileptiform activity in aphasia of childhood: an epiphenomenon, *Epilepsia*, 22: 631–9, 1981.

2207. Hudecki, M.S., Pollina, C.M., Heffner, R.R. and Bhargava, A.K., Enhanced functional ability in drug-treated dystrophic chickens: trial results with indomethacin, diphenylhydantoin and prednisolone, *Exp. Neurol.*, 73: 173-85, 1981.

2208. Jordan, L.S., Receptive and expressive language problems occurring in combination with a seizure disorder: a case report, *J. Commun. Disord.*, 13: 295-303, 1980.

2209. Jubiz, W., Bigler, A.H., Kumagai, L.F. and West, C.D., Estimation of thyroxine production rates in non-steady states, *J. Clin. Endocrinol. Metab.*, 34: 1009-15, 1972.

2210. Jurgenson, J.G. and Brennan, R.W., Stimulus-related myokymia as a manifestation of mild peripheral neuropathy, *Neurology*, 32(2): A204, 1982.

2211. Kaplan, M.M., Breitbart, R., Larsen, P.R., Tatro, J.B. and Appiah, A., Effects of phenytoin (DPH) on thyroxine (T4) 5'-deiodinase in rat liver and anterior pituitary, *Clin. Res.*, 28(2): 261A, 1980.

2212. Kendig, J.J., Courtney, K.R. and Cohen, E.N., Anesthetics: molecular correlates of voltage- and frequency-dependent sodium channel block in nerve, *J. Pharmacol. Exp. Ther.*, 210(3): 446-52, 1979.

2213. Kogure, K., Scheinberg, R., Kishikawa, H. and Bustro, R., The role of monoamines and cyclic AMP in ischemic brain edema, *Dynamics of Brain Edema*, Pappius, H.M. and Feindel, W., Eds., Springer, NY, 1976.

2214. Kong, Y., Heyman, A., Entman, M.L. and McIntosh, H.D., Glossopharyngeal neuralgia associated with bradycardia, syncope, and seizures, *Circulation*, 30: 109-13, 1964.

2215. Krone, R.J., Miller, J.P., Kleiger, R.E., Clark, K.W. and Oliver, G.C., The effectiveness of antiarrhythmic agents on early-cycle premature ventricular complexes, *Circulation*, 63(3): 664-9, 1981.

2216. Kuhn, E., Douwes, O. and Kern R., The action of hydantoin derivatives on the experimental myotonia induced in the isolated rat diaphragm by 2,4-dichlorophenoxyacetate, *Klin. Wschr.*, 47: 278-80, 1969.

2217. Lambert, J.R., Byrick, R.J. and Hammeke, M.D., Management of acute strychnine poisoning, *Can. Med. Assoc. J.*, 124: 1268-70, 1981.

2218. Lang, T.W., Bazika, V., Pappelbaum, S., Gold, H., Bernstein, H., Herrold, G. and Corday, E., Autotransplanted heart-lung and cerebral venous shunt preparations: two new techniques for pharmacologic assay of cardiovascular drugs, *Am. J. Cardiol.*, 16: 695-700, 1965.

2219. Lazar, M.L., Current treatment of tic douloureux, *Oral Surg. Oral Med. Oral Pathol.*, 50(6): 504-8, 1980.

2220. Levin, H.S. and Grossman, R.G., Behavioral sequelae of closed head injury, *Arch. Neurol.*, 35: 720-7, 1978.

2221. Levin, S.R., Driessen, J., Pehlavanian, M., Adachi, R. and Kasson, B., Do "electrolyte pump" enzymes have a role in islet cell function?, *Clin. Res.*, 24: 118A, 1976.

2222. Liewendahl, K., Helenius, T., Majuri, H., Ebeling, P. and Ahlfors, U. G., Effect of anticonvulsant and antidepressant drugs on iodothyronines in serum, *Scand. J. Clin. Lab. Invest.*, 40: 767-74, 1980.

2223. Lipp, H., Pitt, A., Anderson, S.T. and Zimmett, R., Recurrent ventricular tachyarrhythmias in a patient with a prolonged Q-T interval, *Med. J. Aust.*, 1296-9, 1970.

2224. Loh, C.K., Effects of diphenylhydantoin (DPH) on potassium exchange kinetics and transmembrane potentials in amphibian atrium, *Fed. Proc.*, 33: 445, 1974.

2225. Lucchesi, B.R., *Cardiovascular Pharmacology*, Antonaccio, M., Ed., Raven Press, New York, 1977.

2226. Marshall, J. S. and Levy, R. P., Polyacrylanide electrophoretic study of thyroxine binding to human serum, *J. Clin. Endocr.*, 26: 87-98, 1966.

2227. Matsuki, N., Quandt, F.N., Yeh, J.Z. and Eick, R.T., Sodium channel blocking action of phenytoin in mammal neurons in tissue cultures, *Soc. Neurosci. Abstr.*, 7: 811, 1981.

2228. Mayeux, R., Alexander, M.P., Benson, D.F., Brandt, J. and Rosen, J., Poriomania, *Neurology*, 29: 1616-9, 1979.

2229. McCandless, D.W., Feussner, G.K., Lust, W.D. and Passonneau, J.V., Metabolite levels in brain following experimental seizures: the effects of maximal electroshock and phenytoin in cerebellar layers, *J. Neurochem.*, 32: 743-53, 1979.

2230. Melmon, K.L., Ed., *Cardiovascular Drug Therapy*, F.A. Davis, Co., Philadelphia, 1974.

2231. Michalski, F.J., Gala, H.K. and Chen, J., The effect of diphenylhydantoin (Dilantin) on replication of Herpes simplex virus in human fibroblasts *in vitro*, Presented at *20th Interscience Conference on Antimicrobial Agents and Chemotherapy*, New Orleans, 1980.

2232. Moses, L., Postoperative trigeminal neuralgia—case report, *Opthalamic Surg.*, 11: 131-2, 1980.

2233. Nosek, T.M., How valproate and phenytoin affect the ionic conductances and active transport characteristics of the crayfish giant axon, *Epilepsia*, 22: 651-65, 1981.

2234. Neufeld, M.Y., Swanson, J.W. and Klass, D.W., Localized EEG abnormalities in acute carbon monoxide poisoning, *Arch. Neurol.*, 38: 524-7, 1981.

2235. O'Neill, B., Callaghan, N., Stapleton, M. and Molloy, W., Serum elevation of high density lipoprotein (HDL) cholesterol in epileptic patients taking carbamazepine or phenytoin, *Acta Neurol. Scand.*, 65: 104-9, 1982.

2236. Palmer, G.C., Palmer, S.J. and Legendre, J.L., Guanylate cyclase—cyclic GMP in mouse cerebral cortex and cerebellum: modification by anticonvulsants, *Exp. Neurol.*, 71: 601-14, 1981.

2237. Patmas, M.A., Colton, J.S. and Colton, C.A., Modulation of mitochondrial calcium flux by convulsant (diamide) and anticonvulsant (diphenylhydantoin) agents, *Clin. Res.*, 29(1): 62A, 1981.

2238. Pfeiffer, C.C., Observations on the therapy of the schizophrenias, *J. Appl. Nutr.*, 26: 29-36, 1974.

2239. Pincus, J.H., Presynaptic actions of phenytoin and barbiturates, *Neurology*, 31(2): 157, 1981.

2240. Pincus, J.H. and Hsiao, K., Calcium uptake mechanisms affected by some convulsant anticonvulsant drugs, *Brain Res.*, 217: 119-27, 1981.

2241. Pincus, J. H. and Hsiao, K., Phenytoin inhibits both synaptosomal ^{45}Ca uptake and efflux, *Exp. Neurol.*, 74: 293–8, 1981.

2242. Prevot, H., Andrien, J.M., Bounameaux, Y. and Spitaels, J.M., Oral diphenylhydantoin support therapy in arrhythmias, *Rev. Med. de Liege.*, 22(23): 683-7, 1967.

2243. Pritchard, III, P.B. and Gross, J.A., Ictal aphasia, *Electroencephalogr. Clin. Neurophysiol.*, 51: 75P, 1981.

2244. Rall, T.W. and Schleifer, L.S., *The Pharmacological Basis of Therapeutics*, 6th Ed., 454-5, Goodman, L.S. and Gilman, A., Eds., Macmillan, New York, 1980.

2245. Rautio, A., Sotaniemi, E.A., Pelkonen, R.O. and Luoma, P.V., Treatment of alcoholic cirrhosis with enzyme inducers, *Clin. Pharmacol. Ther.*, 28(5): 629-37, 1980.

2246. Reid, C. and Chanarin, I., Effect of phenytoin on DNA synthesis by human bone marrow, *Scand. J. Haematol.*, 20: 237-40, 1978.

2247. Reinckens, W., New drug treatment reported for rare, blistering skin disease, *NIH News & Features*, March, 1981.

2248. Remmer, H., The acceleration of liver regeneration after hepatectomy by phenobarbital and diphenylhydantoin, *Presented at Int. Congress of Gastroenterology*, Prague, July 13, 1968.

2249. Reynolds, E.H., Drug treatment for epilepsy, *Lancet*, 2:721-5, 1978.

2250. Rhee, H., Antiarrhythmic action of phenytoin (DPH) in dogs: inhibition of Ca^{++}-ATPase and Ca^{++} transport, *Fed. Proc.*, 40(3): 645, 1981.

2251. Rocchini, A. P., Chun, P. O., and Dick, M., Ventricular tachycardia in children, *Am. J. Cardiol.*, 47: 1091-7, 1981.

2252. Rogers, M. P., Gittes, R. F., Dawson, D. M. and Reich, P., Giggle incontinence, *JAMA*, 274(10): 1446-8, 1982.

2253. Rushton, J. G., Stevens, C. and Miller, R. H., Glosso-pharyngeal (vagoglossopharyngeal) neuralgia—a study of 217 cases, *Arch. Neurol.*, 38: 201-5, 1981.

2254. Satoh, K., Narimatsu, A. and Taira, N., Effects of an-tiarrhythmic drugs on AV nodal and intraventricular conduc-tion as assessed in the isolated, blood-perfused AV node preparation of the dog, *J. Cardiovasc. Pharmacol.*, 3(4): 753-68, 1981.

2255. Seelig, J. M., Becker, D. P., Miller, D., Greenberg, R. P., Ward, J. D., and Choi, S. C., Traumatic acute subdural hematoma—major mortality reduction in comatose patients treated within four hours, *New Eng. J. Med.*, 304(25): 1511-9, 1981.

2256. Servitz, Z. and Muzil, F., Prophylactic treatment of post-traumatic epilepsy: results of a long-term follow-up in Czechoslovakia, *Epilepsia*, 22: 315-20, 1981.

2257. Stannard, M. and Caplan, H. L., Cardiac arrest due to imipramine hydrochloride, *Med. J. Aust.*, 2(1): 22-4, 1967.

2258. Staple, P.H. and Nakeeb, S.J., Effect of diphenylhydan-toin (phenytoin) on dermal allograft survival in rats, *J. Dent. Res.*, 57: 291, 1978.

2259. Stjernholm, M.R., Alsever, R.N. and Rudolph, M.C., Thyroid-function tests in diphenylhydantoin-treated patients, *Clin. Chem.*, 21(10): 1388-92, 1975.

2260. Swerdlow, M. and Cundill, J.G., Anticonvulsant drugs used in the treatment of lancinating pain. A comparison, *Anaesthe-sia*, 36: 1129-32, 1981.

2261. Terrence, C.F. and Fromm, G.H., Complications of baclo-fen withdrawal, *Arch. Neurol.*, 38: 588-9, 1981.

2262. Trascasa, M.L., Egido, J., Sancho, J. and Hernando, L., Evidence of high polymeric IgA levels in serum of patients with Berger's disease and its modification with phenytoin treatment, *Proc. Eur. Dial Transplant Assoc.*, 16: 513-9, 1979.

2263. Vedernikov, Y.P., Shinskaya, N.E. and Strelkov, R.B., Role of the central monoaminergic structures in the tolerance of animals to extreme hypoxic hypoxia, *Patol. Fiziol. Eksp. Ter.*, 6: 18-25, 1978.

2264. Voorhies, R. and Patterson, R.H., Management of tri-geminal neuralgia (tic douloureux), *JAMA*, 245(24): 2521-3, 1981.

2265. Wagner, P. and Bader, H., Effect of alcohols, chlorproma-zine and diphenylhydantoin on (Ca^{2+})-ATPase of human red blood cells, *Naunyn-Schmied. Arch. Pharmacol.*, 282: R103, 1974.

2266. Walker, M.D. and Strike, T.A., Misonidazole peripheral neuropathy: its relationship to plasma concentration and other drugs, *Cancer Clin. Trials*, 3: 105-9, 1980.

2267. Watson, E.L. and Siegel, I.A., Diphenylhydantoin effects on salivary secretion and microsomal calcium accumulation and release, *Eur. J. Pharmacol.*, 37: 207-11, 1976.

2268. Willow, M., Kuenzel, E. A., Catterall, W. A., Inhibi-tion of voltage-sensitive sodium channels in neuroblastoma cells and synaptosomes by the anticonvulsant drugs diphenyl-hydantoin and carbamazepine, *Mol. Pharmacol.*, 25 (2): 228-35, 1984.

2269. Wohns, R. N. W. and Kerstein, M.D., The role of Di-lantin in the prevention of pulmonary edema associated with cerebral hypoxia, *Crit. Care Med.*, 10(7): 436-43, 1982.

2270. Zaidi, S.M.M., Satsangi, R.K., Nasir, P.K.M., Agarwal, R. and Tiwari, S.S., New anti-myobacterial hydantoins, *Pharmazie*, 35(12): 755-6, 1980.

2271. Aanderud, S., Aarbakke, J., Sundsfjord, J., Metabolism of thyroid hormones in isolated rat hepatocytes: studies on the influences of carbamazepine and phenytoin, *Acta. Endocri-nol.*, 104(4): 479–84, 1983.

2272. Abiko, H., Suzuki, J., Mizoi, K., Oba, M., Yoshimoto, T., Protective effect of phenytoin and enhancement of its ac-tion by combined administration of mannitol and vitamin E in cerebral ischemia, *Brain Nerve*, 38(4): 328–35, 1986.

2273. Abdul-Ghani, A. S., Goutinho-Neito, J., Druce, D., Bradford, H. F., Effects of anticonvulsants on the *in vivo* and *in vitro* release of GABA, *Biochem. Pharmacol.*, 30(4): 363–8, 1981.

2274. Adams, P. R., Constanti, A., Banks, F. W., Voltage clamp analysis of inhibitory synaptic action in crayfish stretch receptor neurons, *Fed. Proc.*, 40(11): 2637–41, 1981.

2275. Adler, E., Yaari, Y., David, G., Selzer, M. E., Use- and frequency-dependent action of phenytoin on the action poten-tial of lamprey spinal axons, *Neurology*, 35(Sup 1): 126, 1985.

2276. Adler, E. M., Yaari, Y., David, G., Selzer, M. E., Fre-quency-dependent action of phenytoin on lamprey spinal axons, *Brain Research*, 362(2): 271–80, 1986.

2277. Ahmad, S. N., Jailkhani, B. L., Jaffery, N. F., A rapid method for separation and estimation of free phenytoin in serum, *Indian J. Exp. Biol.*, 22(11): 605–7, 1984.

2278. Aichele, R., Paik, H., Heller, A. H., Efficacy of phen-ytoin, procainamide, and tocainide in murine genetic my-otonia, *Exp. Neurol.*, 87: 377–81, 1985.

2279. Aldrete, J. A., Cubillos, P., Protection against anoxia by phenytoin and thiopentone in rabbits, *Sixth Eur. Congress of Anaesthesiology*, 248, Sept. 8–15, 1982.

2280. Aldrete, J. A., Cubillos, P., Phenytoin improves hemodynamic tolerance and survival after severe hypoxia, *Anesth. Analg.*, 63: 1021–4, 1984.

2281. Ali, N. N., Harvey, W., Harris, M., Bone matrix turn-over and anticonvulsant drugs, *J. Dent. Res.*, 61: 548, 1982.

2282. Allen, J. K., Whitfield, J. B., Hensley, W. J., The ef-fects of diphenylhydantoin on the relationship between high-density lipoprotein cholesterol and several biochemical assays, *Clin. Chim. Acta*, 102: 111–14, 1980.

2283. Alps, B. J., Hass, W. K., Nicardipine and phenytoin prevention of cerebral ischemic cell change in a new rat sur-vival model of brief four-vessel occlusion, *Neurology*, 35(Sup 1): 141, 1985.

2284. Alvin, J. D., Bush, M. T., Physiological disposition of anticonvulsants, *Anticonvulsants*, Vida, J. A., Ed., Academic Press, New York, 113–50, 1977.

2285. Aly, M. I., Abdel-Latif, A. A., Studies on the effects of acetylcholine and antiepileptic drugs on $^{32}P_i$ incorporation into phospholipids of rat brain synaptosomes, *Neurochem. Res.*, 7(2): 159–69, 1982.

2286. Aman, M. G., Paxton, J. W., Werry, J. S., Fluctuations in steady-state phenytoin concentrations as measured in saliva in children, *Pediatr. Pharmacol.*, 3: 87–94, 1983.

2287. American Medical Association, Drugs used in disor-ders affecting skeletal muscle, *AMA Drug Evaluations, 6th Edition*, AMA, Chicago, 221–37, 1986.

2288. American Medical Association, Antiepileptic drugs, *AMA Drug Evaluations, 6th Edition*, AMA, Chicago, 169–95, 1986.

2289. American Medical Association, Antiarrhythmic Agents, *AMA Drug Evaluations, 6th Edition*, AMA, Chicago, 435–61, 1986.

2290. American Medical Association, Drugs used to treat neuralgias, *AMA Drug Evaluations, 6th Edition*, AMA, Chi-cago, 197–202, 1986.

2291. Amy, B., Legrand, P., Levitzky, M., Welsh, R. A., Schechter, F. G., Suppression of centrineurogenic shock lung by dilantin (DPH) administered early in established hemor-rhagic shock, *J. Trauma*, 21(9) 7628, 1981.

2292. Andoh, B., Idle, J. R., Sloan, T. P., Smith, R. L., Wool-house, N., Interethnic and inter-phenotype differences among Ghanaians and caucasians in the metabolic hydroxylation of phenytoin, *Br. J. Clin. Pharmacol.*, 9: 282–83, 1979.

2293. Anisimov, V. N., The effect of buformin and diphenine on the lifetime, estral function, and frequency of spontaneous tumors in rats, *Vopr. Onkol.*, 26(6): 42–8, 1980.

2294. Anisimov, V. N., Ostroumova, M. N., Dilman, V. N., Inhibition of the carcinogenic effect of 7,12-dimethylbenz (a) anthracene in female rats by buformin, phenytoin, pineal polypeptide extract, and L-dopa, *Bull. Exp. Biol. Med.*, 89(6): 819–22, 1980.

2295. Apple, F. S., Walker, F. C., Dietzler, D. N., Serum creatinine concentration and the discrepancy between EMIT and GLC phenytoin levels, *Clin. Chem.*, 28(7): 1589, 1982.

2296. Aronson, J. K., Digitalis intoxication, *Clin. Sci.*, 64:253–8, 1983.

2297. Asboe-Hansen, G., Treatment of generalized scleroderma with inhibitors of collagen synthesis, *Int. J. Dermatol.*, 21(3): 159–61, 1982.

2298. Ashizawa, T., Butler, I. J., Harati, Y., Roongta, S. M., A dominantly inherited syndrome with continuous motor neuron discharges, *Ann. Neurol.*, 13: 285–90, 1983.

2299. Bachmann, K., Forney, R. B., Voeller, K., Monitoring phenytoin in salivary and plasma ultrafiltrates of pediatric patients, *Ther. Drug Monit.*, 5(3): 325–9, 1983.

2300. Bachmann, K., Schwartz, J., Forney Jr., R., Jauregui, L., Phenytoin as a probe of drug metabolism: predicting clearance with a salivary sample, *Pharmacologist*, 26(3): 207, 1984.

2301. Bachmann, K., Voeller, K., Forney, R., Use of plasma unbound drug concentrations in adjusting phenytoin doses, *Ther. Drug Monit.*, 6(2): 173–8, 1984.

2302. Bady, B., Girard, P. F., Jallade, S., Gaillard, L., A case of pseudomyotonia cured by carbamazepine, *Rev. Neurol.*, 120: 277-86, 1969.

2303. Bailey, E., Farmer, P. B., Hoskins, J. A., Lamb, J. H., Peal, J. A., Determination of Plasma phenytoin by capillary gas chromatography with nitrogen-phosphorus detection and with selective ion monitoring, *J. Chromatogr.*, 310(1): 199–203, 1984.

2304. Balboa De Paz, F., Campos Castello, J., Olivan Palacios, J., Espino Hurtado, P., Vela Bueno, A., Anoretic syndrome associated with convulsive seizures, *Psiquis*, 2(5); 56–61, 1981.

2305. Balogh, E., Mattyus, A., Nemeth, C., Szabadosne, N. M., Transient lowering of the IgA level during diphedan therapy, *Orv. Hetil.*, 120: 2179–82, 1979.

2306. Bandmann, H. J., Perwein, E., Phenytoin in treatment of epidermolysis bullosa hereditaria dystrophica partim inversa (Gedde-Dahl), *Z. Hautkr.*, 57(21): 1587–98, 1982.

2307. Banerjee, A., Turner, A. J., Guha, S. R., GABA dehydrogenase activity in rat brain, *Biochem. Pharmacol.*, 31(20): 3219–23, 1982.

2308. Barba Rubio, J., Diphenylhydantoin in leprosy. Its topical application in ulcers and plantar trophic ulcers, *Presented to XII Mexican Congress of Dermatology*, Oaxaca, Oct. 9–12, 1985.

2309. Barker, J. L., Owen, D. G., Segal, M., Clinically important drugs have opposing actions on the excitability of cultured mammalian neurons, *Neurotransmitters, Seizures, and Epilepsy II*, Fariello, R. G., et al., Eds., Raven Press, New York, 153–66, 1984.

2310. Baron, J. C., Roeda, D., Munari, C., Crouzel, C., Chodkiewics, J. P., Comar, D., Brain regional pharmacokinetics of ^{11}C-labeled diphenylhydantoin: positron emission tomography in humans, *Neurology*, 33: 580–5, 1983.

2311. Barratt, E. S., Faulk, D. M., Brandt, M. E., Bryant, S. G., Effects of phenytoin on N100 augmenting/reducing and the late positive complex of the event-related potential: a topographic analysis, *Neuropsychobiology*, 15: 201–7, 1986.

2312. Barron, S. A., Heffner, R. R., Continuous muscle fiber activity — a case with unusual clinical features, *Arch. Neurol.*, 36: 520–1, 1979.

2313. Bartels, H., Guther, E., Wallis, S., Monitoring therapy by analysis of drug concentration in saliva, *Monatsschr. Kinderheilkd.*, 131(1): 13–16, 1983.

2314. Baruah, J. K., Confusional episode a seizure phenomenon in the elderly, *Epilepsia*, 24: 246, 1983.

2315. Bauer, L. A., Edwards, W. A., Dellinger, E. P., Raisys, V. A., Brennan, C., Importance of unbound phenytoin serum levels in head trauma patients, *J. Trauma*, 23: 1058–60, 1983.

2316. Bechtereva, N. P., Nikitina, L. I., Iliuchina, V. A., Dambinova, S. A., Denisova, V. V., Dilantin: clinical and scientific experience of application, *Eur. J. Clin. Invest.*, 14: 36, 1984.

2317. Behan, P., Migraine: a rational approach to therapy, *Br. J. Clin. Pract.*, 36(10): 359–62, 1982.

2318. Bell, H. H., Dittmeier, G. E., Comparative effects of gemfibrozil, phenytoin, and nicotinic acid on serum HDL, *Arteriosclerosis*, 5(5): 514A, 1985.

2319. Bell, H. H., Dittmeier, G. E., Increase in HDL2 cholesterol with phenytoin therapy, *Arteriosclerosis*, 5(5): 514A, 1985.

2320. Bellak, L., A possible subgroup of the schizophrenic syndrome and implications for treatment, *Am. J. Psychother.*, 30: 194–205, 1976.

2321. Benet, L. Z., Massoud, N., Gambertoglio, J. G., Pharmacokinetic basis and therapeutic concentrations, *Pharmacokinetic Basis for Drug Treatment*, Raven Press, New York, 425–440, 1984.

2322. Berger, J. R., Sheremata, W. A., Melamed, E., Paroxysmal dystonia as the initial manifestation of multiple sclerosis., *Arch. Neurol.*, 41; 747–50, 1984.

2323. Berlit, P., Krause, K. H., Heuck, C. C., Schellenberg, B., Serum lipids and anticonvulsants, *Acta Neurol. Scand.*, 66: 328–34, 1982.

2324. Bernard, P., Wilson, D., Paster, G., Brown, W., Glenn, T. M., Possible involvement of adenosine receptors in the electroshock anticonvulsant effects of carbamazepine, diphenylhydantoin, phenobarbital and diazepam, *Pharmacologist*, 25 (3): 164, 1983.

2325. Bertch, K. E., Norton, J. A., Young, A. B., Rapp, R. P., Tibbs, P. A., A comparative study of laboratory parameters in head-injured patients receiving either phenytoin or placebo for 24 months, *Drug Intell. Clin. Pharm.*, 19: 561–6, 1985.

2326. Besser, R., Schuster, C. J., Possibility of influencing sharp alpha waves in coma by means of drugs: a clinical contribution, *Z. EEG-EMG*, 10: 158–60, 1979.

2327. Bezchlibnyk-Butler, K., New treatment of psychiatric disorders, *On. Contin. Pract.*, 11(2): 13–18, 1984.

2328. Bhandari, A. K., Shapiro, W. A., Morady, F. S., Shen, E. N., Mason, J., Scheinman, M. M., Electrophysiologic testing in patients with the long QT syndrome, *Circulation*, 71(1): 63–71, 1985.

2329. Bhattacharya, S. K., Bhattacharya, D., Effect of restraint stress on anticonvulsant actions of phenobarbitone and diphenylhydantoin in rats, *Indian J. Exp. Biol.*, 20: 406–8, 1982.

2330. Bhise, S. B., Subrahmanyam, C. V., Malhotra, A. K., Srivastava, R. C., Liquid membrane phenomenon in antiepileptic drugs, *Int. J. Pharm.*, 24(2/3): 297–305, 1985.

2331. Bielak, J., Pokora, J., The effect of hydantoinal on cardiac arrhythmias, *Pol. Tyg. Lek.*, 25: 967–9, 1970.

2332. Bigger, J. T., Dresdale, R. J., Heissenbuttel, R. H., Weld, F. M., Wit, A. L., Ventricular arrhythmias in ischemic heart disease: mechanism prevalence significance and management, *Prog. Cardiovasc. Dis.*, 19(4): 255–300, 1977.

2333. Bigger, J. T., Hoffman, B. F., Antiarrythmic drugs, *The Pharmacological Basis of Therapeutics*, 7th edition, Gilman, A. G., Goodman, L. S., Rall, T. W., Murad, F., Eds., Macmillan Publishing Co., New York, 748–83, 1985.

2334. Billings, R. E., Interactions between folate metabolism, phenytoin metabolism and liver microsomal cytochrome P450, *Drug. Nutr. Interact.*, 3(1): 21–32, 1984.

2335. Billings, R. E., Fischer, L. J., Oxygen-18 incorporation studies of the metabolism of phenytoin to the catechol, *Drug Metab. Dispos.*, 13(3): 312–17, 1985.

2336. Billings, R. E., Hansen, D. K., Species differences in phenytoin induction of cytochrome P450 due to pharmacokinetic differences, *Proc. West Pharmacol. Soc.*, 27: 539–42, 1984.

2337. Billings, R. E., Milton, S. G., Chemical nature of reactive metabolites formed with phenytoin in rat liver microsomes, *Fed. Proc.*, 44(4): 1114, 1985.

2338. Bint, A. J., Burtt, I., Adverse antibiotic drug interactions, *Drugs*, 20: 57–68, 1980.

2339. Bird, T. D. Carlson, C. B., Horning, M., Ten year follow-up of paroxysmal choreoathetosis: a sporadic case becomes familial, *Epilepsia*, 19: 129–32, 1978.

2340. Birkmayer, W., Die behandlung der traumatischen epilepsie, *Wein. Klin. Wochenschr.*, 63: 606–9, 1951.

2341. Bittar, E. E., Nwoga, J., Some further observations on the stimulation by high external potassium of the sodium efflux in barnacle muscle fibers, *Pflugers Arch.*, 395: 318–25, 1982.

2342. Bleehen, N. M., The Cambridge glioma trial of misonidazole and radiation therapy with associated pharmacokinetic studies, *Cancer Clin.*, 3: 267–73, 1980.

2343. Block, P. J., Winkle, R. A., Hemodynamic effects of antiarrhythmic drugs, *Am. J. Cardiol.*, 52: 14c–23c, 1983.

2344. Blom, S., Trigeminal neuralgia: its treatment with a new anticonvulsant drug (G-32883), *Lancet*, 1: 839–40, 1962.

2345. Bobrove, A. M., Possible beneficial effects of phenytoin for rheumatoid arthritis, *Arthritis Rheum.*, 26 (1): 118–19, 1983.

2346. Bock, J. L., Ben-Ezra, J., Rapid measurement of free anticonvulsant drugs by direct liquid chromatography of serum ultrafiltrates, *Clin. Chem.*, 31(11): 1884–7, 1985.

2347. Bodewei, R., Hering, S., Schubert, B., Winkler, J., Wollenberger, A., Calcium channel block by phenytoin in neuroblastoma X glioma hybrid cells, *Biomed. Biochim. Acta*, 7/8: 1229–37, 1985.

2348. Boehnert, M., Lovejoy, F. H., The effect of phenytoin on cardiac conduction and ventricular arrhythmias in acute tricyclic antidepressant (TCA) overdose, *Vet. Hum. Toxicol.*, 27: 297, Abst. 32, 1985.

2349. Bowles, A. M., Raines, A., Dretchen, K. L., Protection by phenytoin and verapamil against organophosphate poisoning in the mouse, *Fed. Proc.*, 43(3): 553, 1984.

2350. Bowling, A. C., De Lorenzo, R. J., Anticonvulsant receptors: identification and characterization in brain, *Neurology*, 32 (2): A224, 1982.

2351. Bowling, A. C., De Lorenzo, R. J., Micromolar affinity benzodiazepine receptors: indentification and characterization in central nervous system, *Science*, 216: 1247–50, 1982.

2352. Brady, R. O., King, F. M., Fabry's disease, *Peripheral Neuropathy*, Vol. 2, Dyck, P. J., et al., Eds., W. B. Saunders Co., Philadelphia, 914–27, 1975.

2353. Brandt, L., Ljunggren, B., Andersson, K. E., Hindfelt, B., Uski, T., Effects of indomethacin and prostacylin on isolated human pial arteries contracted by CSF from patients with aneurysmal SAH, *J. Neurosurg.*, 55: 877–83, 1981.

2354. Braun, C. W., Goldstone, J. M., Increased clearance of phenytoin as the presenting feature of infectious mononucleosis, *Ther. Drug. Monit.*, 2(4): 355–57, 1980.

2355. Brodie, M. J., Muir, S. E., Agnew, E., Macphee, G. J., Volo, G., Teasdale, E., Macpherson, P., Protein binding and CSF penetration of phenytoin following acute oral dosing in man, *Br. J. Clin. Pharmac.*, 19(2): 161–8, 1985.

2356. Brodsky, L., Shah, A., Casenas, E., Two distinct "par-

adoxical" reactions to neuroleptics, *Psychiatr. J. Univ. Ottawa*, 9: 61–4, 1984.

2357. Brodsky, L., Zuniga, J. S., Casenas, E. R., Ernstoff, R., Sachdev, H. S., Refractory anxiety: a masked epileptiform disorder?, *Psychiatr. J. Univ. Ottawa*, 8: 42–5, 1983.

2358. Brown, B. S., Akera, T., Brody, T. M., Mechanism of grayanotoxin III-induced afterpotentials in feline cardiac Purkinje fibers, *Eur. J. Pharmacol.*, 75: 271–81, 1981.

2359. Brown, H., Tetanus, *JAMA*, 204(7) 614–16, 1968.

2360. Brown, J. J., Murphy, M. J., Transverse myelopathy in progressive systemic sclerosis, *Ann. Neurol.*, 17: 615–17, 1958.

2361. Brown, M., Liberthson, R. R., Ali, H. H., Lowenstein, E., Perioperative anesthetic management of a patient with long Q-T syndrome (LQTS), *Anesthesiology*, 55: 586–9, 1981.

2362. Brown, S. B., Garcia-Mullin, R., Murai, Y., The Schwartz-Jampel syndrome (myotonic chondrodystrophy) in the adult, *Neurology*, 4 (25): 366, 1975.

2363. Brown, T. J., Isaacs syndrome, *Arch. Phys. Med. Rehabil.*, 65(1): 27–9, 1984.

2364. Browne, T. R., Pharmacologic principles of antiepileptic drug administration, *Epilepsy, Diagnosis and Management*, Browne, T. R., Feldman, R. G., Eds., Little, Brown & Co., Boston, 145–60, 1983.

2365. Bryson, S. M., Kelly, J. C., Kelman, A. W., Whiting, B., Therapeutic free phenytoin monitoring, *Clin. Pharmacokinet.*, 9 (sup 1): 90, 1984.

2366. Burger, L. J., Lopez, R. I., Elliott, F. A., Tonic seizures induced by movement, *Neurology*, 22: 656–9, 1972.

2367. Burke, B. E., De Lorenzo, R. J., Ca^{2+} and calmodulin-dependent phosphorylation of endogenous synaptic vesicle tubulin by a vesicle-bound calmodulin kinase system, *J. Neurochem.*, 38(5): 1205–18, 1982.

2368. Burke, B. E., Delorenzo, R. J., Ca^{2+} and calmodulin-regulated endogenous tubulin kinase activity in presynaptic nerve terminal preparations, *Brain Res.*, 236: 393–415, 1982.

2369. Burnham, W. N., Spero, L., Okazaki, M. M., Madras, B. K., Saturable binding of [^{3}H]-phenytoin to rat brain membrane fraction, *Can. J. Physiol. Pharmacol.*, 59(4): 402–7, 1981.

2370. Butt, O., QT-syndrome includes two symptom complexes, *Med. Klin.*, 76 (6) 38–41, 1981.

2371. Cadnapaphornchai, P., Kellner, D., Mc Donald, F., Role of adrenoceptor in diphenylhydantoin (D)-stimulated renal renin release, *Fed. Proc.*, 44(5): 1570, 1985.

2372. Cadnapaphornchai, P., Kellner, D., Mc Donald, F. D., Inhibition of renal alpha adrenoceptor by diphenylhydantoin, *Fed. Proc.*, 45(4): 1033, 1986.

2373. Cadnapaphornchai, P., Pontes, C., Mc Donald, F. D., Mechanisms of effect of diphenylhydantoin on renal renin release, *Am. J. Physiol.*, 247(3): F418–22, 1984.

2374. Caldwell, K. K., Harris, R. A., Effects of anesthetic and anticonvulsant drugs on calcium dependent efflux of potassium from human erythrocytes, *Eur. J. Pharmacol.*, 107(2): 119–25, 1985.

2375. Calixto, J. B., De-Lima, T. C., Diphenylhydantoin inhibition of drug-induced contractions of isolated rat vas deferens: additional evidence for a calcium-blocking action, *Braz. J. Med. Biol. Res.*, 16: 327–31, 1983.

2376. Campbell, J. W., Frisse, M., *Manual of Medical Therapeutics*, 24th Edition, Little, Brown & Co., Boston, 79 passim 422, 1983.

2377. Cantrill, V., Prophylactic phenytoin in tricyclic overdose, *J. Emerg. Med.*, 1: 169–77, 1983.

2378. Capuano, V., Capobianco, S., Romano, A., Therapeutic approach to arrhythmias in pediatric age, *Osp. Ital. Pediatr.*, 18(5): 769–80, 1983.

2379. Catterall, W. A., Inhibition of voltage-sensitive sodium channels in neuroblastoma cells by antiarrhythmic drugs. *Mol. Pharmacol.*, 20: 356–62, 1981.

2380. Chadda, V. S., Joshi, K. G., Chadda, S., A double-blind crossover study of diphenylhydantoin in irritable bowel syndrome, *J. Assoc. Physicians India,* 31 (7): 425–7, 1983.

2381. Chalfie, M., Hoadley, D., Pastan, S., Perlman, R. L., Calcium uptake into rat pheochromocytoma cells, *J. Neurochem.,* 27: 1405–9, 1976.

2382. Chalk, J. B., Ridgeway, K., Brophy, T. R., Yelland, J. D., Eadie, M. J., Phenytoin impairs the bioavailability of dexamethasone neurological and neurosurgical patients, *J. Neurol. Neurolsurg. Psychiatry,* 47(10): 1087–90, 1984.

2383. Chalmers, R. J., Johnson, R. H., The effect of diphenylhydantoin on metabolic and growth hormones during and after exercise., *J. Neurol. Neurosurg. Psychiatry,* 46(7): 662–65, 1983.

2384. Chambers, D. A., Cohen, R. L., The direct effects of biological response modifiers on epidermal cells, *Br. J. Dermatol.,* 3: 114–22, 1984.

2385. Chang, T., Glasko, A. J., Phenytoin: Biotransformation, *Antiepileptic Drugs,* Woodbury, D. M., et al., Eds., Raven Press, New York, 209–26, 1982.

2386. Chapman, A. G., Meldrum, B. S., Effects of anticonvulsant drugs on brain amino acid metabolism, *Epilepsy: An Update on Research and Therapy,* Nistico, G., et al., Eds., Alan R. Liss Inc., New York, 63–76, 1983.

2387. Chapman, J. R., Roberts, D. W., Schol, H. M., Bagwell, C. B., Hudson, J. L., Flow cytometric analysis of the effects of phenytoin and its major metabolite on mitogen stimulated mouse spleen cells, *Int. J. Immunopharmacol.,* 5(5): 471–8, 1983.

2388. Cheigh, J. S., Reidenberg, M. M., Drug metabolism and dose adjustment in patients with renal failure, *Developments in Nephrology, Vol. 1, Manual of Clinical Nephrology of the Rogosin Kidney Center,* Cheigh, J. S., et al., Eds., Martinus Nijhoff, Boston, 428–52, 1981.

2389. Cheng, S. C., Brunner, E. A., Effects of anesthetic agents on synaptosomal GABA disposal, *Anesthesiology,* 55: 34–40, 1981.

2390. Chiche, P., Benaim, R., Chesnais, F., Phenytoin: Clinical pharmacology. Use in various arrhythmias in 86 cases, *Ann. Cardiol. Angeiol.,* 2: 231–42, 1971.

2391. Chien, C. P., Keegan, D., Diazepam as an oral long-term anticonvulsant for epileptic mental patients, *Dis. Nerv. Syst.,* 33: 100–04, 1972.

2392. Chong-Cheng, X., Occurrence of spontaneous channel sensation in epileptic patients with intracranial damage, *Chin. Med. J.,* 96(1): 33–6, 1983.

2393. Chung, E. K., Unusual form of digitalis-induced triple A-V nodal rhythm, *Am. Heart. J.,* 79(2): 250–53, 1970.

2394. Churchill, P. C., McDonald, F. D., Churchill, M. C., Phenytoin stimulates renin secretion from rat kidney slices, *J. Pharmacol., Exp. Ther.,* 211: 615–19, 1979.

2395. Claesen, M., Moustafa, M. A., Adline, J., Vandervorst, D., Poupaert, J. H., Evidence for an arene oxide-NIH shift pathway in the metabolic conversion of phenytoin to 5-(4-hydroxyphenyl)-5-Phenylhydantoin in the rat and in man, *Drug Metab. Dispos.,* 10(6): 667–71, 1982.

2396. Clifford, D. B., Trotter, J. L., Pain in multiple sclerosis, *Arch. Neurol.,* 41: 1270–2, 1984.

2397. Coers, C., Telerman-Toppet, N., Durdu, J., Neurogenic benign fasciculations, pseudomyotonia and pseudotetany: A disease in search of a name, *Arch. Neurol.* 38: 282–7, 1981.

2398. Cohn, D. F., Avrahami, E., Dalos, E., Thermal epilepsy manifest as fever attacks, *Ann. Intern. Med.,* 101(4): 569–70, 1984.

2399. Connors, B. W., A comparison of the effects of pentobarbital and diphenylhydantoin on the GABA sensitivity and excitability of adult sensory ganglion cells, *Brain Res.,* 207: 357–69, 1981.

2400. Cook, C. E., Christensen, H. D., Amerson, E. W., Kepler, J. A., Tallent, C. R., Taylor, G. F., Radioimmunoassay of anticonvulsant drugs: Phenytoin, phenobarbital, and primidone, *Quantitative Analytic Studies in Epilepsy,* Kellaway, P. and Petersen, I., Eds., Raven Press, New York, 39–58, 1976.

2401. Coodley, E. L., Ofstein, M., Rick, J., Cardiac arrhythmias—an update on identification and therapy, *Postgrad. Med.,* 80(3): 38–55, 1986.

2402. Cook, C. E., Kepler, J. A., Christiansen, H. D., Antiserum to diphenylhydantoin: preparation and characterization, *Res. Commun. Chem. Pathol. Pharm.,* 5(3): 767–74, 1973.

2403. Coombes, E. J., Phenytoin assay on dried blood spots, *Neurology,* 34: 703, 1984.

2404. Coombes, E. J., Gamlen, T. R., Batstone, G. F., Leigh, P. N., A phenytoin assay using dried blood spot samples suitable for domiciliary therapeutic drug monitoring, *Ann. Clin. Biochem.,* 21(6): 519–22, 1984.

2405. Cooper, R. L., Constable, I. J., Davidson, L., Aqueous humor catecholamines, *Curr. Eye Res.,* 3(6): 809–13, 1984.

2406. Cooper, T. W., Bauer, E. A., Therapeutic efficacy of phenytoin in recessive dystropic epidermolysis, *Arch. Dermatol.,* 120 (4): 490–5, 1984.

2407. Cordonnier, M., Delwaide, P. J., Malignant and benign fasciculations. Apropos of a case of neuromyotonia, *Rev. Med. Liege.,* 34: 839–45, 1979.

2408. Cosofret, V. V., Buck, R. P., A poly(vinylchloride) membrane electrode for determination of phenytoin in pharmaceutical formulations, *J. Pharm. Biomed. Anal.,* 4(1): 45–52, 1986.

2409. Cotrufo, R., Di Iorio, G., Ammendola, A., Bravaccio, F., Continuous muscle fiber activity associated with denervation atrophy, *Eur. Neurol.,* 21: 375–9, 1982.

2410. Courtney, K. R., Interval-dependent effects of small antiarrhythmic drugs on excitability of guinea-pig myocardium, *Mol. Cardiol.,* 12: 1273–86, 1980.

2411. Courtney, K. R., Depressant effects of drugs used in myotonia therapy, *Proc. West Pharmacol. Soc.,* 25: 159–61, 1982.

2412. Courtney, K. R., Etter, E. F., Modulated anticonvulsant block of sodium channels in nerve and muscle, *Eur. J. Clin. Pharmacol.,* 88: 1–9, 1983.

2413. Cramer, J., Mattson, R., Gallagher, B., King, D. W., Wannamaker, B., Denio, L., Shellenberger, M. K., Haidukewych, D., Splane, M. L., Whole blood/plasma ratio and clinical performance of a non-instrumented assay for phenytoin., *Neurology,* 36: 84, 1986.

2414. Cranford, R. E., Leppik, I. E., Intravenous administration of phenytoin, *Neurology,* 29: 754, 1979.

2415. Cranford, R. E., Leppik, I. E., Patrick, B., Anderson, C. B., Kostick, B., Intravenous phenytoin: Clinical and pharmacokinetic aspects, *Neurology,* 27(4): 376, 1977.

2416. Cranford, R. E., Leppik, I. E., Patrick, B. K., Anderson, B. B., Kostick, B., Intravenous phenytoin in acute seizure disorders, *Neurology,* 28(4): 351–52, 1978.

2417. Crooks, J., O'Malley, K., Stevenson, I. H., Pharmacokinetics in the elderly, *Handbook of Clinical Pharmacokinetics,* Gibaldi, M., Prescott, L., Eds., ADIS Health Science Press, New York, 169–87, 1983.

2418. Cruz Martinez, A., Arpa, J., Perez Conde, M. C., Ferrer, M. T., Bilateral carpal tunnel in childhood associated with Schwartz-Jampel syndrome, *Muscle Nerve,* 7: 66–72, 1984.

2419. Curcic, M., Preoperative considerations and anesthetic management, University Hospital, Zurich, Switzerland, *Int. Anesthesiol. Clin.,* 20(2): 227–33, 1982.

2420. Curran, A. E., El-Mofty, S. K., Protection of irradiated parotid by phenytoin (DPH), *J. Dent. Res.,* 62: 232, 1983.

2421. Czuczwar, S. J., Turski, L., Kleinrok, Z., Effects of combined treatment with diphenylhydantoin and different benzodiazepines on pentylenetetrazol- and bicuculline-induced seizures in mice, *Neuropharmacology*, 21(6): 563–7, 1982.

2422. D'Arcy, P. F., Drug interactions with new drugs, *Pharm. Int.*, 4: 285–91, 1983.

2423. Dam, M., Phenytoin toxicity, *Antiepileptic Drugs*, Woodbury P. M., Penry, J. K., Pippinger, C. E., Eds., New York, Raven Press, 247–56, 1982.

2424. Dam, M., Summing up of the success so far gained through choice of drugs or combinations of drugs, *Acta Neurol. Scand.*, 69(99): 19–22, 1984.

2425. Dana-Haeri, J., Oxley, J., Richens, A., Pituitary responsiveness to gonadotrophin-releasing and thyrotrophin-releasing hormones in epileptic patients receiving carbamazepine or phenytoin, *Clin. Endocrinol.*, 20: 163–8, 1984.

2426. Danhof, M., Breimer, D. D., Therapeutic drug monitoring in saliva, *Handbook of Clinical Pharmacokinetics*, Gibaldi, M., Prescott, L., Eds., New York, ADIS Health Science Press, 207–27, 1983.

2427. Danielson, D. A., Douglas, S. W., Herzog, P., Jick, H., Porter, J. B., Drug-induced blood disorders, *JAMA*, 252: 3257–60, 1984.

2428. Danilenko, M. V., Ivaniv, Y. A., Corrections of hypoalphacholesterolemia in patients with atherosclerosis by means of diphenine, *Vrach. Delo*, 7: 72–75, 1983.

2429. David, G., Selzer, M. E., Yaari, Y., Suppression by phenytoin of convulsant-induced after-discharges at presynaptic nerve terminals, *Brain Res.*, 330(1): 57–66, 1985.

2430. David, G., Selzer, M. E., Yaari, Y., Activity-dependent depression of nerve action potential by phenytoin, *Neurosci. Lett.*, 66(2): 163–8, 1986.

2431. Davies, J. E., Edmundson, W. F., The effects of phenytoin on human residues of DDT and dieldrin—a compendium, *Epidemiology of DDT*, Davies, J. E., Edmundson, W. F., Eds., Futura Publishing Co., 109–23, 1979.

2432. Davies-Jones, G. A., Antiepileptic medication during pregnancy, *Side Effects of Drugs Annual, Vol. 4, A Worldwide Yearly Survey of New Data and Trends*, Dukes M.N., Ed., Excerpta Medica, Amsterdam, 42–6, 1980.

2433. Davis, C. M., Fenimore, D. C., Rapid microanalysis of anticonvulsants by high performance thin-layer chromatography, *J. Chromatogr.*, 222: 265–270, 1981.

2434. Davis, J. R., Lynam, T. C., Franklyn, J. A., Docherty, K., Sheppard, M. C., Tri-iodothyronine and phenytoin reduce prolactin messenger RNA levels in cultured rat pituitary cells, *J. Endocr.*, 109: 359–64, 1986.

2435. De Belleroche, J., Dick, A., Wyrley-Birch, A., Anticonvulsants and trifluoperazine inhibit the evoked release of GABA from cerebral cortex of rat at different sites, *Life Sci.*, 31: 2875–82, 1982.

2436. De Boer, T., Stoof, J. C., Van Duijn, H., The effects of convulsant and anticonvulsant drugs on the release of radiolabeled GABA, glutamate, noradrenaline, sertonin and acetylcholine from rat cortical slices, *Brain Res.*, 253: 153–60, 1982.

2437. de la Torre, R., Navarro, J. L., Aldrete, J. A., Comparison between phenytoin and conventional treatment for irritable bowel syndrome, *Curr. Ther. Res.*, 38(4): 661–9, 1985.

2438. De Lorenzo, R. J., Antagonistic action of diphenylhydantoin and calcium on the endogenous phosphorylation of specific brain proteins, *Neurology*, 26: 386, 1976.

2439. De Lorenzo, R. J., Calmodulin in neurotransmitter release and synaptic function, *Fed. Proc.*, 41(7): 2265–72, 1982.

2440. De Lorenzo, R. J., Calcium calmodulin protein phosphorylation in neuronal transmission: A molecular approach to neuronal excitability and anticonvulsant drug action, *Advances in Neurology. Status Epilepticus*, Delgado-Escueta, A. V., et al., Eds., Raven Press, New York, 325–38, 1983.

2441. De Lorenzo, R. J., Calmodulin systems in neuronal excitability: a molecular approach to epilepsy, *Ann. Neurol.*, 16: S104–S114, 1984.

2442. De Vane, P. J., Kelly, J. C., Macpherson, P., Whiting, B., Phenytoin prophylaxis in radiological contrast studies, *Br. J. Clin. Pharmacol.*, 17(5): 643p, 1984.

2443. De Wolff, F. A., Vermeij, P., Ferrari, M. D., Buruma, S., Breimer, D. D., Impairment of phenytoin parahydroxylation as a cause of severe intoxication. *Ther. Drug Monit.*, 5(2): 213–15, 1983.

2444. Dearden, N. M., Ischaemic brain, *Lancet*, 2: 255–9, Aug 3, 1985.

2445. Declerck, A. C., Martens, W. L., Wauquier, A., Evaluation of the effects of antiepileptic drugs on sleep-wakefulness patterns following one night total sleep deprivation in epileptic patients, *Neuropsychobiology*, 13: 201–05, 1985.

2446. Delandsheer, E., Guieu, J. D., Bouchez, B., Reant, O., Effect of intravenous diphenylhydantoin on myotonia in myotonic dystrophy, *Lyon Med.*, 252: 279–84, 1984.

2447. Delgado Escueta, A. V., Wasterlain, C., Treiman, D. M., Porter, R. J., Status epilepticus: Summary, *Advances in Neurology. Status Epilepticus*, Delgado-Escueta, A. V., et al., Eds., New York, Raven Press, 537–41, 1983.

2448. Den Hartog Jager, W. A., Hootsmans, W. J., Isaacs' Disease (continuous muscle fiber activity), *Ned. Tijdschr. Geneeskd.*, 122: 1917–20, 1978.

2449. Deutschman, C. S., Haines, S. J., Anticonvulsant prophylaxis in neurological surgery, *Neurosurgery*, 17: 510–7, 1985.

2450. De Vane, P. J., Macpherson, P., Teasdale, E., Volo, G., Casey, M., Kelly, J. C., Whiting, B., The prophylactic use of phenytoin during iopamidol contrast studies of the subarachnoid space, *Eur. J. Clin. Pharmacol.*, 29: 747–9, 1986.

2451. Diamond, I., Gordon, A. S., Davis, C. G., Milfay, D., Phenytoin and phosphorylation of nicotinic receptors, *Advances in Neurology. Status Epilepticus*, Delgado-Escueta, A. V., et al., Eds., Raven Press, New York, 339–44, 1983.

2452. Digregorio, G. J., Barbieri, E. J., Pharmacologic management of pain, *Am. Fam. Physician*, 27: 185–8, 1983.

2453. Dikmen, S., Matthews, C. G., Effect of major motor seizure frequency upon cognitive-intellectual functions in adults, *Epilepsia*, 18(1); 21–9, 1977.

2454. Dilman, V. D., Therapy for aging and diseases of compensation in light of the elevating mechanism of their development, *Diseases of Aging*, Wright, J., Ed., PSG, Inc., Boston, 283–302, 1981.

2455. Dilman, V. M., Cancer susceptibility. *Diseases of Aging*, Wright, J., Ed., PSG, Inc., Boston, 205–33, 1981.

2456. Ding-Guo, S., Investigation in electrophysiology of neuromyotonia, *Electroencephalogr. Clin. Neurophysiol.*, 56(3): S70, 1983.

2457. Dodrill, C. B., Correlates of generalized tonic-clonic seizures with intellectual, neuropsychological, emotional, and social function in patients with epilepsy, *Epilepsia*, 27(4): 399–411, 1986.

2458. Doerner, D., Partridge, L. D., Effects of convulsant and anticonvulsant drugs on potassium inactivation, *Soc. Neurosci. Abstracts*, 9 PT1: 396, 1983.

2459. Doster, S. K., Mc Kinney, L. C., Ferrendelli, J. A., Anticonvulsant specificity and ability to block sodium channels are determined by 5-substitution of hydantoins and alpha-substitution of succinimides, *Soc. Neurosci. Abstracts*, 10: 184, 1984.

2460. Dougherty, R. J., Office management of chronic pain, *Postgrad. Med.*, 76(2): 215–18, 1984.

2461. Drake, Jr., M. E., Coffey, C. E., Complex partial status epilepticus simulating psychogenic unresponsiveness, *Am. J. Psychiatry*, 140: 800–01, 1983.

2462. Dreifus, L. S., Soffer, J., Drug-induced ventricular arrhythmias: prolonged QT interval, *Ann. Emerg. Med.*, 11(10): 597–8, 1982.

2463. Dreifuss, F. E., Adverse effects of antiepileptic drugs, *Epilepsy*, Ward, A. A., et al., Eds., Raven Press, New York, 249–66, 1983.

2464. Dretchen, K. L., Bowles, A. M., Raines, A., Protection by phenytoin and calcium channel blocking agents against the toxicity of diisopropylfluorophosphate, *Toxicol. Appl. Pharmacol.*, 83: 584–9, 1986.

2465. Drew, J. H., Kitchen, W. H., The effect of maternally administered drugs on bilirubin concentrations in the newborn infant, *J. Pediatr.*, 89(4): 657–61, 1976.

2466. Dreyfus, J., *A Remarkable Medicine Has Been Overlooked*, 1st Ed. Simon and Schuster, Inc., New York, 1981; 2nd Ed. Pocket Books, New York, 1982 (Available through Dreyfus Medical Foundation).

2467. Drug Side Effects Bulletin, A review of side effects of antiepileptic drugs over the last eleven years, *Lakartidningen*, 79(28–9): 2646–50, 1982.

2468. Dubick, M. A., Keen, C. L., Alterations in tissue trace element and ascorbic acid metabolism in phenytoin-fed rats and mice, *J. Nutr.*, 115(11): 1481–7, 1985.

2469. Durelli, L., Mutani, R., Sechi, G. P., Traccis, S., Monaco, F., Glorioso, N., Treatment of human myotonia. Double-blind trial carbamazepine and diphenylhydantoin, *Electroencephalogr. Clin. Neurophysiol.*, 54: 5p, 1982.

2470. Dworkin, S. F., Benign chronic orofacial pain. Clinical criteria and therapeutic approaches, *Postgrad. Med.*, 74(3): 239–48, 1983.

2471. Eadie, M. J., Lander, C. M., Tyrer, J. H., Plasma drug level monitoring in pregnancy, *Handbook of Clinical Pharmacokinetics*, Gibaldi, M., Prescott, L., Eds., ADIS Health Science Press, New York, 52–62, 1983.

2472. Editor, Management of trigeminal neuralgia, *Lancet*, 662–3, Mar 24, 1984.

2473. Editor, Antiepileptic drug may enhance attentiveness, *FASEB News*, 1–2, 1984.

2474. Edwards, W. T., Approaches to managing chronic pain, *Med. Times*, 110: 3s–11s, 1982.

2475. Egido, J., Rivera, F., Sancho, J., Barat, A., Hernado, L., Phenytoin in IgA nephropathy: a long-term controlled trial, *Nephron.*, 38: 30–9, 1984.

2476. Eichelbaum, K. M., Polymorphic drug oxidation in humans, *Fed. Proc.*, 43: 2298–2302, 1984.

2477. Eichelbaum, M., Genetic polymorphism of oxidative drug metabolism. Therapeutic and toxicologic implications, *Internist*, 24: 117–127, 1983.

2478. Eldar, M., Motro, M., Yahini, J. H., Neufeld, H. N., Atypical torsade de pointes, *Am. Heart J.*, 106(2): 420–1, 1983.

2479. Elliot, F. A., Neurological factors in violent behavior (the dyscontrol syndrome), *Violence and Responsibility, the Individual, the Family and Society*, Sadoff, R. L., Ed., SP Medical & Scientific Books, New York, 59–86, 1978.

2480. Ellis, D., Effects of stimulation and diphenylhydantoin on the intracellular sodium activity in Purkinje fibres of sheep heart, *J. Physiol.*, 362: 331–48, 1985.

2481. Elwes, R. D., Dellaportas, C., Reynolds, E. H., Robinson, W., Butt, W. R., London, D. R., Prolactin and growth hormone dynamics in epileptic patients receiving phenytoin, *Clin. Endocrinol.*, 23: 263–70, 1985.

2482. Essman, W. B., Essman, E. J., Anticonvulsant effects upon regional synaptosomal GABA uptake: differences in convulsed rats, *Brain Res. Bull.*, 5(2): 821–4, 1980.

2483. Evans, D. E., Gillis, R. A., Effect of diphenylhydantoin and lidocaine on cardiac arrhythmias induced by hypothalamic stimulation, *J. Pharmacol. Exp. Ther.*, 191(3): 506–17, 1974.

2484. Evans, D. E., Gillis, R. A., Effect of ouabain and its interaction with diphenylhydantoin on cardiac arrhythmias in-

duced by hypothalamic stimulation, *J. Pharmacol. Exp. Ther.*, 195: 577–86, 1975.

2485. Evans, P. J., Walker, R. F., Peters, J. R., Dyas, J., Riad-Fahmy, D., Thomas, J. P., Rimmer, E., Tsanaclis, L., Scanlon, M. F., Anticonvulsant therapy and cortisol elimination, *Br. J. Clin. Pharmac.*, 20: 129–32, 1985.

2486. Faber, J., Lumholtz, I. B., Kirkegaard, C., Friis, T., Turnover studies of T_4, T_3 and rT_3 in $L-T_4$ treated hypothyroid subjects receiving phenytoin, *Ann. Endocrinol.*, 44(4): 63a, 1983.

2487. Feldman, M. S., Helfant, R. H., Antiarrhythmic agents. *Bellet's Essentials of Cardiac Arrhythmias*, Helfant, R. H., Ed., W. B. Saunders Company, Philadelphia, 308–29, 1980.

2488. Feldman, R. G., Pippinger, C. E., Florence, M. L., The relation of anticonvulsant drug levels to complete seizure control, *Epilepsia*, 16(1): 203–4, 1975.

2489. Fenimore, D. C., Davis, C. M., Simultaneous determination of phenobarbital and diphenylhydantoin in blood plasma by high performance thin layer chromatography, *J. High. Resolut. Chromatogr, Commun.*, 1: 105–106, 1978.

2490. Ferrendelli, J. A., Daniels-McQueen, S., Comparative actions of phenytoin and other anticonvulsant drugs on potassium- and veratridine-stimulated calcium uptake in synaptosomes, *J. Pharm. Exp. Ther.*, 220(1): 29–34, 1982.

2491. Feurle, G. E., Weidauer, H., Baldauf, G., Schulte-Braucks, T., Anton-Lamprecht, I., Management of esophageal stenosis in recessive dystrophic epidermolysis bullosa, *Gastroenterology*, 87: 1376–80, 1984.

2492. Fields, H. L., Raskin, N. H., Anticonvulsants and pain, *Clinical Neuropharmacology*, Klawans, H. L., Ed., Raven Press, New York, 173–83, 1976.

2493. File, S. E., Lister, R. G., The anxiogenic action of Ro 5-4864 is reversed by phenytoin, *Neurosci. Lett.*, 35: 93–6, 1983.

2494. File, S. E., Pellow, S., RO 5-4864, a ligand for benzodiazepine micromolar and peripheral binding sites: antagonism and enhancement of behavioral effects., *Psychopharmacology*, 80(2): 166–70, 1983.

2495. Fine, A. S., Person, P., Biochemistry of gingival oxidative metabolism: A Review, *J. Oral. Pathol.*, 13: 191–212, 1984.

2496. Fine, W., Post-hemiplegic epilepsy in the elderly, *Br. Med. J.*, 199–201, 1967.

2497. Finkel, M. J., Phenytoin revisited, *Clin. Ther.*, 6(5): 577–91, 1984.

2498. Finn, A. L., Anticonvulsants, *Applied Clinical Pharmacokinetics*, Mungall, D., Ed., Raven Press, New York, 103–26, 1983.

2499. Finucane, J. F., Griffiths, R. S., Effect of phenytoin therapy on thyroid function, *Br. J. Clin. Pharmacol.*, 3, 1041–4, 1976.

2500. Fitzgerald, D. C., Palatal myoclonous. Case report, *Laryngoscope*, 94(2): 217–19, 1984.

2501. Fogoros, R. N., Elson, J. J., Fiedler, S. B., Relative efficacy of phenytoin in suppressing inducible ventricular tachyarrhythmias, *Circulation*, 74(4): II–105, 1986.

2502. Folbergrova, J., Cyclic GMP and cyclic AMP in the cerebral cortex of mice during seizures induced by 3-mercaptopropionic acid: effect of anticonvulsant agents, *Neurosci. Lett.*, 16: 291–6, 1980.

2503. Foong, F. W., Satoh, M., Takagi, H., A newly devised reliable method for evaluating analgesic potencies of drugs on trigeminal pain, *J. Pharmacol. Methods*, 7: 271–78, 1982.

2504. Fortman, C. S., Witte, D. L., Serum 5'-nucleotidase in patients receiving antiepileptic drugs, *Am, J. Clin. Pathol.*, 84(2): 197–201, 1985.

2505. Franceschi, M., Perego, L., Cavagnini, F., Cattaneo, A. G., Invitti, C., Caviezel, F., Strambi, L. F., Smirne, S., Effects of long-term antiepileptic therapy on the hypothalamic-pituitary axis in man, *Epilepsia*, 25(1): 46–52, 1984.

2506. Franklyn, J. A., Davis, J. R., Ramsden, D. B., Sheppard, M. C., Phenytoin and thyroid hormone action, *J. Endocrinol.*, 104: 201–04, 1985.

2507. Franklyn, J. A., Sheppard, M. C., Ramsden, D. B., Measurement of free thyroid hormones in patients on long-term phenytoin therapy, *Eur. J. Clin. Pharmacol.*, 26(5): 633–4, 1984.

2508. Franssen, H., Fortgens, C., Wattendorff, A. R., Van Woerkom, C. A., Paroxysmal kinesigenic choreoathetosis and abnormal contingent negative variation, *Arch. Neurol.*, 40: 381–5, 1983.

2509. Freed, C. R., Gal, J., Manchester, D. K., Increased phenytoin requirement during pregnancy results from an increase in drug metabolism, *Clin. Res.*, 33(1): 91A, 1985.

2510. Frenkel, G. M., Safronova, N. A., Marova, E. I., Lemesheva, S. N., A change in electrical activity of the brain under the effect of diphenylhydantoin in patients with Itsenko-Cushing disease, *Probl. Endokrinol.*, 1: 19–22, 1976.

2511. Friedman, I. M., Litt, I. F., Henson, R. E., Saliva phenobarbital and phenytoin concentrations in epileptic adolescents, *J. Pediatr.*, 98(4): 645–7, 1981.

2512. Friend, D. G., Addiction, psychodelic experimentation and abuse of drugs by the concerned generation, *Md. State Med. J.*, 18: 59–66, 1969.

2513. Frigyesi, T. L., Lombardini, J. B., Augmentation of thalamo–motor cortico–cerebellar epileptogenesis by taurine and its antagonism by diphenlyhydantoin, *Life Sci.*, 24: 1251–60, 1979.

2514. Frisk-Holmberg, M., Hellstrom, L., Holmstrom, M., Dahlberg, E., Jakobsson, A. K., Utilization of blood drug level determinations for therapy monitoring, *Lakartidningen*, 77: 1316–7, 1980.

2515. Fromm, G. H., Chattha, A. S., Terrence, C. F., Glass, J. D., Do phenytoin and carbamazepine depress excitation and/or facilitate inhibition?, *Eur. J. Pharmacol.*, 78: 403–9, 1982.

2516. Fukuda, A., Tabuse, H., Ihara, N., Tanabe, J., Ikeda, H., Kohama, A., Effects of phenytoin on regional cerebral blood flow, electroencephalogram, and electrolyte contents in cerebral blood and cerebral cortex following total cerebral ischemia in dogs, *Circulatory Shock*, 10: 341–50, 1983.

2517. Gaffey, C. M., Chun, B., Harvey, J. C., Manz, H. J., Phenytoin-induced systemic granulomatous vasculitis, *Arch. Pathol. Lab. Med.*, 110: 131–5, 1986.

2518. Gallager, D. W., Mallorga, P., Tallman, J. F., Interaction of diphenylhydantoin and benzodiazepines in the CNS, *Brain Res.*, 189: 209–20, 1980.

2519. Gallagher, J. P., Inokuchi, H., Nakamura, J., Shinnick-Gallagher, P., Effects of anticonvulsants on excitability and GABA sensitivity of cat dorsal root ganglion cells, *Neuropharmacology*, 20: 427–33, 1981.

2520. Gallagher, J. P., Inokuchi, H., Shinnick-Gallagher, P., Actions of anti-convulsants on GABA-depolarizations and action potentials recorded from a mammalian sensory neuron, *Soc. Neurosci. Abstr.*, 5: 588, 1970.

2521. Galvan, M., Actions of 4-aminopyridine on neurones, *Fortschr. Med.*, 101(3), 1983.

2522. Gambertoglio, J. G., Effects of renal disease: altered pharmacokinetics, *Pharmacokinetic basis for drug treatment*, Benet, L. Z., Ed., Raven Press, New York, 149–71, 1984.

2523. Gangarosa, L. P., Mahan, P. E., Pharmacologic management of TMJ-MPDS, *Ear Nose Throat J.*, 61: 670–8, 1982.

2524. Gankina, E. M., Avdulov, N. A., Maisov, N. I., Effects of different psychotropic drugs on ^{14}C-glutamate uptake by rat brain synaptosomes, *Farmakol. Toksikol.*, 45(6): 17–20, 1982.

2525. Garan, H., Ruskin, J. N., Powell, W. J., Centrally mediated effect of phenytoin on digoxin-induced ventricular arrhythmias, *Am. J. Physiol.*, 241: h67–h72, 1981.

2526. Garcia-Bengochea, F., Collins, G. H., Monstrocellular sarcoma of the brain: 6-year postoperative survival, *J. Neurosurg.*, 31: 686–9, 1969.

2527. Garson, A., Ventricular dysrhythmias, *Pediatric Cardiac Dysrhythmias*, Gillette, P. C., Garson, A., Eds., Grune & Stratton, New York, 295–360, 1981.

2528. Garson, A., Gillette, P. C., Treatment of chronic ventricular dysrhythmias in the young, *Pace*, 4: 658–69, 1981.

2529. Garson, A., Kugler, J. D., Gillette, P. C., Simonelli, A., McNamara, D. G., Control of late postoperative ventricular arrhythmias with phenytoin in young patients, *Am. J. Cardiol.*, 46(2): 290–4, 1980.

2530. Garson, A., Randall, D. C., Gillette, P. C., Smith, R. T., Moak, J. P., Mc Vey, P., Mc Namara, D. G., Prevention of sudden death after repair of tetralogy of Fallot: treatment of ventricular arrhythmias, *J. Am. Coll. Cardiol.*, 6: 221–7, 1985.

2531. Gayet-Hallion, T., On the temperature-reducing properties of diphenylhydantoin, *Compt. Rend. Soc. Biol.*, 153: 760–1, 1959.

2532. Gedde-Dahl, T., Sixteen types of epidermolysis bullosa: on the clinical discrimination, therapy and prenatal diagnosis, *Acta Derm. Venerol.*, 95: 74–87, 1981.

2533. Gedik, O., Sayek, I., Raucan, S., Telatar, F., Adalar, N., Usman, A., Akalin, S., Insulinoma. (Clinical, diagnostic and therapeutic features of 3 cases), *Hacettepe Bull. Med. Surg.*, 15: 13–9, 1982.

2534. Geraldini, C., Sideri, G., EMG and nerve conduction velocity in patients treated with antiepileptic drugs, *Electroencephalogr. Clin. Neurophysiol.*, 55(1): 9p, 1983.

2535. Gerson, W. T., Fine, S. P., Sensenbrenner, L. L., Anticonvulsant-induced aplastic anemia: increased susceptibility to toxic drug metabolites *in vitro*, *Blood*, 61(5): 889–93, 1983.

2536. Gilbert, J. C., Wyllie, M. G., Effects of anticonvulsants at the nerve terminal, *Advances in Epileptology*, Meinardi, H., Rowan, A. J., Swets & Zeitlinger, Amsterdam, 172–75, 1978.

2537. Gill, M. W., Connors, M. R., Schaiz, R. A., The effects of diazepam and phenytoin on phospholipid metabolism and ATPase activity: possible correlation with anticonvulsant activity, *Pharmacologist*, 27(3): 230, 1985.

2538. Gillis, R. A., Quest, J. A., The nervous system as an important site of action for drugs affecting cardiovascular function, *Cardiac Pharmacology*, Wilkerson, R. D., Ed., New York, Academic Press, 25–50, 1981.

2539. Gilman, A. G., Goodman, L. S., Rall, T. W., Murad, F., *The Pharmacological Basis of Therapeutics*, 7th Edition, Macmillan Publishing Co., New York, 1985.

2540. Gingrich, S. A., Smith, P. J., Shapiro, L. E., Surks, M. I., 5,5'-diphenylhydantoin (phenytoin) attenuates the action of 3,5,3'-triiodo-l-thyronine in cultured GC cells, *Endocrinology*, 116(6): 2306–13, 1985.

2541. Ginsberg, J., Chen, H. J., Walfish, P. G., Multiple sites of action of diphenylhydantoin on rat thyroid regulation, *Ann. Endocrinol.*, 49a, 1979.

2542. Glueck, C. J., Nonpharmacologic and pharmacologic alteration of high-density lipoprotein cholesterol: therapeutic approaches to prevention of atherosclerosis, *Am. Heart J.*, 110: 1107, 1985.

2543. Gobernado, J. M., Ortin, A., Rodriguez De Castro, A. R., Gimeno, A., Stiffman syndrome, *Prensa Med. Argent.*, 68(15): 613–6, 1981.

2544. Godfrey, J. W., Roberts, M. A., Caird, F. I., Epileptic seizures in the elderly: II. Diagnostic problems, *Age and Ageing*, 11: 29–34, 1982.

2545. Godolphin, W., Trepanier, J., Gas chromatography versus immunoassay (EMIT) for analysis of free phenytoin in serum ultrafiltrate, *Ther. Drug Monit.*, 6(3): 374–5, 1984.

2546. Goerz, G., Merk, H., Progress in dermatology: new biochemical aspects, *Fortschr. Med.*, 100: 1467–71, 1982.

2547. Goldberg, M. A., *The Pharmacology of Phenytoin, H. Houston Merritt Memorial Volume*, Yahr, M.D., Ed., Raven Press, New York, 81–99, 1983.

2548. Goldman, A. S., Biochemical mechanism of glucocorticoid- and phenytoin-induced cleft palate, *Curr. Top. Dev. Biol.*, 19: 217–39, 1984.

2549. Goldman, A. S., Baker, M. K., Piddington, R., Herold, R., Inhibition of programmed cell death in mouse embryonic palate *in vitro* by cortisol and phenytoin: receptor involvement and requirement of protein synthesis, *Proc. Soc. Exp. Biol. Med.*, 174(2): 239–43, 1983.

2550. Grafova, V. N., Danilova, E. I., Kryzhanovskii, G. N., Analgesic effects of antiepileptic agents in pain of spinal origin, *Byull. Eskp. Biol. Med.*, 88(8): 147–51, 1979.

2551. Gram, L., Bentsen, K. D., Hepatic toxicity of antiepileptic drugs: A Review, *Acta Neurol. Scand.*, 68 (sup97): 81–90, 1983.

2552. Grammaticos, P., Mirtsu-Fidant, V., Suslous, C., Paradellis, A., Observations of the action of diphenylhydantoin on the neuromuscular preparation of the rat diaphragm, *Drugs Exptl. Clin. Res.*, 10(4): 235–9, 1984.

2553. Grassa, C., Figa-Talamanca, L., LoRusso, F., Giacanelli, M., Pontesilli, R., Syndrome of continuous muscle fiber activity, *Ital. J. Neurol. Sci.*, 4: 415–8, 1981.

2554. Green, A. R., Grahame-Smith, D. G., The effect of diphenylhydantoin on brain 5-hydroxytryptamine metabolism and function, *Neuropharmacology*, 14: 107–13, 1975.

2555. Greenberg, D. A., Cooper, E. C., Carpenter, C. L., Phenytoin interacts with calcium channels in brain membranes, *Ann. Neurol.*, 16: 616–17, 1984.

2556. Greenway, F. L., Dahms, W. T., Bray, G. A., Phenytoin as a treatment of obesity associated with compulsive eating, *Curr. Ther. Res.*, 21(3): 338–42, 1977.

2557. Grenader, A. K., Ponomareva, V. M., Zurabishvili, G. G., Vasiev, B. N., Changes in the refractoriness of cardiac tissue as a result of a decrease in the fast inward sodium current. Comparison of the atrium and ventricle, *Biofizika*, 27(5): 911–14, 1982.

2558. Griggs, R. C., Davis, R. J., Anderson, D. C., Dove, J. T., Cardiac conduction in myotonic dystrophy, *Am. J. Med.*, 59: 37–42, 1975.

2559. Grindulis, K. A., Nichol, F. E., Oldham, R., Phenytoin in rheumatoid arthritis, *J. Rheumatol.*, 13: 1035–9, 1986.

2560. Guill, M. F., Wray, B. B., Rogers, R. B., Yancey, K. B., Allen, B. S., Junctional epidermolysis bullosa: treatment with phenytoin, *Am. J. Dis. Child.*, 137: 992–4, 1983.

2561. Gupta, C., Katsumata, M., Goldman, A. S., H-2 histocompatibility region influences the inhibition of arachidonic acid cascade by dexamethasone and phenytoin in mouse embryonic palates, *J. Craniofac. Genet. Dev. Biol.*, 5: 277–85, 1985.

2562. Gurevich, V. S., Matveeva, I. M., Ogurechnikov, V. I., Korovkina, G. V., Effect of diphenylhydantoin on taurine binding by subcellular fractions of nerve cells, *Farmakol. Toksikol.* 47(6): 74–7, 1984.

2563. Gurevich, V. S., Razumovskaya, N. I., Molecular mechanisms of the interaction of diphenylhydantoin with biological membranes, *Farmakol. Toksiko.*, 47(1): 114–19, 1984.

2564. Gut, I., Becker, B. A., Diphenylhydantoin stimulation of various pathways of hepatic microsomal drug metabolism in rabbits, *Acta Univ. Carol. Med.*, 26(1–2): 105–14, 1980.

2565. Hagerman, G. A., Hanashiro, P. K., Reversal of tricyclic-antidepressant-induced cardiac conduction abnormalities by phenytoin, *Ann. Emerg. Med.*, 10(2): 82–6, 1981.

2566. Haidukewych, D., Splane, M. L., Vasos, B., Enzyme immunochromatographic assay of phenytoin in capillary and venous blood compared with fluorescence polarization immu-noassay of plasma from epileptic patients, *Clin. Chem.*, 32(1): 204, 1986.

2567. Halmos, P., Molnar, L., Kormos, M., Experiences with anticonvulsants in the treatment of tinnitus, *HNO Praxis*, 7(1): 59–61, 1982.

2568. Hamilton, N. G., Matthew, T., Aphasia: the sole manifestation of focal status epilepticus, *Neurology*, 29: 745–48, 1978.

2569. Hansen, H. W., The treatment of digitalis induced cardiac arrhythmia with diphenylhydantoin, *Med. Klin.*, 65: 101–4, 1970.

2570. Hanson, J. W., Myrianthopoulos, N. C., Harvey, M. A., Smith, D. W., Risks to the offspring of women treated with hydantoins during pregnancy, *Pediatr. Res.*, 10(4): 449, 1976.

2571. Hanstrom, L., The effect of diphenylhydantoin on the metabolism of connective tissue macromolecules in oral mucosa and bone *in vitro*, *University of UMEA, Dissertation*, 1981.

2572. Harik, S. I., Baraka, A. S., Tomeh, G. J., Mire Salman, J., Kronfulk, Z., Afifi, A. K., Autonomic peripheral nerve activity causing generalized muscle stiffness and fasciculations: report of a case with physiological, pharmacological, and morphological observations, *Johns Hopkins Med. J.*, 139: 60, 1976.

2573. Harned, C. L., Nerland, D. E., Sonnenfeld, G., Effects of passive transfer and induction of gamma (type II immune) interferon preparation on metabolism of diphenylhydantoin by murine cytochrome p-450, *J. Interferon Res.*, 2(1): 5–10, 1982.

2574. Harris, M., Goldhaber, P., Root abnormalities in epileptics and the inhibition of parathyroid hormone induced bone resorption by diphenylhydantoin in tissue culture, *Archs. Oral Biol.*, 19: 981–84, 1974.

2575. Harris, R. A., Differential effects of membrane perturbants on voltage-activated sodium and calcium-dependent potassium channels, *Biophys. J.*, 45: 132–4, 1984.

2576. Hartman, G. S., Flamengo, S. A., Riker, W. F., Succinylcholine: mechanism of fasciculations and their prevention by d-tubocurarine or diphenylhydantoin, *Anesthesiology*, 65(4): 405–13, 1986.

2577. Hashimoto, K., Ishii, M., Komori, S., Mitsuhashi, H., Canine digitalis arrhythmia as a model for detecting Na-channel blocking antiarrhythmic drugs: a comparative study using other canine arrhythmia models and the new antiarrhythmic drugs, propafenone, tocainide, and SUN 1165, *Heart Vessels*, 1: 29–35, 1985.

2578. Hashimoto, K., Satoh, H., Shibuya, T., Imai, S., Canine-effective plasma concentrations of antiarrhythmic drugs on the two-stage coronary ligation arrhythmia, *J. Pharmacol. Exp. Ther.*, 223(3): 801–10, 1982.

2579. Hashimoto, K., Shibuys, T., Satoh, H., Imai, S., Quantitative analysis of the antiarrhythmic effect of drugs on canine ventricular arrhythmias by the determination of minimum effective plasma concentrations., *Jpn. Circ. J.*, 47: 92–97, 1983.

2580. Hassell, T., O'Donnell, J., Pearlman, J., Salivary phenytoin levels in institutionalized epileptics, *J. Chronic Dis.*, 36(12): 899–906, 1983.

2581. Hassell, T. M., Evidence for production of an inactive collagenase by fibroblasts from phenytoin-enlarged human gingivae, *J. Oral Pathol.*, 11: 310–17, 1982.

2582. Hawk, G. L., Franconi, L. C., High-pressure liquid chromatography in quantitation of antiepileptic drugs, *Antiepileptic Drugs: Quantitative Analysis and Interpretation*, Pippenger, C. E., et al., Eds., Raven Press, New York, 153–62, 1978.

2583. Hayashi, K., Takemura, N., Inhibition of PCB accumulation in liver and fat of rats by administration of diphenylhydantoin, *Jpn. J. Ind. Health*, 17: 242–3, 1975.

2584. Hayes, M. J., Langman, M. J., Short, A. H., Changes

in drugs metabolism with increasing age: phenytoin clearance and protein binding, *Br. J. Clin. Pharmac.*, 2: 72–9, 1975.

2585. Hegedus, L., Hansen, J. M., Luhdorf, K., Perrild, H., Feldt-Rasmussen, U., Kampmann, J. P., Increased frequency of goitre in epileptic patients on long-term phenytoin or carbamazepine treatment, *Clin. Endocrinol.* (Oxford), 23(4): 423–9, 1985.

2586. Heinemann, U., Franceschetti, S., Hamon, B., Konnerth, A., Yaari, Y., Effects of anticonvulsants on spontaneous epileptiform activity which develops in the absence of chemical synaptic transmission in hippocampal slices, *Brain Res.*, 325: 349–52, 1985.

2587. Heinicke, R. J., Stohs, S. J., Al-Turk, W., Lemon, H. M., Chronic phenytoin administration and the hepatic mixed function oxidase system in female rats, *Gen. Pharmacol.*, 15(2): 85–9, 1984.

2588. Heller, F., Hepatotoxicity caused by antituberculous and antiepileptic drugs, *Louvain Med.*, 101(3): 159–65, 1982.

2589. Herchuelz, A., Lebrun, P., Sener, A., Malaisse, W. J., Ionic mechanism of diphenylhydantoin action on glucose-induced insulin release, *Eur. J. Pharmacol.*, 73 (2–3): 189–97, 1981.

2590. Hernandez, J., Serrano, J. S., Experimental automaticity induced by mechanical lesion in rat isolated right ventricle: the effects of quinidine, phenytoin, and propranolol, *J. Pharmacol. Methods*, 7: 255–61, 1982.

2591. Herschkowitz, N., Mahany, T. M., Baizer, L., Raines, A., Phenytoin reduction of extensor tone and gamma motorneuron activity in the decerebrate cat, *Neurosci. Abstr.*, 4: 297, 1978.

2592. Heuser, D., Possibilities and limitations of brain protections: general survey, *Anasth. Intensivmed*, 23(8): 315–24, 1982.

2593. Hier, D. B., Headache, *Manual of Neurologic Therapeutics*, 2nd Edition, Samuels, M. A., Ed., Little, Brown & Co., Boston, 15–29, 1982.

2594. Himmelhoch, J. M., Major mood disorders related to epileptic changes, *Psychiatric Aspects of Epilepsy*, Blumer, D., Ed., American Psychiatric Press Inc., Washington D.C., 271–94, 1984.

2595. Hinds, J. A., Pincombe, C. F., Smith, S., Duffy, P., The use of a monosaccharide linkage group in a heterologous solid-phase enzyme immunoassay for phenytoin, *J. Immunol. Methods*, 80: 239–53, 1985.

2596. Hinds, J. A., Pincombe, C. F., Smith, S., Duffy, P., Ligand displacement immunoassay—demonstration of its use for the measurement of serum phenobarbital and phenytoin, *Clin. Chim. Acta*, 149(2–3): 105–15, 1985.

2597. Hitchcock, E., Teixeira, M., Anticonvulsant activation of pain-suppressive systems, *Appl. Neurophysiol.*, 45: 582–93, 1982.

2598. Hodson, A. K., Sanders, D. B., Isaac syndrome: a cause of infantile tetany and tremor during sleep, *Neurology*, 33: 74, 1983.

2599. Hoff, H., Hoff, H., Advances in the treatment of epilepsy, *Monatsschr. Psychiatr. Neurol.*, 114: 105–18, 1947.

2600. Hoffman. B. F., Bigger, J. T., Digitalis and allied cardiac glycosides, *The Pharmacological Basis of Therapeutics*, 7th Edition, Gilman, G. A., et al., Eds., Macmillan Publishing Co., New York, 716–747, 1985.

2601. Holland, N. J., Wiesel-Levison, P., McDonnel, M., Nursing care, *Multiple Sclerosis, A Guide for Patients and Their Families*, Scheinberg, L. C., Ed., Raven Press, New York, 111–28, 1984.

2602. Hollander, A., What's new in American dermatology?, *Hautarzt.*, 130–37, 1982.

2603. Hou, H., Chen, D., A report of 25 cases of myotonic congenita, *China Medical Abstracts*, 2(4): 234–5, 1985.

2604. Howrie, D. L., Crumrine, P. K., Phenytoin-induced movement disorder associated with intravenous administration for status epilepticus, *Clin. Pediatr.*, 24(8): 467–9, 1985.

2605. Hrazdira, C. L., Zouhar, A., Hrazdirova, V., Skalova, M., Dynamics of the serum levels of phenytoin and associated EEG changes after a single intravenous dose, *Cesk. Neurol. Neurochir.*, 42: 185–94, 1979.

2606. Hsu, R., Turndorf, H., Mangiardi, J., Fischer, M., Preoperative management and anesthetic considerations, N.Y.U. Med. Center, *Int. Anesthesiol. Clin.*, 20(2): 215–20, 1982.

2607. Iivanainen, M., Savolainen, H., Side effects of phenobarbital and phenytoin during long-term treatment of epilepsy, *Acta Neurol. Scand.*, 68(97): 49–67, 1983.

2608. Ikeda, H., Pharmacologic studies on the central nervous system function of first generation rats of dams administered phenytoin during pregnancy, *Nihon Yakurigaku Zasshi*, 79:65–76, 1982.

2609. Imaizumi, S., Suzuki, J., Kinouchi, H., Yoshimoto, T., Superior protective activity of phenytoin against hypoxia—pharmacological evaluation in a screening test, *Brain Nerve*, 38(2): 135–43, 1986.

2610. Imanaka, S., Matsuda, S., Ito, K., Matsuoka, T., Okada, Y., Studies of pharmacotherapy of inoperable insulinoma. Effectiveness of the combined use of diphenylhydantoin and calcium antagonists, *Nippon Naika Gakkai Zasshi*, 74: 590–6, 1985.

2611. Irace, P., Lesser, R. P., Kutt, H., Winkelman, E., Terrentine, S., Gardner, M., Altered phenytoin clearance in a patient with Crohn's disease, *Neurology*, 33: 232, 1983.

2612. Isaacs, H., Heffron, J. J., The syndrome of continuous muscle-fibre activity cured: further studies, *J. Neurol. Neurosurg. Psychiatry*, 37: 1231–5, 1974.

2613. Ivic, M., Klisic, L., Influence of diphenylhydantoin on the sodium, potassium ATPase activity in thyroid parafollicular cells and on the sodium, potassium-ATPase activity in parathyroid glands, *Stereol. Iugosl.*, 3(1): 593–8, 1981.

2614. Izumi, K., Kishita, C., Nakagawa, K., Huxtable, R. J., Shimizu, T., Koja, T., Fukuda, T., Reduced taurine contents and modification of anticonvulsive effects of phenobarbital and phenytoin by guanidinoethane sulfonate in mice, *Prog. Clin. Biol. Res.*, 179: 425–34, 1985.

2615. Izumi, K., Kishita, C., Nakagawa, K., Huxtable, R. J., Shimizu, T., Koja, T., Fukuda, T., Modification of the antiepileptic actions of phenobarbital and phenytoin by the taurine transport inhibitor, guanidinoethane sulfonate, *Eur. J. Pharmacol.*, 110: 219–24, 1985.

2616. Jacknowitz, A. I., Possible effect of viral infections on drug metabolism, *JAMA*, 251(16): 2084–5, 1984.

2617. Jacobs, A. H., What's new in pediatric dermatology?, *Acta Derm.*, 95: 91–5, 1981.

2618. Jailkhani, B. L., Jaffery, N. F., Comparison of colorimetric, spectrophotometric, and EMIT methods for estimation of phenytoin, *Indian J. Med. Res.*, 79: 679–683, 1984.

2619. Jannetta, P. J., Medical treatment of trigeminal neuralgia, *Neurological Surgery of the Ear and Skull Base*, Brackmann, D. E., Ed., Raven Press, New York, 145–8, 1982.

2620. Januskevicius, Z., Disturbances of cardiac rhythm produced by use of cardiac glycosides, *Kardiologiya*, 10(2): 35–42, 1970.

2621. Janz, D., Pregnancy and development of the embryo in epileptic women, *Geburtshilfe Fraunheilkd.*, 44(7): 428–34, 1984.

2622. Jay, G. W., Epilepsy, migraine, and EEG abnormalities in children: A review and hypothesis, *Headache*, 22: 110–14, 1982.

2623. Jenkins, M. V., Harris, M., Wills, M. R., The effect of phenytoin on parathyroid extract and 25-hydroxycholecalciferol-induced bone resorption: adenosine 3′, 5′ cyclic monophosphate production, *Calcif. Tissue Res.*, 16: 163–7, 1974.

2624. Jenner, P., Marsden, D., Pratt, J., Actions of benzodiazepines and other anticonvulsants on 5HT turnover in mouse brain, *Br. J. Pharmacol.*, 74: 812–3p, 1981.

2625. Johnson, C., Stuckey, M., Mitchell, J., Psychopharmacological treatment of anorexia nervosa and bulimia. Review and synthesis, *J. Nerv. Ment. Dis.*, 524–34, 1983.

2626. Johnson, L. C., Effects of anticonvulsant medication on sleep patterns, *Sleep and Epilepsy*, Sterman, M. B., Shouse, M. N., Passouant, P., Eds., Academic Press, New York, 381–94, 1982.

2627. Johnson, S. W., Riker, W. K., Relationships between the antagonism of electrically-induced maximal seizures by phenytoin (PHT) and central nervous system (CNS) levels of adenosine 3′,5-monophosphate (cAMP) and guanosine 3′,5-monophosphate (cGMP) in frogs and mice, *Soc. Neurosci. Abstr.*, 7, 1981.

2628. Johnson, S. W., Riker, W. K., Phenytoin antagonism of electrically induced maximal seizure in frogs and mice and effects on central nervous system levels of adenosine 3′,5′-monophosphate and guanosine 3′,5′-monophosphate, *J. Pharmacol. Exp. Ther.*, 221(1): 139–45, 1982.

2629. Jones, G. L., Kemp, J. W., Characteristics of the hydrogen bonding interactions of substituted hydantoins with 9-ethyladentine, *Mol. Pharmacol.*, 10: 48–56, 1974.

2630. Jones, G. L., Wimbish, G. H., Hydantoins, *Handbook of Experimental Pharmacology—Antiepileptic Drugs*, Frey, H. H. and Janz, D., Eds., Springer-Verlag, Berlin, 74: 351–419, 1985.

2631. Jones, G. L., Wimbish, G. H., McIntosh, W. E., Phenytoin: Basic and clinical pharmacology, *Med. Res. Rev.*, 3(4): 383–434, 1983.

2632. Jones, G. L., Woodbury, D. M., Biochemistry, *Handbook of Experimental Pharmacology—Antiepileptic Drugs*, Frey, H. H. and Janz, D., Eds., Springer-Verlag, Berlin, 74: 245–263, 1985.

2633. Jubiz, W., Meikle, A. W., Alterations of glucocorticoid actions by other drugs and disease states, *Drugs*, 18: 113–21, 1979.

2634. Juergens, U., Routine determination of eight common anti-epileptic drugs and metabolites by high performance liquid chromatography using a column-switching system for direct injection of serum samples, *J. Chromatogr.*, 310(1): 97–106, 1984.

2635. Jurna, I., Electrophysiological effects of antiepileptic drugs, *Handbook of Experimental Pharmacology—Antiepileptic Drugs*, Frey, H. H., and Janz, D., Eds., Springer-Verlag, Berlin, 74: 611–9, 645–58, 1985.

2636. Jurna, I., Lanzer, G., Inhibition of the effect of reserpine on motor control by drugs which influence reserpine rigidity, *Naunyn-Schmiedebergs Arch Pharmakcol.*, 262: 309–24, 1969.

2637. Kadar, D., Fecycz, T. D., Kalow, W., The fate of orally administered (4–14 C) phenytoin in two healthy male volunteers, *Can. J. Physiol. Pharmacol.*, 61: 403–7, 1982.

2638. Kaeser, H. E., Drug-induced myasthenic syndromes, *Acta Neurol. Scand.*, 70 (Sup. 100): 39–47, 1984.

2639. Kaeser, H. E., Corbat, F., Neuromyotonia or the malady of fasciculations, *Rev. Neurol.*, 120: 430–2, 1969.

2640. Kalff, R., Houtkooper, M. A., Meyer, J. W., Goedhart, D. M., Augusteijn, R., Meinardi, H., Carbamazepine and serum sodium levels, *Epilepsia*, 25(3): 390–7, 1984.

2641. Kallen, B., A register study of maternal epilepsy and delivery outcome with special reference to drug use, *Acta Neurol. Scand.*, 73: 253–9, 1986.

2642. Kalra, V., Transitory IgA deficiency in phenytoin treated epileptics, *Neurology India*, 31(3): 15–17, 1983.

2643. Kaluza, C., Kennedy, B. J., Harman, L., Head and neck complications of epidermolysis bullosa, *Laryngoscope*, 95: 599–600, 1985.

2644. Kaneko, S., Otani, K., Fukushima, Y., Sato, T., Narita,

S., Kurahashi, K., Ogawa, Y., Nomura, Y., Shinagawa, S., Effects of antiepileptic drugs on hGH, TSH, and thyroid hormone concentrations during pregnancy, *Int. J. Biol. Res. Pregnancy*, 3(4): 148–51, 1982.

2645. Kaneko, S., Sato, T., Kirahashi, K., Hill, R. G., Taberner, P. V., Effect of carbamazepine on primary afferent depolarization and gamma-aminobutyric acid metabolism—comparison with phenytoin, *Igaku No. Ayumi*, 121(12): 1030–2, 1982.

2646. Karp, M., Lerman, P., Doron, M., Laron, Z., Effect of diphenylhydantoin on insulin response in the oral glucose tolerance test in children and adolescents, *Helv. Paediatr. Acta*, 28: 617–20, 1973.

2647. Kasai, S., Hachimine, K., Effect of 5,5-diphenylhydantoin sodium on the synthesis of collagen by some fibroblastic cell lines including gingiva derived cells, *Bull. Tokyo Dent. Coll.*, 15: 53–62, 1974.

2648. Kassai, Y., Okishio, Y., Kida, T., Ebisu, S., Okada, H., Immunopathological studies of phenytoin-induced gingival hyperplasia, *Nippon Shishubyo Gakkai Kaishi*, 27: 197–205, 1985.

2649. Kaste, M., Muuronen, A., Nikkila, E. A., Neuvonen, P. J., Increase of low serum concentrations of high-density lipoprotein (HDL) cholesterol in TIA patients treated with phenytoin, *Stroke*, 13: 123, 1982.

2650. Kaste, M., Muuronen, A., Nikkila, E. A., Neuvonen, P. J., Increase of low serum concentrations of high-density lipoproteins (HDL) cholesterol in tia-patients treated with phenytoin, *Stroke*, 14(4): 525–30, 1983.

2651. Katsumata, M., Gupta, C., Baker, M. K., Sussdorf, C. E., Goldman, A. S., Diphenylhydantoin: an alternative ligand of a glucocorticoid receptor affecting prostaglandin generation in A/J mice, *Science*, 218: 1313–15, 1982.

2652. Kaukola, S., Manninen, V., Neuvonen, P. J., Malkonen, M., Ehnholm, C., Effect of phenytoin on serum lipoproteins in middle-aged men, *J. Cardiovasc. Pharmacol.*, 3: 207–14, 1981.

2653. Kauppinen, K., Stubb, S., Drug eruptions: causative agents and clinical types. A series of in-patients during a 10-year period, *Acta Derm. Venereol.*, 64(4): 320–4, 1984.

2654. Kavey, R. E., Blackman, M. S., Sondheimer, H. M., Phenytoin therapy for ventricular arrhythmias occurring late after surgery for congenital heart disease, *Am. Heart J.*, 104: 794–8, 1982.

2655. Kelly, T. E., Teratogenicity of anticonvulsant drugs. I: Review of the literature, *Am. J. Med. Genet.*, 19: 413–434, 1984.

2656. Kennedy, S., Garfinkel, P. E., Anorexia nervosa, *American Psychiatric Association Annual Review*, Vol. 4, Hales, R. E. and Frances, A. J., Eds., American Psychiatric Press, Washington, D.C., 438–63, 1985.

2657. Kepes, E. R., Management of pain, *Fundamentals of Geriatric medicine*, Cape, R. D., et al., Eds., Raven Press, New York, 247–57, 1983.

2658. Kero, M., Palotie, A., Peltonen, L., Collagen metabolism in two rare forms of epidermolysis bullosa, *Br. J. Dermatol.*, 110: 177–84, 1984.

2659. Khan, M. T., The effect of diphenylhydantoin on liver regeneration in partially hepatectomized and on liver growth in normal rats, *Garyounis Med. J.*, 2: 49–53, 1979.

2660. Khan, M. T., Studies on the uterine inhibitory actions of diphenylhydantoins, *Arch. Int. Pharmacodyn. Ther.*, 260: 265–73, 1982.

2661. Kilpatrick, C. J., Wanwimolruk, S., Wing, L. M., Plasma concentrations of unbound phenytoin in the management of epilepsy, *Br. J. Clin. Pharmacol.*, 17(5): 539–46, 1984.

2662. King, R. B., Barnett, J. C., Studies of trigeminal nerve potentials, *J. Neurosurg.*, 14: 617–27, 1957.

2663. Knott, C., Reynolds, F., The place of saliva in antiepileptic drug monitoring, *Ther. Drug Monit.*, 6(1): 35–41, 1984.

2664. Ko, P. T., Gulamhusein, S., Kostuk, W. J., Torsades de pointes, a common arrhythmia induced by medication, *Ann. Emerg. Med.*, 338: 3, 1983.

2665. Koizumi, F., Kumai, M., Ishimori, A., Comparison of i-PiT, TDX and EMIT measurement of serum phenytoin and digoxin levels, *Rinsho Byori*, 33(7): 761–770, 1985.

2666. Koppe, V. I., Klepel, H., Prenatal care and delivery of women having epileptic fits, *Gynakol.*, 105(15): 955–60, 1983.

2667. Kotia, K. C., Haldia, S. S., Gupta, V., Role of oral diphenylhydantoin in angina pectoris, *Clinician*, 44(12): 510–14, 1980.

2668. Kotovskaya, E. S., Erina, E. V., Experiment in the use of neurotropic preparations (diphenylhydantoin and pyrroxan) for the purpose of the crisis-preventive treatment of hypertensive patients, *Biull, Vsesoiuznogo Kardiol. Nauchn. Tsentra AMN SSSR*, 5(1): 75–9, 1982.

2669. Krause, K. H., Rascher, W., Berlit, P., Plasma arginine vasopressin concentrations in epileptics under monotherapy, *J. Neurol.*, 230(3): 193–6, 1983.

2670. Krnjevic, K., GABA-mediated inhibitory mechanisms in relation to epileptic discharges, *Basic Mechanisms of Neuronal Hyperexcitability*, Jasper, H. H. and Van Gelder, N. M., Eds., Alan R. Liss, Inc, New York, 249–80, 1983.

2671. Kruse, K., Kracht, U., Inhibition of calcitonin secretion/synthesis by anticonvulsant drugs, *Acta Endocrinol.*, 96: 38–9, 1981.

2672. Kruse, K., Kracht, U., Gopfert, G., Response of kidney and bone to parathyroid hormone in children receiving anticonvulsant drugs, *Neuropediatrics*, 13(1): 3–9, 1982.

2673. Kugler, J. D., Cheatham, J. P., Gumbiner, C. H., Hofschire, P. J., Latson, L. A., Results of phenytoin and propranolol drug electrophysiology studies for ventricular tachycardia in patients having repaired lesions with tetralogy of Fallot physiology, *Circulation*, 72(4): iii–341, 1985.

2674. Kulig, K., Bar-Or, D., Marx, J., Wythe, E., Rumack, B. H., Phenytoin as treatment for tricyclic antidepressant cardiotoxicity in a canine model, *Vet. Hum. Toxicol.*, 26(5): A–2, 1984.

2675. Kulig, K., Baror, D., Marx, J., Wythe, E., Rumack, B. H., Phenytoin as treatment of the cardiotoxicity of tricyclic antidepressant overdose in experimental animals, *Vet. Hum. Toxicol.*, 25: 285, 1983.

2676. Kulkarni, S. K., Mehta, A. K., Possible mechanism of digoxin-induced convulsions, *Psychopharmacology*, 79(2–3) 287–9, 1983.

2677. Kulpmann, W. R., Gey, S., Beneking, M., Kohl, B., Oellerich, M., Determination of total and free phenytoin in serum by non-isotopic immunoassays and gas chromatography, *J. Clin. Chem. Clin. Biochem.*, 22(11): 773–9, 1984.

2678. Kumps, A., Genin-Ramakers, J., Mardens, Y., Simultaneous determination of anticonvulsant drugs and metabolites in plasma by high-performance liquid chromatography, *J. Chromatogr.*, 342(2): 469–471, 1985.

2679. Kupersmith, J., Monitoring of antiarrhythmic drug levels: values and pitfalls, *Clinical Pharmacology of Cardiac Antiarrhythmic Agents: Classical and Current Concepts Reevaluated*, Garfein, O. B., Ed., N.Y. Acad. Sci., 432: 138–54, 1984.

2680. Kutt, H., Phenytoin: interaction with other drugs, *Antiepileptic Drugs*, Woodbury, D. M., et al., Eds., Raven Press, New York, 227–40, 1982.

2681. Kutt, H., Interactions between anticonvulsants and other commonly prescribed drugs, *Epilepsia*, 25: s118–s131, 1984.

2682. Kwiecinski, H., Myotonia induced with clofibrate in rats, *J. Neurol.*, 219: 107–16, 1978.

2683. Kwiecinski, H., The antimyotonic effect of diphenylhydantoin, *Eur. J. Clin. Invest.*, 14: 37, 1984.

2684. Lai, M. L., Hung, T. P., Pharmacokinetics of a large single dose phenytoin, *J. Formosan Med. Assoc.*, 82: 370–80, 1983.

2685. Lalonde, R., Botez, M. I., Chronic phenytoin and the stereotyped motor response induced by 5-methoxy-N, N-dimethyltryptamine in rats, *Brain Res.*, 326: 388–91, 1985.

2686. Lalonde, R., Botez, M. I., Subsensitivity to muscimol-induced catalepsy after long-term administration of phenytoin in rats, *Psychopharmacology*, 86: 77–80, 1985.

2687. Lamy, P. P., *Prescribing for the Elderly*, PSG Publishing Co., Littleton, Mass., 1980.

2688. Lander, C. M., Smith, M. T., Chalk, J. B., Bioavailability and pharmacokinetics of phenytoin during pregnancy, *Eur. J. Clin. Pharmacol.*, 27(1): 105–10, 1984.

2689. Langer, P., The effects of salicylates and similar acting substances, (diphenylhydantoin, dinitrophenol, etc.) on the hypophyseal-thyroid gland axis, *Vnitr. Lek.*, 30: 48–54, 1984.

2690. Lasker, S. E., Lee, B. Y., Madden, R. E., Jetter, R. B., Topical use of 5,5-diphenyl-2,4-imidazolidinedione (diphenylhydantoin) inducing rapid granulation of chronic skin ulcers, *Clin. Res.*, 31(3): 677a, 1983.

2691. Lason, W., Przewlocka, B., Przewlocki, R., The effect of Gamma-hydroxybutyrate and anticonvulsants on opioid peptide content in the rat brain, *Life Sci.*, 33(1): 599–602, 1983.

2692. Laterza, A., Paolella, P., Valassi, F., Myotonia-like deforming stiffness (a new myo-oculo-skeletal disease sensitive to diphenylhydantoin, *Rev. Otoneuroophtalmol.*, 42 (1): 51–70, 1967.

2693. Lauxerois, M., Pechardre, J. C., Bonnard, M., Colnet, G., Gibert, J., Chabannes, J., Early pre- and postoperative epileptic seizures during operations on osteomeningeal breaches, value of preventive treatment with hydantoins, *Neurochirurgie*, 30(4): 241–4, 1983.

2694. Lazarev, A. V., Chernokhvostov, V. V., Kokoz, Y. M., Calmodulin-dependent regulation of calcium-activated outward current in frog atrial membrane, *Adv. Myocardiol.*, 3: 95–105, 1982.

2695. Lazzara, R., Anomalous atrioventricular conduction and the pre-excitation syndromes, *Bellet's Essentials of Cardiac Arrhythmias*, Helfant, R. H., Ed., W. B. Saunders Co., Philadelphia, 182–96, 1980.

2696. Le Quesne, P. M., Neuropathy due to drugs, *Peripheral Neuropathy by 78 Authorities*, Vol. 2, Dyck, P. J., et al., Eds., W. B. Saunders Co., Philadelphia, 1263–80, 1975.

2697. Lebrun, L. H., Villeneuve, J. P., Hypermetabolism of phenytoin as a cause of treatment failure, *Can. J. Neurol. Sci.*, 9: 277, 1982.

2698. Lee, K. S., Sancesario, L. G., Tetzlaff, W., Kreutzberg, G. W., Post-anoxic treatment with anticonvulsants: electrophysiological and anatomical studies of CA1 pyramidal cells, *Soc. Neurosci. Abstr.*, 12 (Pt 2): 869, 1986.

2699. Lehr, H. A., Zimmer, J. P., Kern, W., Diphenylhydantoin in AIDS, *Dtsch. Med. Wschr.*, 111(44): 1701, 1986.

2700. Lehr, H. A., Zimmer, J. P., Diphenylhydantoin in the prevention and treatment of AIDS?, *Dtsch. Med. Wochenschr.*, 111(25): 1001–2, 1986.

2701. Lemon, H. M., Stohs, S. J., Heinicke, R., Pfeiffer, R., Campbell, J. L., Anti-mammary carcinogenic activity of phenytoin (5,5' diphenylhydantoin), *Proc. Am. Assoc. Cancer Res.*, 25: 128, 1984.

2702. Lennard, M. S., Ramsay, L. E., Silas, J. H., Tucker, G. T., Wood, H. F., Protecting the poor metabolizers: clinical consequences of genetic polymorphism of drug oxidation, *Pharm. Int.*, 4: 53–7 Mar. 1983.

2703. Lepore, V., Di Reda, N., Defazio, G., Pedone, D.,

Giovine, A., Lanzi, C., Tartaglione, B., Livrea, P., Dopamino-mimetic action of diphenylhydantoin in rat striatum: effect on homovanillic acid and cyclic AMP levels, *Psychopharmacology*, 86: 27–30, 1985.

2704. Leppik, I. E., Fisher, J., Kriel, R., Sawchuck, R., Altered phenytoin clearance during febrile illnesses, *Neurology*, 31(2): 158, 1981.

2705. Leppik, I. E., Patrick, B. W., Cranford, R. E., Treatment of acute seizures and status epilepticus with intravenous phenytoin, *Advances in Neurology. Status Epilepticus*, Delgado-Escueta, A. V., Ed., Raven Press, New York, 447–51, 1983.

2706. Leppik, I. E., Ramani, V., Sawchuk, R. J., Cummit, R. J., Seizures and altered phenytoin metabolism in mononucleosis. *Advances in Epileptology: The 10th Epilepsy International Symposium*. Wada, J. A., Penry, J. K., Eds., Raven Press, New York, 506–7, 1980.

2707. Lerner, U., Fredholm, B. B., Hanstrom, L., Diphenyl-hydantoin inhibits parathyroid hormone and prostaglandin E2-stimulated bone resorption in mouse calvaria without affecting cyclic AMP formation, *J. Oral. Pathol.*, 14: 644–53, 1985.

2708. Lerner, U., Hanstrom, L., Influence of diphenylhydantoin on lysosomal enzyme release during bone resorption ·in vitro, *Acta Pharmacol. Toxicol.*, 47: 144–50, 1980.

2709. Levin, R., Lee, S. I., Nonconvulsive status epilepticus following metrizamide myelogram, *Ann. Neurol.*, 17(5): 518–19, 1985.

2710. Levine, D. N., Finklestein, S., Delayed psychosis after right temporoparietal stroke or trauma; relation to epilepsy, *Neurology*, 32: 267–73, 1982.

2711. Levine, M., Toxic reaction to phenytoin following a viral infection, *Can. Med. Assoc. J.*, 128: 1270, 1983.

2712. Levy, G., Protein binding of drugs in the maternal-fetal unit and its potential clinical significance, *Drugs and Pregnancy. Maternal Drug Handling—Fetal Drug Exposure*, Krauer, B., et al., Eds., Academic Press, Orlando, 29–44, 1984.

2713. Levy, R. H., Moreland, T. A., Rationale for monitoring free drug levels, *Clin. Pharmacokinet.*, 9 (sup 1): 1–9, 1984.

2714. Levy, R. H., Schmidt, D., Utility of free level monitoring of antiepileptic drugs, *Epilepsia*, 26(3): 199–205, 1985.

2715. Levy, R. H., Yerby, M. S., Effects of pregnancy of antiepileptic drug utilization, *Epilepsia*, 26(sup1): s52–7, 1985.

2716. Lewin, E., Bleck, V., Electroshock seizures in mice: effect on brain adenosine and its metabolites, *Epilepsia*, 577–81, 1981.

2717. Lewis, D. V., Diphenylhydantoin reduces the outward current of the action potential in Aplasia, *Brain Res.*, 207: 234–8, 1981.

2718. Liedtke, B., Kerschensteiner, M., Manifestation of myotonic disturbances of muscle function under continuous intravenous drip treatment with the beta-adrenergic Th 1165a (fenoterolhydrobromide), *Z. Geburtshilfe. Perinatol.*, 178(4): 297–303, 1974.

2719. Liponi, D. F., Winter, M. E., Tozer, T. N., Renal function and therapeutic concentrations of phenytoin, *Neurology*, 34: 395–7, 1984.

2720. Lisander, B., Jaju, B., Wang, S. C., CNS site of antiar-rhythmic action of diphenylhydantoin (DPH) in the cat, *Eur. J. Pharmacol.*, 31(1): 53–62, 1975.

2721. Lishman, W. A., Symonds, C. P., Whitty, C. W., Willison, R. G., Seizures induced by movement, *Brain*, 85: 93–108, 1962.

2722. Liskow, B. I., Psychiatric disorders, *Conn's Current Therapy*, Rakel, R. E., Ed., W. B. Saunders Company, Philadelphia, 899–902, 1986.

2723. Lisso, C., Mortari, A., Sioli, G., Marked antiar-rhythmic activity of diphenylhydantoin, *Atti Accad. Med. Lombarda*, 22: 385–90, 1967.

2724. Lloyd, K. G., Worms, P., GABA agonists: their potential as anticonvulsant drugs, *Br. Assoc. Psychopharmacol, Monogr.*, 2: 54–61, 1982.

2725. Loh, C. K., McElhinney, A. J., Litwak, R., Peirce, E. C., Effects of antiarrhythmic agents on digitalis and hypoxia induced myocardial K loss, *Fed. Proc.*, 41(4): 1107, 1982.

2726. Loiseau, P., Strube, E., Broustet, D., Battellochi, S., Gomeni, C., Morselli, P. L., Learning impairment in epileptic patients, *Epilepsia*, 24: 183–92, 1983.

2727. Lothman, E. W., Geary, W. A., Wooten, G. F., Perlin, J. B., Absence of specific binding of phenytoin to brain sections *in vitro*, *Neurology*, 36(4): 85, 1986.

2728. Lucchesi, B. R., Patterson, E. S., Antiarrhythmic drugs, *Cardiovascular Pharmacology, 2nd Edition*, Antonaccio, M. J., Ed., Raven Press, New York, 329–414, 1984.

2729. Luckmann, E., Hossmann, H., Dorner, V., Rothenberger, W., Wichert, P. V., Clinical experience with diphenylhydantoin in ventricular and supraventricular extrasystoles, *Aktueller Stand der Pathosphysiologie, Diagnostik und Therapie von Herzrhythmusstorungen*, Haan, D., Runge, M., Eds., Desitin Werk, Hamburg, 165–73, 1973.

2730. Ludewig, R., Otto, G., Therapeutic effect of topical phenytoin application, *Russian Pharmacol. Toxicol.*, 45(3): 101–3, 1982.

2731. Luhdorf, K., Nielsen, C. J., Orbaek, K., Hammerberg, P. E., Motor and sensory conduction velocities and electromyographic findings in man before and after carbamazepine treatment, *Acta Neurol. Scand.*, 67: 103–7, 1983.

2732. Luoma, P. V., Sotaniemi, E. A., Pelkonen, R. O., Arranto, A., Ehnholm, C., Plasma high-density lipoproteins and hepatic microsomal enzyme induction: relation to histological changes in the liver, *Eur. J. Clin. Pharmacol.*, 23: 275–82, 1982.

2733. Luoma, P. V., Myllyla, V. V., Sotaniemi, E. A., Hokkanen, T. E., Plasma HDL cholesterol and growth hormone in epileptics treated with anticonvulsants, *Acta Pharmacol. Toxicol.*, 47: 249–251, 1980.

2734. Luoma, P. V., Myllyla, V. V., Sotaniemi, E. A., Lehtinen, I. A., Hokkanen, E. J., Plasma high-density lipoprotein cholesterol in epileptics treated with various anticonvulsants, *Eur. Neurol.*, 19: 67–72, 1980.

2735. Luoma, P. V., Pelkonen, R. O., Sotaniemi, E. A., Plasma high-density lipoprotein cholesterol and hepatic drug metabolizing enzyme activity in man, *Acta Physiol. Scand.*, 226: 71, 1979.

2736. Luoma, P. V., Reunanen, M. I., Sotaniemi, E. A., Serum lipid levels during long-term therapy with anticonvulsants, *Clin. Pharmacol. Ther.*, 23: 119–20, 1978.

2737. Luoma, P. V., Reunanen, M. I., Sotaniemi, E. A., Changes in serum triglyceride and cholesterol levels during long-term phenytoin treatment for epilepsy, *Acta Med. Scand.*, 206: 229–31, 1979.

2738. Luoma, P. V., Savolainen, M. J., Sotaniem, E. A., Pelkonen, R. O., Arranto, A. J., Enholm, C., Plasma high-density lipoproteins and liver lipids and proteins in man, *Acta Med. Scand.*, 214: 103–9, 1983.

2739. Luoma, P. V., Sotaniemi, E. A., Arranto, A. J., Serum LDL cholesterol, the LDL/HDL cholesterol ratio and liver microsomal enzyme induction evaluated by antipyrine kinetics, *Scand. J. Clin. Lab. Invest.*, 43: 671–75, 1983.

2740. Luoma, P. V., Sotaniemi, E. A., Pelkonen, R. O., Myllyla, V. V., Plasma high-density lipoprotein cholesterol and hepatic cytochrome P-450 concentrations in epileptics undergoing anticonvulsant treatment, *Scand. J. Clin. Lab. Invest.*, 40: 163–67, 1980.

2741. Luoma, P. V., Sotaniemi, E. A., Pelkonen, R. O., Savolainen, M. J., Arranto, A., Enholm, C., Enzyme-inducers reduce the risk of atherosclerotic vascular disease?, *Br. J. Clin. Pharmacol.*, 14(4): 606P, 1982.

2742. Luoma, P. V., Sotaniemi, E. A., Pelkonen, R. O., Inverse relationship of serum LDL cholesterol and the LDL/HDL cholesterol ratio to liver microsomal enzyme induction in man, *Res. Commun. Chem. Pathol. Pharmacol.*, 42(1): 173–6, 1983.

2743. Lust, W. D., Fuessner, G. K., Passonneau, J. V., McCandless, D. W., Biochemical mechanisms of anticonvulsants: studies on cyclic neucleotide systems in brain, *Neuropharmacology of Central Nervous System and Behavioral Disorders*, Palmer, G. C., Ed., Academic Press, New York, 407–31, 1980.

2744. MacDonald, J. T., Childhood migraine—differential diagnosis and treatment, *Postgrad. Med.*, 80(5): 301–6, 1986.

2745. Macdonald, R. L., Barbiturate and hydantoin anticonvulsant mechanisms of action, *Basic Mechanisms of Neuronal Hyperexcitability*, Jasper, H. H. and Van Gelder, N. M., Eds., Alan R. Liss, Inc., New York, 361-87, 1983.

2746. Macdonald, R. L., Anticonvulsant and convulsant drug actions on vertebrate neurones in primary dissociated cell culture, *Electrophysiology of Epilepsy*, Schwartzkroin, P.A. and Wheal, H. V., Eds., Academic Press, London, 353–87, 1984.

2747. Macdonald, R. L., McLean, M. J., Skerritt, J. H., Anticonvulsant drug mechanisms of action, *Fed. Proc.*, 44: 2634–9, 1985.

2748. Macdonald, R. L., Skerritt, J. H., McLean, M. J., Anticonvulsant drug cations on GABA responses and sustained repetitive firing neurons in cell culture, *Neuropharmacology*, 23(7): 843–4, 1984.

2749. Macfarlane, D. G., Clark, B., Panayi, G. S., Pilot study of phenytoin in rheumatoid arthritis, *Ann. Rheum. Dis.*, 45: 954–6, 1986.

2750. MacKinney, A. A., Vyas, R., Lee, S. S., The effect of parahydroxylation of diphenylhydantoin on metaphase accumulation, *Proc. Soc. Exp. Biol. Med.*, 149: 371–5, 1975.

2751. MacKinney, A. A., Vyas, R., Mueller, C., Gorder, C., A comparison of potency of hydantoins in metaphase arrest and inhibition of microtubular polymerization, *Mol. Pharmacol.*, 17: 275–8, 1980.

2752. MacKinney, A. A., Vyas, R., Mueller, C., 1-acetyl-3-acetoxy-5'5-diphenylhydantoin has colchicine-like activity against microtubular protein, *Res. Commun. Chem. Pathol. Pharmacol.*, 44(2): 251–64, 1984.

2753. MacKinney, A. A., Vyas, R., Powers, K., Morphologic effect of hydantoin drugs on mitosis and microtubules of cultured human lymphocytes, *J. Pharmacol. Exp. Ther.*, 204: 195–202, 1978.

2754. MacKinney, A. A., Vyas, R. S., Walker, D., Hydantoin drugs inhibit polymerization of pure microtubular protein, *J. Pharmacol. Exp. Ther.*, 204(1): 189–94, 1978.

2755. Mace, P. F., Hughes, J., The Ames Seralyzer Reagent Strip System evaluated for measuring serum phenytoin, *Clin. Chem.*, 32(2): 391, 1986.

2756. Maciewicz, R., Bouckoms, A., Martin, J. B., Drug therapy of neuropathic pain, *Clin. J. Pain*, 1(1): 1–10, 1985.

2757. Maguire, J. H., Murthy, A. R., Hall, I. H., Hypolipidemic activity of antiepileptic 5-phenylhydantoins in mice, *Eur. J. Pharmacol.*, 117: 135–8, 1985.

2758. Magyarosi, G. H., Therapeutic value of intravenous diphenylhydantoin in digitalis arrhythmia, *Rev. Med. Intern.*, 37(1): 61–6, 1985.

2759. Maitre, M. J., Coltart, J., Diagnosis of digitalis intoxication, *International Symposium on Diagnosis and Treatment of Cardiac Arrhythmias*, Bayes, A. and Cosin, J., Ed., Pergamon Press, New York, 701–24, 1980.

2760. Mann, D. N., Kumara-Siri, M. H., Surks, M. I., Effect of 5-diphenylhydantoin on the activities of hepatic cytosol malic enzyme and mitochondrial alpha-glycerophosphate de-

hydrogenase in athyreotic rats, *Endocrinology*, 112(5): 1732–8, 1983.

2761. Mann, D. N., Surks, M. I., 5,5-diphenylhydantoin decreases specific 3,5,3'-triiodothyronine (T_3) binding by rat hepatic nuclear T_3 receptors, *Endocrinology*, 112(5): 1723–31, 1983.

2762. Marcoli, M., Gatti, G., Ippoliti, G., Lombardi, M., Crema, A., Zocchi, M. T., DePonti, F., Lecchini, S., Frigo, G. M., Effect of chronic anticonvulsant monotherapy on lymphocyte subpopulations in adult epileptic patients, *Hum. Toxicol.*, 4(2): 147–57, 1985.

2763. Maria, G., Pisanelli, S., A case of neuromyotonia—considerations of pathogenesis, *Riv. Neurol.*, 53: 400–09, 1983.

2764. Marshall, J. B., Forker, A. D., Cardiovascular effects of tricyclic antidepressant drugs: therapeutic usage, overdose, and management of complications, *Am. Heart J.*, 103 (3): 401–14, 1982.

2765. Martin, M. L., Pharmacologic therapeutic modalities: phenytoin, dimethyl sulfoxide, and calcium channel blockers, *Crit. Care Quart.*, 5: 72–81, 1983.

2766. Marx, K. A., Anastasi, N. C., Hernandez, Y. M., Fivozinsky, K. B., Protection by phenytoin against the toxic effects of organophosphate on central respiratory centers, *Soc. Neurosci. Abstracts*, 10: 709, 1984.

2767. Mason, D. T., Zelis, R., Lee, G., Hughes, J. L., Spann, J. F., Amsterdam, E. A., Current concepts and treatment of digitalis toxicity, *Am. J. Cardiol.*, 27: 546–59, 1971.

2768. Massei, R., DeSilva, E., Grosso, P., Robbiati, B. R., Infuso, L., Ravagnati, L., Altamura, C. A., Cerebral protection with diphenylhydantoin during disobliterating surgery of the sovra-aortic branches, *J. Neurosurg. Sci.*, 27(2): 107–10, 1983.

2769. Mathur, K. S., Wahal, P. K., Seth, H. C., Intermittent anomalous atrioventricular excitation (W.P.W. aberation)—an unusual manifestation of digitalis toxicity, *Indian Heart J.*, 21: 249–52, 1969.

2770. Matsuki, N., Quandt, F. N., Ten Eich, R. E., Yeh, J. Z., Characterization of the block of sodium channels by phenytoin in mouse neuroblastoma cells, *J. Pharmacol. Exp. Ther.*, 228(2): 523–30, 1984.

2771. Matsumoto, Y., Hiramatsu, M., Mori, A., Effects of phenytoin on convulsions and brain 5-hydroxytryptamine levels in E1 mice, *IRCS Med. Sci. Biochem.*, 11(9): 837, 1983.

2772. Matsumoto, Y., Hiramatsu, M., Mori, A., Effects of chronic administration of phenytoin on its metabolism and brain monoamine level, *Neurosciences* (Kobe, Jpn), 10: 183–9, 1984.

2773. Matsuo, A., Yajima, T., Cell proliferation and collagen fibrogenesis of cultured fibroblasts, *Jpn. J. Oral Biol.*, 27: 53–63, 1985.

2774. Matthews, W. D., McCafferty, G. P., Anticonvulsant activity of muscimol against seizures induced by impairment of GABA-mediated neurotransmission, *Neuropharmacology*, 18: 885–9, 1979.

2775. Mattson, R. H., Cramer, J. A., Epilepsy, sex hormones, and antiepileptic drugs, *Epilepsia*, 26(sup1): S40–51, 1985.

2776. Maurya, A. K., Boyle, S., Mutagenic potential of anticonvulsant diphenylhydantoin (DPH) on human lymphocytes in vitro, *Meth. Find. Exp. Clin. Pharmacol.*, 7(3): 109–12, 1985.

2777. Maxion, H., Jacobi, P., Schneider, E., Kohler, M., Effect of the anticonvulsant drugs primidone and diphenylhydantoin on night sleep in healthy volunteers and epileptic patients, *Sleep 1974. 2nd Europ. Congr. on Sleep Research*, Koella, W. P. and Levin, P. Eds., Karger, Basel, 510–13, 1975.

2778. Mayron, R., Ruiz, E., Phenytoin: does it reverse tricyclic-antidepressant-induced cardiac conduction abnormalities?, *Ann. Emerg. Med.*, 14(5): 505, 1985.

2779. McClanahan, J. S., Maguire, J. H., Human stereoselective production of phenytoin (5,5-diphenylhydantoin) dihydrodiol and phenol metabolites, *Pharmacologist*, 27(3): 148, 1985.

2780. McGuire, S. A., Tomasovic, J. J., Ackerman, N., Hereditary continuous muscle fiber activity, *Arch. Neurol.*, 41: 395–6, 1984.

2781. McKinney, L. C., Diphenylhydantoin reduces veratridine-induced sodium permeability in frog skeletal muscle, *Neurosci. Lett.*, 55(2): 173–8, 1985.

2782. McLean, M., Carbamazepine and phenytoin limit rapid firing of action potentials of dorsal root ganglion neurons in cell culture, *Soc. Neurosci. Abstr.*, 12 (Pt 2): 1015, 1986.

2783. McLean, M. J., Macdonald, R. L., Multiple actions of phenytoin on mouse spinal cord neurons in cell culture, *J. Pharmacol. Exp. Ther.*, 227(3): 779–89, 1983.

2784. Mehta, M., Chronic pain, *Recent Advances in Anaesthesia and Analgesia*, Atkinson, R. S. and Hewer, L. C., Eds., Churchill Livingstone, New York, 157–77, 1982.

2785. Meldrum, B., Griffiths, T., Evans, M., Hypoxia and neuronal hyperexcitability—a clue to mechanisms of brain protection, *Protection of Tissues Against Hypoxia*, Wauquier, A., et al., Eds., Elsevier Biomedical Press, New York, 275–86, 1982.

2786. Meldrum, B. S., Anlezark, G. M., Ashton, C. G., Horton, R. W., Sawaya, C. B., Neurotransmitters and anticonvulsant drug action, *Post-Traumatic Epilepsy and Pharmacological Prophylaxis*, Majokowski, J., Ed., Polish Chapter of the Int. League Against Epilepsy, 139–53, 1977.

2787. Melten, J. W., Wittebrood, A. J., Willems, H. J., Faber, G. H., Wemer, J., Faber, D. B., Comparison of equilibrium dialysis, ultrafiltration, and gel permeation chromatography for the determinations of free fractions of phenobarbital and phenytoin, *J. Pharm. Sci.*, 74(6): 692–694, 1985.

2788. Mendiola-Gonzalez, J. F., Espejo-Plascencia, I., Chapa-Alvarez, J. R., Rodriguez-Noriega, E. Sodium diphenylhydantoin in burns: effects of pain and healing, *Invest. Med. Int.*, 10: 443–7, 1983.

2789. Mercer, H. P., McGill, J. J., Ibrahim, R. A., Envenomation by sea snake in Queensland, *Med. J. Aust.*, 1: 130–2, 1981.

2790. Messing, R. O., Carpenter, C. L., Greenberg, D. A., Mechanism of calcium channel inhibition by phenytoin: comparison with classical calcium channel antagonists, *J. Pharmacol. Exp. Ther.*, 235(2): 407–11, 1985.

2791. Messing, R. O., Carpenter, C. L., Greenberg, D. A., Phenytoin (DPH) inhibits calcium flux through voltage-gated calcium channels in cultured cells, *Neurology*, 35(sup 1): 157, 1985.

2792. Meulenhoff, J. S., Phenytoin and the liver, *Pharm. Weekbl.*, 117(39): 916–17, 1982.

2793. Meyer, J., Epidermolysis Bullosa—Phenytoin, *Schweiz. Med. Wochensch.*, 111(4): 1662–3, 1981.

2794. Michenfelder, J. D., Barbiturates for brain resuscitation: yes and no, *Anesthesiology*, 57(2): 74–75, 1982.

2795. Miller, J. A., Richter, J. A., Effects of anticonvulsants *in vivo* on high affinity choline uptake *in vitro* in mouse hippocampal synaptosomes, *Br. J. Pharmacol.*, 84(1): 19–25, 1985.

2796. Miller, T. D., Pinkerton, T. C., Determinations of free phenytoin in plasma by ultra-filtration and high-performance liquid chromatography, *Anal. Chim. Acta*, 170(2): 295–300, 1985.

2797. Mimaki, T., Deshmukh, P. P., Yamamura, H. I., Effect of phenytoin on benzodiazepine receptors in rat brain, *Advances in Epileptology: 12th Epilepsy International Symposium*, Dam, M., et al., Eds., Raven Press, New York, 73–9, 1981.

2798. Minchin, M. C., Iversen, L. L., Release of [3H] gamma-aminobutyric acid from glial cells in rat dorsal root ganglia, *J. Neurochem.*, 23: 533–40, 1974.

2799. Missri, J. C., Shubrooks, S. J., Torsade de pointes: an atypical form of ventricular tachycardia, *Conn. Med.*, 46: 69–70, 1982.

2800. Mitchell, J. E., Pyle, R. L., Eckert, E. D., Bulimia, *American Psychiatric Association Annual Review*, vol. 4, Hales, R. E. and Frances, A. J., Eds., American Psychiatric Press, Washington, D. C., 464–80, 1985.

2801. Mohr, J. P., Facial pain, *Manual of Clinical Problems in Neurology*, Little, Brown and Co., Boston, 97–8, 1984.

2802. Monroe, R. R., *Episodic Behavioral Disorders, a Psychodynamic and Neurophysiologic Analysis,* Harvard University Press, Cambridge, 1–517, 1970.

2803. Monson, R. R., Heinonen, O. P., Shapiro, S., Slone, D., Diphenylhydantoin and epilepsy in relation to congenital malformations and mental development, *Am. J. Epidemiol.*, 100(6): 509, 1974.

2804. Moore, S. L., Rakes, S. M., Binge eating—therapeutic response to diphenylhydantoin: case report, *J. Clin. Psychiatry*, 43: 385–6, 1982.

2805. Morello, R. S., Begenisich, T., Form and site of action of diphenylhydantoin on the sodium channel of squid axons, *Biophys. J.*, 25: 135a, 1979.

2806. Morganroth, J., Comparative evaluation of antiarrhythmic agents, *Drugs*, 29 (Sup 4): 14–20, 1985.

2807. Moss, A. J., Schwarz, P. J., Delayed repolarization (QT or QTU prolongation) and malignant ventricular arrhythmias, *Mod. Concepts Cardiovasc. Dis.*, 51: 85–90, 1982.

2808. Moss, G., Stein, A. A., Cerebral etiology of the acute respiratory distress syndrome: diphenylhydantoin prophylaxis, *J. Trauma*, 15(1): 39–41, 1975.

2809. Mount, L. A., Reback, S., Familial paroxysmal choreoathetosis, *Arch. Neurol. Psychiatry*, 44: 841–7, 1940.

2810. Moustafa, M. A., Claesen, M., Adline, J., Vandervorst, D., Poupaert, J. H., Evidence for an arene-3,4-oxide as a metabolic intermediate in the meta- and para-hydroxylation of phenytoin in the dog, *Drug Metab. Dispos.*, 11(6): 574–80, 1983.

2811. Moy, L. S., Tan, E. M., Holness, R., Uitto, J., Effects of phenytoin on collagen metabolism and growth of skin fibroblasts in culture, *Clin. Res.*, 31(1): 22A, 1983.

2812. Mullen, P. W., Queiroz, M. L., The humoral immunotoxicological effects of phenytoin, an anticonvulsant drug with nonlinear pharmacokinetics, *Immunotoxicology*, NATO ASI Ser., Vol. G2, Mullen, P. W., Ed., Springer-Verlag, Berlin, 89–95, 1984.

2813. Murphy, J. V., Reddy, M. N., Marquardt, K., High-density lipoprotein cholesterol concentrations in the plasma of children receiving anticonvulsants, *Ann. Neurol.*, 10(3): 292, 1981.

2814. Muuronen, A., Kaste, M., Nikkila, E. A., Tolppanen, E. M., Mortality from ischaemic heart disease among patients using anticonvulsive drugs: a case-control study, *Br. Med. J.*, 291: 1481–3, 1985.

2815. Nagatomo, T., Effects of spartein and diphenylhydantoin on the sarcolemmal (Na$^+$ + K$^+$)-ATPase activity of rat skeletal muscle, *Niigata Yakka Daigaku Kenkyu Hokoku*, 2: 1–4, 1982.

2816. Nakamura, H., Kadokawa, T., Nakatsuji, K., Nakamura, K., Pharmacological studies of a new anti-inflammatory drug, 1-phenylsulfony 1–5,5-diphenylhydantoin (PC-796) in experimental animals, *Arzneim. Forsch.*, 20(8): 1032–46, 1970.

2817. Nakayama, K., Nakagawa, S., Sato, J., Kasahara, H., Sasaki, M., Mori, A., A clinicopharmacological study on a seizure-controlled group with low serum concentrations of diphenylhydantoin, *Acta Neurol. Scand.* suppl 79, 62: 103, 1980.

2818. Narr, H., New aspects in the treatment of dermatogenous contractures of the hand in epidermolysis bullosa, *Handchir. Mikrochir. Plast. Chir.*, 16: 48–51, 1984.

2819. Nau, H., Kuhnz, W., Egger, H. J., Anticonvulsants during pregnancy and lactation. Transplacental, maternal and neonatal pharmacokinetics, *Clin. Pharmacokinet.*, 7: 508–43, 1982.

2820. Nemoto, E. M., Shiu, G. K., Nemmer, J. P., Bleyaert, A. L., Pharmacologic attenuation of brain free fatty acid liberation during complete global ischemia as a measure of therapeutic efficacy, *Protection of Tissues Against Hypoxia*, Wauquier, A., Borgers, M., Eds., Elsevier Biomedical Press, New York, 211–21, 1982.

2821. Nencini, P., Phenytoin induces cyclic-AMP accumulation and free fatty acids release in rat brown adipose tissue, *Pharmacol. Res. Commun.*, 14(7): 593–604, 1982.

2822. Neppe, V. M., The neuroleptic malignant syndrome, *S. Afr. Med. J.*, 65: 523–5, 1984.

2823. Nicoletti, I., Mariotti, G., Filipponi, P., Serena Lungarotti, M., Hydantoin-induced fetopathy: description of one case, *Minerva Pediatr.*, 32: 61–4, 1980.

2824. Niedermeyer, E., Interactions of anticonvulsant drugs, *Epilepsy Guide, Diagnosis and Treatment of Epileptic Seizure Disorders*, Niedemeyer, E., Ed., Urban & Schwarzenberg, Baltimore, 208–11, 1983.

2825. Niedermeyer, E., Prevention of epileptic seizures, *Epilepsy Guide, Diagnosis and Treatment of Epileptic Seizure Disorders*, Niedermeyer, E., Ed., Urban & Schwarzenberg, Baltimore, 199–202, 1983.

2826. Niewiadomski, J. S., The hypothalamic and neurohypophysial vasopressin content as influenced by diphenylhydantoin in dehydrated rats, *Acta Physiol. Pol.*, 30(3): 351–8, 1979.

2827. Nikkila, E. A., Kaste, M., Ehnholm, C., Viikari, J., Increase of serum high-density lipoprotein in phenytoin users, *Br. Med. J.*, 99, 1978.

2828. Nishikawa, T., Kubo, H., Saito, M., Competitive nephelometric immunoassay method for antiepileptic drugs in patient blood, *J. Immunol. Methods*, 29(1): 85–9, 1979.

2829. Nishimura, S., Imazawa, M., Miyamoto, K., Possible existence of loosely membrane-bound specific binding sites for phenytoin, *Folia Psychiatr. Neurol. Jpn.*, 37(3): 303–5, 1983.

2830. Nissimov, R., Weiss, S., Zaavi, I., Mozes, K., Cardiac arrhythmias and electrocardiographic abnormalities in amitriptyline poisoning, *Harefuah*, 105–8 142–43, 1981.

2831. Noachtar, S., Roder, U. U., Wolf, P., The influence of long-term medication with diphenylhydantoin (DPH) on polygraphic sleep of epileptic patients, *16th Epilepsy International Congress*, Abstracts, Hamburg, Sept. 6–9, Ciba-Geigy, Basel, 1, 1985.

2832. Norris, B., Saez, C., Comparison of the effects of carbamazepine and of diphenylhydantoin on the electrical properties of isolated toad skin, *IRCS Med. Sci.*, 12: 164–5, 1984.

2833. North, J. B., Penhall, R. K., Hanieh, A., Frewin, D. B., Taylor, W. B., Phenytoin and postoperative epilepsy—a double-blind study, *J. Neurosurg.*, 58: 672–7, 1983.

2834. Nosek, T. M., The effects of valproate and phenytoin on the cAMP and cGMP levels in nervous tissue, *Proc. Soc. Exp. Biol. Med.*, 178(2): 196–9, 1985.

2835. Nosek, T. M., Crosland, M. B., Csukas, S., Calcium-activated neutral protease: activation and inhibition in striated muscle, *Fed. Proc.*, 42(4): 1088, 1983.

2836. Notani, M., Kawamura, H., Amano, K., Tanikawa, T., Kawabatake, H., Iseki, H., Shiwaku, T., Nagao, T., Kakinoki, Y., Kitamura, K., The incidence of postoperative epilepsy and prophylactic anticonvulsants in patients with intracranial aneurysm, *No Shinkei Geka*, 12(3): 269–74, 1984.

2837. O'Callaghan, A. C., Normandale, J. P., Morgan, M., The prolonged Q-T syndrome. A review with anaesthetic implications and a report of two cases, *Anaesth. Intensive Care*, 10: 50–5, 1982.

2838. O'Neill, B., Callaghan, N., Stapleton, M., Molloy, W., Serum elevation of high density lipoprotein (HDL) cholesterol in epileptic patients taking carbamazepine or phenytoin, *Acta Neurol. Scand.*, 65: 104–9, 1982.

2839. Oellerich, M., Muller Vahl, H., The EMIT free level (TM) ultrafiltration technique compared with equilibrium dialysis and ultracentrifugation to determine protein binding of phenytoin, *Clin. Pharmacokin.*, 9 (Sup. 1) 61–70, 1984.

2840. Ogura, C., Kunimoto, N., Kishimoto, A., Takeshita, H., Mizukawa, R., Tsutsui, T., Hazama, H., Ryoke, K., Kurooka, S., Diphenylhydantoin concentrations in whole saliva, parotid saliva and plasma measured by enzyme immunoassay kit, Markit, *Yonago Acta Med.*, 26(2–3): 55–64, 1983.

2841. Okabe, H., Lehrer, M., Karmen, A., Effects of anticonvulsants on fatty acid metabolism in human serum, *Tohoku J. Exp. Med.*, 148: 267–73, 1986.

2842. Oldenkott, P., Lehr, H. A., Raisbeck, A. P., Ungerechtfe-tigter ausschlub von spendernieren nach phenytoin behandlung?, *Dtsch. Med. Wschr.*, 110: 1834–5, 1985.

2843. Oneal, J. S., Sloan, K. B., Schulman, S. G., Substrate-labelled fluorescence immunoassay of phenytoin, *J. Pharm. Biomed. Anal.*, 4(1): 103–6, 1986.

2844. Osawa, Y., The protective action of diphenylhydantoin (DPH) on the brain, *J. Tokyo Med. Coll.*, 41(1): 3–14, 1983.

2845. Oxley, J., Janz, D., Meinardi, H., *Chronic Toxicity of Antiepileptic Drugs*, Raven Press, New York, 1983.

2846. Oyama, Y., Minagawa, K., Miura, H., Koshimizu, T., Effects of long-term administration of antiepileptic drugs on the pituitary-thyroid system in children, *Acta Paediatr. Jpn.*, 21(1): 68–9, 1979.

2847. Pagni, C. A., Trigeminal neuralgia, *Panminerva Med.*, 24: 113–36, 1982.

2848. Painter, M. J., David, R., Alvin, J., The use of a stable isotope to study phenytoin metabolism in the newborn, *Ann. Neurol.*, 16(3): 379, 1984.

2849. Parsons, J. M., Sapse, A. T., Significance of hypercortisolism in anorexia nervosa, *J. Orthomol. Psychiatry*, 14(1): 13–18, 1985.

2850. Partanen, V. S., Soininen, H., Saksa, M., Riekkinen, P., Electromyographic and nerve conduction findings in a patient with neuromyotonia, normocalcemic tetany and small-cell lung cancer, *Acta Neurol. Scand.*, 61: 216–26, 1980.

2851. Patsalos, P. N., Lascelles, P. T., Changes in regional brain levels of amino acid putative neurotransmitters after prolonged treatment with the antiepileptic drugs diphenylhydantoin, phenobarbitone, sodium valproate, ethosuximide, and sulthiame in the rat, *J. Neurochem.*, 36(2): 688–95, 1981.

2852. Paule, M. G., Killam, E. K., The effects of chronic phenytoin administration on incremental repeated acquisition (learning) tasks in the epileptic baboon, papio papio, *Fed. Proc.*, 43(4): 1035, 1984.

2853. Paule, M. G., Killam, E. K., Serum anticonvulsant levels during chronic administration in the immature epileptic baboon, Papio papio, *Proc. West. Pharmacol. Soc.*, 38: 169–72, 1985.

2854. Pedersen, J. G., An evaluation of the changes in bone turnover in an *in vitro* system: the direct effect on bone turnover of diphenylhydantoin, *Acta Orthop. Scand.*, 53 (4): 703, 1981.

2855. Pedersen, J. G., Lund, B. J., Reimann, I., Influence of diphenylhydantoin on isotope release and bone enzymes *in vitro*, *Acta Orthop. Scand.*, 53: 885–88, 1982.

2856. Peerless, S. J., Pre- and postoperative management of cerebral aneurysms, *Clin. Neurosurg.*, 26: 209–30, 1979.

2857. Pei, Y. Q., Development and clinical application of antiepileptic drugs, *Sheng Li Ko Hsueh Chin Chan*, 12: 228–33, 1981.

2858. Perez-Ruvalcabaga, J. A., Quintero-Perez, N. P.,

Campa-Uribe, G., Chapa-Alvarez, R., Rodriguez-Noriega, E., The multiple uses of phenytoin in a general hospital setting, *Eur. J. Clin. Invest.*, 14: 37, 1984.

2859. Perucca, E., Anticonvulsant drug interactions, *Psychopharmacology of Anticonvulsants*, Sandler, M., Ed., Oxford University Press, New York, 122–28, 1982.

2860. Perucca, E., Crema, A., Therapeutic monitoring of serum antiepileptic drug levels, *Epilepsy: An Update on Research and Therapy*, Nistico, G., et al., eds., Alan R. Liss, Inc., New York, 267–83, 1983.

2861. Perucca, E., Richens, A., Drug interactions with phenytoin, *Epilepsy Abstracts*, 15(5): 189, 1982.

2862. Perucca, E., Richens, A., Antiepileptic drug interactions, *Handbook of Experimental Pharmacology, Antiepileptic Drugs*, Frey, H. H. and Janz, D., Eds., Springer-Verlag, Berlin, 831–855, 1985.

2863. Perwein, E., Diphenylhydantoin therapy of a Gedde-Dahl Inverse (recessive) hereditary dystrophic bullous epidermolysis, *Hautarzt.*, 34(4): 188, 1983.

2864. Petersen, E. N., DMCM: a potent convulsive benzodiazepine receptor ligand, *Eur. J. Pharmacol.*, 94: 117–24, 1983.

2865. Peterson, D. I., Phenytoin absorption following Jejunoileal bypass, *Bull. Clin. Neurosci.*, 48: 148–9, 1983.

2866. Peterson, G. M., McLean, S., Monitoring free plasma concentrations of phenytoin, *Br. J. Clin. Pharmacol.*, 18(6): 971–2, 1984.

2867. Pettengell, K. E., Spitaels, J. M., Simjee, A. E., Dysphagia and dystrophia myotonica: a case report, *S. Afr. Med. J.*, 68: 113–14, 1985.

2868. Phillips, T. L., Wasserman, T. H., Johnson, R. J., Levin, V. A., Vanraalte, G., Final report on the United States phase 1 clinical trial of the hypoxic cell radiosensitizer, misonidazole (Ro-07-0582; NSC 261037), *Cancer*, 48: 1697–1704, 1981.

2869. Phillis, J. W., Wu, P. H., The effect of various centrally active drugs on adenosine uptake by the central nervous system, *Comp. Biochem. Physiol.*, 72c: 179–87, 1982.

2870. Pincus, J. H., Weinfeld, H. M., Acetylcholine release from synaptosomes and phenytoin action, *Brain Res.*, 296: 313–17, 1984.

2871. Pippenger, C. E., Bastiani, R. J., Schneider, R. S., Evaluation of an experimental homogeneous enzyme immunoassay for the quantitation of phenytoin and phenobarbitone in serum or plasma, *Clinical Pharmacology of Anti-epileptic Drugs*, Schneider, H., et al., Eds., Springer-Verlag, New York, 331–41, 1975.

2872. Piredda, S., Yonekawa, W., Whittingham, T. S., Kupferberg, H. J., Potassium, pentylenetetrazol, and anticonvulsants in mouse hippocampal slices, *Epilepsia*, 26(2): 167–74, 1985.

2873. Pirttiaho, H. I., Sotaniemi, E. A., Pelkonen, R. O., Pitkanen, U., Hepatic blood flow and drug metabolism in patients on enzyme-inducing anticonvulsants, *Eur. J. Clin. Pharmacol.*, 22: 441–5, 1982.

2874. Pisciotta, A. V., Phenytoin: hematological toxicity, *Antiepileptic Drugs*, D. M. Woodbury, J. K. Penry, C. E. Pippenger, Eds., Raven Press, New York, 257–8, 1982.

2875. Plant, G., Focal paroxysmal kinesigenic choreoathetosis, *J. Neurol. Neurosurg. Psychiatry*, 46: 345–8, 1983.

2876. Pollack, S. V., Wound healing: a review—systemic medications affecting wound healing, *J. Dermatol. Surg. Oncol.*, 8: 667–72, 1982.

2877. Pond, S. M., Pharmacokinetic drug interactions, *Pharmacokinetic Basis for Drug Treatment*, Benet, L. Z., et al., Eds., Raven Press, New York, 195–220, 1984.

2878. Pozdeev, V. K., The effect of diphenylhydantoin on the function of the brain transmitter systems, *Mediator Processes in Epilepsy*, Nauka, Leningrad, 85–92, 1983.

2879. Prasad, S., Kumari, P., Effect of diphenylhydantoin (DPH) sodium on some neurotransmitters of central nervous system, *Indian J. Pharmacol.*, 14: 25, 1982.

2880. Pratt, J. A., Jenner, P., Marsden, C. D., Benzodiazepines, anticonvulsants, epilepsy and myoclonus, *Neurotransmitters, Seizures, and Epilepsy*, Morselli, P. L., et al., Eds., Raven Press, New York, 227–38, 1981.

2881. Pratt, J. A., Jenner, P., Marsden, C. D., Comparison of the effects of benzodiazepines and other anticonvulsant drugs on synthesis and utilization of 5-HT in mouse brain, *Neuropharmacology*, 24(1): 59–68, 1985.

2882. Pritchard, P. B., O'Neal, D. B., Nonconvulsive status epilepticus following metrizamide myelography, *Ann. Neurol.*, 16: 252–4, 1984.

2883. Puccinelli, G., Ceccarelli, C., Mucci, G., Landucci, C., Phenytoin utilization as a possible treatment of torsade de pointe ventricular tachycardia, *Minerva Cardioangiol.*, 29: 423–30, 1981.

2884. Quandt, F. N., Narahashi, T., Internal perfusion of neuroblastoma cells and the effects of diphenylhydantoin on voltage-dependent currents, *Neurosci. Abstr.*, 6: 97, 1980.

2885. Quandt, F. N., Yeh, J. Z., Slow inactivation of single Na channels induced by diphenylhydantoin, *Soc. Neurosci. Abstr.*, 12 (Pt 1): 45, 1986.

2886. Quattrone, A., Crunelli, V., Samanin, R., Seizure susceptibility and anticonvulsant activity of carbamazepine, diphenylhydantoin and phenobarbital in rats with selective depletions of brain monoamines, *Neuropharmacology*, 17: 643–7, 1978.

2887. Quest, J. A., Breed, C. R., Gillis, R. A., Effect of phenytoin on cardiac slowing induced by cholinergic stimulation, *J. Cardiovasc. Pharmacol.*, 4: 629–34, 1982.

2888. Rahwan, R. G., Piascik, M. F., Witiak, D. T., The role of calcium antagonism in the therapeutic action of drugs, *Can. J. Physiol. Pharmacol.*, 57(5): 443–60, 1979.

2889. Raines, A., Mahany, T. M., Baizer, L., Swope, S., Hershkowitz, N., Description and analysis of the myotonolytic effects of phenytoin in the decerebrate cat: implications for potential utility of phenytoin in spastic disorders, *J. Pharmacol. Exp. Ther.*, 232(1): 283–94, 1985.

2890. Rall, T. W., Schleifer, L. S., Drugs effective in the therapy of the epilepsies, *The Pharmacological Basis of Therapeutics*, 7th edition, Gilman, A. G., et al., Eds., Macmillan Publishing Co., New York, 446–72, 1985.

2891. Rane, A., Peng, D., Phenytoin enhances epoxide metabolism in human fetal liver cultures, *Drug Metab. Dispos.*, 13(3): 382–5, 1985.

2892. Rapport, R. L., Harris, A. B., Friel, P. N., Ojemann, G. A., Human epileptic brain: Na, K, ATPase activity and phenytoin concentrations, *Arch. Neurol.*, 32(8); 549–54, 1975.

2893. Rashid, S., Waterfall, J. F., Effect of antiarrhythmic and analgesic drugs on the effective refractory period of guinea pig isolated atria and ventricular strips, *J. Pharm. Pharmacol.*, 31: 411–2, 1979.

2894. Rating, D., Nau, H., Kuhnz, W., Antiepileptic drugs in the newborn clinical and pharmacological data, *Monatsschr. Kinderheilkd.*, 131(1): 6–12, 1983.

2895. Ratshin, R. A., Hunt, D., Russel, R. O., Rackley, C. E., QT-interval prolongation, paroxysmal ventricular arrhythmias, and convulsive syncope, *Ann. Intern. Med.*, 75: 919–24, 1971.

2896. Rau, J. H., Struve, F. A., Green, R. S., Electroencephalographic correlates of compulsive eating, *Clin. Electroencephalogr.*, 10: 180–9, 1979.

2897. Reddy, M. N., Effect of anticonvulsant drugs on plasma total cholesterol, high-density lipoprotein cholesterol, and apolipoproteins A and B in children with epilepsy, *Proc. Soc. Exp. Biol. Med.*, 180(2): 354–63, 1985.

2898. Reeves, S. E., Hanyok, J. J., Amon, S. A., Cooley, P. J., Discrepancy in serum phenytoin concentrations determined by two immunoassay methods in uremic patients., *Am. J. Hosp. Pharm.*, 42: 359–361, 1985.

2899. Reisecker, J., Markut, H., Tulzer, W., Problems with diagnosis and therapy of myotonia dystrophica, *Wien. Med. Wochenschr.*, 133 (12): 319–21, 1983.

2900. Requena, R., Forte, R., Knopf, M., Scherrer, J., Kirschner, J., Levowitz, B. S., Intracellular potassium and vitamin A in the prevention of stress ulcers. *Surg. Forum*, 23: 388–9, 1972.

2901. Resnekov, L., Das Gupta, D. S., Prevention of ventricular rhythm disturbances in patients with acute myocardial infarction, *Am. Heart J.*, 98(5): 653–9, 1979.

2902. Reynolds, E. H., Travers, R. D., Serum anticonvulsant concentrations in epileptic patients with mental symptoms, *Br. J. Psychiat.*, 124: 440–5, 1974.

2903. Reynolds, E. H., Adverse haematological effect of antiepileptic drugs, *Chronic Toxicity of Antiepileptic Drugs*, Oxley, J., et al., Eds., Raven Press, New York, 91–99, 1983.

2904. Rhee, H. M., Effects of some antiarrhythmic agents on $^{45}Ca^{++}$ transport in dog heart membrane vesicles and $^{86}Rb^{+}$ transport in specialized cardiac tissues, *Calcium-Binding Proteins 1983*, DeBernard, B., et al., Eds., Elsevier Science Publishers, Amsterdam, 293–5, 1983.

2905. Rhee, H. M., Evidence against an involvement of Na^{+}, K^{+}-ATPase in antiarrhythmic mechanism of phenytoin, *Naunyn. Schmiedebergs. Arch. Pharmacol.*, 323(1): 78–84, 1983.

2906. Ribares, R. G., Miller, R. J., Phenytoin inhibits voltage-dependent and dihydropyridine-stimulated calcium uptake by NG108cc15, *Soc. Neurosci. Abstr.*, 11: 596, 1985.

2907. Ricevuti, G., Mazzone, A., Danesino, M., Toscano, M., Rizzo, S. C., Phenytoin to prevent or control granulocyte transfusion reactions, *Lancet*, 37, Jul 7, 1984.

2908. Rimmer, E. M., Buss, D. C., Routledge, P. A., Richen, A., Should we routinely measure free plasma phenytoin concentration?, *Br. J. Clin. Pharmacol.*, 17(1): 99–102, 1984.

2909. Rodenkirchen, R., Bayer, R., Mannhold, R., Specific and non-specific Ca antagonists. A structure-activity analysis of cardiodepressive drugs, *Prog. Pharmacol.*, 5(1): 9–23, 1982.

2910. Rodin, E., Subramanian, M. G., Gilroy, J., Investigation of sex hormones in male epileptic patients, *Epilepsia*, 25(6): 690–4, 1984.

2911. Rodriguez-Noriega, E., Esparza-Ahumada, S., Andrade-Perez, J. S., Espejo-Plascencia, I., Chapa-Alvarez, R., Treatment of ulcerations in soft tissues with topical diphenylhydantoin, *Invest. Med. Int.*, 10: 184–6, 1983.

2912. Rodriguez-Noriega, E., Chapa-Alvarez, R., Perez-Ruvalcaba, J. A., The many in-hospital indications of diphenylhydantoinate, *Invest. Med. Int.*, 10: 443–7, 1983.

2913. Rodriguez-Noriega, E., Perez-Ruvalcaba, J. A., Quintero-Perez, N. P., Hernandez-Bugarin, O., Macias-Hernandez, O., Chapa-Alvarez, J. R., Andrade-Perez, J. S., The effect of phenytoin on muscle spasms and the hyperactive sympathetic syndrome of tetanus, *Eur. J. Clin. Invest.*, 14: 36, 1984.

2914. Rosen, T., Schimmel, M. S., A short review of perinatal pharmacology, *Bull. N.Y. Acad. Med.*, 59(7): 669–77, 1983.

2915. Rosman, N. P., Oppenheimer, E. Y., O'Connor, J. F., Emergency management of pediatric head injuries, *Emerg. Med. Clin. North Am.*, 1: 141–74, 1983.

2916. Rothstein, P., Dornbusch, J., Shaywitz, B. A., Prolonged seizures associated with the use of viscous lidocaine, *J. Pediatr.*, 101: 461–3, 1982.

2917. Rousso, I., Pharmakiotis, A., Gatzola, M., Karatza, E., Tourkantonis, A., Sklavounou-Tsouroutsoglou, S., Effects of phenobarbital, diphenylhydantoin and carbamazepine on thyroid function in epileptic children, *Acta Endocrinol.*, 107(265): 48–9, 1984.

2918. Rowe, D. J., Harris, M., Effects of anticonvulsant drugs on bone resorption induced by parathyroid extract *in vitro, Anticonvulsant Drugs and Enzyme Induction*, Richens, A. et al., Eds., Associated Scientific Publ., Amsterdam, 113–121, 1976.

2919. Russel, J. M., Harvey, S. C., Effects of diphenylhydantoin on canine atria and A-V conduction system, *Arch. Int. Pharmacyodyn.*, 182(1): 219–31, 1969.

2920. Sakai, T., Hosokawa, S., Shibasaki, H., Goto, I., Kuroiwa, Y., Sonoda, H., Murai, Y., Syndrome of continuous muscle-fiber activity: increased CSF GABA and effect of dantrolene, *Neurology*, 33: 495–8, 1983.

2921. Saladini, M., Gabana, M. A., Bracco, F., Effect of antiepileptic drugs on the cerebral amino acid uptake *in vitro*, *Ital. J. Neurol. Sci.*, 2(4): 351–9, 1981.

2922. Sanchez-Chapula, J., Josephson, I. R., Effect of phenytoin on the sodium current in isolated rat ventricular cells, *J. Mol. Cell Cardiol.*, 58(8): 515–22, 1983.

2923. Satoskar, R. S., Bhandakar, S. D., Pharmacotherapy of cardiac arrhythmias, *Pharmacology and Pharmacotherapeutics*, Bombay Popular Prakashan, Bombay, 316–30, 1983.

2924. Sayk, J., Kmietzyk, H. J., Survival time of glioma/glioblastoma patients under antiepileptic medication, *Nervenarzt*, 52: 611–15, 1981.

2925. Scandellari, C., Zaccaria, M., Sicolo, N., Casara, D., Erle, G., Federspil, G., Medical treatment of endogenous organic hyperinsulinism, *Horm. Metab. Res.*, 6: 46–54, 1976.

2926. Schachner, E. R., Oster, Z. H., Cicale, N. R., The effect of diphenylhydantoin (Dilantin) on thallium-201 chloride uptake, *Epilepsy Abstracts*, 15(6): 202, 1982.

2927. Schaerrer, W. C., The use of Dilantin in the treatment of chronic ulcerative colitis, *Personal Communication*, 1–3, 1963.

2928. Schaffler, L., Karbowski, K., Relapsing paroxysmal abdominal pains of cerebral origin, *Schweiz. Med. Wochenschr.*, 111(37): 1352–60, 1981.

2929. Scheinberg, L., Giesser, B. S., Drug therapy, *Multiple Sclerosis a Guide for Patients and Their Families*, Scheinberg, L., Ed., Raven Press, New York, 45–55, 1984.

2930. Scherber, A., Richter, K., Schaps, P., Distribution of antiepileptic drugs between plasma, plasma water, cerebrospinal fluid, saliva and brain, *Epilepsy: a Clinical and Experimental Research*, Majkowski, J., Ed., Karger, Basel, 208–12, 1980.

2931. Scheuer, T., Kass, R. S., Phenytoin reduces calcium current in the cardiac Purkinje fiber, *Cir. Res.*, 53: 16–23, 1983.

2932. Schless, G. L., Functional hypoglycemia: diagnosis and treatment, *Diabetes*, 31(2): 167a, 1982.

2933. Schmidt, D., Phenytoin, *Adverse Effects of Antiepileptic Drugs*, Raven Press, New York, 134–40, 1982.

2934. Schmidt, D., Adverse effects, *Handbook of Experimental Pharmacology, Antiepileptic Drugs*, Springer-Verlag, Berlin, 791–829, 1985.

2935. Schmidt, D., Seldon, L., *Adverse Effects of Antiepileptic Drugs*, Raven Press, New York, 1982.

2936. Schorer, R., Brain protection, *Anaesthesiol. Intensivmed.*, 23(8): 3, 1982.

2937. Schottelius, D. D., Homogeneous immunoassay system [EMIT] for quantitation of antiepileptic drugs in biological fluids, *Antiepileptic Drugs: Quantitative Analysis and Interpretation*, Pippenger, C. E., et al., Eds., Raven Press, New York, 95–108, 1978.

2938. Schreiner, C. A., Holden, H. E., Mutagens as teratogens: a correlative approach, *Teratogenesis and Reproductive Toxicology*, Johnson E. M. and Kochhar D. M., Eds., Springer-Verlag, Berlin, 135–68, 1983.

2939. Schwarz, M., Sontag, K. H., Phenytoin potentiates the antispastic action of diazepam in spastic Han-Wistar mutant rats, *Naunyn-Schmied. Arch. Pharmacol.*, 321: r42, 1982.

2940. Sechi, G. P., Traccis, S., Durelli, L., Monaco, F., Mutani, R., Carbamazepine versus diphenylhydantoin in the treatment of myotonia, *Eur. Neurol.*, 22: 113–18, 1983.

2941. Seeman, P., The membrane actions of anesthetics and tranquilizers, *Pharamacol. Rev.*, 24(4): 583–655, 1972.

2942. Seipel, L., Breithardt, G., Medical treatment of sinus node disease: antiarrhythmic drugs and sinoatrial conduction, *International Symposium on Diagnosis and Treatment of cardiac Arrhythmias*, Bayes, A., and Cosin, J., Eds., Pergamon Press, New York, 636–61, 1980.

2943. Selby, G., Diseases of the fifth cranial nerve, *Peripheral Neuropathy*, Vol. 1, Dyck, P. J., et al., Eds., W. B. Saunders Co., Philadelphia, 533–69, 1975.

2944. Selzer, M. E., David, G., Yaari, Y., Phenytoin reduces frequency potentiation of synaptic potentials at the frog neuromuscular junction, *Brain Res.*, 304(1): 149–53, 1984.

2945. Selzer, M. E., David, G., Yaari, Y., On the mechanism by which phenytoin blocks post-tetanic potentiation at the frog neuromuscular junction, *J. Neurosci.*, 4(11): 2894–9, 1985.

2946. Serra, S., Gallito, G., DeDomenico, P., Morgante, L., Bianchi, L., Ajello, L., Musolino, R., Arena, A., DiPerri, R., Influence of antiepileptic drugs on plasma lipid levels, *Acta Neurol.*, 38(3): 190–7, 1983.

2947. Shah, D. S., Chambon, P., Guidotti, A., Binding of [^{3}H]-5,5 Diphenylhydantoin in rat brain membranes, *Neuropharmacology*, 20: 1115–9, 1981.

2948. Sheppard, M. C., Davis, J. R., Lynam, T. C., Franklyn, J. A., Docherty, K., Phenytoin effects on prolactin release and synthesis, *J. Endocrinol.*, 107 sup:abs 113, 1985.

2949. Shiba, D. A., Weinkam, R. J., The *in vivo* cytotoxic activity of procarbazine and procarbazine metabolites against L1210 ascites leukemia cells in CDF-1 mice and the effects of pretreatment with procarbazine phenobarbital, diphenylhydantoin and methylprednisolone, *Cancer Chemother. Pharmacol.*, 11(2): 124–9, 1983.

2950. Shibuya, T., Hashimoto, K., Imai, S., Effective plasma concentrations of antiarrhymic drugs against sustained halothane-adrenaline arrhythmia in dogs, *J. Cardiovasc. Pharmacol.*, 5(4): 538–45, 1983.

2951. Shrivastava, S., Tandon, R., The long QT interval: clinical significance and therapeutic implications, *Indian J. Chest Dis. Allied Sci.*, 25: 60–8, 1983.

2952. Seigel, E. G., Janjic, D., Wollheim, C. B., Phenytoin inhibition of insulin release: studies on the involvement of Ca$^+$ fluxes in rat pancreatic islets, *Diabetes*, 31: 265–9, 1982.

2953. Siegel, R. C., Scleroderma (systemic sclerosis), *Conn's Current Therapy*, Rakel, R. E., Ed., W. B. Saunders Co., Philadelphia, 627–30, 1986.

2954. Simmonds, M. S., Distinction between the effects of barbiturates, benzodiazepines and phenytoin on responses to gamma-aminobutyric acid receptor activation and antagonism by bicuculline and picrotoxin. *Br. J. Pharmacol.*, 73(3): 739–47, 1981.

2955. Simpson, C. F., Taylor, J., Neurotoxic and antihypertensive effects of phenytoin in turkeys, *J. Pharmacol. Exp. Ther.*, 233(3): 853–6, 1985.

2956. Singer, H. S., Slesinger, P., Effect of anticonvulsants on a neuroblastoma X glioma hybrid cell line: cell growth and synaptic neurochemistry, *Epilepsia*, 26(5): 519, 1985.

2957. Singer, P. A., Crampton, R. S., Bass, N. H., Familial Q-T prolongation syndrome, *Arch Neurol.*, 31: 64–6, 1974.

2958. Sirgo, M. A., Green, P. J., Rocci, M. L., Vlasses, P. H., Interpretation of serum phenytoin concentrations in uremia is assay-dependent, *Neurology*, 34: 1250–1, 1984.

2959. Sironi, V. A., Ravagnati, L., Ettorre, G., Cabrini, G. P., Marossero, F., Differences between the concentrations of antiepileptic drugs in normal and pathological human brain, *Eur. J., Clin. Pharmacol.*, 22: 447–9, 1982.

2960. Skerritt, J. H., Davies, L. P., Johnston, G. A., A Purinergic component in the anticonvulsant action of carbamazepine?, *Eur. J. Pharmacol.*, 82: 195–7, 1982.

2961. Skerritt, J. H., Johnston, G. A., Inhibition of amino acid transmitter release from rat slices by phenytoin and related anticonvulsants, *Clin. Exp. Pharmacol. Physiol.*, 10: 527–33, 1983.

2962. Skerritt, J. H., Johnston, G. A. Modulation of excitant amino acid release by convulsant and anticonvulsant drugs, *Neurotransmitters, Seizures, and Epilepsy II*, Fariello, R. G. et al., Eds., Raven Press, New York, 215–26, 1984.

2963. Skillrud, D. M., Goldstein, N. P., Paroxysmal limb hemiataxia with crossed facial paresthesias in multiple sclerosis, *JAMA*, 250(20): 2843–4, 1983.

2964. Smith, P. J., Surks, M. I., Multiple effects of 5,5-diphenylhydantoin on the thyroid hormone system, *Endocr. Rev.*, 5(4): 514–24, 1984.

2965. Smith, R. G., Daves, G. D., Lynn, R. K., Gerber, N., Hydantoin ring glucuronidation: characterization of a new metabolite of 5,5-diphenylhydantoin in man and the rat, *Biomed. Mass Spectrom.*, 4(4): 275–9, 1977.

2966. Snow, R. W., Hasan, Z., Dudek, F. E., Effects of phenytoin on field bursts of rat hippocampal slices in low-calcium solutions, *Neuropharmacology*, 24(9): 915–17, 1985.

2967. Snyder, C. H., Epileptic equivalents in children, *Pediatrics*, 21: 308–18, 1958.

2968. Solomon, G. E., Kutt, H., Plum, F., Special management problems. Complications of anti-epileptic drug therapy, *Clinical Management of Seizuers. A guide for the Physician*, 2nd edition, W. B. Saunders Co., Philadelphia, 292–304, 1983.

2969. Solomon, G. E., Plum, F., Seizure types, *Clinical Management of Seizures: A Guide for the Physician*, W. B., Saunders Co., Philadelphia, 20–53, 1976.

2970. Sonnenfeld, G., Harned, C. L., Nerland, D. E., Effects of interferon on drug metabolism, *Tex. Rep. Biol. Med.*, 41: 363–9, 1981.

2971. Sordillo, P., Matarese, R. A., Novich, R. K., Zabetakis, P. M., Michelis, M. F., Specific modalities of therapy for inappropriate antidiuretic hormone secretion, *Clin. Nephrol.*, 15(3): 107–10, 1981.

2972. Spark, R. F., Wills, C. A., Royal, H., Hypogonadism, hyperprolactinaemia, and temporal lobe epilepsy in hyposexual men, *Lancet*, 413–7 Feb. 25, 1984.

2973. Spiehler, V., Sun, L., Miyada, D. S., Sarandis, S. G., Walwick, E. R., Klein, M. W., Jordan, D. B., Jessen, B., Radioimmunoassay, enzyme immunoassay, spectrophotometry and gas-liquid chromatography compared for determination of phenobarbital and diphenylhydantoin, *Clin. Chem.*, 22(6): 749–53, 1976.

2974. Spielberg, S. P., Gordon, G. B., Blake, D. A., Goldstein, D. A., Predisposition to phenytoin hepatotoxicity assessed *in vitro*, *N. Eng. J. Med.*, 305(13): 722–27, 1981.

2975. Spinelli, W., Rosen, M., Developmental and use-dependent effects of phenytoin on neonatal and adult Purkinje fibers, *J. Am. College Cardiol.*, 7(2): 123A, 1986.

2976. Spinelli, W., Rosen, M. R., Frequency-dependent actions of phenytoin in adult and young canine Purkinje fibers, *J. Pharmacol. Exp. Ther.*, 238(3): 794–801, 1986.

2977. Sprague, G. L., Craigmill, A. L., Control of ethanol withdrawal symptoms in mice by phenytoin, *Res. Commun. Chem. Pathol. Pharmacol.*, 15: 721–31, 1976.

2978. St. John, J. N., Glossopharyngeal neuralgia associated with syncope and seizures, *Neurosurgery*, 10: 380–3, 1982.

2979. Staple, P. H., Eisenberg, G. M., Slosey, J. L., Waterhouse, J., Schofield, J., Patel, M., Effect of phenytoin on adjuvant arthritis (AA) in the rat, *Arthritis Rheum.*, 24(4): s98, 1982.

2980. Staple, P. H., Wigdor, H. A., Phenytoin and proteoglycans of rabbit cartilage, *J. Dent. Res.*, 63; 269, 1984.

2981. Steen, B., Rane, A., Lonnerholm, G., Phenytoin excretion in human breast milk and plasma levels in nursed infants, *Ther. Drug. Monit.*, 4(4): 331–4, 1982.

2982. Stein, E., Kleinfeld, M., Diphenylhydantoin on sinoatrial pacemaker cells, *Circulation* 35,36: 242, 1967.

2983. Stone, T. W., Studies with excitatory amino acid antagonists in rat CNS: 2-amino-5-phosphonovaleric acid, phenytoin, and benzodiazepines, *Adv. Biochem. Psychopharmacol.*, 23: 223–30, 1981.

2984. Stone, W. E., Javid, M. J., Effects of anticonvulsants and other agents on seizures induced by intracerebral L-glutamate, *Brain Res.*, 264(1): 165–67, 1983.

2985. Stopfkuchen, H., Gilfrich, H. J., Jungst, B. K., Gempp, W., Massive digoxin intoxication in childhood, *Intensive Care Med.*, 4:199–201, 1978.

2986. Striano, S., Meo, R., Bilo, L., Vitolo, S., Sleep apnea syndrome in Thomsen's disease. A case report, *Electroencephalogr. Clin. Neurophysiol.*, 56: 323–5, 1983.

2987. Strickler, S., Dansky, L., Andermann, E., Spielberg, S., Pharmacogenetic predisposition to phenytoin-induced birth defects, *Pediatr. Res.*, 19(4 pt. 2): 180a, 1985.

2988. Strickler, S. M., Miller, M.A., Andermann E., Dansky, L. V., Seni, M. H., Spielberg, S. P., Genetic predisposition to phenytoin-induced birth defects, *Lancet*, 746–9, Oct. 5, 1985.

2989. Subik, M., Robinson, D. S., Phenytoin overdose with high plasma levels (case report), *W. Va. Med. J.*, 78(11): 281–2, 1982.

2990. Sugaya, E., Matsuo, T., Takagi, T., Kajiwara, K., Kidokoro, Y., Phenytoin inhibition of hyperexcitability induced by low calcium in frog nerves, *IRCS Med. Sci.*, 12: 1109–10, 1984.

2991. Sugaya, E., Onozuka, M., Furuichi, H. A., Kishii, K., Imai, S., Sugaya, A., Effect of phenytoin on intracellular calcium and intracellular protein changes during pentylenetetrazole-induced bursting activity in snail neurons, *Brain Res.*, 327(1985) 161–8, 1985.

2992. Sung, M. L., Liang, Y. H., Wang, C. S., Shieh, C. C., Lu, S. A., Torsade de pointes—an unusual multiform ventricular tachycardia: a case report, *Chin. Med. J.*, 29(6): 455–8, 1982.

2993. Surawicz, B., Pharmacologic treatment of cardiac arrhythmias: 25 years of progress, *J. Am. Coll. Cardiol.*, 1: 365–81, 1983.

2994. Surks, M. I., Ordene, K. W., Mann, D. N., Kumara-Siri, M. H., Diphenylhydantoin inhibits the thyrotropin response to thyrotropin-releasing hormone in man and rat, *J. Clin. Endocrinol. Metab.*, 56: 940–5, 1983.

2995. Surman, O. S., Parker, S. W., Complex partial seizures and psychiatric disturbance in end-stage renal disease, *Psychosomatics*, 22: 1077–80, 1981.

2996. Suzuki, H., Yamazake, N., Suzuki, Y., Hiraiwa, M., Shimoda, S., Mori, K., Miyasaka, M., Lowering effect of diphenylhydantoin on serum free thyroxine and thyroxine binding globulin (TBG), *Acta Endocrinol.*, 105 (4): 477–81, 1984.

2997. Swerdlow, M., Anticonvulsant drugs and chronic pain, *Clin. Neuropharmacol.*, 7 (1): 51–82, 1984.

2998. Taguchi, K., Watanabe, M., Ioku, M., A case of syringomyelia: electrophysiological analysis and treatment for attacks of periodical spasms and intractable pain, *Neurol. Med. Chir.*, 21: 135–42, 1981.

2999. Takagi, T., Kajiwara, K., Komatsubara, J., Sugaya, E., Inhibitory effect of phenytoin on hyperexcitability induced by low calcium in frog nerves, *Kanagawa Shigaku.*, 20(3): 394–401, 1985.

3000. Takayasu, S., Maeda, M., Tsuji, A., Chemiluminescent enzyme immunoassay using β-D-galactosidase as the label and the bis(2,4,6-trichlorophenyl)oxalate-fluorescent dye system, *J. Immunol. Methods*, 83(2): 317–25, 1985.

3001. Takeya, K., Hotta, Y., Yajima, M., Effect of phenytoin on the positive inotropic actions of grayanotoxin-I and G-strophanthin in the isolated guinea pig atria under contraction-frequency change, *J. Aichi Med., Univ. Assoc.*, 8(2): 96–104, 1980.

3002. Talesnik, E. G., Rivero, S. D., Gonzalez, B. M., Low serum concentrations of IgA and IgM in epileptic children treated with phenytoin, *Rev. Chil. Pediatr.*, 56(2): 76–80, 1985.

3003. Tang, X., Isaacs syndrome: report of a Chinese case with clinical and electrophysiologic study, *China Med., Abstr.*, 2(3): 183, 1985.

3004. Tappaz, M., Pacheco, H., Effects of convulsant and anticonvulsant drugs on the spontaneous and induced release of GABA (^{14}C) from slices of rat cerebral cortex, *J. Pharmacol.*, 4: 433–52, 1973.

3005. Tasse, D. P., Protective value of diphenylhydantoin and vitamin A against stress ulcer, *Can. J. Surg.*, 25(2): 194–5, 1982.

3006. Taylor, J. W., Murphy, M. J., Rivey, M. P., Clinical and electrophysiologic evaluation of peripheral nerve function in chronic phenytoin therapy, *Epilepsia*, 26(5): 416–20, 1985.

3007. Taylor, R. G., Layzer, R. B., Davis, H. S., Fowler, W. M., Continuous muscle fiber activity in the Schwartz-Jampel syndrome, *Electroencephalogr. Clin. Neurophysiol.*, 33: 497–509, 1972.

3008. Teasdale, E., Macpherson, P., Guidelines for cervical myelography: lumbar versus cervical puncture technique, *Br. J. Radiol.*, 57: 789–93, 1984.

3009. Tesseraud, F., Puissant, A., Epidermolysis bullosa, *Rev. Prat.*, 33(15): 751–8, 1983.

3010. Theodore, W. H., Bairamian, D., Newmark, M. E., DiChiro, G., Porter, R. J., Larson, T., Fishbein, D., Effect of phenytoin on human cerebral glucose metabolism, *J. Cereb. Blood Flow Metab.*, 6(3): 315–20, 1986.

3011. Theodore, W. H., Yu, L., Price, B., Yonekawa, W., Porter, R. J., Kapetanovic, I., Moore, H., Kupferberg, H., The clinical value of free phenytoin levels, *Ann. Neurol.*, 18: 90–3, 1985.

3012. Thomas, M., Verges, B., Treatment of diabetic diarrhoea with phenytoin, *Presse Med.*, 15: 11–14, 1986.

3013. Thompson, P. J., Phenytoin and psychosocial development, *Antiepileptic Drug Therapy in Pediatrics*, Morselli, P. L., Pippinger, C. E., Penry, J. K., Eds., Raven Press, New York, 193–200, 1983.

3014. Thompson, P. J., Huppert, F. A., Trimble, M. R., Phenytoin and cognitive function: effects on normal volunteers and implications for epilepsy, *Br. J. Clin. Psychol.*, 20: 155–62, 1981.

3015. Thompson, P. J., Trimble, M. R., Comparative effects of anticonvulsant drugs on cognitive functioning, *Br. J. Clin. Pract.*, 154–6, 1981.

3016. Thompson, P. J., Trimble, M. R., Anticonvulsant drugs and cognitive functions, *Epilepsia*, 23: 531–44, 1982.

3017. Tilson, H. A., Hong, J. S., Mactutus, C. F., Effects of 5,5-diphenylhydantoin (phenytoin) on neurobehavioral toxicity of organochlorine insecticides and permethrin, *J. Pharmacol. Exp. Ther.*, 233(2): 285–9, 1985.

3018. Timiras, P. S., Hill, H. F., Hormones and epilepsy, *Antiepileptic Drugs: Mechanisms of Action*, Glaser, G. H., et al., Eds., Raven Press, New York, 655–66, 1980.

3019. Todd, M. M., Chadwick, H. S., Shapiro, H. M., Dunlop, B. J., Marshall, L. F. Dueck, R., The neurologic effects of thiopental therapy following experimental cardiac arrest in cats, *Anesthesiology*, 57: 76–86, 1982.

3020. Tongia, S. K., Antagonism of frusemide diuresis by diphenylhydantoin sodium, *Indian J. Med. Res.*, 74: 572–4, 1981.

3021. Toone, B., Wheeler, M., Fenwick, P., Effects of anticonvulsant drugs on male sex hormones and sexual arousal, *Psychopharmacology of Anticonvulsants*, Sandler, M., Ed., Oxford University Press, New York, 136–42, 1982.

3022. Toone, B. K., Wheeler, M., Nanjee, M., Fenwick, P., Grant, R., Sex hormones, sexual activity and plasma anticonvulsant levels in male epileptics, *J. Neurol. Neurosurg. Psychiatry*, 46: 824–6, 1983.

3023. Trimble, M., Anticonvulsant drugs, behavior, and cognitive abilities, *Curr. Dev. Psychopharmacol.*, 65–91, 1981.

3024. Trimble, M. R., Corbett, J. A., Behavioural and cognitive disturbances in epileptic children, *Irish Med. J.*, 73(10): 21–8, 1980.

3025. Trimble, M. R., Thompson, P., Corbett, J., Anticonvulsant drugs, cognitive function, and behavior, *Psychopharmacology of Anticonvulsants*, Sandler, M., Ed., Oxford University Press, New York, 106–21, 1982.

3026. Trimble, M. R., Thompson, P. J., Anticonvulsant drugs, cognitive function and behavior, *Epilepsia*, s55–s63, 1983.

3027. Troupin, A. S., Shaw, L. M., A new centrifugal filtration device for free drug separation, *Epilepsia*, 26(5): 455–9, 1985.

3028. Tsuchiya, J., Experimental studies on stress ulcer pathogenically related to subarachnoid hemorrhage, *Gifu Daigaku Igakubu Kiyo*, 29(5): 929–72, 1981.

3029. Tsuru, M., Erickson, R. R., Holtzman, J. L., The metabolism of phenytoin by isolated hepatocytes and hepatic microsomes from male rats, *J. Pharmacol. Exp. Ther.*, 222(3): 658–61, 1982.

3030. Tuffanelli, D. L., Scleroderma (systemic sclerosis), *Conn's Current Therapy*, Rakel, R. E., Ed., W. B. Saunders Co., Philadelphia, 681–83, 1984.

3031. Tunnicliff, G., Smith, J. A., Ngo, T. T., Competition for diazepam receptor binding by diphenylhydantoin and its enhancement by gamma-aminobutyric acid, *Biochem. Biophy. Res. Commun.*, 91: 1018–24, 1979.

3032. Turk, J. W., Ladenson, J. H., Phenytoin and phenobarbital concentrations in renal insufficiency, *Ann. Intern. Med.*, 101(4): 568–9, 1984.

3033. Turley, C. P., Milligan, T., Rapid protein determinations on ultrafiltrates prepared for free phenytoin quantification, *Ther. Drug Monit.*, 7(3): 313–14, 1985.

3034. Turnbull, D. M., Rawlins, M. D., Weightman, D., Chadwick, D. W., "Therapeutic" serum concentration of phenytoin: the influence of seizure type, *J. Neurol. Neurosurg. Psychiatry*, 47(3): 231–4, 1984.

3035. Twombly, D., Narahashi, T., Phenytoin suppresses calcium channel currents in neuroblastoma cells, *Soc. Neurosci. Abstr.*, 11: 518, 1985.

3036. Twombly, D. A., Narahashi, T., Phenytoin block of low threshold calcium channels is voltage- and frequency-dependent, *Soc. Neurosci. Abstr.*, 12 (Pt 2): 1193, 1986.

3037. Uhl, H. A., Phenytoin: the drug choice in tricyclic antidepressant overdose?, *Ann. Emerg. Med.*, 10(5): 270–4, 1981.

3038. Umstead, G. S., McKernan, T. M., Salivary phenytoin concentrations in geriatric patients, *Epilepsy Abstracts*, 15(9): 340, 1982.

3039. Uram, M., Nemoto, E. M., Winter, P. M., A comparison of the effects of cerebral protective drugs and nonprotective drugs on monolayers of phospholipids, *Anesthesiology*, 59(3): A301, 1983.

3040. Urbaniak, J. R., Roth, J. H., Office diagnosis and treatment of hand pain, *Orthop. Clin. North Am.*, 13: 477–95, 1982.

3041. U.S. Pharmacopeia Drug Information, *Drug Information for the Health Care Provider*, U.S. Pharmacopeial Convention, Inc., Rockville.

3042. Valimaki, M., Effects of drugs and nonthyroid disorders on thyroid hormones, *Duodecim.*, 98(17): 1247–56, 1982.

3043. Valli, G., Barbieri, S., Cappa, S., Pellegrini, G., Scarlato, G., Syndromes of abnormal muscular activity: overlap between continuous muscle fiber activity and the stiff man syndrome, *J. Neurol. Neurosurg. Psychiatry*, 46: 241–7, 1983.

3044. Van der Molen, H. L., Phenytoin: pharmacology of seizure control, *Hormonal Factors in Fertility, Infertility and Contraception*, Van der Molen, H. J., et al., Eds., Excerpta Medica, Princeton, 71–82, 1982.

3045. Van Hoeck, G. M., Comparison study between anticonvulsants assays and their free fractions in serous blood,

saliva and capillary blood in man, *J. Pharmacol.*, 15(1): 27–35, 1984.

3046. Varotto, M., Roman, G., Battistin, L., Pharmacological influences on the cerebral level and transport of GABA. Effect of some antiepileptic drugs on the cerebral level of GABA, *Boll. Soc. Ital. Biol. Sper.*, 57(8): 904–8, 1981.

3047. Vasilescu, C., Florescu, A., Peripheral neuropathy with a syndrome of continuous motor unit activity, *J. Neurol.*, 226: 275–82, 1982.

3048. Vernadakis, A., Neurotoxic effects of phenytoin: the developing organism, *Mechanisms of Actions of Neurotoxic Substances*, Prasad, K. N., Vernadakis, A., Eds., Raven Press, New York, 155–79, 1982.

3049. Vincent, P. C., Drug-induced aplastic anaemia and agranulocytosis, incidence and mechanisms, *Drugs*, 31: 52–63, 1986.

3050. Vizi, E. S., Pasztor, E., Release of acetylcholine from isolated human cortical slices: inhibitory effect of norepinephrine and phenytoin, *Exp. Neurol.*, 73: 114–53, 1981.

3051. Von Albert, H. H., Phenytoin infusion in the treatment of epilepsy, *Advances in Epileptology: 14th Epilepsy International Symposium*, Parsonage, M, Ed., Raven Press, New York, 307–12, 1983.

3052. Von Demers, H. G., Cardiac therapy in the intensive care unit, *Intensivbehandlung*, 6(1): 28–33, 1981.

3053. Wada, A., Izumi, F., Yanagihara, N., Kobayashi, H., Modulation by ouabain and diphenylhydantoin of veratridine-induced 22 Na influx and its relation to 46 Ca influx and the secretion of catecholamines in cultured bovine adrenal medullary cells, *Arch. Pharmacol.*, 328(3): 273–8, 1985.

3054. Wagner, J. H., Another report of nonconvulsive status epilepticus after metrizamide myelography, *Ann. Neurol.*, 18(3): 369–70, 1985.

3055. Wald, R. W., Waxman, M. B., Downar, E., The effect of antiarrhythmic drugs on depressed conduction and undirectional block in sheep Purkinje fibers, *Circ. Res.*, 46: 612–9, 1980.

3056. Wallin, B. G., Westerberg, C. E., Sundlof, G., Syncope induced by glossopharyngeal neuralgia: sympathetic outflow to muscle, *Neurology*, 34: 522–4, 1984.

3057. Walsh, J. C., Neuromyotonia: an unusual presentation of intrathoracic malignancy, *J. Neurol. Neurosurg. Psychiatr.*, 39: 1086–91, 1976.

3058. Wang, B. J., Chang, Y. C., Therapeutic blood levels of phenytoin in treatment of paroxysmal choreaoathetosis, *Ther. Drug. Monit.*, 7(1): 81–2, 1985.

3059. Wang, S. T., Peter, F., The Abbott TDx fluorescence polarization immunoassay and liquid chromatography compared for five anticonvulsant drug serum, *Clin. Chem.*, 31(3): 493–4, 1985.

3060. Wasserman, T. H., Stetz, J., Phillips, T. L., Radiation therapy oncology group clinical trials with misonidazole, *Cancer*, 47: 2382–90, 1981.

3061. Wasserstrom, J. A., Ferrier, G. R., Effects of phenytoin on digitalis oscillatory afterpotentials, aftercontractions, and inotropy, *Fed. Proc.*, 39: 1001, 1980.

3062. Wasserstrom, J. A., Ferrier, G. R., Effects of phenytoin and quinidine on digitalis-induced oscillatory afterpotentials, after-contractions, and inotropy in canine ventricular tissues, *J. Mol. Cell Cardiol.*, 14: 725–36, 1982.

3063. Watanabe, A. M., Bailey, J. C., The role of the autonomic central nervous system in mediating and modifying the action of cardiac antiarrhythmic drugs, *Ann. N.Y. Acad. Sci.*, 432: 90–102, 1984.

3064. Wehrmann, W., Reichl, W., Bauer, R., Phenytoin treatment in hereditary bollous epidermolysis, *Therapiewoche*, 34(39): 5571–5, 1984.

3065. Weidauer, H., Feurle, G. E., Baldauf, G., Anton-Lamprecht, I., Therapy of esophageal stenoses in recessive epidermolysis bullosa dystrophica, *Laryngol. Rhinol. Otol.*, 64: 552–6, 1985.

3066. Wellens, H. J., Brugada, P., Abdollah, H., Drug therapy of patients with arrhythmias associated with bypass tracts, *Clinical Pharmacology of Cardiac Antiarrhythmic Agents: Classical and Current Concepts Reevaluated*, Garfein, O. B., Ed., Ann. New York Academy of Science, 432: 272–8, 1984.

3067. Westveer, D. C., Gadowski, G. A., Gordon, S., Timmis, G. C., Amiodarone-induced ventricular tachycardia, *Ann. Intern. Med.*, 97(4): 561–2, 1982.

3068. White, B. C., Penry, J. K., Bracket, C. F., Lisco, M., Art, D., Nemore, J., Mann, T., Mumaw, L., Whitley, L., Study on pharmacological prophylaxis of posttraumatic epilepsy in severely head injured patients utilizing therapeutic serum levels of antiepileptic drugs. *NINCDS*, Bethesda, Md. & Kansas Univ. Med. Center, Ka., 1982.

3069. White, H. S., Chen, C. F., Kemp, J. W., Woodbury, D. M., Effects of acute and chronic phenytoin on the electrolyte content and the activities of Na^+, K^+-, Ca^{2+}, Mg^{2+}-, and HCO_3^--ATPases and carbonic anhydrase of neonatal and adult rat cerebral cortex, *Epilepsia*, 26(1): 43–57, 1985.

3070. White, H. S., Yen-Chow, Y. C., Chow, S. Y., Kemp, J. W., Woodbury, D. M., Effects of phenytoin on primary glial cell cultures, *Epilepsia*, 26(1): 58–68, 1985.

3071. White, J. C., Sweet, W. H., *Trigeminal Neuralgia Tic Douloureux Pain and the Neurosurgeon. A Forty-year Experience*, Charles C. Thomas, Springfield, 1969.

3072. Willow, M., Pharmacology of diphenylhydantoin and carbamazepine action on voltage-sensitive sodium channels, *Trends in Neurosciences*, 147–9, 1986.

3073. Willow, M., Gonoi, T., Catterall, W. A., Voltage clamp analysis of the inhibitory actions of diphenylhydantoin and carbamazepine on voltage-sensitive sodium channels in neuroblastoma cells, *Mol. Pharmacol.*, 27(5): 549–58, 1985.

3074. Wilson, J. F., Marshall, R. W., Williams, J., Richens, A., Comparison of assay methods used to measure antiepileptic drugs in plasma, *Ther. Drug. Monit.*, 5(4): 449–60, 1983.

3075. Wirth, H., Nesch, A., Ostapowicz, B., Anton-Lamprecht, I., Phenytoin therapy of recessive dystrophic epidermolysis bullosa hallopeau siemens and epidermolysis bullosa inversa, *Z. Hautkr.*, 58(8): 555–74, 1983.

3076. Wit, A. L., Hoffman, B. F., Modification of the cardiac action potential by pharmacologic agents, *Cell Pharmacol. Excitbl. Tiss.*, 408–84, 1975.

3077. Witchitz, S., Giudicelli, J. F., Diphenylhydantoin, *International Symposium on Diagnosis and Treatment of Cardiac Arrhythmias*, Bayes A., and Cosin, J., Eds., Pergamon Press, New York, 871–7, 1980.

3078. Wohns, N. W., Colpitts, M., Clement, T., Karuza, A., Blackett, W. B., Foutch, R., Larson, E., Phenytoin and acute mountain sickness on Mount Everest, *Am. J. Med.*, 80: 32–36, 1986.

3079. Wolf, P., Influence of the anti-epileptic drugs on sleep, *16th Epilepsy Congress, Abstracts*, Hamburg, Ciba-Geigy, 1985.

3080. Wolf, P., Roder-Wanner, U. U., Brede, M., Influence of therapeutic phenobarbital and phenytoin medication on the polygraphic sleep of patients with epilepsy, *Epilepsia*, 25(4): 467–75, 1984.

3081. Woodbury, D. M., Metabolites and the mechanisms of action of antiepileptic drugs, *Advances in Epileptology*, Meinardi, H., Rowan, A. J., Eds., Swets & Zeitlinger, Amsterdam, 134–50, 1978.

3082. Woodbury, D. M., Antiepileptic drugs—phenytoin: introduction and history, *Antiepileptic Drugs—Mechanisms of Action*, Glaser, G. H., Penry, J. K., Woodbury, D. M., Eds., Raven Press, New York, 305–13, 1980.

3083. Woodbury, D. M., Phenytoin: Mechanisms of action, *Antiepileptic Drugs*, Woodbury, D. M., Penry, J. K., Pippinger, C. E., Eds., Raven Press, New York, 269–81, 1982.

3084. Woodbury, D. M., Engstrom, F. L., White, H. S., Chen, C. F., Kemp, J. W., Chow, S. Y., Ionic and acid-base regulation of neurons and glia during seizures, *Ann. Neurol.*, 16: s135–s144, 1984.

3085. Woodbury, D. M., Kemp, J. W., Chow, S. Y., Mechanism of action of antiepileptic drugs, *Epilepsy*, Ward, A. A., et al., Eds., Raven Press, New York, 179–223, 1983.

3086. Woolhouse, N. M., Adjepon-Yamoah, K. K., Critchley, J. A., Prescott, L. F., Reduced capacity for diphenylhydantoin hydroxylation in Ghanaians, *Br. J. Clin. Pharmacol.* 18(2): 287p–8p, 1984.

3087. Woscoff, A., Paz, A., Abulafia, J., Jaimovich, L., Grinspan, D., Dystrophic epidermolysis bullosa. Urogenital manifestation and phenytoin treatment, *Med. Cutan. Iber. Lat. Am.*, 12(2): 129–35, 1984.

3088. Yaari, Y., Carbone, E., Phenytoin reduces the number of Na channel openings in inside-out patches of avian sensory neurons, *Pflugers. Arch.*, 405 (sup 2): 47, 1985.

3089. Yaari, Y., David, G., Selzer, M. E., Use- and frequency-dependent depression of nerve action potentials by phenytoin, *Personal Communication*, 1985.

3090. Yaari, Y., Devor, M., Phenytoin suppresses spontaneous ectopic discharge in rat sciatic nerve neuromas, *Neurosci. Lett.*, 58(1): 117–22, 1985.

3091. Yaari, Y., Pincus, J. H., Argov, Z., Depression of synaptic transmission by diphenylhydantoin, *Ann. Neurol.*, 1: 334–8, 1977.

3092. Yaari, Y., Selzer, M. E., David, G., Frequency-dependent effects of phenytoin on frog junctional transmission, *Brain Res.*, 345(1): 102–110, 1985.

3093. Yaari, Y., Selzer, M. E., Pincus, J. H., Phenytoin: mechanisms of its anticonvulsant action, *Ann. Neurol.*, 20: 171–84, 1986.

3094. Yatani, A., Hamilton, S. L., Brown, A. M., Diphenylhydantoin blocks cardiac calcium channels and binds to the dihydropyridine receptor, *Circ. Res.*, 59: 356–61, 1986.

3095. Yi, S. J., Seitz, P. K., Cooper, C. W., Inhibition of *in vitro* secretion of rat calcitonin by phenytoin, *Fed. Proc*, 46(3): 393, 1987.

3096. Young, H. G., Becker, D. P., Treatment of tic douloureux: current concepts, *Va. Med.*, 108: 718–20, 1981.

3097. Younger, L. E., Silverman, H., Chronic phenytoin administration alters the metabolic profile of superficial gastrocnemius muscle fibers in dystrophic mice, *Exp. Neurol.*, 84: 140–52, 1984.

3098. Zacchetti, O., Sozzi, G., Zampollo, A., Paroxysmal kinesigenic choreoathetosis. Case report, *Ital. J. Neurol. Sci.*, 3: 345–7, 1983.

3099. Zimmer, J. P., Lehr, H. A., Kornhuber, M. E., Breitig, D., Montagnier, L., Gietzen, K., Diphenylhydantoin (DPH) blocks HIV-receptor on lymphocyte surface, *Blut*, 53: 447–50, 1986.

3100. Zisfein, J., Sivak, M., Aron, A. M., Bender, A. N., Isaac's syndrome with muscle hypertrophy reversed by phenytoin therapy, *Arch. Neurol.*, 40: 241–2, 1983.

Index

Page numbers that appear in *italics* refer to laboratory information—
all other page numbers refer to clinical information.

Medical Journals in Which Many of the Clinical Uses of PHT Have Been Reported

Acta Dermato-Venereologica
Acta Endocrinologica
Acta Medica Scandinavica
Acta Medica Venezolana
Acta Neurologica
Acta Neurologica Scandinavica
Actualités Odonto-
  Stomatologiques
American Heart Journal
American Journal of Cardiology
American Journal of Diseases of
  Children
American Journal of Digestive
  Diseases
American Journal of the Medical
  Sciences
American Journal of Medicine
American Journal of Physiology
American Journal of Psychiatry
American Journal of
  Psychotherapy
American Journal of Surgery
Anales de Medicina de Barcelona
Anaesthesia and Intensive Care
Anesthesia and Analgesia
Anesthesiology
Angiology
Annales de Cardiologie et
  d'Angeiologie
Annales de Dermatologie et de
  Syphiligraphie
Annales de Medecine Interne
Annals of Emergency Medicine
Annals of Internal Medicine
Annals of Neurology
Annals of Rheumatic Diseases
Antiseptic
Archiv für Ohren-, Nasen- und
  Kehlkopfheilkunde
Archives of Dermatology
Archives of General Psychiatry
Archives of Internal Medicine
Archives des Maladies du Coeur et
  des Vaisseaux
Archives of Neurology
Archives of Neurology and
  Psychiatry
Archives of Otolaryngology
Archives of Pediatrics
Archives of Physical Medicine and
  Rehabilitation
Archives of Surgery
Archivos del Instituto de
  Cardiologia de México
Arquivos de Neuro-Psiquiatria

Arteriosclerosis
Arthritis and Rheumatism
Arztliche Wochenschrift
Australian Journal of Dermatology
Biulleten Vsesoiuznogo
  Kardiologicheskogo
  Nauchnogo (Moscow)
Blut
Brain
British Heart Journal
British Journal of Addiction
British Journal of Clinical
  Pharmacology
British Journal of Dermatology
British Journal of Radiology
British Medical Journal
Bulletin of the Los Angeles
  Neurological Societies
Bulletin of the New York Academy
  of Medicine
California Medicine
Canadian Anaesthetists Society
  Journal
Canadian Medical Association
  Journal
Canadian Psychiatric Association
  Journal
Ceskoslovenska Neurologie
Chest
Child's Brain
China Medical Abstracts
Chinese Medical Journal
Circulation
Clinical Electroencephalography
Clinical Journal of Pain
Clinical Medicine
Clinical Nephrology
Clinical Neurology
Clinical Neuropharmacology
Clinical Neurophysiology
Clinical Pharmacology and
  Therapeutics
Clinical Research
Clinical Science
Clinical Science and Molecular
  Medicine
Clinical Therapeutics
Clinician
Comprehensive Psychiatry
Connecticut Medicine
Criminal Psychopathology
Critical Care Medicine
Current Therapeutic Research
Cutis
Delaware Medical Journal

Dental Hygiene
Deutsche Medizinische
  Wochenschrift
Deutsche Stomatologie
Diabetes
Diseases of the Chest
Diseases of the Nervous System
Ear, Nose and Throat Journal
Electroencephalography and
  Clinical Neurophysiology
Epilepsia
European Journal of Clinical
  Investigation
European Journal of Clinical
  Pharmacology
European Neurology
Experimental Medicine and
  Surgery
Fertility and Sterility
Folia Psychiatrica et Neurologica
  Japonica
Fortschritte der Neurologie-
  Psychiatrie
Gaceta Medica Española
Gastroenterologie Clinique et
  Biologique
Gastroenterology
Geriatrics
Giornale de Psichiatria e di
  Neuropatologia
Handchirurgie, Mikrochirurgie,
  Plastische Chirurgie
Harefuah
Hautarzt
Headache
HNO-Praxis
Indian Journal of Chest Diseases
Intensive Care Medicine
International Journal of
  Dermatology
International Journal of
  Neuropsychiatry
International Surgery
Investigacion Medica
  Internacional
Israel Journal of Medical Sciences
Italian Journal of Neurological
  Sciences
Johns Hopkins Medical Journal
Journal of American College of
  Cardiology
Journal of the American Geriatrics
  Society
Journal of the American Medical
  Association

Journal of the American
    Osteopathic Association
Journal of the Association of
    Physicians in India
Journal of Cardiovascular Surgery
Journal of Clinical Endocrinology
    and Metabolism
Journal of Clinical Investigation
Journal of Clinical Pharmacology
Journal of Clinical Psychiatry
Journal of Dermatologic Surgery
    and Oncology
Journal of Diabetic Association of
    India
Journal of the Egyptian Medical
    Association
Journal of Emergency Medicine
Journal of the Florida Medical
    Association
Journal of Formosan Medical
    Association
Journal of the Indian Medical
    Association
Journal of the Kansas Medical
    Society
Journal of Laboratory and Clinical
    Medicine
Journal of Laryngology and
    Otology
Journal of Mental Science
Journal of the Michigan State
    Medical Society
Journal of the Mississippi State
    Medical Association
Journal of Nervous and Mental
    Disease
Journal of the National Proctologic
    Association
Journal of Neurology
Journal of Neurology,
    Neurosurgery and Psychiatry
Journal of Neurosurgery
Journal of Neurosurgical Sciences
Journal of Oral Surgery
Journal of Orthomolecular
    Psychiatry
Journal of Pediatrics
Journal of Reproductive Medicine
Journal of Rheumatology
Journal of Surgery
Journal of Urology
Kardiologiia
Klinische Wochenschrift
Lancet
Laryngoscope
Lyon Medical

Maryland Medical Journal
Medical Clinics of North America
Medical Journal of Australia
Medicina Cutanea Ibero-Latino-
    Americana
Medicina Experimentalis
Medizinische Klinik
Medizinische Monatsschrift
Metabolism
Michigan Medicine
Minerva Cardioangiologica
Modern Concepts of
    Cardiovascular Disease
Monatsschrift Psychiatric and
    Neurologie
Mount Sinai Medical Journal
Münchener Medizinische
    Wochenschrift
Muscle and Nerve
Nebraska State Medical Journal
NederlandsTijdschrift Voor
    Geneeskunde
Nervenarzt
Neurologia i Neurochirurgia
    Polska
Neurologia Medico-Chirurgica
Neurology
Neuropadiatrie
Neuropsychobiology
Neurosurgery
Neurosurgical Science
New England Journal of Medicine
New York State Journal of
    Medicine
New Zealand Medical Journal
Pacing and Clinical
    Electrophysiology
Pediatrics
Physician's Drug Manual
Pittsburgh Medical Bulletin
Polish Medical Journal
Polski Tygodnik Lekarsky
Portsmouth Journal of Psychology
Postgraduate Medical Journal
Postgraduate Medicine
Practitioner
Prensa Medica Argentina
Presse Medicale
Problemy Endokrinologii
Proceedings of American
    Association of Cancer
    Research
Proceedings of the Australian
    Association of Neurologists
Proceedings of the Symposium on
    Aggressive Behavior

Progress in Cardiovascular
    Disease
Psychiatric Journal of the
    University of Ottawa
Psychopharmacologia
Psychophysiology
Psychosomatic Medicine
Psychosomatics
Rational Drug Therapy
Revista Argentina de Cardiologia
Revista Brasileira de
    Anestesiologia
Revista Clinica Española
Revista Española de
    Pediatria
Revista Iberica de Endocrinologia
Revista de Medicina Interna
Revue de Laryngologie
Revue Medicale de Liege
Revue de Médecine Aeronautique
    et Spatiale
Revue Neurologique
Revue d'Odonto-Stomatologie
Revue d'Oto-Neuro-
    Ophthalmologie
Revue Roumaine de Medecine
    Serie Neurologie et
    Psychiatrie
Rivista di Neurologia
Russian Pharmacology and
    Toxicology
Schweizerische Medizinische
    Wochenschrift
Semaine dex Hospitaux
South African Journal of
    Laboratory and Clinical
    Medicine
South African Medical Journal
Southern Medical Journal
Stomatologie der DDR
Stroke
Svensk Larkartidningen
Therapeutic Archives
Therapeutic Drug Monitoring
Therapeutische Umschau
Therapiewoche
Transactions of the American
    Neurological Association
Vrachebnoe Delo
Virginia Medical Monthly
Vnitrni Lekarstvi
Western Medicine
Wiener Klinische Wochenschrift
Zeitschrift fur Hautkrankheiten
Zhurnal Nevropatologii i
    Psikhiatrii Korsakova

PRINTED BY R. R. DONNELLEY & SONS COMPANY
CRAWFORDSVILLE, INDIANA DIVISION
A QUALITY PRINTER OF BOOKS, MAGAZINES, CATALOGS,
DIRECTORIES AND OTHER PRINTED PRODUCTS